Guides to Information Sources

Information Sources in the
Medical Sciences

Guides to Information Sources

Other titles available include:

Information Sources in Sport and Leisure
  edited by Michele Shoebridge

Information Sources for the Press and Broadcast Media
  edited by Selwyn Eagle

Information Sources in Patents
  edited by C.P. Auger

Information Sources in Information Technology
  edited by David Haynes

Information Sources in Grey Literature (Second edition)
  by C.P. Auger

Information Sources in Pharmaceuticals
  edited by W.R. Pickering

Information Sources in Metallic Materials
  edited by M.N. Patten

Information Sources in the Earth Sciences (Second edition)
  edited by David N. Wood, Joan E. Hardy and Anthony P. Harvey

Information Sources in Cartography
  edited by C.R. Perkins and R.B. Barry

Information Sources in Polymers and Plastics
  edited by R.T. Adkins

Information Sources in Science and Technology (Second edition)
  edited by C.C. Parker and R.V. Turley

Information Sources in Physics (Second edition)
  edited by Dennis Shaw

Information Sources in Economics (Second edition)
  edited by John Fletcher

Information Sources in the Life Sciences (Third edition)
  edited by H.V. Wyatt

Information Sources in Engineering (Second edition)
  edited by L.J. Anthony

Information Sources in the
Medical Sciences

Fourth Edition

Editors
L.T. Morton and Shane Godbolt

Bowker-Saur

London • Melbourne • Munich • New York

British Library Cataloguing in Publication Data
Information sources in the medical sciences
   I. Morton, L.T. II. Gobolt, Shane
   610.7

   ISBN 0 86291 596 1

Library of Congress Cataloging-in-Publication Data
Information sources in the medical sciences / editors, L.T.
  Morton and S. Godbolt. — 4th ed.
     p. cm. — (Guides to information sources)
  Includes bibliographical references and index.
  ISBN 0-86291-596-1 (alk. paper) :
    1. Medical literature. 2. Medicine — Bibliography. I.
  Morton, Leslie T. (Leslie Thomas), 1907– . II. Gobolt S. III.
  Series: Guides to information sources (London, England)
   [DNLM: 1. Bibliography of Medicine. ZWB 100 I43]
  R118.I56 1991
  610'.7 — dc20
  DNLM/DLC
  for Library of Congress
                    91-40653
                       CIP

Bowker-Saur is part of the REED REFERENCE PUBLISHING which
specializes in publishing database reference works for the international library
and legal communities. Other REED REFERENCE imprints are R. R. Bowker,
Martindale-Hubbell, Marquis Who's Who, K. G. Saur and D. W. Thorpe.

Cover design by Calverts Press
Printed on acid-free paper
Typeset by SunSetters
Printed and bound in Great Britain by Antony Rowe Ltd, Chippenham,
Wiltshire

Series editors' foreword

As is obvious, any human being, faced with solving a problem or with understanding a task, reacts by thinking, by applying judgement and by seeking information. The first two involve using information from the most readily available source, namely one's memory, though searching this and retrieving what is wanted may be conducted below the level of consciousness. If this source does not provide all that is needed then the information searcher may turn to all or any of three external sources: observation (which can consist simply of 'going and looking' or can involve understanding sophisticated research); other people, who may be close colleagues or distant experts; and stores of recorded information, for example a local filing system or an electronic databank held on a computer network or even a book or journal in a national library.

The order (observation; other people; recorded information), is not significant though it is often a common sequence. Certainly it is not intended to impute an order of importance. Which of the three or what combination of them one uses depends on a number of factors including the nature of the problem and one's personal circumstances. Suffice to say that all three have their place and all three are used by every literate person.

Nowadays the amount of information in any field, even if one can exclude that which has been superseded, is so large that no human being or small group of people can hope to know it all. Thus, company information systems, for example, get bigger and bigger even when there are efficient means of discarding unwanted and out-of-date information. Managing these systems is a complex and full time task.

Many factors contribute to the huge information growth and overload. Throughout the world, large amounts of research continue to be undertaken and their results published for others to use or follow up. New data pours out of the financial markets. Governments keep passing new legislation. The law courts keep generating new rulings. Each organization and everyone in it of any significance, it seems, is in the business of generating new information. Most of it is recorded and much of it is published.

Although there is a growing tendency to record information in electronic media and to leave it there for distribution via electronic networks of one sort or another, the traditional media are still in use. Even tablets of stone are still used in appropriate circumstances but, of course, it is paper that predominates. The electronic age has not yet led to any reduction in the amount of printed material being published.

The range of types of published or publicly available information sources is considerable. It includes collections of letters, monographs, reports, pamphlets, newspapers and other periodicals, patent specifications, standards, trade literature including both manufacturers' product specifications and service companies' descriptions of their services, user manuals, laws, bye-laws, regulations and all the great wealth of leaflets poured out by official, semi-official and private organizations to guide the public. Then there are all those publications that present their information in other than verbal form; maps; graphs; music scores; photographs; moving pictures; sound recordings; videos. Nor, although their main content is not published information, should one forget as sources of information collections of artefacts.

In an attempt to make some of the more frequently needed information more easily accessible, these sources of primary information are supplemented with the well-known range of tertiary publications, and text books, data books, reviews and encyclopaedias.

To find the information source one needs, another range of publications has come into being. To find experts or organizations or products there are directories, masses of them, so many that directories of directories are published. To find a required publication there are library catalogues, publishers' lists, indexes and abstracting services, again a great many of them.

For librarians and information specialists in the industrialized countries, access to abstracting services is now normally achieved online, i.e. from a computer terminal over the telephone lines to remote computer-base database host. Since 1960 the use of libraries by information and even document seekers has changed considerably and can be expected to change further as the British Library study *Information 2000* indicates. More and more primary information is being stored electronically and more and more copies of printed documents are supplied via telephone or data networks. Sets of newspapers or other major publications can be acquired on optical discs for use in-house. Scientists in different universities, perhaps working on a common project, are sharing their results via the medium of electronic bulletin boards. The use of electronic messaging systems for disseminating information is now commonplace. Thus the combination of computer technology with telecommunications engineering is offering new ways of accessing and communicating information. Nevertheless, the old ways continue to be important and will remain so for many years yet.

The huge wealth of sources of information, the great range of resources, of means of identifying them and of accessing what is wanted increase the need for well-aimed guides. Not all sources are of equal value even when only those well focused on the required topic are considered. The way new journals proliferate whenever a new major topic is established, many it seems just trying to 'climb on the bandwagon' and as a consequence substantially duplicating each other, illustrates this. Even in an established field the tendency of scientists, for example, to have a definite 'pecking order' for selecting journals in which to publish their research is well known. Some journals submit offered articles to referees; some others publish anything they can get. Similar considerations apply to other publications. The degree of reliance that can be placed on reports in different newspapers is an illustration. Nor is accuracy the only measure of quality. Another is the depth to which an account of a given topic goes.

The aim of this series *Guides to Information Sources*, is to give within each broad subject field (chemistry, architecture, politics, cartography etc.) an account of the types of external information source that exist and of the more important individual sources set in the context of the subject itself. Individual chapters are written by experts, each of whom specializes in the field he/she is describing, and give a view based on experience of finding and using the most appropriate sources. The volumes are intended to be readable by other experts and information seekers working outside their normal field. They are intended to help librarians concerned with problems of relevance and quality in stock selection.

Since not only the sources but also the needs and interests of users vary from one subject to another, each editor is given a free hand to produce the guide which is appropriate for his/her subject. We, the series editors, believe that this volume does just that.

Douglas Foskett
Michael Hill

Preface

This book is intended to serve as an evaluative guide to the most important sources of information that each contributor has recommended from experience of the subject, rather than as a directory of sources.

For this fourth edition each chapter has been revised to take account of important new publications and information services that have become available since the appearance of the previous edition. Most contributors have designed their chapters to be self-contained guides to their respective subjects, but overlapping has been reduced as much as possible by cross-referencing.

A new chapter on radiology and medical imaging has been added. This was originally to have been prepared by Jennifer Wade, but after her illness and death in April 1990 her place was taken by Maureen Forrest. Other new contributors are Robin Adams, Susan Bloomfield, Anne Collins, Catherine Deering, Brian Furner with Gaynor Messenger, Martin Guha, Stan Jenkins, and Peter Morgan. Margaret Hammond has been joined by Professor Pereira Gray.

Coverage of the following subject areas had been introduced or expanded within the appropriate chapters: AIDS and sexually transmitted diseases, alternative medicine, CD-ROM, geriatrics, intensive care, the National Health Service, ophthalmology, otorhinolaryngology, and parasitology. The chapter on personal files, published in previous editions, has been omitted; it is now covered by Christopher Norris's chapter on online information sources, reflecting the increasing use of personal database software by medical practitioners and scientists.

We are indebted to all our contributors who have collaborated to produce this book. Thanks are also due to the series editors, Douglas Foskett and Michael Hill, who gave us invaluable advice during the planning stage of this work, and to the staff of Bowker-Saur, particularly Geraldine Turpie and Val Skelton, for their help and guidance during its preparation for publication.

L.T.M.
S.G.

About the contributors

Robin Adams

Has recently been appointed as Deputy Librarian at Trinity College, Dublin. Prior to this he headed the Physical and Life Sciences Division at Glasgow University Library where he was also responsible for development of electronic information service and office automation. His earlier career was in the field of medical librarianship at Queen's University, Belfast and Cambridge University.

Suzanne P. Bates

Graduated from the University of Hull in 1984. She studied Librarianship and Information Studies at the Polytechnic of North London in 1986 and became an Associate member of the Library Association in 1991. For the last four years she has worked with the Oncology Information Service at the University of Leeds as Managing Editor for the current awareness journal *Aids Information*.

Susan Bloomfield

Graduated in Applied Biology before qualifying as a librarian. She was Chief Librarian at the Public Health Laboratory Service from 1982 to 1990. Prior to this she held posts in polytechnic libraries, the most recent being that of Science Librarian at Hatfield Polytechnic. She is currently a member of the Registration Board of the UK Library Association.

Elaine Brooke

Has been Librarian of the Institute of Child Health, London since 1971. She was previously Librarian at the Royal Free Hospital, London. She is an Associate of the Library Association.

Derek Calam

Is Head of the Chemistry Division at the National Institute for Biological Standards and Control. He was educated at Oxford University and subsequently worked with the Medical and Agricultural Research councils. He is a member of the European and British Pharmacopoeia Commissions and of a WHO Expert Panel. His interests include application of chemical methods to biological standardization and exploitation of information sources.

Margaret A. Clennett

Was appointed Chief Librarian of the Public Health Laboratory Service in 1991. She was formerly Librarian at the British Dental Association, having taken up this post in 1981 after several years as Librarian at the Institute of Dental Surgery. She is the author of *Keyguide to information sources in dentistry*, published in 1985.

Anne Collins

Has been Medical Sub-Librarian at the University of Leeds since 1974. A graduate of University College, Wales, she attended the then Manchester College of Commerce to obtain her professional qualifications. She is the author of a number of papers about CD-ROM services and a member of the SCONUL Advisory Committee on medical materials. She has been involved with the establishment and development of the Oncology Information Service at Leeds University.

Catherine M. Deering

Originally qualified at the University of Manchester where she gained a BA and a PhD. She worked as a writer in an advertising agency before becoming Education Faculty Librarian at the University of Manchester. She is now Head of Library and Information Services at the Liverpool School of Tropical Medicine.

Maureen Forrest

Is Librarian of the Cairns Library, John Radcliffe Hospital, Oxford, which is jointly funded by Oxford University and the Regional Health Authority. She has served on the Committee of the Library Association Medical, Health and Welfare Libraries Group and is currently Secretary to the Medical Information Working Party and the University Medical School Librarians Group. She has made various contributions to the literature and has given a number of papers at conferences, including the first European Conference of Medical Libraries, held in Brussels in 1986.

Eric J. Freeman

Is a professional librarian currently in charge of the Library of the Wellcome Institute for the History of Medicine. He is also Director

(History of Medicine) for the Wellcome Trust, a leading British charity in the field of medical research.

Brian Furner

Is a chartered librarian with a degree in South East Asian languages. He worked abroad with VSO and the British Council before taking up his current post as Librarian of the London School of Hygiene and Tropical Medicine.

Robert Gann

Is Director of The Help for Health Trust, a registered charity established by Wessex Regional Health Authority with the aim of promoting the active involvement of people in their own health care through the provision of information. He qualified as a librarian in 1976 and worked in the NHS for 15 years before setting up The Help for Health Trust. He has been a consultant on health information to the British Council and the World Health Organization.

Shane Godbolt

Is Regional Librarian, North-West Thames Regional Health Authority, British Postgraduate Medical Federation. She was formerly librarian of Charing Cross and Westminster Medical School. She began her career in 1969 at St Bartholomew's Hospital Medical College, moving in 1970 to Charing Cross Hospital Medical School Library as Deputy and later as Librarian. She has been active for many years in the Library Association's Professional Group for Medical and Health-care Librarians and is the Editor of the official Group journal *Health Libraries Review*.

Martin Guha

Graduated in International Relations from the University of Keele, and undertook postgraduate studies in librarianship at Manchester Polytechnic and in European Studies at the University of Sussex, before becoming social sciences librarian at North East London Polytechnic. For the past eight years he has been Librarian of the University of London Institute of Psychiatry. He has published innumerable book reviews in the fields of psychiatry and clinical psychology but has hitherto evaded any pressure put upon him to publish anything longer.

Howard Hague

Is Reader Services Librarian at Charing Cross and Westminster Medical School in London. Previously he worked as Medical Librarian at Ahmadu Bello University in Nigeria. He represents medical, health and welfare libraries on the standing committeee on Official Publications (SCOOP) and has recently compiled a *Core collection of medical books and journals* published by the Medical Information Working Party.

Margaret Hammond

Joined the Royal College of General Practitioners in 1963 as Manager/Librarian intending to stay for a year only. She is still there. She trained in library work at St Bartholomew's and Guy's Hospitals, escaped the medical scene to *The Times* newspaper. Trained in a parallel discipline as an indexer. Member and registered Indexer of that Society. Failed to make 'others' understand the information aspect of library and ancillary types of work, but has been rewarded by the involvement in the growth of a College and its literature.

Stan Jenkins

Obtained a degree in Hispanic Studies from the University of Liverpool in 1962 and worked for a brief period as an assistant in Birmingham Reference Library. In January 1964 he joined the staff of the Barnes Medical Library and the University of Birmingham planning to stay for only a short period as he felt it was too early in his career to specialize. He has been there ever since and is now Deputy Medical Librarian. He has written a number of articles on information retrieval in medicine and is the author of *Medical libraries: a user guide*, published by the British Medical Association in 1987.

Gaynor Messenger

Is Library Services Manager at the King's Fund Centre for Health Services Development, and has been closely involved in enquiry service there for a number of years. She has worked in the medical and health care field since graduating in 1983, and is currently contributing to a bibliography on the changing role of the acute care hospital.

Robert Moore

Is Librarian of the National Institute for Medical Research, which he joined in 1962. He is a chartered librarian, Member of the Institute of Information Scientists, Member of the Institute of Biology, and has a BA in science, history of science, and philosophy. He coordinates the provision of library and information services covering the basic biomedical sciences and is also involved, when time allows, in historical and archive work. His personal interests include the post-1800 history of medicine and the allied sciences.

Peter Morgan

Has been Medical Librarian at Cambridge University since 1975, and holds qualifications from Leeds and Sheffield Universities. He is closely involved with professional activities in medical librarianship, and has held representative offices within the Library Association, SCONUL, and the NHS Regional Librarians Group. He has also worked in collaboration with the British Council on various activities in Britain and the developing world.

Leslie T. Morton

Began his library career in 1923. He was Librarian at St Thomas's Hospital Medical School (1935-43), Information Officer, *British Medical Journal* (1946-59) and Librarian, National Institute for Medical Research (1959-72). After retiring in 1972 he returned the following year to serve as Library Adviser to North-East and North-West Thames Regional Health Authorities until 1980, when he became Consultant Librarian to the British Postgraduate Medical Federation. He is the author of *A medical bibliography* (4th edition, 1983).

Christopher Norris

Graduated in Natural Sciences from Cambridge University. He is Manager of the Medical Information Service of the British Library, where he has worked as an indexer/searcher and reviser since 1968, apart from a spell of six years as a freelance indexer.

Denis Pereira Gray

Is a general practitioner in Exeter where he has followed his father and grandfather. He works in a four-partner training practice with about 7000 patients. He is Professor of General Practice and Director of the Postgraduate Medical School of the University of Exeter and Regional Adviser in General Practice for the South Western Region. His books include *Training for general practice* and *Running a practice* (written jointly) and he delivered the 1988 McConaghey Memorial Lecture on 'The literature of general practice'.

Alex Rodger

Is the Librarian at the Royal College of Physicians and Surgeons of Glasgow, a post he has held since 1969. Prior to his present appointment he was a district librarian in Lanark County Library service.

Fytton Rowland

Currently runs the Computers in Teaching Initiative Centre for Library and Information Studies and Loughborough University as well as his own freelance scientific editing business, Dovecote Editorial Services. He read Biochemistry at Cambridge University and qualified in Information Science from the City University. For almost twenty years he was a member of the staff of the Royal Society of Chemistry, latterly as Publications Production Manager.

David Stewart

Is Librarian of the Royal Society of Medicine, London. He joined the Society on graduating from Dublin University in 1963 and has held various posts at the RSM from junior assistant to Librarian. He has been involved in professional activities in the UK, Europe and USA.

Patricia Want

Is Librarian of the Royal College of Obstetricians and Gynaecologists where she has worked for more than twenty years. Her main area of interest is the history of medicine particularly within the specialty of obstetrics and gynaecology. She has made various contributions to the literature.

Contents

CHAPTER ONE

Medical libraries and their use

L.T. MORTON AND SHANE GODBOLT

Today's doctor, physician, surgeon, or medical scientist requires more information than ever before. Medical education and training have increased in complexity and are followed by specialization and possibly also research. The need for both the researcher and the practitioner to keep abreast of current developments necessitates using libraries and being conversant with the literature.

The technology revolution of the 1980s has seen the widespread introduction of the PC microcomputer in libraries, offices and homes. This crucial development and the many changes afforded by the confluence of computing and telecommunications technologies, which offer new and powerful ways of finding and managing information, have brought many benefits to library users. The pace of change is rapid and is set to remain so. The advent of the CD-ROM (Compact Disc — Read-only-Memory) laserdisc technology, the development of interactive video disc technology, the emergence of many new products including software for personal database management, advances in electronic telecommunications systems and the appearance of distributed knowledge networks are all part of a new framework for the way information is organized. This developing infrastructure offers users the potential to access a vast array of knowledge from desks or research offices as well as from the library (Godbolt, 1991).

A good example is provided by one of the largest and most exciting experiments ever launched when, in 1991, a major citation database was mounted over an academic network (Law, 1991). The potential user base consists of academics in the UK, with their own personal computers, and students who have access free at the point of use. Following negotiations with the Institute for Scientific Information agreement was reached to allow their data to be leased, for an initial 5-year period, and made available to the academic community over JANET (Joint Academic Network) (Stone, 1990) which links all British universities. This pattern, bringing information directly to the end user, in addition to access via the library, has important implications and users will find support and training courses offered by libraries to assist them in exploiting these developments. Initial experience, notably at Newcastle, suggests that users have received the new service enthusiastically (O'Donovan, 1991). The ISI service is likely to be the first of a series of data deals, including MEDLINE intended to bring information direct to academic users.

The 1980s have also seen widespread and drastic budget cuts in many libraries but it is encouraging that the technology has brought changes and benefits. Many users perceive the period as one of improvements in library services, despite the problems experienced. It may therefore be noted that despite upheavals and financial stringency the modern medical library, large or small, provides the key to a network of sophisticated and comprehensive services. The user may expect to find information in a variety of non-print formats, such as tape-slide, microform, video and compact disc. CD-ROM is now standard equipment in many libraries and is usually available for searching by readers themselves. Equipment consists of a microcomputer, software, compact disc drive, and a printer (if hard copy of the search result is required). Most versions of databases on compact disc (CD) are menu-driven. In larger libraries a terminal, through which many databases may be interrogated, is now essential equipment, and smaller libraries can provide advice on access and availability of computerized information retrieval services.

Computer or microfiche library catalogues and the transformation of reference tools such as *British Books in Print* (UK) or *Books in Print* (USA) into microfiche and CD-ROM formats necessitate machines for their use. This equipment is well designed and easy to use. Reader printers are likely to be available in these and libraries may have journal runs as well as catalogues in microfiche and CD form.

Even the smallest library will possess a photocopier and larger libraries may have several.

Use of the library is free to its membership but a charge may be made for certain services, such as photocopying, interlibrary loans and online searching. However, many hours of work in manual searching may be saved by having an online search at a relatively small cost. Photocopying, too, is cheap and offers the convenience of copies for personal files or perusal when the library is closed. The restrictions imposed by the Copyright Designs and Patents Act 1988 should be observed when making photocopies. The circumstances in which it is necessary to seek prior permission before photocopying Crown and Parliamentary material have been clarified by Penn (1990). The Copyright Licensing Agency Ltd representing rights owners (33–34 Alfred Place, London WC1E 7DP) has been set up to oversee and regulate copying from books, periodicals, etc. When copying, readers should, for their own convenience, check that the article reference on the copy is complete.

Great emphasis has been placed in recent years, formally and informally, on the importance of reader services and user education. The staff are the most valuable resource in any library and getting to know library staff members with special responsibilities for reference and advisory functions so that they are aware of particular interests and needs is an important aspect of good library use.

Library publications designed to assist users to exploit available services are numerous and range from lists of the library's periodicals to newsletters and/or accessions lists, bulletins and other information leaflets.

A thorough and lucid review of the biomedical literature and its use is provided by *Coping with the biomedical literature: a primer for the scientist and clinician* (Warren, 1981). It contains contributions from 12 distinguished U.S. biomedical scientists and librarians and deals with the structure, production, utilization and sources of biomedical information. *How to use a medical library* (Morton and Wright, 1990) is intended as an introduction to the subject for medical practitioners and research workers. *Medical libraries: a user guide* (Jenkins, 1987) describes the practical aspects of using a medical library and the wide range of services now provided by librarians. *Medical librarianship in the eighties and beyond* (Picken and Kahn, 1986) takes a look at how the world's medical librarians have approached present-day problems and their use of new technologies offering new opportunities for satisfying the information needs of their users. It includes papers from 57 contributors worldwide.

Medical libraries in Great Britain and Ireland

Britain is well equipped with medical libraries. The royal colleges, the medical societies and the teaching and research institutes have between them accumulated a rich storehouse of literature probably unsurpassed elsewhere. In recent years this has been substantially augmented by the British Library. A key to this storehouse is provided by the *Directory of medical and health care libraries in the United Kingdom and Republic of Ireland* (1990), which provides information on about 650 libraries.

London

The greatest concentration of libraries is in London and includes those of the Royal Society of Medicine, the Wellcome Institute for the History of Medicine, the British Medical Association and the royal colleges.

The Royal Society of Medicine was founded as the (Royal) Medical and Chirurgical Society in 1805. In 1907 it was combined with other UK medical societies (and their libraries) and assumed its present name. Its library is one of the largest postgraduate medical collections in Europe, with about 600 000 volumes and taking 2030 current journals. The library is available to Fellows of the Society; others may have reference facilities on the introduction of a Fellow. The Society has a Library (Scientific Research) Section intended to accommodate employees of private and public companies and of certain other organizations, who wish to use the library to assist their employers in the furtherance of medical research. The library provides full reference and postal services. It is a back-up library for the British Library Document Supply Centre.

The British Medical Association is the representative body of the medical profession in Britain. Its library, founded in 1887, now has over 30 000 volumes and takes 1200 current journals. Reference and postal services are available to its members; others may use it at the discretion of the Librarian. It also offers institutional membership, on subscription, and service facilities to libraries in National Health Service hospitals, royal colleges, universities and their institutes, and is also open to commercial institutions.

One of the finest collections of medico-historical material in the world is in the Wellcome Institute for the History of Medicine, founded about 1890 through the generosity of Henry S. Wellcome (1853–1936) and opened to the public in 1949. It has some 300 000 volumes, besides manuscripts, incunabala, prints, autograph letters, etc. It frequently stages exhibitions on medico-historical topics. It is available for reference purposes to all interested in the history of medicine and science. Readers' tickets are available on application to the Librarian. Further details of the holdings of the Wellcome Library are given on pp 578-9.

The formation of the British Postgraduate Medical Federation (University of London) in 1945 led to the establishment of a number of specialist postgraduate institutes. The Federation also incorporated two existing institutes — the Institute of Cancer Research and the (Royal) Postgraduate Medical School at Hammersmith Hospital (875 current periodicals). The latter has since become an independent school of London University. Both these establishments already had good libraries and the majority of the new institutes have assembled sound, specialized collections in the care of experienced librarians. They include the National Heart and Lung Institute and the Institutes of Child Health, Dental Surgery, Neurology, Ophthalmology and Psychiatry. Another postgraduate school of the University is the London School of Hygiene and Tropical Medicine, founded under another name in 1899, which possesses some 85 000 volumes and takes 1200 current periodicals. All these libraries are intended primarily for the use of the institutes or associated hospital staff, although other people are usually allowed reference facilities.

The undergraduate medical schools in London have good libraries which also cater for the hospital medical staff and for the postgraduate research staff. The majority of the librarians, like their provincial colleagues, give instruction in the use of the library and full exploitation of the literature, and by so doing make an important contribution to the early training of research workers.

The combined library resources of the University of London Library at Senate House and those of its constituent schools and colleges are vast. The University of London is a federal university with no centralized library system. The task of co-ordination is carried on by the Federal Library Co-ordinating Services (FLCS), formally constituted in 1973, whose staff are based at the University Library. Initiatives of major importance have been undertaken by the implementation of LIBERTAS, working in co-operation with the librarians throughout the University. LIBERTAS is a suite of software programs designed by Swalcap Library Services Ltd to handle library routine procedures. Access to LIBERTAS is over JANET (Joint Academic Network)(Stone, 1990). It provides both cataloguing and issue modules. Interlibrary software is available but is not yet in use in London. Acquisitions software is being developed. A number of the larger colleges in the university have acquired the same software in order to provide a common approach to library systems. For example, the LONDON UNIVERSITY LIST OF SERIALS (ULS) database is coordinated by FLCS and has ensured more effective utilization of academic library resources for the user. It is available over JANET.

In the Bloomsbury Science Library (incorporating the Thane Medical Sciences Library) at University College there is an important collection covering the basic medical sciences, with 70 000 volumes and 400 current periodicals on anatomy, physiology, biochemistry, biophysics and pharmacology. It is designed for the use of its academic and research staff and its students.

The royal colleges maintain valuable libraries. The Royal College of Physicians of London was founded in 1518 but most of its original library was lost in the Great Fire of 1666. Its present collection of about 50 000 volumes is rich in historical material; it also has a working collection of modern books and periodicals. Fellows and Members of the College and all bona fide workers may use it.

The Royal College of Surgeons of England (1800) has a fine specialist collection, including 650 current journals and 160 000 books. It is a reference library and does not lend to individuals although books and journals less than 50 years old may be lent to other libraries.

The Royal College of Obstetricians and Gynaecologists, founded in 1929, has developed a library of both historical and contemporary publications in its subject field. It has about 4000 volumes and takes 180 current journals dealing with its specialties. It is available to Fellows and Members and to suitably introduced and qualified persons for reference only.

The Royal College of General Practitioners (1952) inaugurated a medical recording service (now the Graves Medical Audiovisual Library, an independent charity) and maintains a bibliographical service on general practice publications. Since 1985 its library has been building up a machine-readable database of literature on general practice, GP-LIT, and now has over 10 000 records available. It is investigating ways of making this database available to a wider public.

The Royal College of Pathologists (1962) is building up a historical library covering pathology, microbiology and related subjects.

The principal medical research institute in Britain is the Medical Research Council's National Institute for Medical Research at Mill Hill, London. Its library (1920) of 75 000 volumes, books and 500 current journals serves the scientific staff of the MRC at the Institute and elsewhere. Others wishing to use it may apply to the Director. The MRC has smaller libraries in a number of its research units in various parts of the country. Its Clinical Research Centre at Northwick Park, Harrow, with a library of clinical material, is to be closed in 1994.

The library of the (former) Department of Health and Social Security was founded in 1834. It is concerned with all aspects of public health and social welfare and is available to staff, postgraduate students and accredited research workers, for reference only. The main library at Hannibal House, Elephant & Castle, London, covers material on health and social services. Branch libraries are: Richmond House Library, Whitehall (general health and social services policy), Social Security Library, Adelphi (social security and pensions), Medicines Library, Nine Elms Lane (safety of medicines), Health Building Library, Euston Tower (health building, architecture), Supply Library, 14 Russell Square (health equipment and supplies), MED TEH Information Unit, Hannibal House (deals with queries on chemical hazards in the environment, food, consumer goods, radiation and smoking). The Department of Health Library now takes 2000 current journals and contains a total of over 200 000 volumes. It has developed (1983) and maintains DHSS-DATA, an online database publicly available on Data-Star and containing records of books, pamphlets, journal articles, departmental publications and circulars, standards, conference proceedings, research documents and annual reports.

About 12 000 records are added each year. The library produces several current-awareness bulletins, including *Health Service Abstracts* (monthly), *Social Service Abstracts* (monthly), *Quality Assurance Abstracts* (bi-monthly, produced in conjunction with the King's Fund Centre Quality Assurance Information Service), *Nursing Research Abstracts* (quarterly) and *Social Security Library Bulletin* (monthly). It is a back-up library of the British Library Document Supply Centre.

The library of the Office of Population Censuses and Surveys has a comprehensive range of British and foreign publications concerned with population and medical statistics, censuses, social surveys, etc. The Office is responsible for a number of relevant official publications. Some account of these publications will be found on p. 83.

Under a scheme of specialization operated by the public libraries of London, the Marylebone Road branch of Westminster City Libraries maintains a collection of all medical books published in the UK (for both professional and lay users) and such foreign publications as are within its means. It has a selection of about 120 periodicals and also offers an inquiry service. This library is, appropriately, near Harley Street. It is open to the public and lends (books only).

Other research establishments, such as the Imperial Cancer Research Fund, the National Institute for Biological Standards and Control, and several of the pharmaceutical houses, maintain specialized libraries of good standing.

Besides the postgraduate institute libraries already mentioned, some other London libraries dealing with particular specialties are worth noting. The British Dental Association (founded 1920) has the principal library in the country covering this subject, with 11 000 books and 200 current journals. It lends books and journals to members and (journals only) to other libraries. The Institute of Dental Surgery at the Eastman Dental Hospital is a postgraduate institute of the University of London and has a good representative collection of books and journals.

The most important pharmaceutical library is that of the Royal Pharmaceutical Society of Great Britain, founded in 1841 and now possessing 65 000 volumes and taking 500 current journals. Fellows, Members and other bona fide qualified persons may use it; books may be borrowed only by Fellows and Members. The School of Pharmacy (University of London) has a good library in its field.

The need for continuing medical education has led in recent years to the establishment of a number of postgraduate medical centres, sited mainly in non-teaching hospitals in the provinces. Their aim is to provide a suitable adequately-equipped location for the postgraduate teaching of hospital staff and general medical and dental practitioners, and at the same time to cater for consultants, junior hospital staff and general practitioners who wish to meet to discuss problems of common interest. The first purpose-built postgraduate medical centre was opened in 1963. Many of these centres have only small libraries; in most cases a regional network has been developed (see p.14) covering all libraries within the area administered by the Regional Health Authority and backed up by the university medical library.

The Royal College of Nursing established its library in London in 1921. It now possesses some 45 000 volumes and receives over 200 current journals. The Library holds the Steinberg collection of nursing research theses; it is responsible for the publication of the monthly *Nursing Bibliography.*

Provinces

Excellent medical libraries are maintained in the provincial medical schools and in Wales: Birmingham (Barnes Library, 66 000 books, 1300 current journals), Bristol, Cambridge, Cardiff (University of Wales College of Medicine), Leeds, Leicester, Liverpool, Manchester (John Rylands University Library, 135 000 medical books, 1000 current journals includes the library of the Manchester Medical Society), Newcastle upon Tyne, Nottingham, Oxford, Sheffield, Southampton.

Medical societies, too, are active in the provinces, but most of their libraries have now been incorporated in local hospital or university medical libraries. An important exception is the Liverpool Medical Institution founded about 1779 and now containing more than 30 000 volumes and about 150 current journals.

Scotland

The University of Edinburgh has a medical library (Erskine Medical Library) of about 43 000 volumes and 950 current sets of periodicals. Notable medical collections are available in the other universities — Aberdeen, Dundee, Glasgow and St Andrews. The younger Strathclyde University (1964) is building up a library covering the biological sciences.

The Royal College of Physicians of Edinburgh (1681) has a fine library of both historical and modern material amounting to about 250 000 volumes. The smaller, more specialized library at the Royal College of Surgeons of Edinburgh contains about 32 000 volumes. In Glasgow the

Royal College of Physicians and Surgeons (1690) has a good modern library supported by a rich historical collection, together totalling 200 000 volumes and 300 current journals. The college libraries are available to Fellows and Members, with restricted use by others. For further information on medical libraries in Scotland, see Jamieson (1986).

Ireland

In Belfast, the Queen's University Medical Library is housed in the Institute of Clinical Science. The Northern Ireland Health and Social Services Library is incorporated with it and the medical library provides a province-wide service for the social services' teaching units, nursing schools, district hospital medical collections and postgraduate medical schools, besides catering for the needs of the medical staff and students of the University and members of the medical profession in Northern Ireland. Its stock amounts to 120 000 volumes and 1200 current journals.

In Eire the Royal College of Surgeons in Ireland, University College Dublin and the Irish Dental Library, all in Dublin, have notable collections.

National Libraries

The British Library was formed in 1973. Two sections are of particular usefulness in medicine and science — the British Library Document Supply Centre (BLDSC) and the Science Reference and Information Services (SRIS) (see also Cannell, 1990).

BLDSC

The BLDSC at Boston Spa, Yorkshire, is the largest library in the world devoted to the supply of documents. It is the national centre for library interlending in the UK and between the UK and overseas. It supplies material only to other libraries and not directly to individuals. Applications for loans and photocopies are made through libraries registered as borrowers.

The stock of the BLDSC includes most significant serials in all subjects and languages (55 000 titles are currently received), most important English-language and foreign monographs, report literature and conference proceedings. It makes use of a number of 'back-up' libraries, including the Royal Society of Medicine and the Department of Health, to supply material not on its own shelves, as a result of which some major libraries not previously able to take much part in interlibrary lending can now make a useful contribution.

The *Current List of Serials* in the BLDSC records titles but not holdings. It is frequently updated. *Serials in the British Library*, a quarterly listing with annual cumulations, gives title, place of publication, date of commencement and frequency of issue. It is published by the bibliographic services of the British Library, London.

SRIS

The British Library's Science Reference and Information Service was formed by expanding the former Patent Office Library with scientific literature from the British Museum Library and with newly-acquired material. Life science subjects, including a medical collection, are housed in its Aldwych building in Kean Street, Drury Lane, London WC2. The Scottish Science Library, a unit of the National Library of Scotland, was opened at 33 Salisbury Place, Edinburgh EH9 1SL in 1989.

Organization

The professional organization for medical librarians in Britain is the Medical, Health and Welfare Libraries Group of the Library Association. Its meetings include an annual weekend conference, usually in one of the large cities or towns with well-established medical libraries. It is responsible for several publications including the quarterly *Health Libraries Review*, inaugurated in 1984, and the *Directory of medical and health care libraries* (1990), and in other ways does its best to promote the interests of medical libraries and their users.

There is a companion Scottish group, the Association of Scottish Health Sciences Librarians, set up in 1970, and a Welsh Group.

For language and other reasons British medical libraries have a close affinity with their North American counterparts.

North American libraries

USA

The United States has a wealth of medical libraries. Developments have been reported by Walker and Due (1986) and more recently an overview of on going work in the USA on the development of programmes for Integrated Academic Information Management Systems has been described (Matheson, 1988). The most important medical library in the world is the National Library of Medicine, at Bethesda, Maryland.

Founded in 1836 as the Library of the Surgeon General's Office, U.S. Army, the National Library of Medicine now possesses nearly 2 000 000 volumes and over 2 000 000 items of non-book material (microforms, audio-visual, manuscripts, etc.). It receives some 23 000 serial publications, of which 2750 are selected for indexing in *Index Medicus* and other publications. It is rich in historical material: its catalogues of incunabula and early printed books and its other publications are described elsewhere in this volume (p. 581). It is responsible for the compilation of the *Index Medicus* (p. 51) and for MEDLARS (p. 91), perhaps the two most valuable services to medical information in the world today. It has generously arranged the decentralization of MEDLARS, which is made available to suitably equipped centres in the USA and elsewhere. One of these centres is the British Library Medical Information Service. The National Library of Medicine also offers the usual reference and interlibrary loan facilities. Its functions and responsibilities are outlined by Mehnert and Leiter (1988) and its long and fascinating history has been fully documented by Miles (1982). Its long-range plans were published in 1987 (NLM, 1987; Tabor, 1988).

The second largest American medical library is the Francis A. Countway Library at Harvard Medical School. This was formed by the amalgamation in 1965 of Harvard Medical School Library (1783) with the Boston Medical Library (1807). This amalgamation resulted in a library of more than 600 000 volumes and 5000 current periodicals.

The library of the New York Academy of Medicine has an exhaustive collection of contemporary medical literature and is richly endowed with historical material covering all branches of medicine, together with a collection of portraits, manuscripts, letters, medals, stamps, etc. It contains over half a million volumes.

Other U.S. libraries

Other important American medical collections that may be mentioned here are those of the College of Physicians of Philadelphia, Yale Medical Library, the Mayo Clinic, Johns Hopkins School of Medicine, the State University of New York Downstate Medical Center, the Biomedical Library at the Center for the Health Sciences, University of California at Los Angeles, the National Institutes of Health at Bethesda, the Cleveland Health Sciences Library and the medical section of the John Crerar Library at Chicago. Some recent developments in health sciences libraries in North America are described by Doran (1990).

Canada

Canada's principal medical libraries are at the Academy of Medicine (Toronto), McGill Medical Library (Montreal), the Department of National Health and Welfare (Ottawa), the W.K. Kellogg Health Sciences Centre Library at London (Ontario) and the McMaster University Health Sciences Library at Hamilton (Ontario) (see Groen, 1986). The

Canadian Health Libraries Association (Association des Bibliothèques de la Santé du Canada) has its offices in Toronto.

Organization

The professional organization for medical librarians in North America is the Medical Library Association (MLA) founded in 1898. Its objectives are to foster medical libraries and to encourage the training and continuing education of medical librarians. It publishes the quarterly *Bulletin of the Medical Library Association* and the *Handbook of medical library practice* (Darling *et al.*, 1982–88). The MLA holds an annual meeting for the presentation of papers and the discussion of its organizational affairs.

Other countries

Recent development in the medical libraries of Finland, France, Germany, Greece, Italy, Norway, Portugal and Yugoslavia are reviewed in Picken and Kahn (1986).

France

In France, medical libraries are usually funded by government, either academic libraries in universities and teaching hospitals, or libraries of important national institutions such as the Centre Nationale de la Recherche Scientifique (CNRS) or the Institut National de la Santé et de la Recherche Médicale (INSERM). The French host Télésystèmes-Questel offers a number of medical databases. It was established under a contract with the Ministère de l'Industrie et de la Recherche with INSERM and CNRS to permit the loading of MEDLINE. The former Bibliothèque de la Faculté de Médecine, Paris, now renamed Bibliothèque Interuniversitaire de Médecine, acts as the national interlibrary lending centre in medicine (Deschamps, 1986). INIST (Institut de l'Information Scientifique et Technique), the French national library of scientific and technical information, collects, analyses, indexes and distributes worldwide literature in all the scientific and technical fields; it provides various accesses to the PASCAL database (see p. 57).

Belgium

In Belgium the library of the University of Louvain Faculty of Medicine, Brussels, has designed a programme (TELEDOC) that automates interlibrary loan requests between libraries. When a request has been typed in by the user, TELEDOC consults the BIOMED union catalogue of biomedical periodical subscriptions in Belgium and, according to a pre-established order of priority, automatically selects from the 40 libraries listed one that holds the document; requests are then forwarded by electronic mail or telex (Walckiers *et al.*, 1988).

Germany

In Germany large medical libraries are established at Cologne, Heidelberg, Göttingen and Munich. The Deutsches Institut für Medizinische Dokumentation und Information (DIMDI) at Cologne has numerous foreign and domestic databases for information retrieval, including MEDLARS. The Zentralbibliothek für Medizin, Cologne, represents the national library for medical sciences in the country (see Kühnen, 1986).

Switzerland

Switzerland is fortunate in being the home of the World Health Organization, in which the need for an adequate library and reference service to support the technical work of WHO was recognized at its foundation. The first books and periodicals were acquired by 1946, since when the collection has grown steadily. The WHO library in Geneva now contains more than 100 000 volumes, having inherited at an early stage the library of the Office International de l'Hygiène Publique. It currently receives about 3000 periodicals on an exchange, gift or subscription basis. Its special collections include one on the history of international health and an extensive collection of WHO unpublished documents and reports.

A distinguishing feature of the WHO library has been its use as a training centre for future medical and scientific librarians. In 1974 it initiated a global health literature programme for the improvement of medical library services and, particularly, the development of regional medical libraries. A MEDLARS service is operated by the library (Ruff, Rhee and Senadhira, 1986).

There is a modern library for the Faculté de Médecine of the University of Geneva. The universities of Basle and Zürich have extensive medical collections.

Scandinavia

In Scandinavia the Karolinska Institutet, Stockholm, has the largest collection of current medical literature. Its Biomedical Documentation Centre operates a MEDLARS service for Scandinavia; the Biomedical Department of Göteborg is also well provided. An outstanding medical library in Norway is that in the Biomedical Department of the University Library, Oslo. The State Hospital and Ullevål Hospital in Oslo and

Haukeland Hospital in Bergen are also well equipped. The largest collection of medical literature in Denmark is in the Second Department of the University Library, Copenhagen. The most important medical library in Finland is the Central Medical Library at Helsinki.

Fine collections exist in Italy, Russia and elsewhere. Tabor (1990) should be consulted for information on these and other foreign libraries. The problems of libraries in the Third World have been discussed by McCarthy (1981).

Fine collections exist in Italy, Russia and elsewhere. Taylor (1990) should be consulted for information on these and other foreign libraries. The problems of libraries in the Third World have been discussed by McCarthy (1981).

Co-operation

The continuous growth of scientific literature, the proliferation of the periodical literature and the interconnection of one discipline with another make it almost impossible for any one library to be completely self-sufficient; other sources must be tapped.

The most recent trend in Britain and in the United States has been similar — the development of library networks; approaches are varied but the objectives are common. On both sides of the Atlantic standards of service to the user have been raised through co-ordination and co-operation to make more effective use of local and regional resources. In the UK, regionally organized library services to National Health Service staff began, effectively, with the appointment of a Regional Librarian in the Wessex Region in 1967. The NHS Regional Librarians Group was formally instituted in 1976. Today 14 Regions into which the NHS in England is administratively divided, together with Scotland, Wales and Northern Ireland, are all represented in the Group, either by holders of the designated post of Regional Librarian or by the librarian of a major library having Regional contact and support (Forrest and Carmel, 1987).

Crossing national boundaries

The first International Congress on Medical Librarianship was held in London in 1953. Others have followed in Washington (1963), Amsterdam (1969), Belgrade (1980), Tokyo (1985) and Delhi (1990). The seventh is planned for Washington in 1995.

The first European Congress of Medical Libraries took place in Brussels in 1986, the second in Bologna in 1988 and the third is planned for

Montpellier in 1992. The European Association of Health Information and Libraries was founded during the first European Congress and formally constituted in August 1988 at IFLA's Brighton conference.

Arrangement within the library

A large part of the stock of a modern medical library consists of periodicals. These are usually kept together, arranged in subject or alphabetical order. Current issues are often segregated for the benefit of readers who regularly monitor the incoming literature. Besides the usual catalogue, most libraries provide a hand list of their current periodicals.

Catalogues

A catalogue may be in the form of:

1 *an author catalogue*, with entries arranged under the names of authors, institutions, and sometimes series titles;

2 *a subject catalogue*, with its entries grouped together under subject headings, arranged alphabetically or in a classified order; most libraries have both author and subject catalogues of their books, pamphlets, etc. *MeSH (Medical Subject Headings)*, a thesaurus compiled by the National Library of Medicine, may be used as a subject authority list (see p. 92);

3 *a dictionary catalogue*, in which both author and subject entries are assembled in one alphabetical sequence.

Main entries in catalogues usually include a classification symbol or shelf mark to indicate the location of the item concerned. The catalogue of periodicals is usually separate. Computer-produced catalogues are essentially databases, with retrieval on certain specified fields. For example, the names of authors, subjects or keywords, titles, publishers and dates would be placed in retrieval fields, but the collation is usually placed in a non-retrieval field. The process for retrieval varies from system to system but is usually via a menu.

Classification schemes

NLM SCHEME

The National Library of Medicine has introduced a classification scheme developed from that of the Library of Congress, Washington, the *National Library of Medicine Classification*, 1981. This scheme permits specific entry, bringing together in one place material on all aspects of a particular topic. A combination of letters and figures is employed in the notation. Material concerning the preclinical sciences is arranged under the letters QS–QZ and material on medicine and related subjects under the letter W. The synopsis of classes is as follows:

Preclinical Sciences

QS	Human Anatomy	QW	Microbiology and Immunology
QT	Physiology	QX	Parasitology
QU	Biochemistry	QY	Clinical Pathology
QV	Pharmacology	QZ	Pathology

Medicine and Related Subjects

W	Medical Profession	WI	Gastrointestinal system
WA	Public health	WJ	Urogenital system
WB	Practice of medicine	WK	Endocrine system
WC	Communicable diseases	WL	Nervous system
WD 100	Nutrition disorders	WM	Psychiatry
WD 200	Metabolic diseases	WN	Radiology
WD 300	Immunologic diseases; diseases of hypersensitivity	WO	Surgery
		WP	Gynecology
		WQ	Obstetrics
WD 400	Animal poisoning	WR	Dermatology
WD 500	Plant poisoning	WS	Pediatrics
WD 600	Diseases and injuries caused by physical agents	WT	Geriatrics. Chronic disease
		WU	Dentistry. Oral surgery
WD 700	Aviation and space medicine	WV	Otorhinolaryngology
		WW	Ophthalmology
WE	Musculoskeletal system	WX	Hospitals and other health facilities
WF	Respiratory system	WY	Nursing
WG	Cardiovascular system	WZ	History of medicine
WH	Hemic and lymphatic systems		

An example of subdivision WG (Cardiovascular system) is:

WG	Cardiovascular system
WG 200	Heart, general works
WG 201	Anatomy, Histology, Embryology
WG 202	Physiology, Mechanism of the heart beat
WG 205	Cardiac emergencies
WG 220	Congenital heart disease

One advantage of this scheme is its simplicity. Another is that the National Library of Medicine publishes *NLM Current Catalog*, quarterly, with annual cumulations (see p. 52) in which entries are given NLM classification numbers and subject headings. New medical books published in the USA sometimes contain the NLM classification number on the reverse of the title page.

DDS/UDC

Some medical libraries in Britain use the Dewey Decimal System or the Universal Decimal Classification (UDC). In these schemes the whole field of knowledge is divided into ten main classes:

000	Generalities	600	Technology, applied sciences
100	Philosophy	700	The arts. Fine and
200	Religion		decorative arts
300	Social sciences	800	Literature
400	Languages	900	Geography and history,
500	Natural sciences and mathematics		and auxiliary disciplines

These classes are subdivided by adding figures to the right of the main number, giving decimal subdivision. A decimal point is added after the third figure. An advantage of these two decimal systems is that they permit infinite expansion within each subject field to accommodate new subjects or to expand existing ones in UDC by synthesis, which is not possible in Dewey. A disadvantage is that they separate material dealing with different aspects (anatomy, physiology, disease, etc.) of an organ, system or region. In UDC the user library can bring together subjects as it wishes by using the colon. In the Dewey system the class 600 is devoted to Technology, applied sciences, and its first subdivision, 610, is devoted to medicine. Examples of subdivision are:

600	Technology
610	Medical sciences. Medicine
611	Human anatomy, cytology, histology
611.1	Cardiovascular organs
611.11	Pericardium
611.12	Heart
612	Human physiology
612.1	Blood and circulation
616	Diseases
616.1	Diseases of cardiovascular system
616.11	Diseases of the endocardium and pericardium
616.12	Diseases of the heart

The subdivisions .1 to .8 are the same in Anatomy (611), Physiology (612) and Diseases (616).

The UDC has the same framework as Dewey. It is particularly useful for large collections or where very detailed classification is necessary.

BLISS CLASSIFICATION

The Bliss classification is a very detailed general scheme, covering all branches of knowledge and suitable for large libraries. It has an alphabetical notation, for example:

H	Anthropology, Human biology and Health sciences	
HWE	Respiratory system	
HWF	Pharynx	
HWFT	Tonsils	
HWFT GL		Surgery
HWFT GNG		Tonsillectomy
HWG	Larynx	
HWG GL		Surgery
HWG GNG		Laryngectomy

LIBRARY OF CONGRESS CLASSIFICATION

The Library of Congress scheme is a general scheme devised specially for that library but used very widely. A mixed notation is employed. The various fields of knowledge are indicated by letters of the alphabet, with a second letter to indicate the principal subdivision of each field. Further subdivision is by the use of figures. An example is:

R	Medicine (general)	
RC	Internal medicine	
RC 666-701	Diseases of the circulatory (cardiovascular) system	
RC 681-687	Diseases of the heart	
RC 685	Individual diseases of the heart, A–Z;	
	then divided alphabetically, e.g.	
RC 685.A6	Angina pectoris	
A65	Arrhythmias	
C6	Coronary heart disease	
I	Psychiatry	
Q	People with learning difficulties	

OTHER SCHEMES

A few other classification schemes may be met in medical libraries — for example the Barnard scheme (1955), once popular in the UK but now rather out of date and being replaced in some libraries by the National Library of Medicine classification. Some libraries have designed their own scheme to meet their particular needs.

References

Cannell, S. (1990) The role of the British Library for medical and health information. *Health Libraries Review*, **7**, 14-19.

Copyright, Designs and Patents Act 1988. London: HMSO.

Darling, L. *et al.* (eds) (1982-88) *Handbook of medical library practice*, 4th edn. (3 vols). Chicago: Medical Library Association.

Deschamps, C. (1986) 'France'. In *Medical librarianship in the eighties and beyond*, ed. F.M. Picken and A.M.C. Kahn, pp. 192-198. London: Mansell.

Directory of medical and health care libraries in the United Kingdom and the Republic of Ireland (1990) 7th edn., compiled by D.J. Wright. London: Library Association.

Doran, B. (1990) North American medical libraries: report of a study tour. *Health Libraries Review*, 7, 145-154.

Forrest, M. and Carmel, M. (1987) The NHS Regional Librarians Group. *Health Libraries Review*, 4, 160-163.

Godbolt, S. (1991) Electronic publishing, the end user, and medical education. *Annals of the Rheumatic Diseases*, 50, 411-414.

Groen, F. (1986) 'Canada'. In *Medical librarianship in the eighties and beyond*, ed. F.M. Picken and A.M.C. Kahn, pp. 229-236. London: Mansell.

Jamieson, A.H. (ed.) (*c.* 1986) *Directory of health library resources in Scotland*. Edinburgh: Association of Scottish Health Sciences Librarians.

Jenkins, S. (1987) *Medical libraries: a user guide*. London: British Medical Association.

Kühnen, J.F. (1986) 'German Federal Republic'. In *Medical librarianship in the eighties and beyond*, ed. F.M. Picken and A.M.C. Kahn, pp. 198-201. London: Mansell.

Law, D. (1991) Databases free at the point of use: a unique opportunity for academics and students. *Health Libraries Review*, 8, 61-62.

McCarthy, C. (1981) 'Third world medical libraries'. In *Medical librarianship*, ed. M. Carmel, pp. 297-309. London: Library Association.

Matheson. N. (ed.) (1988) Integrated Academic Information Management Systems. *Bulletin of the Medical Library Associations*, 76, 221-267.

Mehnert, R.B. and Leiter, J. (1988) 'The National Library of Medicine'. In *Handbook of medical library practice*, 4th edn. ed. L. Darling *et al.*, pp.143-176. Chicago: Medical Library Association.

Miles, W.D. (1982) *A history of the National Library of Medicine*. Washington DC: U.S. Government Printing Office.

Morton, L.T. and Wright, D.J. (1990) *How to use a medical library*, 7th edn. London: Library Association.

National Library of Medicine (1987) *Long-Range Plan (Report of the Board of Regents). Panel Reports 1-5*. Bethesda, MD: National Library of Medicine.

O'Donovan, K. First experiences with BIDS. *Health Libraries Review*, **8**, 94-97.

Penn, C. (1990) Photocopying Crown and Parliamentary publications. *Library Association Record*, **92**, 117-118.

Picken, F.M. and Kahn, A.M.C. (eds) (1986) *Medical librarianship in the eighties and beyond*, London: Mansell.

Ruff, B., Rhee H. and Senadhira, A. (1986) 'The World Health Organization'. In *Medical librarianship in the eighties and beyond*, ed. F.M.C. Picken and A.M.C. Kahn, pp. 310-320. London: Mansell.

Stone, P. (1990) *JANET: a report on its use for libraries* (British Library Research Paper 77). London: British Library.

Tabor, R. (1988) Planning for the future? National Library of Medicine long-range plan. *Health Libraries Review*, **5**, 248-251.

Tabor, R. (1990) 'Medical libraries of today'. In *Thornton's medical books, libraries and collectors*, ed. Besson, 3rd edn. Aldershot: Gower.

Walckiers, M., Blitz, D. and Soree, G. (1988). TELEDOC – automated document ordering between libraries in Belgium. *Health Libraries Review*, **5**, 178-180.

Walker, W.D. and Due, K.M. (1986) 'The United States'. In *Medical librarianship in the eighties and beyond*, ed. F.M. Picken and A.M.C. Kahn, pp. 236-248. London: Mansell.

Warren, K.S. (ed.) (1981) *Coping with the biomedical literature: a primer for the scientist and clinician*. New York: Praeger.

CHAPTER TWO

Primary sources of information

R. J. DANNATT[*]; revised by D.R.H. ADAMS

One of the earliest large-scale surveys of a representative group of scientists (Halbert and Ackoff, 1959) showed that, on average, more time was spent on scientific communication than on any other activity. The mean 33 per cent of total time identified in the survey included time spent in both oral and print communication. As a prelude to this chapter on primary sources of information, it seems worthwhile to consider first the importance of oral communication, so far as it is known, and how it relates to communication mechanisms which operate through the published literature. The work done in this field has usually considered communication in science and technology, but much of it carries significance for medicine as well.

Personal contacts

De Solla Price (1963) postulated the existence of 'invisible colleges': informal groupings of 100–200 scientists, active in research, who communicate verbally with each other at conferences, colloquia, summer schools and by long-distance telephone while adding to the cumulating structure of the scientific literature only belatedly and more from convention than need. The colleges clearly have much in common with the

---

* Formerly Librarian, University of Wales College of Medicine, Cardiff

Information Exchange Groups (IEG) sponsored by the National Institutes of Health in the early 1960s whose aim was the free circulation of unrefereed memoranda among members and the encouragement of informal comment, without prejudice to later publication of the same material in the literature. The subject scope of the seven experimental IEGs was quite limited, as for instance Haemostasis and Immunopathology, but even so memberships were generally between 500 and 1000. More recent examples of invisible colleges are the informal networks using electronic mail which are assuming growing importance.

A recurrent theme in studies in communication has been that it is a complex and often idiosyncratic process in which the individuals are concerned to safeguard their sense of autonomy and creativity against the pressure of both other people's words and other people's writings. Information discovered by chance, whether during casual conversation with colleagues or while browsing in the literature, may be valued more highly than information sought specifically or deliberately because it seems to have been elicited spontaneously. It is possible that communication studies carried out by means of interviews emphasize the importance of personal contacts and chance because this is a natural response in the interview situation, whereas studies carried out by questionnaire, often associated with libraries, emphasize the systematic scanning and searching of the literature.

Other studies of the invisible college concept (Meadows, 1974) have shown that it, too, is a complex process which varies according to the subject field in which communication is taking place. These studies emphasize the importance of local research groups, often based on one scientific centre, whose 'internal' communication system provides a necessary backing to the longer-range contacts between individuals. While the existence of certain individuals, often prominent members of research teams, is fundamental to the invisible college, the same individuals also have a range of contacts outside the college, facilitated now by the emergence of electronic networks and in addition communicate extensively by means of the literature.

These findings seem to confirm work that has been done on the diffusion of information in industrial R & D Laboratories (Allen, 1969) and on the communication of drug information to physicians (Herman and Rodowskas, 1976). Allen showed that certain individuals in each organization function as 'gatekeepers' — intermediaries through whom other members of the staff contacted individuals outside the organization and kept in touch with the published literature. The implication here is that though much of the flow of information in industrial laboratories is through personal contacts, the literature is being monitored nevertheless by means of the gatekeepers. In an analogous way, surveys of the process by which drug information is disseminated in communities of physicians have tended to show that in respect of new drugs at least, the process is dependent on a few individuals who advise their colleagues while at the same time keeping in touch with both professional (including published) sources of information and commercial ones.

As already mentioned, the concept of the 'invisible college' has a more recent manifestation in the growth in the use of electronic mail via networks such as EARN, BITNET and JANET for rapid communication within a group of researchers with a common interest. While communication is not oral, the immediacy of electronic exchanges has some of the characteristics of conversation. The ability to disseminate or request information to a world community, or to individuals, has produced a large volume of unprocessed information exchange. There are signs that unmediated systems generate so much information that they may become personally unmanageable.

In biomedical fields such as cancer research, where the pace of investigation and achievement is at its most rapid, communication by means of personal contacts has been described as both 'instantaneous' and accurate (Thomas, 1978). This is due to the greater openness of present-day research, which is in itself due to a heightened awareness on the part of researchers that so much still awaits discovery. Communication in technology is of interest because it is possible that medicine has more affinities with technology than with science. De Solla Price (1965, 1970) has distinguished between science and technology on the basis of the pattern of citation in scientific and technological papers. Bibliographies in science are longer and exhibit a higher proportion of references to the recent literature than those in technology — a measure of this being the percentage of references to papers less than five years old in the total number of references included in a bibliography. This value may range from 70 to 90 per cent for a science with a rapidly accumulating literature such as biochemistry (where the number of references per paper is normally about 30) to figures of less than 40 per cent in engineering. In an analysis of papers published in *The Lancet* and *British Medical Journal* between 1900 and 1970, Liepa (1971) showed that the increase in the proportion of scientifically orientated papers during the period was matched by an increase in the 'immediacy' of the references listed in the bibliographies published during this period.

In a large-scale survey of British publications in all fields, Earle and Vickery (1969) showed that bibliographies in medical books and periodicals are, on average, five times longer that those in engineering, and some two-and-a-half times longer than those in other technologies, such as agriculture. It can therefore be argued that by De Solla Price's test much of the present-day laboratory and clinical medicine, as well as anaesthetics, pathology, obstetrics, epidemiology and pharmacology, is akin to science. In surgery, and especially its various branches such as orthopaedic or plastic surgery, bibliographies are both shorter and conform to the technological pattern. One senses, too, that in these fields the paper being written is less important than the particular prothesis or technique of skin grafting under discussion. Another of the distinctions between science and technology made by De Solla Price is that in the former, it is the literature that develops and cumulates, while in the latter the literature is subservient and it is a 'state of the art' that cumulates. There may be some significance in the fact that the *Journal of Bone and Joint Surgery* is published in two sections, an American and a British, with the implication that the journals contribute towards a national art rather than international knowledge.

Making use of Wood and Hamilton's survey of mechanical engineers working in the UK (1967), it seems likely that the surgeons rate personal contacts higher as an information source than the documentary sources, such as original papers or reviews, while workers in other branches of medicine rate personal contacts relatively lower. The success of the various 'clinical librarian' experiments during the 1970s seems to indicate the readiness of doctors in the typical clinical setting to accept verbal information, either from a clinical librarian or from a colleague, and also their ultimate reliance on the published literature. Greenberg (1978) reports that no significant differences were found in the experiment at Yale–New Haven Hospital between the use made of clinical librarian services across a range of medical fields, which included surgery, paediatrics and psychiatry. The results of a clinical librarian experimental project in Britain are reported by Childs (1972), Moore (1982) and Wilkin (1982).

The periodical literature

One of the most valuable and largely unforeseen consequences of our increased awareness of oral communication in science and technology has been increased understanding of the way the literature operates and the ends it serves. The view that the function of the periodical literature is the communication of information was put by Bernal (1939) in his now classic *The social function of science*. He voiced quite clearly the indifference of science to linguistic or national barriers and the need of practitioners, at all levels, for the data, information on techniques, conceptual frameworks and new ideas that the literature conveys (Bernal, 1959).

Characteristically, he saw the literature as part of a system having properties such as 'sluggishness' and 'waste' and was one of the first to propose ways by which the system could be improved. This is in contrast to the view (Ziman, 1968) that the fact of publication is less important than the process of comment, modification and evaluation that each account of new work passes through during publication (the refereeing process) and thereafter, and that ends with assimilation into the corpus of scientific knowledge. While allowing that the literature embodies great quantities of data and information, this view allows also for the fact that much of it may be unimportant or unoriginal; value resides not in the literature but in the consensus of ideas that experienced scientists create out of it. De Solla Price (1965, 1967) has described the periodical literature as having merely an archival function in contrast to the function of primary communication performed verbally and through agencies such as the invisible colleges. Hence his view that scientists are motivated to add to the published literature but not any longer to read it. The literature, while accounting only for about 20 per cent of overall reviewing the relationships and significance of new advances, partly as a means whereby the inexperienced can obtain access to problems of current research and partly as a record of achievement which interacts with technology and the general culture of the time. This view of the periodical literature as archive emphasizes the permanent need of all scientists for access to it.

Publication in the periodical literature has been the prime way scientists claim priority for their work; the public availability of this literature is the chief guarantee that the recognition awarded them, however much or little it may amount to, emanates from their peers and is real (Hagstrom, 1965). The growth of team research, often giving rise to multiple authorship, and the custom of publishing a description of a research project for accounting purposes has undoubtedly eroded this particular aspect of the literature, but it still exists. It was assumed at their inception that memoranda distributed within IEGs would eventually be published in the normal way, thus safeguarding the right of authors to recognition. Whether the circulation of a memorandum gave priority or not was an early cause of embarrassment, but what ended the IEG experiment, apart from its cost, was the refusal of a number of important biochemical journals to accept any paper for publication that had previously existed as an IEG memorandum (Thorpe, 1967). In the same way, the indifference which most scientists feel for the research report literature is due not so much the 'open' literature. One may note in passing that in medicine and in engineering there are ways of establishing priority, and of thereby obtaining recognition, that are additional to the way established within science of first publishing in the literature. These are, in medicine, the first accurate description of a disease or physical condition and, in engineering, the successful patenting of a new mechanism or process.

It has been left to the journal editors such as Fox (1965), Maddox (1967) and Ingelfinger (1974) to emphasize that periodicals, in addition to their other functions, must stimulate their readers and provide an outlet for argument, criticism, speculation and comment. In medicine, especially, they must also meet the needs of the developing specialty and of education in general, which means the publication of papers with a factual rather than an experimental content addressed by the expert to the less well qualified. *The Lancet, Nature* and the *New England Journal of Medicine* have deliberately set out to combine the function of 'recorders' of advances in knowledge with the function of medical or scientific 'newspapers'. Review periodicals are covered in Chapter 3, but the point is perhaps worth making here that they can be grouped with the 'newspapers' rather than the 'recorders'.

The Council of Biology Editors accepted (Zwemer, 1970) a formal definition of the scientific periodical which stresses, among others, the following characteristics:

1   It should contain first disclosures, i.e. first accounts of new work.
2   Papers should provide sufficient detail for observations to be assessed, experiments repeated and ideas evaluated.
3   It should be permanent.

Developments in biomedical communication

In biomedicine, as in other fields, it seems clear that the historical development of periodicals has been in the direction of perfecting them as a means by which knowledge can be enlarged and consolidated while at the same time providing a mechanism for the reward, through peer recognition, of individual contributing authors. The outcome of this historical process is the primary journal as we know it — a package made up of a varying number of the basic and now perfected units of information, or scientific papers. It seems equally clear that the orientation of periodicals towards what Ziman aptly called 'public knowledge', with the attendant concern to prefer the publication of first disclosures and to aim at archival permanence, has meant that the other important function of the literature — communication — has become neglected. What seems to have happened is that the immense strength of the scientific tradition, as demonstrated in a widespread feeling that papers with a different aim — that of education, or speculation, or case report — must still be as self-contained and formal as the archival literature proper. We may smile at the drug advertisements, each with its carefully composed list of references but were it not for the strength of the archive tradition they could dispense with them and get on with the business of telling doctors how good the drugs are!

Wyatt (1972) has taken this line of argument a stage further and, in a detailed analysis of the events, discussions and publications leading up to the discovery of the helix structure of DNA in 1953, suggests that the process of discovery itself was slower and more erratic that it need have been had an earlier paper on DNA in 1948 been less reticent, or the reviews of it less cautious. He has also analysed the network of citations linking the various papers published between 1948 and 1953 and shows that there are several serious discontinuities; he concludes, pessimistically, that new information is unrecognized until it has transformed into knowledge. Perhaps the often documented part played by chance in the process of discovery is so large simply because the literature as a source of events is so unresponsive. An account of the events, some accidental, leading up to the discovery of the mechanism of poliomyelitis infection (Bodian, 1976) gives some support to this. Shephard (1973) has documented the history of a paper reporting some unusual cases of poisoning in the USA which was refused publication by four major national journals (some refereed) before being accepted, unchanged, by a local medical journal. It appears that the paper was not well written in the first place, and it seems likely that a further reason for the rejections was the paper's limited scope. Nevertheless, it was, as Shephard points out, the first original case report in America of this particular type of poisoning. The continuing importance of case reports in clinical medicine is shown by the fact that research into a new method of publishing and storing them forms one of the recommendations of the report of the Medical Information Review Panel (Cockerill, 1981).

The IEGs were a significant experiment in communication because they were devised by scientists rather than by documentalists or scientific management. The proposal that unrefereed and unedited communications should be circulated to loosely defined groups of coworkers was both made and received with enthusiasm (Green, 1964). Memberships of the groups rose rapidly, as did the number of memoranda in circulation. There is an interesting parallel here with the informal distribution of preprints, reprints and reports of research, in addition to discussions of work in progress at meetings and seminars, which exists on an extensive scale in psychology (Garvey and Griffith, 1965). Posen and Posen (1969) have shown that the demand for reprints for some quite representative papers published in the earliest years of *Current Contents, Life Sciences* and long before the appearance of *Current Contents, Clinical Medicine* can run well into three figures, while requests for a reprint of a particular review on alkaline phosphatase were as high as 1246. A reprint, once received, can be thought of as a personal communication and it may be that the demand for reprints is higher than the demand, within an equivalent time, for the same papers as part of the normal periodical literature. If so, this and the popularity of reprint and memorandum circulation systems, such as the IEG, may be due to the individual scientist's wish to participate both as a giver and receiver, in an informal — even personal — information system within which a degree of inefficiency and waste of time is taken for granted.

The traditional communication system in science is held together by two groups of people: the authors, who generate new information but who as readers equally consume it, and the referees. The traditional rewards of recognition and status can only be given by the consumers of new information and, therefore, the referee's function is really to distance and screen new information during its transmission from author to consumer. This preliminary validation is nevertheless essential for the health of the system, but there is also a basic rule underpinning the whole — that of the 'first disclosure'. It follows, therefore, that any weakening of the reporting tradition shows itself either in a weakening of the basic rule or in a weakening of the author–consumer and referee relationship. In biomedicine especially there are now indications that the rule is not being observed, or rather that its importance to the system is no longer understood. Relman (1977) describes two occasions in which a paper submitted to the *New England Journal of Medicine* was already being considered by two other journals. The two papers were both in effect published three times over a short period without any of the editors, or referees, having been apprised of the situation.

One aspect of these two instances of triplicate publication that Relman does not discuss is the part that may have been played by the co-authors, since both papers had several authors. It seems likely that co-authorship now so common dilutes 'authorship' to the point at which the first disclosure rule loses significance. Any recent issue of *New England Journal of Medicine* or *The Lancet* shows a list of original articles with an average of six or more authors for each. Durack (1978) showed that the number of papers with a single author published in the *New England Journal of Medicine* had declined to 4 per cent by 1977 and that the average authorship in this journal for that year was between four and five per paper. The question that needs to be asked is whether the multiple publication of new work is a help or a hindrance to its dissemination. This question is not answered definitively by referring to the danger of choking the communication system; it is well known, for instance, that the same information is multiplied many times in the prepublication mode of communication in science.

It may also be significant that the role of referees in biomedicine is being questioned and especially their traditional anonymity (Ingelfinger, 1974). Furthermore, certain journals of high standing such as *The Lan-*

cet make little use of referees. The significance of this development is that it seems to show a weakening of the referee role. The editor of the *British Medical Journal* criticizes refereeing from the point of view of its unreliability and merit (Lock, 1985). In contrast to what appears to be a trend in medicine towards publishing for dissemination, the trend in science seems strongly towards preserving the traditional system of publishing for knowledge through the quality control mechanism of first disclosure, refereeing and peer review. A study of the scientific information system in the UK conducted by the Royal Society (Rowland, 1982) showed that nearly all British scientists were in favour of refereeing and that most thought that the important characteristic of a journal chosen for publication purposes was its scientific standard and reputation. There was little enthusiasm for the developments which, potentially at least, dilute the first disclosure principle by two-part publication, i.e. synopsis journals or 'letters' journals — and still less for the publication of all new papers as separates. This study of the scientific information system was conducted by means of questionnaire. Ziman (1982) reiterates his belief in the communication system as the 'core institution' of science and in its absolute dependence on the 'public social apparatus' of authoritative refereeing, open publication and collective review.

A challenge to this view and to the author–referee relationship has come from access to personal computers capable of producing camera-ready text for publishing and from the ability to transmit documents electronically. The dilemma for the author is that recognition still rests on refereed articles in the journal literature, while the pace of research will rely increasingly on electronically disseminated research results.

Medical journals

Journals comprising the primary literature of medicine are basically of three types: journals devoted to news, opinion and comment; journals devoted to original contributions; and review journals. Original contributions in medicine are normally reported once only and full length but journals publishing preliminary communications (normally about 2500 words), such as *Biochemical and Biophysical Research Communications* have become well established in recent years. The three basic types of journal are not mutually exclusive; the *New England Journal of Medicine* contains, for example, original contributions as well as case reports and editorial comment, while a high percentage of the review articles listed in *Bibliography of Medical Reviews* do not appear in review journals. Certain journals with, primarily, a review function such as *Obstetrical and Gynecological Survey* and the *Year Book* series, also publish extended abstracts of original papers appearing elsewhere. English-language review journals in medicine are comparatively recent in origin, the earliest *Year Books* appearing in the mid-1930s and the first formal review journals, *Progress in Allergy* and *Advances in Internal Medicine,* several years later. German journals in the *Ergebnisse* series were first published between 1892 and 1902.

The Lancet, one of the oldest medical journals, first appeared in 1823. Liepa (1971) sampled issues from this and the *British Medical Journal* decennially from 1900 to 1970 and has shown that the decline of 16 per cent in the number of clinical studies being published by the end of this period was matched by an increase of 22 per cent on the number of experimental studies. More specifically, she found that surgical and pathological papers diminished by 19 per cent and 15 per cent, respectively, while papers in biochemistry and drug therapy increased by 12 per cent and 18.5 per cent. Articles in the field of social medicine increased during the period by 7 per cent. In addition to the apparent change in orientation, there has been a great increase in the volume of periodical publishing in medicine, particularly in the 1960s and 1970s. Webb (1970) analysed papers in 19 primary journals in biochemistry between 1958 and 1967 and found that the doubling time for the total number of papers in this field was 6.9 years. The doubling time for pages or words was 5.2 years — a more realistic figure from the point of view of the reader wishing to keep up to date and one which shows, incidentally, that in spite of editorial policies, papers are tending to become longer rather than shorter. A sample year (1977) of the Source Data listing in *Journal Citation Reports* shows that nearly half of the world's journals that publish more than 1000 articles a year, general journals such as *Nature* excluded, were biomedical ones.

The volume of publishing in medicine is giving rise, inevitably, to change in the proportion of primary literature devoted to original contributions, to commentary and to review. The review journals have grown relative to the recorders because, especially in the more clinical fields, they play such an active and essential part in promulgating therapy and in advancing the 'state of the art'. If scientific knowledge cumulates, only occasionally to be reformed, it is probably truer of knowledge in medicine to say that it constantly updates. De Solla Price (1981) makes the point that the clinical literature, unlike the scientific, is not self-validating (since revising a 'state of the art' is an end in itself) and that the functions of evaluation and validation must therefore be performed separately. It is noticeable that in medicine there are a number of newer journals, for instance *Cancer Surveys* or *Life Chemistry Reports* whose aim is to review a section of the overall field in depth and thereby arrive at a definitive update. These publications represent a further development in the traditional review journal, a further development being the creation of knowledge bases. The *Hepatitis Knowledge Base*, for instance (Bernstein, 1980), is more authoritative than any single review since it is based on a large number of them (40), with additional input from other experts, yet it still maintains links with the contributing papers by quoting data from them and citing them in full. Developing the medical journal in this direction necessitates computer storage of the material and interrogation of it online.

The electronic journal

The concept of the electronic journal, introduced in the past decade, is one still to arrive at a workable model. Lancaster (1978) outlined a state where the processes of submission and reviewing of articles, publication, storage and retrieval would all be part of a single electronic system. A number of experiments have explored the application of this model. One of the earliest was in the biomedical field, the International Research Communications System. In this the basic unit of information was a paper of 1000 words (more if no tables were included) with a bibliography of not more than ten references. Papers were submitted electronically, refereed and 'published' online on two online host systems. The project did not attract sufficient contributions to succeed, perhaps due to the lack of development of a word-processing/electronic network infrastructure at the time. Other electronic journal projects experienced similar results, as reported by Turoff and Hiltz (1982) and Shackel (1983). Piternick (1989) postulates that the development of electronic publishing may in fact continue as a parallel rather than a substitute technology. The issues raised remain those of refereeing, problems in 'handling' information stored electronically and the economics of publishing. The practice of subscribing to a title in advance does not appear appropriate to a system where the reader selectively extracts articles from a database. Publishers may have to come to terms with a system of retrospective payment for use of an electronic journal. It is possible that the private Bulletin Board, or online conference-lists developed by some learned societies, will develop as a challenge to commercial publishers.

Guides to journals

General guides are often presented from the viewpoint of the availability of periodicals on subscription while other guides cover particular applications, such as inter-library borrowing. There are two useful general guides to medical periodicals now available. *Ulrich's International Periodicals Directory* is published every year and there is also *Irregular Serials and Annuals*, a separate biennial publication listing less frequent periodicals and annuals. A supplement to both of these is entitled *Ulrich's Quarterly*. The *Directory* is confined to periodicals currently in print and now incorporates an International Standard Serial Number (ISSN) for each title. Periodicals in *Ulrich* are listed under general headings such as Medical Sciences and Biology, divided to cover special areas such as Dentistry or Genetics. The other, more recent, general guide is *The Serials Directory; an International Reference Book*, published by EBSCO. This includes a listing of recently ceased periodical titles and an ISSN index. *World Medical Periodicals* is a listing of all medical, dental and veterinary journals in print at the time of the latest edition (1961, plus Supplement, 1968) with the addition of a number of journals which ceased publication between 1900 and 1950. Unlike *Ulrich* it is an alphabetical listing, but there is an index to the entries by subject. *World medical periodicals* and its *Supplement* indicate that about 6000 periodicals were being published during the 1960s in medicine generally. *Medical and Health Care Books and Serials in Print* from Bowker provides a listing of current medical journals by title and subject in its second volume. A more selective list of journals is the *List of Journals Indexed in Index Medicus*. This is published each year with the January issue of *Index Medicus* (also separately) and comprises currently about 2750 titles. In addition to subject representation, other criteria used in drawing up the *List* are: sponsorship of a journal by a recognized professional organization or national academy, existence of an active and high-level editorial board and freedom from sectional or promotional bias. BIOSIS (BIOSciences Information Service) and *Excerpta Medica* also publish lists of the journals from which papers are chosen and abstracted. The BIOSIS list, published annually, includes an American Standard abbreviation for each title plus a coden (further abbreviation to six upper case letters), if available.

While all these tools include listings of journals according to subject, the separately published version of the *Index Medicus* list and the Bowker *Medical and Health Care Books and Serials* guide are more detailed and carried out at the level of specialties such as orthopaedics or nephrology. Subject guidance to medical periodicals may also be obtained from the list of journals held by a library specializing in the field, for instance the *Periodical holdings* of the Institute of Psychiatry, or by consulting the subject index of *World Medical Periodicals* or a national listing such as *British Medical Periodicals*. The latter covers current British journals of repute and includes notes on subject scope, with additional information on subscription costs, date of first publication, frequency, and publishers and their addresses. The last edition appeared in 1980.

Guides to abstracts journals and indexes in medicine are dealt with in Chapter 3. Review articles, as noted earlier, tend to be dispersed throughout the medical literature, but a list of review journals proper can be found in *List of annual reviews of progress in science and technology*, published by Unesco: 53 review journals are identified in medicine and a further 45 in special fields such as surgery and paediatrics. Apart from obscure journals, the one category less easily covered by lists is new journals. *Ulrich* gives coverage in the *Directory* and the information is updated in the *Quarterly*. The National Library of Medicine *Current Catalog* lists new journals quarterly.

The first issue of all new UK periodicals is listed in the weekly *British national bibliography*, where details of publisher, subscription and frequency are given. *Serials in the British Library* lists new periodicals, British and foreign, with details which include publisher, price, frequency, abbreviated key title, location and holdings. It has wider coverage than indicated by its title as it includes new periodicals held in a number of British libraries.

Usage

Because periodicals are not themselves units of information, but merely packages, comparative studies of the use of periodicals are of little interest to first-hand readers. Few doctors or biomedical scientists work in isolation and the 'pecking order' of the current journals in a research field is one of the least disputed of its characteristics (Royal Society, 1981). Use studies are, however, of great interest to librarians since their work is, to a considerable extent, the management and handling of information packages, not that of units of information — or papers — themselves.

Records of the consultation of periodicals either in or between libraries form the usual material for studies of use, though the scale of consultation must obviously be large enough to sustain any subsequent comparisons between titles of ranking. The alternative material for studying use is a very different record of consultation of a periodical: the citation. In the search for quantifiable acts of use from which generalizations can be made, it is extremely easy to lose sight of the basic fact that a citation is a rather specific linking of one unit of information with another. The consultation of periodicals in or between libraries on the other hand includes other linkings of equal importance from the usage point of view. It covers the use of the package directly, for instance to look up a particular periodical's instructions to authors. It also covers a wider spectrum of the readers of periodicals since use studies based on citation are necessarily limited to readers who are also authors; often, indeed, authors writing from some interdisciplinary viewpoint. From the librarian's point of view it is not unfair to say that the overall ranking of periodicals based on frequency of citation in the *Science Citation Index* source journals and reported in *Journal Citation Reports* and elsewhere (Garfield, 1972, 1976a) are of limited use precisely because the database is so general. The more specific studies that have been published from time to time such as the analysis of citations in a number of pathology journals (Garfield, 1976b) are of more practical interest. It may well be of course that an overall ranking based on interdisciplinary citation turns out *not* to be so different from one based on citation in one particular field of one particular discipline!

The phenomena of 'self-citation' and 'self-derivation' play a part in all use studies based on citation since they vary considerably from one discipline to another. Earle and Vickery (1969) showed that self-citation in medicine, the extent to which medical publications (books excluded) cite publications in medicine, is quite high (61 per cent), but less high than in science generally (70 per cent) and much less so than in technology (81 per cent). Self-derivation in medicine, the extent to which medical references derive from medical sources, was 70 per cent, again lower than in science (78 per cent), but higher than in technology (62 per cent). The implication is that medicine is not less but more interdisciplinary than science and therefore that a ranking of periodicals by interdisciplinary citation in science favours general periodicals slightly less than should be the case for medicine.

The closest equivalent to a usage study based on borrowing from a British medical library is a survey carried out at the then National Lending Library for Science and Technology (NLLST) in 1967 (Wood and Bower, 1969). The assumption is made in this survey, as in other NLLST and British Library Lending Division (BLLD) — now the British Library Document Supply Centre (BLDSC) — surveys, that borrowing within a certain field from a national library can be equated with borrowing within the same field from a local library. In the context of medicine this assumption seems questionable, one reason being an apparent disparity between the population of borrowers from the national library and the population of borrowers in a normal medical library. Less than a quarter of the libraries requesting items from the NLLST at the time of this survey were medical ones, the majority being industrial, research establishment and general university libraries. It is well known that in medicine the availability of libraries (and hence the availability to practitioners of the national library) is generally poor; in this field, more perhaps than in any other today, an older tradition of buying the literature either oneself or through one's employer still persists.

Scales (1976) has compared rankings of most frequently cited periodicals obtained from the *Science Citation Index* database with rankings of periodicals carrying similar dates of publication as most frequently borrowed from NLLST. She found many differences between the two rank lists so produced. Titles common to both the 50 most borrowed and the 50 most cited totalled 16 only. The conclusion is drawn that since inter-library borrowing is a measure of 'actual' use, citation frequency must therefore be unreliable as such a measure. Some consideration is, however, given in this paper to the question of whether the pattern of borrowing from a national library through inter-library loan is a true reflection of literature needs generally. This question has been taken up in a later survey of the usage of periodicals at the BLDSC in 1980 (Clarke, 1981) in which rank lists of titles most frequently borrowed was found to be substantially different from one produced five years earlier. The point is conceded that 'core lists' of periodicals do not seem to have any lasting validity and that this may be due to the effect of changing local circumstances on the demand relationship between client libraries and a central inter-lending one. The Clarke survey reported in passing that medical libraries accounted in 1980 for 14 per cent of overall requests for periodicals at BLDSC. Since this figure excluded some university medical libraries it may well be that the total demand on BLDSC from medical libraries exceeds 20 per cent. One wonders what proportion of the total usage at BLDSC is represented by medicine as a subject. It is probably safe to assume that this usage is greater than that represented by the social sciences (13 per cent), but there is no breakdown in this paper (nor in the British Library *Annual Reports*) of the overall science and technology figure of 80 per cent approximately.

A refinement of the citation method of estimating usage was employed by Raisig (1966) to produce a rank list of all biomedical periodicals being published between 1951 and 1960. In this the final ranking was not derived from numbers of citations as such, but from the number of citations per article published in the given period, essentially the same method as the one used in *Journal Citation Reports* under the heading 'impact factor'. The advantage of ranking periodicals by impact factor is that it eliminates the bias introduced by periodicals which publish a large tally of papers every year (since more papers means potentially more citations) and at the same time the bias introduced by the existence in some years of a few papers in a few journals carrying very high citation counts. These papers may well be the first ones to describe a promising technique, for instance in pathology, or a new statistical method as in epidemiology. The disadvantage of ranking by impact factor is that it unduly favours review periodicals, since these inevitably contain a number of very frequently cited articles. A further point is that ranking by impact factor lends itself to viewing the usefulness of periodicals in terms of cost effectiveness, but this in turn raises the question of 'cost effectiveness to whom?'

Research reports

As a form of primary communication, reports are of much less significance in medicine than in other areas of science, or in technology. Not only is there a long-standing tradition of publication in the conventional literature, but the somewhat less government-controlled institutional research in medicine than, for instance, in atomic energy or space research, has meant less demand for the 'instant publication' that reports provide. The Medical Research Council's research reports and the American Public Health Service's equivalents are published not as communications directly from a research establishment, with merely an identifying code and serial number, but as normal publications of the respective state publishing systems. As such they are better organized bibliographically and much more easy to acquire. The beginnings of a research report literature can, however, be seen in the field of aerospace medicine particularly in the USA. Documents in this field carry prefixes such as ARU (U.S. Army Aeromedical Research Unit) and SAM-TR (USAF School of Aerospace Medicine, Technical Report) and are often available only on microfiche.

Theses

Theses, like conference papers, must be considered primary sources of information since the research projects written up in them may not receive publication in any other form. Part or parts of a thesis are sometimes rewritten and published as a periodical article or monograph, but the thesis remains a first and often fuller statement of results. As such it may be of great importance to a research worker commencing study in a new field and to others as a source of ideas. It is said that both Germany and Japan have a blanket order for copies of all theses handled by University Microfilms, amounting to about 90 per cent of all american doctoral dissertations. A copy of all theses submitted and accepted for higher degrees is deposited in the university, faculty of medicine or medical school library, as appropriate, where it is normally available on inter-library loan. Some universities also deposit a copy of each of their doctoral theses with the British Library Document Supply Centre. In the

UK about 8000 theses a year are accepted for the award of higher degrees and a guide to these is Aslib's *Index to Theses Accepted for Higher Degrees by the Universities of Great Britain and Ireland and the Council for National Academic Awards.* Theses are listed by subject with an index by author.

An indirect guide to theses in progress is *Current Research in Britain*, since this lists research projects under the names of academic staff immediately responsible. It is a national register of current research being carried out in universities, colleges and other institutions. It appears annually in four parts, one of which — *Biological Sciences* — includes medicine. There is a subject index, by study area and a name and keyword index.

Dissertation Abstracts International is still basically a guide to American and Canadian doctoral theses, though a larger number of theses accepted by European universities is now being included. It is published in two parts, the second being science and engineering, including biology and health science. The details of theses entered include a summary of 400–600 words and the names of both the author and supervisor of the thesis. *Dissertation Abstracts International* is now available online through commercial host systems and in CD-ROM format. Both University Microfilms and Aslib are making attempts to improve bibliographical access to British theses, chiefly by proposing ways in which the abstracts submitted with theses can be collected and published separately. Abstracts of British theses are now usually available from the Aslib Library.

Translation facilities

The significance of foreign-language publications in academic work generally has been examined by Hutchins, Pargeter and Saunders (1971) and some interesting conclusions were arrived at regarding this significance in medicine as distinct from science and other non--humanities subjects. Surveys of borrowing, both local and non-local, photocopying, library consultation and citation were carried out at Sheffield University and these were backed by a number of interviews. It was found that the use made of foreign-language materials was lower in the faculty of medicine than, on average, in other non-humanities publications, either in the original or in cover-to-cover translation. It was also found that the tendency for French-language publications to be most frequently used after those in English was not confirmed in medicine. German-language publications proved slightly more important here than French.

Both Aslib and the International Translations Centre at Delft maintain indexes of translations complete and in progress from most languages into the chief European ones, and can put individuals interested in a translation of a particular item in touch with the library or other organization which has undertaken it. The International Translations Centre publishes a monthly *World Transindex* and the American equivalent of this, published by the U.S. National Translations Center, is *Translations Register-Index*. The Aslib index of translations into English covers both British and American work and is at present growing by about 10 000 items a year.

Both Aslib and the Institute of Linguists maintain lists of qualified and experienced translators in all fields including medicine. The Institute's list is published as *Index of Members of the Translators' Guild* and is arranged primarily by subject, but also has a list of translators by geographical location.

Current awareness

The prime importance of current awareness for doctors and other hospital medical staff, for dentists and for general practitioners was established in a survey conducted in the UK (Ford, 1980). Not only was 'keeping up to date' mentioned most often by respondents to the survey questionnaire as a reason for seeking information, but, more significantly, it was ranked as the most important among a list of information needs by all groups except hospital dentists. Second place in terms of the importance of information needs was occupied by most respondents by 'clinical problems'. The Ford report included an account of a separate survey of the information needs of some paramedical hospital staff (physiotherapists) in which the paramount importance of keeping up to date was again emphasized, clinical problems coming second in the ranking.

Medical libraries often issue bulletins listing references of current interest which makes it easier for their readers to keep up to date. Inevitably, the coverage of the primary literature in these is dependent on the range of journals received in the library, while compilation is dependent on prompt receipt of current issues. The advantage of locally produced current-awareness bulletins is that they may select from the medical literature papers of special interest, as for instance in dentistry, or carry out some editing of the titles which are not self-explanatory. Current awareness is a small and fairly self-contained segment of the total communication field and in it the publications and methods recommended by librarians, more perhaps than in other segments such as retrieval, seem out of step with the methods favoured and used by biomedical scientists, if not also by doctors. We recommend using the secondary literature (see Chapter 3) — a surrogate literature designed to facilitate handling and scanning, yet reasonably complete. In the past our scientific clients have preferred the primary (Royal Society, 1981), though the availability of current awareness products, such as *Current Contents* and sections of the *Excerpta Medica* database, on disk may help to win them over. The reason for this can only be a difference in what is held to be the most important characteristic of 'current' information. As librarians, we believe this relates to scope, since all librarians aim at completeness in some sense or other, but our users are more concerned that current information should provide stimulus.

References

Allen, T.J. (1969) *Administration Science Quarterly*, **14**, 12.

Bernal, J.D. (1939) *The social function of science*. London: Routledge.

Bernal, J.D. (1959) In *Procedings of the international conference on scientific information*, vol. 1. New York: National Academy of Sciences.

Bernstein, L.M. (1980) *Annals of Internal Medicine*, **93**, 169.

Bodian, D. (1976) *Johns Hopkins Medical Journal*, **138**, 130.

Childs, S. (1982) *The experiences of a clinical librarian in medicine*. London: British Library.

Clarke, A. (1981) *Interlending Review*, **9**. 111.

Cockerill, P.E. (1981) *Information and the practice of medicine: report of the Medical Review Information Panel*. London: British Library.

De Solla Price, D.J. (1963) *Little science, big science*. New York: Columbia University Press.

De Solla Price, D.J. (1965) *Technology Culture*, **6**, 553.

De Solla Price, D.J. (1967) In *Communication in science* Boston: Little, Brown.

De Solla Price, D.J. (1970) In *Communication among scientists and engineers*. Lexington: D.C. Heath & Co.

De Solla Price, D.J. (1981) In *Coping with biomedical literature*, ed. K.S. Warren. New York: Praeger.

Durack, D.T. (1978) *New England Journal of Medicine*, **298**, 773.

Earle, P. and Vickery, B. (1969) *Aslib Proceedings*, **21**, 237.

Ford, G. (1980) *The use of medical literature*. London: British Library.

Fox, T. (1965) *Crisis in communication*. London: Athlone Press.

Garfield, E. (1972) *Science*, **178**, 471.

Garfield, E. (1976a), *Nature*, **264**, 609.

Garfield, E. (1976b) *Pathology Annual*, **11**, 335.

Garvey, W.D. and Griffith, B.C. (1965) *American Psychology*, **20**, 175.

Godbolt, S. (1991) Electronic publishing, the end user, and medical education. *Annals of the Rheumatic Diseases* **50**, 411-414

Green, D.E. (1964) *Science*, **148**, 1543.

Greenberg, B. (1978) *Bulletin of the Medical Library Association*, **66**, 319.

Hagstrom, W.O. (1965) *The scientific community*. New York: Basic Books.

Halbert, M.H. and Ackoff, R.L. (1959) In *Proceedings of the international Conference on scientific information*, vol. 1. New York: National Academy of Sciences.

Herman, C.M. and Rodowskas, C.A. (1976) *Journal of Medical Education*, **51**, 189.

Hutchins, W.J., Pargeter, L.J. and Saunders, W.L. (1971) *The language barrier: a study in depth of the place of foreign language materials in the research activity of an academic community*. Sheffield University.

Ingelfinger, F.J. (1974) *American Journal of Medicine*, **56**, 686.

Lancaster, F.W. (1978) *Towards paperless information systems*. New York: Academic Press.

Liepa, D. (1971) MSc Thesis. Postgraduate School of Librarianship and Information Science, Sheffield University.

Lock, S. (1985) *A difficult balance. Editorial peer review in medicine*. London: Provincial Hospitals Trust.

Maddox, J. (1967) *Nature*, **214**, 1077.

Meadows, A.J. (1974) *Communication in science*. London: Butterworths.

Moore, A. (1982) *The clinical librarian in the department of surgery*. London: British Library.

Piternick, A.B. (1989) *Canadian Library*, **46**, 93.

Posen, S. and Posen J.S. (1969) *Journal of Medical Education*, **44**, 648.

Raisig, L.M. (1966) *Bulletin of the Medical Library Association*, **54**, 108.

Relman, A.S. (1977) *New England Journal of Medicine*, **297**, 724.

Rowland, J.F.B. (1982) *Journal of Documentation*, **38**, 94.

Royal Society (1981) *A study of the scientific information system in the United Kingdom*. London: The Royal Society.

Scales, P.A. (1976) *Journal of Documentation*, **32**, 17.

Shackel, B. (1983) *Journal of the American Society for Information Science*, **34**, 22.

Shepard, D.A.E. (1973) *IEEE Transactions and Professional Communications*, **PC 16**, 143.

Thomas, L. (1978) *Science*, **200**, 1459.

Thorpe, W.V. (1967) *Nature*, **213**, 132.

Turoff, M. and Hiltz, R.S. (1982) *Journal of the American Society for Information Science*, **33**, 195.

Webb, E.C. (1970) *Nature*, **225**, 132.

Wilkin, A. (1982) *The evaluation of a clinical library experiment.* London: British Library.

Wood, D.N. and Bower, C.A. (1969) *Bulletin of the Medical Library Association*, **57**, 47.

Wood, D.N. and Hamilton, D.R.L. (1967) *The information requirements of medical engineers.* London: Library Association.

Wyatt, H.V. (1972) *Nature*, **235**, 86.

Ziman, J.M. (1968) *Public knowledge.* Cambridge: Cambridge University Press.

Ziman, J.M. (1982) *Times Higher Education Supplement*, No. 518.

Zwemer, R.L. (1970) *Federation Proceedings*, **29**, 1595.

CHAPTER THREE

Indexes, abstracts, bibliographies and reviews

F.M. SUTHERLAND[*]; revised by S.R. JENKINS

Since the fifteenth century, the printed book, and subsequently the periodical, have been the principal means for communicating scientific knowledge over the barriers of space and time. Until the mid-nineteenth century the number of publications in the field of medicine was comparatively small, and individual doctors were able, by personal contact with their fellows, and by their own reading, to keep abreast of current developments. Bibliographies and guides to the literature had been compiled since the sixteenth century, but they were private efforts by enthusiasts and would not have been regarded by the ordinary medical practitioners as publications essential to their needs.

In the early years of the nineteenth century, the changes wrought on the political and economic scenes by the French and Industrial Revolutions were matched by equally fundamental changes in the sphere of science. In medicine, the pace and scope of research quickened, and the communication of the results of that research led, inevitably, to an increase in the volume of publications. The growth of specialization in medicine produced a like effect, with the proliferation of books and journals devoted to particular subjects. By the 1860s it was no longer possible for the individual worker to read all the literature which might

---

[*] Formerly Librarian, British Medical Association

be of interest. By the same token it was no longer possible for the individual bibliographer, working alone, to compile and publish guides to that literature. The production of such guides required, to an ever-increasing degree, resources in finance, manpower, and, ultimately, in machines, which could only be deployed by organizations and governments. The indexing of medical publications not only became essential for medical progress, but also developed into the institutional and commercial affair which it is today.

The guides to medical literature which have evolved during the past hundred years fall into two distinct categories. The first, in the form of indexes, catalogues and book lists, draw attention to the existence of publications without elaborating on their contents. The primary test of their efficiency is the comprehensiveness of their coverage of the literature and the speed with which they announce its publication; a secondary test is the ease with which the information contained in them can be made available by retrospective searching. In the earliest form they sought to cover both books and journals, but the differing techniques involved in indexing the two types of literature meant that the marriage was never an entirely happy one, and this led ultimately to the physical separation of journal indexes and booklists, which, at present, is more or less complete.

The second category of guide to the literature goes beyond the mere listing of titles, and, in the form of abstracts or reviews, provides a summary of content to a varying degree of detail. The summary may be quite brief, and be meant purely as an indication to the reader of the importance of the publication and whether the original should be consulted; alternatively, it may seek to be a substitute for that original by outlining its salient features. Review articles, which collect together and summarize recent information on specific subjects, are a collective form of abstract; if they are based on adequate coverage of the literature and are the product of expert and critical authorship, they can perform an extremely useful function. As with indexes and book lists, the effectiveness of abstracts and reviews is dependent on their comprehensiveness, the rapidity of their production and their adaptability for retrospective searching. A full account of mechanized sources of information retrieval is to be found in Chapter 5.

Indexes

The detailed story of the modern indexing of medical literature begins in 1865, when John Shaw Billings, a U.S. army doctor, was given responsibility for the Library of the Surgeon General's Office in Washington. It is perhaps, a strange fact that modern medical bibliography owes much of its origin to the USA where, in the nineteenth century, resources in medical literature were meagre as compared with those in the countries of Western Europe. It was, however, this very lack of resources which Billings himself experienced when writing his graduation thesis that convinced him of the necessity, not only for adequate libraries, but also for adequate bibliographical procedures to exploit the contents of those libraries. With the same energy that was being used to develop all other aspects of American life at the time, Billings proceeded to create, out of the comparatively small library at the Surgeon General's Office, one of the greatest collections in the world, and his first step to exploit the contents of that collection, for the benefit of the medical profession at large, was the *Index-Catalogue.*

Index-Catalogue of the Library of the Surgeon General's Office (1800–1950)

A detailed history of the *Index-Catalogue* and the *Index Medicus* can be found in Miles (1982). To obviate possible confusion later in this chapter, it must be emphasized that the Library of the Surgeon General's Office has undergone several changes of title, being called, at a later date, the Army Medical Library and the Armed Forces Medical Library, and it is known today as the National Library of Medicine.

In 1876 Billings had outlined his intentions by issuing an author and subject catalogue of his library in dictionary form under the title of *Specimen Fasciculus of a Catalogue of the National Medical Library*, but the first volume of the *Index-Catalogue* proper did not appear until 1880, when Congress appropriated the necessary funds.

As the name *Index-Catalogue* implies, both book and periodical literature were covered. Books were listed under authors' names and under subject headings; journal articles were listed under subject headings only. Under subject headings useful cross-references were made to kindred topics and sub-headings were provided where the amount of material justified it.

The main author and subject entries were arranged alphabetically in dictionary form, the first volume of 1880 covering the letters 'A' to 'Berlinski'. Volumes appeared annually until 1895, when the alphabet was completed in 16 volumes. Some 679 669 subject references had been published, and the Surgeon General's Library itself had grown to 308 000 volumes. It is important to note, however, that much of the older literature had still to be acquired by the Library, and references to these older books must be sought in later series of the *Index-Catalogue* .

Billings himself retired from the Library in 1895, but the work was carried on by his successors in the form of further series:

1st Series: vols 1–16 (1880–1895)
2nd Series: vols 1–21 (1896–1916)
3rd Series: vols 1–10 (1918–1932)
4th Series: vols 1–11 (A-Mn) (1936–1955)
5th Series (Selected Monographs): vols 1–3 (1959–1961)

Nearly 540 000 books and pamphlets and 2 556 000 journal articles are recorded in these different series. As to the extent to which the *Index-Catalogue* covered the whole field of medical literature, Billings was careful to emphasize, in his preface to the first volume of the 1st Series, that it was not a complete medical bibliography but rather a catalogue of a single collection, and indeed as an index to that one collection it had certain limitations. All books, pamphlets and theses receive entries, but the indexing of periodicals was selective, aiming to include the principal original papers in medical journals and transactions'. Secondary material, which was regarded as worthless, was omitted. It must not be forgotten then, however, that the Surgeon General's Library had already become one of the world's greatest medical libraries, and that, even with the selective indexing of periodicals, the *Index-Catalogue* forms a published guide to the medical literature of its day that was as comprehensive as could reasonably be expected.

It suffered, however, from the fundamental defects of being arranged alphabetically and of covering both book and periodical literature. The alphabetical arrangement meant that insertions or supplements were not possible, and that publication in series was inevitable. Even in the 1st Series, authors and subjects, whose entries began with the letter 'A' and which had just missed inclusion in the first volume, had to wait some 15 years before they appeared in the 2nd Series. The inexorable increase in the volume of publication, particularly in periodical form after 1900, made such delay ever worse and, ultimately, unacceptable.

By the 1920s, the number of entries awaiting publication had become so large that, in 1926, the decision was taken, beginning with volume 6 of the 3rd Series, to omit subject entries for material published after 1925. In 1932 the decision was reversed, and some of the missing material from the period 1926–1932 under the letters Ge-Z, is to be found in the volumes of the 4th Series. For complete coverage of those years, however, use of the *Index-Catalogue* must be supplemented with *Index Medicus* and *Quarterly Cumulative Index Medicus* (see below).

The final crisis for the *Index-Catalogue* came immediately after World War II. The effects of the increase in publication of scientific literature were exacerbated by the inflow of a backlog of overseas publications from the war years. By 1950 there were 1 750 000 subject entries from the period 1920–1950 still awaiting publication, and it was estimated that by 1958 the *Index-Catalogue* would be withholding from publication more references than it had published over the whole period since 1880. The prudent decision was made to cease publication with volume 11 (Mh-Mn) of the 4th Series. Entries for monographs published up to 1950 were subsequently published, under both authors and subjects, in a 5th Series of three volumes.

Although, by its design, the *Index-Catalogue* proved inadequate to meet the needs of the medical community for up-to-date indexing, it is now an invaluable mine of historical information, recording, as it does, a total of about 3 000 000 journal articles, books and pamphlets from the earliest times up to 1950. It forms a bibliographical tool without equal in any other subject field. But above all it established in the USA a pioneering tradition for the comprehensive indexing of medical literature, which has been carried forward to the present day.

Index Medicus (1879–1927)

Before describing the successors to the *Index Catalogue* and their role in the present-day indexing of medical literature, it is necessary to retrace one's steps to 1879, when the first issue of *Index Medicus* was published. If the format of the *Index-Catalogue* was incapable of coping with the rapid indexing of current literature, it was largely because Billings had not intended it for such a purpose. It was to be the repository catalogue of the Surgeon General's Library, and it was *Index Medicus* which was intended for the role of current indexing. In the prospectus contained in the first issue of *Index Medicus* of 31 January 1879, Billings declared that it would:

> 'record the titles of all new publications in medicine, surgery and the collateral branches received during the preceding month [and that they] will be followed by the titles of valuable original articles upon the same subject, found, during the like period, in medical journals and transactions of medical societies. The periodicals thus indexed will comprise all current medical journals and transactions of value, so far as they can be obtained.'

The odd fact about *Index Medicus* is that, although it was based on material already prepared for the *Index-Catalogue*, Billings did not seek public funds for its publication. It was a private commercial venture and, as such, was beset by financial difficulties from the start. Three separate publishers undertook responsibility for it at different times during the early years, and in 1899 publication was entirely suspended. In 1903 it was resumed with financial help from the Carnegie Institution of Washington, and publication continued until 1927, when *Index Medicus* was merged with the American Medical Association's *Quarterly Cumulative Index to Current Medical Literature* to form the *Quarterly*

Cumulative Index Medicus. For some years thereafter, the Army medical Library's only bibliographical publication was the *Index-Catalogue* and it was not until 1960, under quite new circumstances, that it reintroduced the title *Index Medicus.*

The earlier *Index Medicus* was published in three separate series: Series 1: 1879–1899; Series 2: 1903–1920; Series 3: 1921–1927. The first two series were issued monthly in classified form, with subject headings that were more general and less subdivided than those in the *Index-Catalogue.* Under each subject, books and theses were listed by authors, followed by an author listing of journal articles. An annual index was provided for both authors and subjects, but in these, as reference was made only to the number of the page on which a particular item occurred, the finding of that item could be a time-consuming business. In the third series (1921–1927), *Index Medicus* became a quarterly instead of a monthly, the subject arrangement became alphabetical instead of classified, and the annual indexes were limited to authors only. The prime importance of *Index Medicus* is that, for the period 1879–1927, it is an author guide to periodical literature, and, as such, is an indispensable supplement to the *Index-Catalogue.*

For the years 1899–1902, when *Index Medicus* was not published, there are two substitute bibliographical aids. *Bibliographia Medica (Index Medicus)*, 1–3, 1900–1902, was published monthly by the Institut de Bibliographie in Paris. As with *Index Medicus*, both books and journal articles were listed under subjects in a classified arrangement; an annual author index was provided, but an abbreviated index to the classification formed the only annual guide to subjects. *Bibliographia Medica* supplies a bridge to the gap in *Index Medicus* but the literature for late 1899 is not covered and the indexing is neither as comprehensive nor as accurate. *Index Medicus Novus* was published in Vienna between 15 June 1899 and 10–25 February 1900, and is another source of bibliographical information for the missing years of *Index Medicus.* Its classified arrangement and lack of annual indexes, however, make it of very limited value.

In the years following 1927, after *Index Medicus* ceased publication, the main instruments for indexing contemporary medical literature were the *Quarterly Cumulative Index Medicus* and, at a later date, the *Current List of Medical Literature*

Quarterly Cumulative Index Medicus

In 1916 the American Medical Association had begun publication of a *Quarterly Cumulative Index to Current Medical Literature*, an index which was intended primarily for the general practitioner, and its coverage of the literature was, accordingly, very selective and restricted in the main to the clinical field. In 1926, for example, only 326 periodical tit-les were indexed. From 1916 to 1925 the quarterly issues were cumulated annually; for 1926 there are two semi-annual cumulations. At the start of each volume are to be found lists of new books arranged by authors, of new books arranged by subject, of book publishers, of U.S. government publications and of the journal titles indexed in the main text. This main index of journal articles is one of authors and sub-jects in a single alphabetical sequence, a form that is extremely simple to use. The titles of foreign-language articles are translated into English.

By 1926 this publication had run into financial difficulties, and was merged with *Index Medicus* to form the *Quarterly Cumulative Index Medicus*, which, from 1927 to 1931, was sponsored jointly by the American Medical Association and the Army Medical Library; from 1932 until it ceased publication in 1956 it was the responsibility of the American Medical Association alone.

All the features of the previous *Quarterly Cumulative Index* were maintained, with the exception of the list of U.S. Government publica-tions. Coverage of journal literature was much more complete; in 1956, the final year of publication, 933 biomedical periodicals were indexed. It remained a quarterly publication, with semi-annual cumulations, until 1948; from 1949 to 1956 it was published in the form of semi-annual volumes only. Entries under authors' names in the main index are given in the original language, if that is English, French, German, Spanish, Italian, or Portuguese; other languages are translated into English. The titles of all subject entries are in English.

The fact that full details of each reference are to be found with every entry, and that those entries are arranged in a self-indexing sequence of authors and subjects makes the *Quarterly Cumulative Index Medicus* the easiest of all medical bibliographies to use. The format, however, was not a suitable one for rapid production. Delays in publication were made worse by the effects of World War II, with the result that, by the 1950s, volumes were appearing over two years late. For purposes of medical research this meant that they were of little value, and that radical change was necessary.

Current List of Medical Literature

The imperative need for a more rapid indexing service had first become apparent during the early years of World War II, and in 1941, in re-sponse to that need, the *Current List of Medical Literature* was first issued. Although based on cards already prepared for the *Index-Cata-logue*, it was initially a private venture and was not formally taken over by the Army Medical Library until 1945. It was intended as a service primarily for U.S. Army medical officers serving overseas by providing them with an up-to-date weekly list of the contents of some of the more important journals in the Army Medical Library. From 1950 onwards it appeared monthly.

The arrangement of each number of the *Current List* constitutes an alphabetical sequence of journal titles, and under each title are to be found the contents of one or more issues of that title. Each entry provides details of author and title of the article, together with a translation of items in foreign languages, and inclusive pagination. Each article is numbered for indexing purposes, and semi-annual indexes for both authors and subjects were published.

The strength of the *Current List* was its speed of publication; a survey in 1954 showed that 56 per cent of all material published was less than one year old. Its great weakness is that its format makes it a laborious work to consult; it cannot be used without referring first to an index, and, as entries in that index can refer to several numbered items in the main text, location of a particular item is rarely straightforward. Up to the end of 1956 the *Quarterly Cumulative Index Medicus* and the *Current List* should be used as complementary indexes, as each covered some part of the literature not dealt with by the other; following the demise of the *Quarterly Cumulative Index Medicus* at the end of 1956, the *Current List* is the only guide to medical periodical literature for the years 1957 to 1959. At the end of the latter year it also ceased publication and 1960 saw the introduction of an entirely new look to medical indexing in general.

The new arrangements were based initially on a return to the co-operation between the National Library of Medicine and the American Medical Association, which had existed between 1927 and 1931 for the publication of the *Quarterly Cumulative Index Medicus*. There were two new features in 1960 which must be stressed. In all the principal indexes which have been mentioned up to this time, both book and periodical literature were listed within the same framework to a greater or lesser degree. From 1960 onwards the fundamental difference between the techniques required for indexing the two types of literature is finally recognized, and the published guides to each type, issued by the National Library of Medicine, went their separate ways. Periodical literature is henceforth indexed in *Index Medicus* and *Cumulated Index Medicus*; new books and monographs are listed in the *National Library of Medicine Catalog* and the *National Library of Medicine Current Catalog*.

The second innovation, in 1960, was mechanization. Up to that time, all the published indexes, including the *Quarterly Cumulative Index Medicus* and the *Current List*, had been compiled basically by the manual manipulation of cards. For compiling the new *Index Medicus* of 1960 the National Library of Medicine introduced mechanization which was further developed in 1964, when *Index Medicus* was produced for the first time by the National Library of Medicine's automated medical literature analysis and retrieval system (MEDLARS) and was composed for printing, binding and distribution by the Library's Photon 900 graphic arts composing equipment (GRACE). These technical developments were timely in the extreme in the face of the mounting volume of medical literature. They made possible, in 1989, the coverage of approximately 3000 journal titles and the publication of more than 250 000 citations to articles; the listing of those articles could appear as little as three months after their original publication; and the *Cumulated Index Medicus* is published about four months after the close of the year which it covers.

In the selection of materials for indexing, the National Library of Medicine is advised by a committee of physicians, medical editors and medical librarians. The Library indexes the literature that has been judged most useful to *Index Medicus* users, but, while it is not possible to include every journal that might contain useful articles, an effort is made to maintain a reasonable subject balance. A historical account of the system by which journals are evaluated for inclusion in *Index Medicus* has been given by Karel (1967).

Index Medicus (1960–) and *Cumulated Index Medicus*

Since January 1960, *Index Medicus* has been published in monthly parts, each part being divided into subject and author sections arranged alphabetically. Citations are given in full in every entry. In the subject section, under each heading, entries are grouped according to the original language of the articles, with the English-language items first, followed by citations for articles in other languages arranged alphabetically by language. Titles in foreign languages are translated into English and shown in square brackets, together with an indication of the language concerned. Since 1972 each citation to a foreign-language article includes the phrase 'Eng. Abstr.' if the original article is accompanied by an English-language abstract. The increasing size of the monthly issues of *Index Medicus* led to the decision in January 1989 to publish each issue in two separately bound parts. Part 1 now contains the Subject section, and Part 2 the Author section and the *Bibliography of Medical Reviews,* which is discussed later in this chapter.

Up to ten authors' names are included in citations in the author section and a cross-reference is given from each author to the first author. The citations in the subject index include only the first author.

In the indexing process each article is given as many subject headings as are necessary to describe adequately its content. Only those subject headings which represent the most important concepts are cited in *Index Medicus*, but all subject headings are stored in MEDLARS, the National Library of Medicine's computer-based file of citations for use in computer retrieval. As a guide to the choice of the correct headings when a search is made, a list of headings currently in use is published annually as a supplement to the January issue of *Index Medicus* under the title *Medical Subjects Headings*, usually referred to as *MeSH*. This includes an alphabetical list of headings with cross-references, categorized lists of headings, and full information on new, deleted, and altered headings.

Issued with the January issue of *Index Medicus* is a publication which lists, by both full and abbreviated titles, the journals which are currently being indexed. This section is also published separately as *List of Journals Indexed in Index Medicus* in which the journals concerned are given additional listings under subjects and countries.

In 1976 *Index Medicus* introduced coverage of selected non-serial monographs containing papers presented at congresses and symposia. In 1981, however, this was discontinued in order to devote the entire capacity of *Index Medicus* to an expanding journal literature. To trace such material one can now turn to the *Index to Scientific and Technical Proceedings* which is described later in this chapter.

The monthly issues of *Index Medicus* are cumulated annually into *Cumulated Index Medicus*. This brings together the subject and author sections of *Index Medicus*, the *List of Journals Indexed*, *Medical Subjects Headings* (since 1966) and *Bibliography of Medical Reviews* (since 1967). In the early years, volumes of *Cumulated Index Medicus* tended to be heavy and unwieldy; between 1977 and 1989 it was published in 14 volumes of more reasonable size. In 1990 the number was increased to 16 volumes.

Since January 1970 the National Library of Medicine has also issued a monthly *Abridged Index Medicus* which cites articles from 117 English-language journals, using the same subject headings as in *Index Medicus*. The issues are brought together annually into *Cumulated Abridged Index Medicus*. The low cost of this index makes it an attractive proposition for the individual practitioner or smaller library, but the selection of such a limited number of journals for indexing, together with a bias towards American titles, must inevitably limit its value in the UK.

National Library of Medicine Current Catalog

Index Medicus is a guide only to periodical literature; detailed information on monographs must be sought in the *National Library of Medicine Current Catalog*, which was first published in 1966 as an additional product of MEDLARS.

We have seen that the *Index-Catalog*, when it finally ceased publication, had listed monographs published up to 1950. The details of books published between that date and the appearance of the *National Library of Medicine Current Catalog* in 1966 are to be found in the following: *Armed Forces Medical Library Catalog*, 1950–1954, 6 vols, 1955 *National Library of Medicine Catalog*, 1955–1959, 6 vols, 1960 *National Library of Medicine Catalog*, 1960–1965, 6 vols, 1966.

These furnish comprehensive author and subject guides to books of worldwide imprint reflecting, as they do, the international acquisitions policy of the National Library of Medicine.

As from January 1966, *National Library of Medicine Current Catalog* was computer-generated. It began as a twice-monthly publication, with quarterly and annual cumulations. The biweekly parts contained entries for books catalogued by the Library which had been published during the current or two previous years. The cumulations cited all books catalogued by the Library with the exception of those printed before 1801.

Until the end of 1969 each issue of the *Current Catalog* contained:

1   A subject section in which the headings are taken from *MeSH*.

2   A name section listing authors and titles, providing guidance on subject headings and cross-references, and giving information on prices when available.

3   A technical reports section listing reports under both subjects and names.

Beginning with January 1970 the biweekly issues were replaced by monthly ones, which contained a name section only and listed imprints for the current and two previous years only; there were quarterly and annual cumulations which had both name and subject sections, and which listed all imprints. The monthly issues ceased in December 1973 and the *Current Catalog* is now published quarterly with an annual cumulation.

In 1971 subject and name sections for audio-visual material were introduced, but after 1977 these were cumulated annually in an entirely separate publication, *National Library of Medicine Audiovisuals Catalog*. In 1973 serials, subject and name sections were brought in and became permanent features.

A sexennial cumulation of the *Current Catalog*, covering the years 1965 to 1970, has been published, and further quinquennial cumulations for the years 1971 to 1976 onwards have also appeared, although since the one for 1976 to 1980 they have been issued on microfiche only.

National Library of Medicine Catalog

The *NLM Catalog* was published on microfiche in 1985; it contains citations to approximately 585 000 printed monographs, serials, and audiovisual serials with an imprint year of 1984 or earlier, including many of the materials housed in the National Library of Medicine's History of Medicine Division. It cumulates all the citations previously included in the *Current Catalog 1965–* and many of those which appeared in the *National Library of Medicine Current Catalog 1955–1965*, the *Armed Forces Medical Library Catalog 1950–1955* and the *Armed Forces Medical Library Catalog Cards 1948 and 1949*. The *NLM Catalog* was kept up to date with quarterly cumulations by the *NLM Catalog Supplement* until this ceased in December 1988. The *Supplement* included titles which had been catalogued or converted to machine readable form up to that date.

Discussion of the indexes to current medical literature has so far been confined to those published by the National Library of Medicine. There are, however, a number of guides published elsewhere which deserve attention. Three such, published by the Institute for Scientific Information in Philadelphia, are *Current Contents, Science Citation Index* and *Index to Scientific and Technical Proceedings*.

Current Contents, Clinical Medicine

Current Contents is a weekly publication which contains photographically-reproduced copies of the contents pages of journals. For the medical worker the most important are *Current Contents: Clinical Medicine* which covers over 850 journals, and *Current Contents: Life Sciences* which covers over 1200. There is a certain overlap between the two. In addition to the contents pages each issue contains a title-word index taken from every article appearing in that issue, and an author index, together with addresses. A further section, *Current Book Contents*, lists the contents pages of new multi-authored books, including many titles which are issued in series. The producers aim to deal with every journal issue within two weeks of receipt, making it an extremely up-to-date current-awareness tool.

Science Citation Index

The concepts behind the *Science Citation Index* have been described by Garfield (1979), the founder of the Institute for Scientific Information. Essentially it consists of a list of references (cited works) in which each reference is followed by a list of the sources (citing works) which quote it. The main purpose behind the index is to lead the searcher from a key article to others which have referred to it on the basic assumption that they will be relevant.

Science Citation Index indexes both journals and non-journal items and a list of source material is included in each issue. In 1989 around 3 000 journals and other publications were covered. The most important journals in each subject area are selected for inclusion based on citation analysis of their contents and are regarded as those that have the highest impact in their subject. Every substantive item is indexed, including original research articles, corrections, discussions, editorials, biographical items, letters, meeting abstracts, technical notes and reviews. It is published six times a year. There is an annual cumulation; five-year cumulations from the years 1965 to 1984 have been published as have ten-year cumulations covering the years 1945 to 1964. It is available online as SCISEARCH (see p. 105).

Science Citation Index is particularly useful in information retrieval when a key reference, rather than a key word, is known. From such a key reference it is possible to trace more easily subsequent developments in a particular field. It can also be claimed, with justification, that it provides a novel link between literatures of different scientific disciplines. *Science Citation Index* consists of a number of separate parts: the 'Citation Index' itself; the 'Source Index' (equivalent to an author index); the 'Permuterm Subject Index' (which acts like a keyword index); and the 'Corporate Index' (which lists authors by institution).

The basic principle of the *Science Citation Index* is that a scientific paper cites other articles which are relevant to its own subject content. By the same token a paper will itself be cited by later papers dealing with the same topic. Thus *Science Citation Index* can move the user *forward* in time to relevant references, whereas other indexing and abstracting publications move the user *backwards* to older material. Although useful as a supernumerary tool, *Science Citation Index* cannot provide the coverage in depth of the conventional medical indexes and abstracts.

Index to Scientific and Technical Proceedings

First issued in 1978, the *Index to Scientific and Technical Proceedings* is a monthly publication with annual cumulations, which indexes the contents of proceedings of meetings, whether they have been published in books, as parts of journals, or separately as reprints. In 1989 it indexed 137 449 papers which had been presented at over 4000 conferences. It can usefully be consulted as an adjunct to more conventional indexes which tend to neglect conference proceedings, although these are often an extremely important source of information on new developments in a subject.

Abstracts

Attention must now be turned from publications of the index type, which point solely to the existence of particular medical literature, to abstracting publications which provide greater detail of the content of that literature. Their purpose may be to indicate briefly the importance of the original articles or to give more complete summaries of those articles for the benefit of those readers unable to obtain them without difficulty. In their coverage of the literature, abstracting services may seek to be either selective or comprehensive. Abstracts have been a feature of medical literature since the earliest times, both as separate publications and as an integral part of conventional medical journals. A nineteenth-century example of the former type was *Braithwaite's Retrospect of Practical Medicine and Surgery* which was published in 123 volumes from 1840 to 1901. From the early years of the twentieth century, the *Berichte* and *Zentralblätter*, published by the firm of Springer, provided German abstracts with the set intention of furnishing complete coverage in many areas of medicine and surgery. A typical example of abstracts included in ordinary medical journals was the *Epitome of Current Medical Literature*, which was a supplement to the *British Medical Journal* from 1892 to 1939. Abstracts sections are a feature, at the present time, of *JAMA: Journal of the American Medical Association*.

In the years immediately following World War II, a number of comprehensive abstracting services, covering the field of general medicine, were developed as one means of combating the problems caused by the increasing amount of medical literature, and by the language barrier, which hindered the flow of medical information. Among these was *Abstracts of World Medicine* (British Medical Association, 1947–1977), which scanned 1500 journals and published about 3000 informative abstracts a year.

Excerpta Medica

The Excerpta Medica Foundation, an international non-profit organization, was founded in 1946 with headquarters in Amsterdam and with, as its principal aim, the furthering of 'the progress of medical knowledge by making information available to the medical and related professions on all significant basic research and clinical findings reported in any language, anywhere in the world'. The abstracting publication, *Excerpta Medica*, the main instrument for carrying out this aim, first appeared in 1947. It is divided into different sections, each of which covers a special subject field and may be purchased separately; the number of sections in 1991 totalled 41. The individual issues in each section appear at varying intervals and the abstracts, all in English, are arranged in classified order. Subject and author indexes are provided with each issue and for the cumulated volumes which also appear at varying times throughout the year for different sections.

In 1991 more than 3500 journals from over 110 countries were being screened by Excerpta Medica. Compiled by experts in the relevant subject fields, the abstracts are well written but are of the informative rather than the indicative type. They usually appear in *Excerpta Medica* within sixty days of publication of the original articles.

Pascal

Pascal is the successor to the *Bulletin Signalétique* which had been published in Paris by the Centre National de la Recherche Scientifique, from 1940. In its present format, which began in 1984, it indexes the contents of over 5000 periodicals published worldwide. It is published in 65 sections, each covering a very specific subject, of which approximately one-third deal with medicine and related topics.

In view of the increasingly interdisciplinary nature of the study of medicine, brief mention must be made of two important abstracting services in allied subject fields.

Chemical Abstracts

Chemical Abstracts, the first volume of which appeared in 1907, provides as near to complete coverage of the chemical literature as could be desired. The literature covered includes journal articles, patents, conference proceedings, research reports, books and dissertations. The abstracts, which are classified in 80 subject groups or sections, provide brief informative summaries. A substantial proportion of the material published is of biochemical interest. *Chemical Abstracts* is published weekley in two 26-issue volumes per year. Each issue is provided with indexes to authors, substances, formulae and patents. Collective indexes are also published at regular intervals. The computer-base for the Chemical Abstracts Service is also used to produce a current-awareness service in the form of *Chemical Titles*, a biweekly index to approximately 750 journals. A detailed account of *Chemical Abstracts* is given by Bottle (1992).

Biological Abstracts

Biological Abstracts, which has been in existence since 1926 and which is published by BIOSIS of Philadelphia, is important for the medical research worker who is interested in such subjects as genetics, biophysics, biochemistry, immunology and nutrition. In 1990, 8585 serials were screened and 535 000 items were added.

The abstracts in *Biological Abstracts* are generally well written and informative. Issues appear fortnightly and abstracts are arranged in classified order with author, biosystematic, generic and subject indexes, which are cumulated semi-annually. The subject indexes to *Biological Abstracts* have a complicated history, an account of which is to be found in Bottle and Wyatt (1971).

A number of useful lists of abstracting services are available. Blake and Roos (1967) and the supplements to their work (see p. 9) give detailed information, on a considerable number of current and discontinued medical abstracting journals. The third edition of *World Medical Periodicals*, published by the World Medical Association in 1961, and its *Supplement* published in 1968, list over 100 titles with the publishers' addresses. A comprehensive guide to medical abstracting and indexing journals was published by Dalby in 1975; for current information on abstracting and indexing journals in all subjects, including medicine, the best list is that published in *Ulrich's International Periodicals Directory* (now also available on CD-ROM).

Bibliographies

Information on monograph publications in medicine can be obtained from a number of sources. It is helpful to distinguish between those sources which provide current-awareness information on recently published works and those which aim simply to list those titles which are currently in print. A full set of the former type can also constitute a very valuable record of published works over a long period of time and is therefore an indispensable aid to retrospective searching.

One useful source for current awareness is book reviews in medical journals. Most such reviews have the great advantage of giving an authoritative assessment of the value of individual books, although the prospective purchaser needs to be aware of occasional bias on the part of some reviewers. They may not, however, appear until long after the books themselves have been published and, except in journals of a very specialized nature, reviews can provide only limited coverage of the total number of books published.

Conventional reviews tend to ignore new editions of textbooks but this area is covered by a useful feature in the *British Medical Journal* entitled 'What's new in the new editions?' In this, Dr. Clifford Hawkins, a retired physician, provides brief reviews of new editions of textbooks and standard medical works.

For further guidance to what is being published there are, in the first instance, the various advertising methods employed by publishing firms, varying from leaflets describing individual books to lists devoted to special subject areas and recent publications. To co-ordinate this ill-assorted material is a difficult and time-consuming task and it is often more useful to use other published book lists, among which can be included the following.

Cumulative Book Index

Published by the H. W. Wilson Co. of New York, this seeks to include the majority of books in the English language, wherever published. Excluded, however, are government documents, most pamphlets, cheap paperbacks and, in general, all material of a local, fugitive and ephemeral nature. Entries are arranged alphabetically by authors, subjects and titles. It is published monthly, except in August, with a bound cumulation each year.

British Book News

British Book News is published monthly by the British Council and is a very useful survey of new and forthcoming UK titles. Each issue contains a listing of some 1000 titles due to be published the following month, with a brief annotation about content and a guide to readership level. It is arranged by broad subject groupings, of which medicine is one; the sections on social sciences and pure sciences may also be of interest. In addition, each issue contains a review of the literature on a topical subject and notes about new periodicals and book-trade developments.

Index of Conference Proceedings

The Index of Conference Proceedings is issued monthly, with an annual cumulation, by the British Library Document Supply Centre, and is of considerable assistance in tracing recent conference proceedings; such proceedings can be valuable but difficult to locate as they are often poorly treated by other indexes and bibliographies. Publication began in 1964 and a 25-year cumulation is now available on microfiche for the years 1964 to 1988. Arrangement is by keyword taken from the title of the conference. Details of 16 000 conferences covering all subject fields are added annually and there are over 260 000 conferences on the index to date.

A list of 363 older congress proceedings is to be found in Bishop (1958).

British Reports, Translations and Theses

British Reports, Translations and Theses is a monthly publication, with annual cumulations, issued by the British Library Document Supply Centre. It lists semi-published or 'grey' literature, such as reports and translations produced by UK government organizations, local government, universities and learned institutions, and most doctoral theses accepted at UK universities during and after 1970. It also covers reports and unpublished translations from the Republic of Ireland and selected official publications of a report nature that are not published by HMSO.

Index to Theses

Index to Theses lists all theses accepted for higher degrees by the universities of Great Britain and Ireland and the Council for National Academic Awards. It was first published by Aslib in 1950 and from 1986 it was expanded to include abstracts. It is published quarterly and provides abstracts of around 9000 theses a year.

Health Science Books 1876–1982

Health Science Books was published in New York by Bowker in 1982 and lists 132 000 books published in the USA and catalogued by the Library of Congress. It is an extremely useful source for checking the bibliographical details of books published during the period covered.

Whitaker's Books in Print

Whitaker's is an annual list of UK books in print listed by author, title and subject in one alphabetical sequence. The latest edition is published in four volumes and gives details of 500 000 titles issued by 14 500 publishers.

Books in Print

Published annually by the American company, Bowker, *Books in Print* lists by author, title and subject, over 800 000 titles in print from 30 000 U.S. publishers. It is currently published in eight volumes.

Medical and Health Care Books and Serials in Print

Material in this work is derived from *Books in Print*. The latest edition (1991), has entries for 59 728 books under author, title and Library of Congress subject headings. It lists books which are currently in print which are either published or distributed in the USA. A separate section includes a subject listing of 13 252 current serials published worldwide, giving details of publishers, subscription rates, frequency of publication and an indication as to which indexes and abstracts cover their contents.

Booksellers' catalogues

After the closure of H.K. Lewis's Library and Bookshop in October 1989, its stock was incorporated into Dillons, making this the largest medical bookshop in the UK. It adds all new medical books in English to its stock and its *Quarterly Medical Catalogue*, though not cumulative, is a very useful source of full bibliographical information on recent medical titles. Haigh and Hochland, the Manchester booksellers, produce a similar catalogue.

Medical Textbook Review by V.G. Daniels (Cambridge Medical Books)

Medical Textbook Review is a guide principally to current medical textbooks, with full bibliographical details, together with a brief review, the purpose of which is to help medical students, hospital doctors, general practitioners and paramedical staff in the selection of textbooks. It is arranged in broad subject categories and has an author index. A separate section is a compilation of books which may be regarded as standard works for medical libraries. It is an excellent aid to selection of current books for a personal or a library collection. The latest, 9th, edition (1987) has an update (September 1990). There are plans to issue it in loose-leaf format. A similar list of books and journals suitable for American libraries is published regularly by Brandon and Hill (1989) in the *Bulletin of the Medical Library Association*. The latest includes 607 books and 141 journals arranged in broad subject groups.

Reviews

Reviews are a more sophisticated version of abstracts. They bring together, summarize and critically annotate information on a special subject which has been published over a period of time. If they are compiled with expert knowledge, give adequate coverage of the literature and are well written, with full bibliographical detail, they are of inestimable value, as they can save much time in tracking down and consulting references.

Review articles have always been a feature of scientific journals and, since the beginning of the nineteenth century, the number of periodicals which confine themselves entirely to reviewing has steadily increased. A detailed account of reviews and yearbooks is included in Chapter 4 and references to those in special subjects are in the appropriate chapters. In the sphere of general medicine the following titles are among the most useful of those currently being published.

Advances in Internal Medicine

Advances in Internal Medicine first appeared in 1942 and is now published annually by Year Book Medical Publishers of Chicago and London. Each volume contains articles of reasonable length which synthesize from the literature 'those areas of progress so significant that those who practise advanced internal medicine, subspecialized or comprehensive, cannot afford to be unaware of them'. Substantial bibliographies are appended to the articles. Each volume includes a cumulative subject index to the five most recent volumes.

Annual Review of Medicine; Selected Topics in Clinical Sciences

Published by Annual Reviews Inc. of Palo Alto, California, the *Annual Review of Medicine* seeks to treat in depth topics in internal medicine in which there have been remarkable recent advances. In general, the articles are not as lengthy as those in *Advances in Internal Medicine*, but the bibliographies are more extensive. Each volume contains a subject index to that volume and an author index and a classified list of chapter titles covering the previous five years.

Advanced Medicine

Advanced Medicine which began in 1964 as *Symposium on Advanced Medicine*, now consists of papers presented at the annual Advanced Medicine Conference held at the Royal College of Physicians in London. The aim of each conference is to present information on a wide variety of clinical topics, emphasizing new and recent advances. Not all subjects are covered each year, priority being given to those areas of clinical medicine in which rapid progress is being made. Each chapter is concise but provides a good overview of a subject and includes a well-selected brief bibliography.

Medical Annual

Medical Annual has been published continuously by John Wright of Bristol since 1883–1884. It comprised a selection of special articles on topics of current interest and a section devoted to reviews of the past year's work covering the whole field of medicine. It was for a century an invaluable work of reference, particularly for those practitioners with no ready access to medical literature. After the appearance of the hundredth volume in 1982, however, a decision was made that its content should change and that it should thereafter be targeted specifically at general practitioners and other professionals in primary medical care (see p. 70).

Recent Advances in Medicine

Published by Churchill Livingstone, *Recent Advances in Medicine* first appeared in 1924, and subsequent volumes have been issued at irregular intervals, the most recent being Number 20 in 1987. It seeks to provide readable and critical surveys of subjects in which there have been significant advances since the previous edition; the authors are active workers in the subjects concerned. It is designed for senior students, generalists, and specialists with interests outside their field. Each chapter has a good bibliography, and there is a subject index but no name index. Other books in the *Recent Advances* series are described in their appropriate chapters.

Year Book of Medicine

Year Book of Medicine published annually since 1901 by Year Book Medical Publishers, Inc. of Chicago, contains abstracts of individual articles selected from around 70 major medical journals. They are arranged in broad subject groups and each article is annotated and commented on by the section editor. Thirty-six *Year Books* are published, mostly devoted to major medical disciplines, and over 700 journals are surveyed for the complete series (see p. 69).

Bibliography of Medical Reviews

For tracing up-to-date review articles, workers in the medical field are fortunate in having a comprehensive reference tool in the *Bibliography of Medical Reviews*, which is published in Washington by the National Library of Medicine. The articles included in the *Bibliography* are indexed from the journals covered for *Index Medicus*. It was an annual publication from 1955 to 1966 and a monthly from 1967 to 1977 after which it ceased to appear as a separate publication. It continued as a section within the monthly issues of *Index Medicus*, a practice which was introduced in March 1965. When the monthly issues of *Index Medicus* were split into two in January 1989, the *Bibliography* was included with the Author section in Part 2.

Annual cumulations have been included in *Cumulated Index Medicus* since 1967. Volume 6 of 1960 consolidated the reviews for the period 1955 to 1960 and further cumulations covering 1966 to 1970, 1971 to 1975, and 1976 to 1980 have been published.

From 1955 to 1987 the National Library of Medicine defined medical reviews as well-documented surveys of the recent biomedical literature. This was broadened in 1988 to encompass reviews of current thinking on a given subject, regardless of the age of the literature cited, and to include categories of material previously excluded. Types of articles now considered to be reviews include academic or classical reviews, tutorial or didactic reviews, multicase or epidemiologic reviews, consensus conferences, reviews of known or published cases, and state-of-the-art reviews.

As with *Index Medicus*, the arrangement of each issue is a dual one of subjects and authors; the subject headings are taken from *MeSH* but are somewhat broader than those used in *Index Medicus*. A very useful feature is that the number of references cited by each article is given.

Current Bibliographies in Medicine

Current Bibliographies in Medicine is a series of bibliographies on specific biomedical topics compiled by the Reference Section of the National Library of Medicine. Around 20 such bibliographies are issued each year and it is possible to subscribe to the entire series or to order individual items as required. The *Specialised Bibliography* Series appears less frequently but is comprehensive in scope and is usually the result of a combination of manual and computerized searching, including non-MEDLARS databases. Details of the bibliographies in both series are published in the monthly issues of *Index Medicus*.

Conclusions

Can it be said that the indexes, abstracting services and reviews which have evolved since John Shaw Billings launched the *Index-Catalogue* constitute adequate guides to the medical literature of 1990 and of the past hundred years? Despite the prodigious volume of that literature, it can fairly be said that the tools are available for the medical worker to keep up to date with current developments and to retrieve past information in a reasonably comprehensive and efficient way. It cannot be denied, however, that there are some flies in the bibliographical ointment. Subscription rates to the more important reference works are so high that the maintenance of a complete collection is possible only for libraries with substantial financial resources. The haphazard manner in which the various bibliographical aids have been developed to meet particular situations has resulted in the large number of publications which are involved. This is one of the factors responsible for high cost, and has also led to a considerable duplication of effort by the different services.

As we enter the 1990s, the amount of literature being published continues to increase and shows no signs of abating. While one can accept the need for a new book describing recent events and updating information in a subject, one cannot help questioning the necessity for yet another basic text in a field already more than adequately covered by existing publications. The same holds true for journals. There seems to be no limit at present to the number of new titles deemed essential to meet the needs of those who wish to publish in rapidly expanding subject areas.

All this puts considerable pressure both on librarians, who must inevitably be the principal purchasers of and subscribers to such material and on the medical worker for whom it is vital to keep up to date with what is being published. For librarians the problem, if they wish to meet the needs of their readers adequately, can be solved mainly by adequate funding or, where this fails, by co-operative measures. For the researcher this means greater application and determination to obtain access to the literature.

The advent of computerization has done a great deal to alleviate the problem for the researcher. The introduction of online services in the 1970s was a great step in this direction although the need for searchers to be experienced always meant that access to the literature was made through a skilled intermediary such as a librarian. The latest development has been the arrival of CD-ROMs which are described in Chapter 5. This means that the research worker can now obtain literature with greater rapidity, and (provided adequate training has been given) with greater accuracy than ever before.

References

Bishop, W.J. (1958) *Bibliography of international congress of medical sciences*. Oxford: Blackwell.

Blake, J.B. and Roos, C. (1967) *Medical reference works, 1679–1966; a selected bibliography*. Chicago: Medical Library Association.

Bottle, R.T. (1992) *Use of chemical literature*, 4th edn. London: Butterworths.

Bottle, R.T. and Wyatt, H.V. (1971) *The use of biological literature*, 2nd edn. London: Butterworths.

Brandon, A.N. and Hill, D.R. (1989) Selected lists of books and journals for the small medical library. *Bulletin of the Medical Library Association*, **77**, 139.

Dalby, A.K. (1975) *Medical abstracts and indexes, 1975; a bibliography of abstracting, indexing and current awareness services in medicine and related subjects* (Cambridge University Library, Librarianship Series 2). Cambridge: University Library.

Garfield, E. (1979) *Citation indexing: its theory and application in science, technology and humanities.* New York: John Wiley.

Karel, L. (1967) Selection of journals for *Index Medicus:* a historical review. *Bulletin of the Medical Library Association,* **55**, 259.

Miles W.D. (1981) *A history of the National Library of Medicine.* Washington DC: US Government Printing Office.

CHAPTER FOUR

Standard reference sources

H. R. HAGUE

It is sometimes assumed that reference librarians have the answer to all possible queries in their heads. This is, of course, far from the truth, but what librarians should have is a good idea of where to start looking for the answer. Experience tells which particular source is likely to produce a good result, and consequently which should be consulted first. To this end even the smallest library should have available a basic stock of reference and bibliographical sources. Even a specialized library is expected to provide the answers to many general questions.

The most comprehensive guide to medical reference material is *Medical reference works 1679-1966: a selected bibliography* edited by J.B. Blake and C. Roos (Medical Library Association (MLA), 1967), which contains 2700 entries. Arranged alphabetically by subdivisions of medicine, each section has lists of material under subheadings such as indexes and abstracts, reviews, bibliographies, dictionaries, lists of periodicals, directories and histories. *Supplement I, 1967-1968* compiled by M.V. Clark (MLA, 1970) contains 315 items. *Supplement II, 1969-1972* compiled by J. S. Richmond (MLA, 1973), lists some 500 items, and *Supplement III, 1973-1974* (MLA, 1975) includes 244 annotated entries. No further supplements have been issued. Instead the role of updating Blake and Roos has been taken over by entries in the *National Library of Medicine Current Catalog*. There is now a separate section in both the quarterly issues and the annual volume, entitled 'Medical Reference Works'. The 1988 annual cumulation devoted 20 pages to reference works, many of them provided with a brief annotation.

Volume one of *Walford's Guide to reference material* (5th edn., Library Association, 1989) covers science and technology in general, with

55 pages devoted to medicine. It is arranged according to the Universal Decimal Classification. Although *Walford's Guide* is inevitably selective, many important works are listed, and the section devoted to dictionaries is particularly helpful. It is also useful for fringe subjects.

Encyclopaedias

It must be admitted that encyclopaedias are now of little value in the medical field. Even when updated by means of annual supplements, they are unsatisfactory for finding information on particular topics when compared with other sources, such as textbooks, monographs and reviews. Medical encyclopaedias should be regarded mainly as recording the state of knowledge on a particular subject at the time of writing, and are therefore primarily of historical interest.

The *McGraw-Hill Encyclopedia of science and technology* (6th edn., 20 vols, 1987) is of little relevance for clinical medicine, though it may be of some value in the basic sciences and for related fields such as biophysics and computing. Also available is the *McGraw-Hill Concise encyclopedia of science and technology* (2nd edn., 1989), though smaller libraries may find the *Chambers Science and technology dictionary* (1989) more affordable.

A small, but valuable, work is the *Penguin Medical encyclopedia* by P. Wingate (3rd edn., 1988). This is aimed at patients or anyone concerned with the care of sick people. Entries range in size from a few lines to over a page, and explain diseases, organs and bodily processes in straightforward, non-technical language. On a larger scale is the *British Medical Association Complete family health encyclopedia* (Dorling Kindersley, 1990). Its 5000 entries are well illustrated, clear and informative.

Although rather difficult to categorize, the *Oxford Companion to medicine* (2 vols, Oxford University Press, 1986) is more an encyclopaedia than anything else. It has a wide, if unpredictable, range of entries, but is particularly useful for the history of a subject, for its descriptions of the health services of certain countries, and for biographical information. The reviewer in *Nature* called it curious and 'almost quirky' in its choice of entries, but it can make fascinating reading. It is available on CD-ROM.

Handbooks

Before World War II, a number of multi-volumed works were published in Germany as *Handbücher*. These were usually issued in parts, bound or unbound, sometimes out of numerical sequence, so that often several years elapsed before volumes were completed. These *Handbücher* were expensive yet of great importance, because they consisted of authoritative surveys by writers of international repute and reviewed the literature historically and bibliographically. Despite a modern tendency to regard any scientific literature more than five to ten years old as obsolete, there is a persistent demand for reliable reviews surveying progress to date and evaluating the material. This is particularly so when theses are being written and prior to research work being undertaken. A surprising number of these handbooks are still being issued today, and an interesting trend in recent years has been the adoption of English as the language of publication for some of them.

Examples include W. von Möllendorff's *Handbuch der mikroskopischen Anatomie des Menschen* (Springer), which was started in 1929 and is still appearing; the *Handbuch der speziellen pathologischen Anatomie und Histologie* (Henke/Lubarsch) in 40 volumes (Springer, 1925-1978); the *Handbook of experimental pharmacology* (Springer, 1950-), which from volume 36, 1973, is entirely in English; and the *Handbook of sensory physiology* (Springer, 1971-1981) which was completed upon publication of the 23rd part, all volumes being in English. Individual volumes in these series can normally be bought separately, and they can usually be borrowed from the British Library Document Supply Centre at Boston Spa.

The *Handbook of physiology* published by the American Physiological Society and now distributed by Oxford University Press (USA) commenced in 1959 and appeared in nine sections. A new edition is now in progress (from 1977), with some changes in the titles of sections, and this will maintain its place as a work of great significance. Equally important is P.J. Vinken and G. W. Bruyn's *Handbook of clinical neurology* (North-Holland–Elsevier), which started publication in 1969 and is still appearing (volume 53 being published in 1989). Other examples are the *Handbook of neurochemistry* edited by A. Lajtha (7 vols, Plenum Press, 1969–1972) and the *Handbook of psychopharmacology* edited by L.L. Iversen *et al*. (14 vols, Plenum Press, 1975–1978).

Year books, annual reviews

Individual items in these series are detailed in other chapters and are many and varied in scope, reliability and coverage. Generally, they survey the literature of the previous year, evaluating it in chapters contributed by experts.

The *Year Book* series is published regularly by Year Book Medical

Publishers (Chicago) and currently covers 38 areas of medicine. Recent additions to the series are the volumes devoted to *Occupational and Environmental Medicine* (1990–) and *Speech, Language and Hearing* (1990–). A number of the earlier volumes have changed their titles over the years. Academic Press (New York) publishes *Recent progress in hormone research* and also issues the *Advances* series, of which more than 20 titles are in the biomedical field, including the well known volumes for *Cancer research, Clinical chemistry and Immunology*.

Year Book Medical Publishers produce another *Advances* series including *Internal medicine, Pediatrics, Sports medicine and fitness* and two new titles *Cardiac surgery* (1989–) and *Urology* (1988–). Grune and Stratton publish the *Progress* series, which appear irregularly. The subjects covered include *Clinical pathology, Diseases of the skin, Hematology* and *Liver diseases*.

The *Annual reviews* series (Palo Alto, Annual Reviews Inc.) now contains some 12 titles of medical interest, and include *Immunology* (1983–), *Neuroscience* (1978–), *Nutrition* (1981–) and *Public Health* (1980–). The various chapters in all these volumes normally contain extensive lists of references. Many libraries treat these annual volumes as bound periodicals, rather than as books.

One British publication which did not always receive the recognition it deserved was the *Medical Annual* (John Wright), published regularly from 1883 until 1987. Each volume included one or more special, original articles, with the remainder devoted to a review of the year's work, arranged under broad headings. The *Medical Annual* was re-launched in 1991 by the Clinical Press of Bristol, under new editorship but with similar content and purpose.

Volumes in Churchill Livingstone's *Recent advances* series are issued irregularly. Some 35 different titles are now available, covering most branches of medicine and surgery. Recent additions to the series include the volumes for *Psychogeriatrics* (No.1, 1985) and *Tropical medicine* (No. 1, 1985). These volumes are now numbered serially rather than being designated as editions. Earlier issues provide a guide to the historical development of the subject, and may be worth retaining for this reason.

The series of *Clinics*, previously published by W.B. Saunders and latterly by Harcourt Brace Jovanovich, are issued bound as separate symposia, usually in three, four or six parts each year. Their publication was revamped with effect from 1987, and those titles published in Britain now carry the Baillière Tindall imprint. Their seven current titles include *Baillière's clinical gastroenterology* and *Baillière's clinical rheumatology*. The series on *Clinical oncology* ceased publication at the end of 1988. The 40 titles published from North America still appear under the W.B. Saunders imprint, and include *Clinics in chest medicine* and *Clinics in geriatric medicine* as well as the well-known *Medical, Pediatric* and *Surgical clinics of North America*.

The *Modern trends* series published by Butterworths covered many areas of medicine in volumes issued every few years, but gradually ceased publication during the 1970s. To some extent they were replaced by the *Butterworths international medical reviews*, which covered 16 different subject areas. Individual volumes within each subject focused on a single topic or major theme of current interest rather than attempting to survey the whole field. However, this series itself appears to have been discontinued during the 1980s.

Directories

There is available a wide range of directories — national and international — and only a brief selection can be given here. The *Medical Register* has been published annually since 1859 by the General Medical Council, and is the official register of doctors qualified to practise in this country. More detailed information is given in the *Medical Directory* (Churchill Livingstone) which has been issued annually since 1845. This provides names, addresses, telephone numbers, qualifications, past and present posts held and a list of up to three publications. Information is also given on hospitals (including the names of consultants in each department), societies, medical schools, postgraduate medical centres, geographical listing of doctors and other topics. Directories for other countries include the *Medical Directory of Australia* (Sydney, 1935), the *Canadian Medical Directory* (Toronto, 1955–) and the *American Medical Directory* (Chicago, 1906–), published irregularly by the American Medical Association (31st edn., 1988). This also lists the chief medical societies, hospitals and medical journals, while the *Directory of medical specialists* (24th edn., 3 vols, Marquis, 1989) includes details of 220 000 American specialists. The *Dentists Register* (London) has been published since 1879 by the General Dental Council, and the American Dental Association has issued the *American Dental Directory* since 1947.

The General Medical Council publishes every two years a *List of hospitals and house officer posts in the United Kingdom which are approved or recognised for pre-registration service* (14th edn., 1991). The *Hospitals and Health Services Year Book* (Institute of Health Service Administrators, annual) provides a wealth of information on government departments, statutory bodies, health authorities, all types of hospitals, circulars and statutory instruments, important reports and hospital suppliers. Also available is the *Directory of hospitals 1990/91* (Churchill Livingstone, 1990), which includes the names of consultants in each specialty but has less general information. Further details of the organization of the National Health Service will be found in the National Association of Health Authorities' *NHS handbook* (5th edn., Macmillan, 1991), while the *Directory of schools of medicine and nursing* issued by the International Hospital Groups (2nd edn., Kogan Page, 1984) provides more information about the training and qualifications of the professions supplementary to medicine than is elsewhere available. Brian Watkins's *Documents on health and social services 1834 to the present day* (Methuen, 1975) is a very useful source for older official reports and legislation.

The annual *World of Learning* (Europa Publications) is arranged alphabetically by country and provides information on universities, colleges, research institutes, museums and libraries. It also has a section listing international organizations. *The Commonwealth Universities Yearbook* (Association of Commonwealth Universities) gives very detailed information about the universities in the countries it covers, including historical background, courses offered and full lists of staff by department. The World Health Organization issues the *World directory of medical schools* (6th edn. 1988). For the UK and Ireland, courses are listed in the *Guide to postgraduate degrees, diplomas and courses in medicine*, published annually by Intelligene in association with the National Advice Centre for Postgraduate Medical Education at the British Council. Advisory, governmental and semi-official bodies in British public life are listed in *Councils, committees and boards* (7th edn., C.B.D. Research, 1989).

Keyguide to information sources in the paramedical sciences, edited by J. Hewlett (Mansell 1990) provides an overview of the paramedical sciences and their literature, a bibliographical listing of sources of information, and a list of selected organizations concerned with chiropody, dietetics, occupational therapy, physiotherapy and speech therapy.

Details of ongoing research are provided by *Current research in Britain*, published by the British Library in four parts: *Physical sciences* (5th edn., 1990). *Biological sciences* (5th edn., 1990), *Social sciences* (5th edn., 1990) and *Humanities* (3rd edn., 1989). The first three parts are revised annually, while the *Humanities* volume appears in a new edition every two years. This data can be accessed online via Pergamon INFOLINE. The Medical Research Council *Handbook* (MRC, annual) provides details of research sponsored by the Council, while the *DH Yearbook of Research and Development* (HMSO, annual) lists projects sponsored by the Department of Health.

Information about grants available in this country can be found in the *Grants register* 1989–1991 (Macmillan, 1988) and the *Directory of grant-making trusts 1989* (CAF Publications, 1991). On a smaller scale are the free *Handbook of British medical research charities* (Association of Medical Research Charities, annual) which is restricted to the major trusts and foundations, and the British Medical Association's *Research funds guide* (3rd edn., BMA, 1976). The Association of Commonwealth Universities publishes *Awards for Commonwealth university academic staff 1990–92* (ACU, 1989), giving details of fellowships, visiting professorships and grants, and *Scholarships guide for Commonwealth postgraduate students 1989-91* (ACU, 1988), providing information on scholarships, grants, loans and assistantships for postgraduate study outside the home country. More general information about trusts and foundations is found in the *International Foundation Directory* (5th edn., Europa Publications, 1990).

In addition to the directories listed above, university and medical school calendars and the annual reports of institutions often provide additional information. This section would not be complete, however, without mention of *Whitaker's Almanack*, published annually since 1868, which contains a vast amount of information of all kinds. An up-to-date copy should be available in every library, however small.

Dictionaries

The most comprehensive British medical dictionary is *Butterworths medical dictionary* with Macdonald Critchley as editor-in-chief (2nd edn., Butterworths, 1978), first published in 1961 as the *British medical dictionary* and edited by Sir Arthur MacNalty. This contains biographical and eponymous material, as well as abbreviations, and includes as an appendix an 80-page anatomical nomenclature. More up to date is *Churchill's illustrated medical dictionary* (Churchill Livingstone, New York, 1989). Although this claims to be the first entirely new medical dictionary to be published in the USA this century, it is in fact based on the three-volume *International dictionary of medicine and biology* (Wiley, 1986). An interesting feature is that British spellings and terminology are offered as cross-references. However it received rather mixed reviews on publication. Two good, small British dictionaries are the *Heinemann medical dictionary* (2nd edn., 1988) and the *Concise medical dictionary* (3rd edn., Oxford University Press, 1990), the latter covering nearly 10 000 terms and including some illustrations.

There are several large American dictionaries of long standing which are popular in this country. *Dorland's Illustrated medical dictionary* (27th edn., Saunders, 1988) has been published since 1900, though successive editions have tended to include fewer illustrations. It contains biographical and eponymous material and, because of its reliability, is included in the bibliography accompanying the list of Medical Subject Headings used by *Index Medicus*. An abridged version is published as

Dorland's pocket medical dictionary (24th edn., Saunders, 1989). *Stedman's medical dictionary* (25th edn., Williams and Wilkins, 1990) was first issued in 1911 and has some 100 000 entries. It is easy to use and contains a number of additional tables and appendices, including a 30-page section on medical etymology. *Blakiston's Gould medical dictionary* (4th edn., McGraw-Hill, 1979), first compiled by G.M. Gould in 1894, has very full coverage of terms and many extra tables. On a smaller scale is *Taber's cyclopedic medical dictionary* now edited by C.L. Thomas (16th edn., F.A. Davies, 1989) with some 47 000 entries and 150 good illustrations.

Foreign-language dictionaries

Three polyglot dictionaries are worth noting, as smaller medical libraries may stock one of these in preference to multiple foreign-language dictionaries: E. Veillon and A. Nobel's *Medical dictionary* (6th edn., Huber, 1977), which contains over 40 000 numbered terms, the main section being English with references back from German and French words; *Elsevier's encyclopaedic dictionary of medicine in five languages*, compiled by A.F. Dorian and appearing in several parts. Part A (1987) covers general medicine, and the first section is an alphabetical listing of over 11 000 English-language entries with concise definitions, and their equivalents in French, German, Italian and Spanish. There are indexes for these languages, referring back to the numbered entries in the English section. Part B (1988) covers anatomy, Part C (1989) biology, genetics and biochemistry, and Part D is to cover therapeutic substances. Parts B, C and D include some 7500 terms each. A new arrival in 1991 is the *Radcliffe European medical dictionary* (Radcliffe Medical Press), in which 3000 key medical terms are translated into English, French, German, Italian and Spanish. A smaller, pocket reference edition will also be published.

Foreign-language medical dictionaries are numerous. The following are suggested as examples.

FRENCH

> *English–French dictionary of medical and paramedical sciences* by W.J. Gladstone (Maloine, 1978), with 83 000 entries
>
> *Dictionary, French–English, English–French, of medical and biological terms* by P. Lepine (Flammarion, 1984) with 25 000 French terms
>
> *Dictionary, French–English, of medical terms* by J. Delamare and T. Delamare-Riche (2nd edn., Maloine, 1986) with 35 000 entries in each half; more balanced sections than Lepine

GERMAN

Medical dictionary of the English and German languages by D.W. Unseld (8th edn., Wissenschaftliche Verlag's Gesellschaft, 1982), containing 25 000 entries in each section in one small volume

Medical and pharmaceutical dictionary, English–German by W.E. Bunjes (4th edn., Thieme, 1981) with a *Supplement* comprising more than 17 000 new entries; also *German-English* volume (3rd edn., Thieme, 1981) with 50 000 entries

Dictionary of medicine, English–German by J. Nohring (Elsevier, 1984) containing 55 000 terms; also *German–English* volume (Elsevier, 1987) with some 60 000 entries

Dictionary of clinical medicine by S. Dressler (VCH Publishers, 1990) in two volumes, *English–German* and *German–English*

RUSSIAN

English–Russian medical dictionary by M.P. Multanovsky and A.Y. Ivanova (Collets, 1969)

Russian–English biological and medical dictionary by E.A. Carpovich (2nd edn., Technical Dictionaries Co., 1960) containing over 32 000 entries

S. Jablonski's Russian–English medical dictionary edited by B.S. Levine (Academic Press, 1958) with 29 000 entries

Russian–English medical dictionary (Russian Language Publishers, 1975), containing 50 000 terms and using American spelling

SPANISH

Spanish–English/English–Spanish medical guide by H.H. Hirschhorn (Bailey Bros, 1968)

Diccionario Inglés–Español y Español–Inglès de medicina by F. Ruiz Torres (3rd edn., Editorial Alhambra, 1965, reprinted 1979) which contains over 50 000 entries, with eponyms and abbreviations

OTHER

Hitti's medical dictionary: English–Arabic, with an Arabic–English vocabulary by Y.K. Hitti (4th edn., Librairie du Liban, 1982) with some 40 000 English entries and 31 coloured anatomical plates

A short English–Swahili medical dictionary by T.H. White (Churchill Livingstone, 1978)

Specialist dictionaries

Dictionaries dealing with a particular subject are referred to in the relevant chapters. A useful and necessary addition to the literature is the *Dictionary of medical ethics* edited by A. S. Duncan *et al.* (2nd edn., Longman and Todd, 1981), which contains entries on such important topics as abortion, bereavement, embryo transfer, psychosurgery, etc. It also includes the texts of some declarations.

Nomenclature, terminology and abbreviations

Medical terminology is of vital importance and the clear description of a clinical condition assumes a standard nomenclature. The *Nomenclature of disease* was drawn up by a committee of the Royal College of Physicians (8th and final edition, HMSO, 1960). It has two sections: the first is an aetiological classification which, in the second section, is applied to the body as a whole and to its systems. It is a nomenclature only, concerned with absolute specificity in the description of disease, and cannot be used to code or classify. E. T. Thompson and A. C. Hayden prepared the *Standard nomenclature of diseases and operations* for the American Medical Association (5th edn., McGraw-Hill, 1961). This incorporates a classification and is intended primarily as a diagnostic code for record-keeping and for statistical purposes — as such it is readily adaptable for use in machine-readable data-handling systems.

Standardization is particularly necessary for international co-operation and for statistical purposes. The World Health Organization manages the *International classification of diseases (ICD)*, the 9th revision of which was published in the *Manual of the international statistical classification of diseases, injuries and causes of death* (2 vols, WHO, 1977, 1978). The first volume gives a tabular list of diseases and causes of death, and the second volume is an alphabetical index to the first. The classification is widely used in the recording of pathological conditions and forms the basis of many national mortality and morbidity statistical compilations. The 10th revision of *ICD* is due to appear in 1992. The *International classification of procedures in medicine* (2 vols, WHO, 1978) was published for trial purposes following a resolution at the Twenty-Ninth World Health Assembly in May 1976 and is intended to present, in a systematic fashion, the many procedures used in the different branches of medicine. The *International classification of impairments, disabilities and handicaps* (WHO, 1980) is concerned with the consequences of disease and has also been issued in an experimental first edition. Both these volumes are intended to supplement the *ICD* itself.

The Committee on Nomenclature and Classification of Disease of the College of American Pathologists has produced two important classifications: *Systematized Nomenclature of pathology (SNOP)* (College of American Pathologists, 1965) and *Systematized nomenclature of medicine (SNOMED)* (2nd edn., 2 vols, 1979). Both these publications aim to help pathologists and clinicians organize and utilize their material, and the codings are sufficiently comprehensive and flexible to have many applications in the storage and retrieval of clinical information. A supplement to *SNOMED* containing several hundred additions and amendments was issued in 1982. Anatomical nomenclature is covered by the International Anatomical Nomenclature Committee's *Nomina anatomica* (6th edn., Churchill Livingstone, 1989); this now incorporates the *Nomina Histologica* and the *Nomina Embryologica*. Also relevant is T. Donath's *Anatomical dictionary with nomenclatures and explanatory notes*; the English edition is by G.N.C. Crawford (Pergamon Press, 1970). This brings together the *Basle Nomina anatomica* (1895), the *Jena Nomina anatomica* (1935) and the *Nomina anatomica parisiensia* (1955) in a comparative dictionary, and also contains a list of eponymous authors, with dates of birth and death, nationality and subject specialty. First published in Hungarian in 1958, this has also been translated into German (1960) and Russian. The *Enzyme nomenclature 1984* (Academic Press, 1984) comprises the recommendations of the Nomenclature Committee of the International Union of Biochemistry on the nomenclature and classification of enzymes.

Guides to the derivation, construction and meaning of medical terms include: H.A. Skinner's *The Origin of medical terms* (2nd edn., Williams and Wilkins, 1961), which contains about 4000 terms and has been updated by W.S. Haubrich's *Medical meanings: a glossary of word origins* (Harcourt Brace Jovanovich, 1984) with 500 terms; F. Roberts' *Medical terms: their origin and construction*, revised by B. Lennox (6th edn., Heinemann Medical, 1980); P.M. Davies' *Medical terminology; a guide to current usage* (4th edn., Heinemann Medical, 1985), which is aimed especially at the professions supplementary to medicine; and D. Anderson and R. Buxton's *A pocket etymology of medical terms — an introduction to the Greek and Latin roots of medical terminology* (Bristol Classical Press, 1981) aimed primarily at medical students. M.A. Collins' *Medical terminology and the body systems* (Harper and Row, 1974) is arranged by systems, while *Henderson's dictionary of biological terms*, now edited by E. Lawrence (10th edn., Longman, 1989), provides definitions of over 22 000 terms in related fields. J. Parkinson's *Manual of English for the overseas doctor* (4th edn., Churchill Livingstone, 1991) is concerned mainly with language and terminology, but is also one of the few books to contain a sample curriculum vitae.

Medical and scientific abbreviations appear in some of the dictionaries referred to earlier, but two separate compilations are *Baillière's abbreviations in medicine* (5th edn., by E.B. Steen, Baillière Tindall, 1984), listing over 15 000 items and *Dictionary of medical acronyms and abbreviations* by S. Jablonski (Hanley and Belfus, 1987).

Eponyms, syndromes and quotations

The use of eponyms in medical literatures has been criticized because some diseases, syndromes, etc., may have more than one eponymous name associated with them and this can lead to confusion. However they are undoubtedly here to stay, and it can be argued that they do have a mnemonic quality. Several guides to this kind of terminology have been produced and the most comprehensive is the *Dictionary of medical syndromes* by S.I. Magalini (3rd edn., Lippincott, 1990) with some 3700 entries. This is arranged alphabetically, and under each syndrome are listed synonyms, symptoms, signs, aetiology, pathology, diagnostic procedures, therapy, prognosis and bibliography — the way that a doctor might approach a particular medical problem. Several references are given in the bibliography, including the original reference, but where books are quoted page references are seldom given. *Jablonski's Dictionary of syndromes and eponymic diseases* (2nd edn., R.E. Krieger, 1991) is arranged alphabetically by personal names, with dates of birth and death where appropriate, followed by synonyms, definition and original source. Cross-references and numerous illustrations are included. Two older compilations are R.H. Durham's *Encyclopaedia of medical syndromes* (Hoeber-Harper, 1960), which includes a classification of syndromes by system or type, but which does not always refer to the original description, and E.C. Kelly's *Encyclopedia of medical sources* (Williams and Wilkins, 1948), which provides full references to the original source and often gives brief biographical information. J. Lourie's *Medical eponyms: who was Coude?* (Churchill Livingstone, 1982) is a small work intended for the laboratory coat pocket, and comprises some 900 entries, concentrating on biographical information. B.G. Firkin and J.A. Whitworth's *Dictionary of medical eponyms* (Parthenon Publishing, 1987) also concentrates on biographical details and includes some illustrations. With under 2000 entries it is not as comprehensive as Magalini, but it is a useful addition to the literature.

The field of anatomy is adequately served by J. Dobson's *Anatomical eponyms: being a biographical dictionary of those anatomists whose fames have become incorporated into anatomical nomenclature ...* (2nd edn., Livingstone, 1962), while *Notable names in medicine and surgery* by H. Bailey and W.J. Bishop (4th edn., H.K. Lewis, 1983) is also useful for eponymous material. C. Allan Birch's *Names we remember* (Ravenswood Publications, 1979) consists of 56 short eponymous medical biographies. A vital source for tracing original descriptions, as well as sign-posting the development of medicine, is *Morton's Medical bibliography* (Garrison-Morton) (5th edn., ed. J.M. Norman, Gower, 1991).

The texts of the various declarations and codes of ethics are often sought, and a useful source for these is *Decision-making in medicine: the practice of its ethics*, edited by G. Scorer and A. Wing (Arnold, 1979, p.189–200). Amongst others this includes the text of the Declarations of Geneva, Helsinki, Oslo and Tokyo, as well as the Hippocratic Oath.

Medical quotations are frequently requested, as are their sources, and these can be traced in *Familiar medical quotations* edited by M.B. Strauss (Little, Brown, 1968). This is arranged by subjects, and dates of birth and death are appended to names, but few of the sources are provided with dates or other bibliographical details, making it difficult to trace original sources (for example, if one wants to place a quotation in its original context). Strauss provides some 7500 quotations, and there are indexes of authors and keywords. A welcome addition to the literature is J. Daintith and A. Isaacs' *Medical quotes: a thematic dictionary* (Facts on File, 1989), a compilation of over 1750 medical sayings. It is arranged by subjects, with name and keyword indexes. More general in coverage, but equally fascinating, is A.L. Mackay's *The harvest of a quiet eye* (Institute of Physics, 1977), a delightful and stimulating collection of scientific quotations.

Medical writing and research

Most members of the medical profession become involved in formal writing at some stage during their careers, whether for a thesis, a book or a journal article. The following are suggested as general guides: E.J. Huth's *How to write and publish papers in the medical sciences* (2nd edn., ISI Press, 1987); P. Morgan's *An insider's guide for medical authors and editors* (ISI Press, 1986); and *Research: how to plan, speak and write about it*, edited by C. Hawkins and M. Sorgi (Springer, 1985). Also useful are C.J. Partridge and R.E. Barnitt's *Research guidelines: a handbook for therapists* (Heinemann, 1986), *How to obtain Biomedical research funding*, edited by J.T. Dingle (Elsevier, 1986) and J. Calnan's *Coping with research: the complete guide for beginners* (Heinemann, 1984).

Technical guidance is provided by the Royal Society of Medicine's *Units, symbols and abbreviations* edited by D.N. Baron (4th edn., RSM, 1988), which is intended for biological and medical editors and authors, and by three British Standards: BS 1629: 1976, *Recommendations for bibliographical references*; BS 4821: 1972, *Recommendations for the presentation of theses*, and BS 5261c: 1976, *Marks for copy preparation and proof correction*. The Institute of Medical and Biological Illustration's *Charts and graphs: guidelines for the visual presentation of statistical data in the life sciences* edited by D. Simmonds (MTP Press, 1980) is a practical guide for anyone concerned with preparing charts and graphs either for teaching or for publication. The *Sourcebook of medical illustrations*, edited by P. Cull (Parthenon Publishing, 1989) includes over 400 anatomical, medical and scientific illustrations which are available for re-use or adaptation on a non-copyright basis. Copyright itself is often an area of concern, and assistance is provided by M.F. Flint's *A user's guide to copyright* (3rd edn., Butterworths, 1990).

A number of compilations give advice to authors about the requirements of particular journals, though it should be remembered that instructions are revised from time to time. N.D. Lane and K.L. Kammerer's *Writer's guide to medical journals* (Ballinger, 1975) gives publication data and instructions for over 300 journals, while D.B. Ardell and J.Y. James' *Author's guide to journals in the health field* (Haworth, 1980) covers 260 titles. Many eminent journals in both Europe and North America have decided to adopt the so-called 'Vancouver style', which proposes uniform requirements for manuscripts submitted to biomedical journals. Details will be found in the *British Medical Journal* for 9 February 1991, **302**, 338–341. A list of those periodicals currently using the new style is in *British Medical Journal*, 1988, **296**, 401–405. It should be noted that this code requires the titles of journals to be abbreviated according to the *List of journals indexed in Index Medicus*, which is published each year.

In addition to writing, many doctors are also required to address meetings of various kinds. Sound advice is provided by J. Calnan and A. Barabas' *Speaking at medical meetings: a practical guide* (2nd edn., Heinemann Medical, 1981), which ranges from classroom teaching to giving a paper at an international conference and is very humorously illustrated. Finally, the *British Medical Journal* has issued a most useful series of compilations entitled, *How to do it* (No. 1 — 2nd edn., 1985; No. 2 — 1987, No. 3 — 1990). These give guidance on many topics, including writing an MD thesis, planning a research project, giving a lecture, writing a paper, using slides, appearing on television, etc.

Data books

Data books are intended to provide basic scientific data in concise form and they include such information as mathematical, statistical, chemical and physical tables, dosages, toxicities, normal values, etc. Devoted mainly to subjects connected with scientific medicine, they embrace chemistry and biochemistry, biology and allied topics. Organic chemistry boasts a most comprehensive tool in Beilstein's *Handbuch der organischen Chemie* (4th edn., Springer, 1918–), a monumental work listing all known compounds. *Beilstein* is described in *Information sources in chemistry*, edited by R.T. Bottle and J.F.B. Rowland (Bowker-Saur, 1992), and sources of biological data are indicated in R.T. Bottle and H.V. Wyatt's *The use of biological literature* (2nd edn., Butterworths, 1972, chapter 8). A few standard reference books are mentioned below.

Geigy scientific tables should be available in every medical library. Volumes 1–4 of the 8th edition appeared between 1981 and 1986 (Geigy Pharmaceuticals, Horsham), and further volumes are in preparation. The series provides basic scientific information in concise form, and includes sections devoted to body fluids, statistics, physical chemistry, haematology, biochemistry and metabolism. Another popular source is *The Merck index: an encyclopedia of chemicals and drugs* (11th edn., Merck, 1989), providing information on the chemical and physical properties, dosages and toxicities of about 10 000 compounds, with references to the literature.

The *Biology data book* edited by P.L. Altman and D.S. Dittmer and published by the Federation of American Societies for Experimental Biology (2nd edn., 3 vols, 1972–1974) contains evaluated reference data for the life sciences, and is particularly useful because full details of the original sources are given. The FASEB series of *Biological handbooks* includes *Blood and other body fluids* (1961, reprinted 1971), *Environmental biology* (1966), *Respiration and circulation* (1971), *Cell biology* (1976), *Human health and disease* (1977) and *Inbred and genetically defined strains of laboratory animals* (2 vols, 1979).

Compounds, reagents and techniques used in biochemistry are described in *Data for biochemical research* by R.M.C. Dawson *et al.* (3rd edn., Clarendon Press, 1986). G.D. Fasman has edited the *Handbook of biochemistry and molecular biology* (3rd edn., 8 vols, CRC Press,, 1976), while R.C. Weast edits the regularly revised *Handbook of chemistry and physics* (71st edn., CRC Press, 1990). G.W.C. Kaye and T.H. Laby's *Tables of physical and chemical constants* (14th edn., revised by A.E. Bailey *et al.* (Longman, 1986) covers general physics, chemistry, atomic and nuclear physics and some mathematical functions. All tabulated volumes are expressed in SI units. Statistical tables are often in demand, and a suitable small compilation is F.C. Powell's *Cambridge mathematical and statistical tables* (Cambridge University Press, 1976), while A.M. Bold and P. Wilding's *Clinical chemistry companion*

(Blackwell, 1978) is a handy source of information on normal reference values and standard laboratory tests in medicine.

Vital statistics and statistical tables

For further information on this topic, see Chapter 9, p. 207. Statistical information is often hard to find in the format required. Workers may ask for more up-to-date figures than are available, or else they need them broken down in different ways from their published form. It may be that a recent journal article, located through *Index Medicus*, is the only source for a certain subject. However, a good starting point for many enquiries is the *Guide to official statistics* compiled by the Central Statistical Office (No. 5, HMSO, revised 1990). This is a detailed source of reference, not only to published statistical tables, but also to the journal articles and to reports. Also useful are: M. Alderson and R. Dowie's *Health surveys and related studies* (Pergamon Press, 1979) which forms volume 9 of that publisher's *Reviews of United Kingdom statistical sources* series; B. Benjamin's *Population statistics: a review of UK sources* (Gower, 1989), which is broader in scope than the title suggests; and A. Cowie's article 'Medical statistical information – a guide to sources' which appeared in *Health Libraries Review*, 1986, **3**, 203–221. A quick source of basic information about the incidence of particular types of illness and disease in this country is J. Fry's *Common diseases: their nature, incidence and care* (4th edn., MTP, 1985), which gives figures gathered mainly from general practice. G.M. Howe's *The national atlas of disease mortality in the United Kingdom* (2nd edn., Nelson, 1970) was compiled on behalf of the Royal Geographical Society, and indicates by means of maps the varying pattern of disease mortality in the UK.

On the international level, the World Health Organization published *Annual epidemiological and vital statistics* from 1939 to 1951, which was then succeeded by the *World health statistics annual* (Geneva, 1952–). This now appears in one volume per year, covering vital statistics and life tables, environmental health, causes of death and with a global overview. Since 1948 the United Nations has issued the *Demographic yearbook* (New York), providing statistics from over 220 countries or areas on population, births, mortality, marriage and divorce and international migration. M. Alderson's *International mortality statistics* (Macmillan, 1981) is an important source of information, giving serial mortality tables for European and other selected countries by sex, calendar period and cause of death. It is valuable both for analysing long-term mortality trends within a particular country and for comparing patterns of mortality in different countries during this century.

The Registrar-General's *Statistical Review of England and Wales* came to an end with the three volumes for 1973 (published 1975–1976), and this has been replaced by a series of smaller annual volumes, each dealing with one topic or a number of related topics (HMSO, 1974-). The volumes issued include: *Birth statistics, Mortality statistics — cause*; *Mortality statistics — childhood*; *Mortality statistics — accidents and violence*; *Mortality statistics — area*; *Cancer statistics*; *Communicable disease statistics*; and *Abortion statistics*. This is a selection only, and full details are found in *Sectional List No. 56: Office of Population Censuses and Surveys* (OPCS), revised every two years or so and available free from HMSO. Each main subject carries a colour and reference code; for example, volumes in the morbidity series are pale blue and carry the reference number MB. The aim is to publish figures more quickly than was possible before. The annual reference volumes are supplemented by a series of OPCS *Monitors*, designed for the quick release of selected information as it becomes available. The *Monitors* are divided into the same colour and reference codes as the annual volumes, and their frequency may be monthly, quarterly or 'occasional'. The Registrar-General's *Weekly Return for England and Wales* is published as one of the *Monitors*, and includes notifications of infectious diseases for each administrative area. It is issued about ten days after the end of the week to which figures relate. The *Monitors*, formerly free, are now available on subscription from OPCS, whereas the annual reference volumes must be bought from HMSO. *Population Trends*, the quarterly journal of OPCS, contains regular and up-to-date tables on vital statistics, births, marriages, divorces, migration, deaths and abortions.

Figures relating to the management of the National Health Service (NHS) are found in *Health and Personal Social Services Statistics for England, Scottish Health Statistics*, and *Health and Personal Social Services Statistics for Wales* (all HMSO, annual). The Office of Health Economics' *Compendium of health statistics* (7th edn., OHE, 1989) contains information on the costs of the NHS, staffing, hospital services, family practitioner services, mortality and morbidity. This includes particularly clear tables and graphs. Another important title is the OPCS *Classification of occupations* (HMSO, 1980), not least for its explanation of social classes and socioeconomic groups, while *Social trends* (No. 21, HMSO, 1991) gives a great deal of statistical and other information about British society today.

Texts for research workers in the statistical field include: *Medical statistics: a commonsense approach* by M.J. Campbell and D. Machin (Wiley, 1990); *Mortality, morbidity and health statistics* by M. Alderson (Macmillan, 1988); *Statistics for health management and research* by N. Woodward and L.M.A. Francis (Arnold, 1988); *Introduction to medical statistics* by M. Bland (OUP, 1987); *Statistical methods in medical research* by P. Armitage and G. Berry (2nd edn., Blackwell Scientific, 1987); *Interpretation and uses of medical statistics* by G.J. Bourke *et al.* (Blackwell, 3rd edn., 1985; 4th edn., 1991); *Short textbook of medical statistics* by A. Bradford Hill (11th edn., Hodder and Stoughton, 1984); *Survey methods in community medicine* by J.H. Abramson (3rd edn., Churchill Livingstone, 1984).

Conferences

It is estimated that some 10 000 scientific meetings take place each year and that three-quarters of these result in some kind of published record of the papers given. The proceedings of congresses, conferences and symposia are notoriously difficult to trace, and references to them may appear in many forms. Some proceedings are published separately, though not always by the well-known commercial publishers, some appear as supplements to journals or as reports, and individual papers may appear as articles in journals. The British Library Document Supply Centre at Boston Spa aims to acquire conference proceedings on a comprehensive basis, and issues the monthly *Index of Conference Proceedings* (1964-), which is arranged by keywords. This cumulates annually, some 20 000 conferences now being listed each year. A 25-year cumulation covering 1964–1988 is available on microfiche and in printed form (26 vols, K.G. Saur). This data is also available online as the *Conference proceedings index* via the British Library's BLAISE-Link service, and a compact disc version called *Boston Spa Conferences on CD-Rom* is to be released in 1991. The foregoing titles index only the proceedings of a conference as a whole, while the Institute for Scientific Information's *Index to Scientific and Technical Proceedings* (1978–) indexes the individual papers given. This appears monthly, with semi-annual cumulations, and covers some 3600 published proceedings each year, of which it is estimated that 35 per cent are in the field of the life sciences and clinical medicine. Some earlier congresses can be traced in W.J. Bishop's *Bibliography of international congresses of medical sciences* (Blackwell, 1958), listing 363 congresses. *Index Medicus* indexed certain selected conference proceedings between 1976 and 1981.

Future meetings are listed by Aslib's *Forthcoming International Scientific and Technical Conferences*, issued quarterly, and the *International Congress Calendar*, published quarterly by K.G. Saur. On the medical side, *World Meetings: Medicine*, published quarterly by the World Meetings Information Centre, Chestnut Hill, MA (1978–) covers more than 1000 meetings a year in considerable detail, and the *Calendar of Congresses of Medical Sciences*, issued annually by The Council for International Organizations of Medical Sciences (CIOMS, Geneva), lists meetings up to five year hence. One of the main tasks of the CIOMS since its establishment in 1949 has, indeed, been to assist with the co-ordination of international medical congresses, and to offer advice on their planning and organization. For the USA, forthcoming meetings are listed regularly in the *Journal of the American Medical Association*, monthly in the case of home meetings and twice a year for foreign meetings.

Societies

Information on current medical and scientific societies can be obtained from their own handbooks and annual reports, or from more general reference books. The *Medical directory* and the *American Medical Directory* both contain lists of medical societies, and the *World of learning* has broader coverage of this material under the heading 'learned societies'. The *Directory of British associations and associations in Ireland* (10th edn., C.B.D. Research, 1990) covers some 8500 organizations and is updated every two to three years. It is arranged alphabetically by the name of the association, with subject and abbreviation indexes. Although general in scope it covers a considerable number of medical and scientific societies. The same firm has also issued *Pan-European associations* (1983), which lists over 2000 multi-national organizations in Europe, and the *Directory of European professional and learned societies* (revised edn., 1989).

For the USA a useful compilation is the *Encyclopedia of medical organizations and agencies* (3rd edn., Gale Research Co., 1990), a subject guide to more than 11 000 societies and institutions in the health-care field. The names, addresses and chief office-holders of medical societies are also listed quarterly in the *Journal of the American Medical Association*. An older source is *Scientific and learned societies of the United States*, published by the National Academy of Sciences (9th edn., Washington, 1971), which covers over 500 organizations and gives details of their history and activities.

Current biographical sources

Information on contemporary medical men and women is difficult to acquire except for the brief details of address, posts held, qualifications, etc. to be found in the *Medical directory* and equivalent publications for other countries. A few very eminent people have books and issues of journals dedicated in their honour, and are written about on the occasion of their retirement or when awards are bestowed on them. But these are few, as are those who achieve the pages of *Who's Who*, which inevitably contains only a small percentage of medical people. *Who's Who in science in Europe: a reference guide to European scientists* (revised edn., 4 vols, Longman, 1989) contains over 44 000 entries for the whole of Europe and includes medicine in its coverage. The *Who's Who of British Scientists 1980-81* (3rd edn., Simon Books, 1980) is a revised edition of a work formerly published by Longman, while the *International medical who's who* (2 vols, Longman, 1980) aims to be a biographical guide to those engaged in medical research.

American men and women of science (16th edn., 8 vols, Bowker, 1986) contains entries for 130 000 active U.S. and Canadian scientists in the physical and biological sciences, and cross-references are provided for those listed in previous editions, but not in the current one. This compilation is available as an online database via the Lockheed Dialog information system. Historical biographical sources are described in Chapter 24.

CHAPTER FIVE

Online and CD-ROM sources of information retrieval

C. NORRIS

The most significant development in mechanized information retrieval in the past five years has been the growth in use of CD-ROM (compact disc, read-only memory) as a medium for database provision. While the total number of online biomedical databases has continued to increase, many files are now available in CD-ROM and as floppy disc versions for use with personal computers.

Where a database is offered by several online hosts and as CD-ROM systems, a choice between different versions is often difficult to make. Many factors will have to be considered in the choice — convenience, frequency of use, familiarity of the search language, and cost, as well as the range of databases available, and which one might wish to use, on any particular host.

Developments have also taken place in the provision of full text from journals and textbooks both online and in CD-ROM. Over 100 medical journals are already available in full text online and many medical textbooks and reference works are available as online files and on compact discs. A commercial ADONIS operation is planned for 1991 which will make available the full text of articles from over 400 medical journals on weekly CD-ROM discs as an alternative to photocopying.

User-friendly 'front-end' searching, downloading and record management systems have also been developed, including GRATEFUL MED, which will dial the National Library of Medicine (NLM) computer, run a search against a number of databases and download the resulting references for examination automatically, without any expert knowledge on the part of the user.

Online, CD-ROM or manual searching?

Bibliographic searches for a small number of recent references which require the scanning of only a few subject headings can be carried out quickly and effectively manually, using an abstracting or indexing journal. The main drawback to manual searches is the time required to scan more than a few pages of indexes or abstracts to select items, and to write out a list of citations. A search covering many years is very time-consuming and tedious compared with the other methods. However, for a literature search covering material published before 1964 there is no alternative to searching manually.

Now that many indexing and abstracting journals are available in the form of CD-ROM databases, it is possible for searches of combinations of subject headings, keywords or authors' names to be carried out without the open-ended expense of online searches. Once the initial investment in equipment and the expense of hiring the CD-ROM database has been made by a library, there is little additional cost other than consumables (printer, paper, ribbons and floppy discs), maintenance, and training of staff and readers. Training is necessary to operate the equipment efficiently and to improve searching skills. Most CD-ROM systems can be operated in either menu-driven or search command mode, depending on the level of experience and skills of the user. The main disadvantages of CD-ROM are in comparison with online searching and in the incompatibility of CD-ROM products and software from different suppliers. Large databases like MEDLINE or EMBASE usually require one or sometimes two compact discs for each year's records. Changing discs and re-running searches for a number of years can become tedious. One solution is to link several CD-ROM players together in series, or to use a multi-disc player. This allows a number of discs to be searched in sequence, minimising disc changes and increasing the capital cost of the equipment, but a search may still take an appreciable length of time to perform.

The time taken to retrieve and assemble records from the compact disc is dependent on the retrieval software as well as the processing power of the microcomputer. These both vary considerably between different computer models and software systems. Until recently no CD-ROM system could match the speed and capacity of the mainframe computers used for providing access to online databases.

However, a workstation with eight CD drives and a 650 Mbyte hard disc designed to run CD PLUS/MEDLINE and other databases has recently been developed which claims to match the speed and response times of online systems.

The main disadvantage of CD-ROM compared with printed abstracts or indexes is the restriction to use by one reader unless the system is networked. A CD-ROM searching session may take each reader up to an hour to complete, and in most libraries an appointments system for booking time is essential. In contrast, printed bibliographies are available for use by several readers using different parts or volumes simultaneously.

Online searches scan very large numbers of records selected from the whole database, or portions of it, retrieving all the relevant citations within seconds. Enlarging or narrowing a search in response to what one finds is available to manual searchers and CD-ROM users, but neither can match the speed and flexibility available with online searching. Online databases are often updated with new records six weeks or more before the corresponding printed and CD-ROM versions appear, and some are updated with new records at weekly intervals. Online databases frequently carry additional data which is not available in the printed or CD-ROM version, and may have a greater variety of access points to information than is available from CD-ROM.

'False drops'

All lists of citations produced by CD-ROM or online searches are liable to contain some items that are irrelevant. These are called 'false drops' or 'noise'. Such citations contain all the descriptors or parameters required for the citation to be retrieved but the relationship between the headings is not that implied by the searcher. For example, if I wished to retrieve citations to articles on the brain in liver disease I might use the three textwords 'brain', 'liver' and 'disease' linked by the operator 'AND'. I instruct the computer to search for the co-occurrence of 'brain AND liver AND disease'. This will retrieve citations on the brain in liver disease as I wished, but will also find records on the liver in brain disease which I would consider to be 'false drops'. The citations have been correctly retrieved by the computer in response to the given strategy. The number of 'false drops' can be reduced by altering search strategies in various ways to make them more specific. However, there is a trade-off between precision and recall in every search, and relevant citations may be lost in the attempt to improve precision. Most searches aim to achieve a reasonable balance.

Choosing a database

All online hosts produce lists of the databases they offer for searching, and most provide detailed information about the size and scope of each file and the structure of its records. For example, Data-Star and Dialog both provide 'blue sheets' of information for each database they host, while NLM provides extensive documentation about its databases and searching software in the form of an *Online Reference Manual*.

A number of directories of databases are published which draw the information together into a single source, and provide updated information at regular intervals. Multi-disciplinary guides include the Cuadra/Elsevier Directory of Online Databases, completely revised every half-year and updated with quarterly supplements between revisions, which lists over 4400 databases and files, the *Directory of Online Information Resources*, updated annually, and the *Eusidic Database Guide*, also annual.

A specific guide for medicine, *Online* medical databases 1989 by Elizabeth Lyon (1988), lists over 130 bibliographic or full-text online databases which cover medical subjects or contain material related to medicine. It provides information on the content and subject coverage of each database, the producer, online hosts and charges. It also contains a list of host, producer and supplier addresses with telephone numbers.

Directories of CD-ROM databases have also been published. Over 600 CD-ROM and diskette and magnetic tape databases in all subject fields are listed in the *Directory of Portable Databases*, a semi-annual publication from Cuadra/Elsevier. Armstrong and Large (1990) list over 500 CD-ROM products in all subject areas including medicine, while the *CD-ROM Directory 1990* has full descriptions of over 800 titles and contains information about CD-ROM drives, as well as listing books, journals and exhibitions where the different CD-ROM products may be seen.

The two major biomedical databases are MEDLINE and EMBASE. Both databases claim to give reasonably comprehensive coverage of the most important biomedical literature. Surprisingly, the amount of overlap is only 40 per cent overall. This is due to differences in selection policy and the journal lists of the database producers. EMBASE (Excerpta Medica) scans more journals and adds citations more selectively from them, whereas MEDLINE includes all original articles and all substantive editorials and letters from a somewhat smaller list of journals. EMBASE has a bias towards drugs, pharmaceutical and environmental health literature and to European journals. MEDLINE includes nursing, dentistry and veterinary medicine, which are not indexed by EMBASE, and has a bias towards American journals. MEDLINE is cheaper, more widely available and more widely used than EMBASE.

BIOSIS, a major database covering biology and the life sciences, also includes considerable amounts of material on experimental medicine and preclinical research, and is worth considering for comprehensive coverage of this type of literature. A more detailed account of each database is given below.

There are also many smaller databases and databanks covering a wide range of specialized subject fields or types of material, and these can be valuable sources of additional information or specialist material. A selection of smaller databases is also described below.

MEDLINE

The world's first computerized bibliographic database was MEDLARS (MEDical Literature Analysis and Retrieval System) which was begun in mid-1963. The database is a by-product of the compilation of *Index Medicus*, the *Index to Dental Literature* and the *International Nursing Index*. The online files of the database are called MEDLINE (MEDlars onLINE).

Coverage

MEDLINE covers the whole field of biomedicine from 1964 to date, although most online hosts offer files from 1966 onwards, the date when subject heading qualifiers were first introduced. 3200 journals published in over 70 countries are indexed, amounting to 250 000 citations each year, and the total file size now exceeds six million citations. The *List of Serials Indexed for Online Users*, published annually, gives details of the journals indexed for MEDLINE and other National Library of Medicine files, and indicates those titles which are selectively indexed to include only articles of medical interest, for example, *Nature*.

Substantive editorials, letters, biographies and obituaries are indexed in addition to articles, but short abstracts and summaries of proceedings are not indexed. Selected book chapters and monographs were included from 1976 to 1981 but are no longer added. (NLM has a separate file of books and monographs, CATLINE, available for searching this type of material.)

Major clinical journals receive priority treatment and are indexed with an average of 10–12 subject descriptors per article. Experimental and preclinical journals are indexed in similar detail, but articles from lighter-weight clinical and paramedical journals are indexed in less depth with an average of four to five descriptors. Three or four descriptors are applied to editorials and letters taken for indexing. Of the descriptors used for indexing, only three on average are used as headings to cite the article in *Index Medicus*. These correspond to the main point of the article. The remaining descriptors covering secondary points and other details are available only on the MEDLINE files.

Since 1975 author abstracts have been added to the MEDLINE records, and these are available for textword searching. However, very long abstracts are truncated at 400 words. Over 60 per cent of records have abstracts. All published author abstracts have been included since 1990, including short abstracts and those from lower priority journals which were previously excluded.

MeSH

The descriptors used to index MEDLINE are taken from *Medical Subject Headings (MeSH)*. *MeSH* is available in four versions and is updated and revised each year. The first version of *MeSH*, sometimes referred to as public *MeSH*, is for use with *Index Medicus*. The second, *Medical Subject Headings — Annotated Alphabetic List (Annotated MeSH)* is a thesaurus of the 16 000 descriptors used in indexing, arranged in alphabetical order. Each heading is annotated with information and instructions useful for indexing and searching, cross-references from synonyms and related headings, and the date of introduction of the heading into *MeSH*. *Medical Subject Headings — Tree Structures (MeSH Trees)* is an arrangement of the headings into hierarchies based on subject categories. Category A contains anatomical headings, B contains organism headings, C disease headings, D drugs and chemicals, and so on, each category being subdivided (A1 — body regions, A2 — musculoskeletal system, etc.) and having an hierarchical arrangement in up to nine levels of specificity within each subcategory.

Individual headings may be in more than one category or subcategory and can have different relations and arrangements in each. Since indexing is carried out by using the most specific heading for a concept, with no posting-on of entries to higher levels, the trees are important in tracing the relationships of headings and are used extensively in gathering together groups of related headings for searching.

Permuted Medical Subject Headings (Permuted MeSH) is a keyword out-of-context index to the *MeSH* headings, often found useful by searchers for discovering overlooked or obscure headings.

Annotated MeSH contains geographical headings, check tags and qualifiers within the alphabetical listing. Check tags include concepts such as age groups of patients, common experimental animals, types of study, for example, case reports and *in vitro* experiments, and publication types, for example, journal articles, news items, subject reviews and biographies, These are minor concepts looked for routinely during indexing, and are checked off automatically if they occur. These types of descriptors do not appear in *Index Medicus* but are available for searching on MEDLINE both in the online and CD-ROM versions. The list of publication types was greatly increased in 1991.

Qualifiers

81 qualifiers or subheadings are available to modify *MeSH* headings. *Annotated MeSH* includes qualifiers within the alphabetical listing of headings but also gives a separate list of them in the introductory pages, with definitions, an outline of their scope, date of introduction, and the subject categories and subcategories of headings to which, broadly speaking, each may be applied. The individual descriptors in *Annotated MeSH* list the qualifiers which are forbidden or have restricted use with the particular heading.

Qualifiers were first introduced in 1966 to break up the list of citations printed under each heading in *Index Medicus* into convenient groups for reading. They are also useful in searching, since they can be used tied to descriptors to increase specificity or used free-floating to give blanket retrieval of all subject headings modified by the particular qualifier. For example, 'adverse effects' as a free floating qualifier in conjunction with the combination ASTHMA/drug therapy would retrieve citations to any drug having adverse effects during its use in the treatment of asthma.

Co-ordination of headings

The most common form of co-ordination in MEDLINE is the combination of a *MeSH* heading with a qualifier. For example, 'X-ray diagnosis of osteoporosis' is indexed as OSTEOPOROSIS/radiography. The combination is physically linked when co-ordinated in this way. Sometimes no suitable qualifier is available to modify a heading and two separate headings are used. For example, 'biophysics of the hip joint' is indexed by HIP JOINT and BIOPHYSICS.

The use of some combinations of headings and qualifiers is forbidden due to the existence of pre-co-ordinated headings. LEAD POISONING is used in preference to the main heading/qualifier combination LEAD/poisoning. Other combinations are restricted to avoid ambiguous choices, for example, ENZYMES/blood is always used instead of BLOOD/enzymology to avoid confusion.

Individual qualifiers are restricted in use to particular categories or part categories of headings to which they are appropriate, and not to any others. The allowed categories are listed as part of the definition in *Annotated MeSH*. For example, /drug therapy may be applied only to the disease headings in categories C and F3 and not to other categories of headings.

In recent years the use of some qualifiers has been extended to groups and part categories of headings to which they were formerly un-available. For example, the qualifier /blood may now be used with the group of headings related to 'PREGNANCY' in Category G3. The headings to which qualifiers have been extended in this way are usually annotated with the information. Changes in policy of this kind can give rise to unexpected failures in retrieval prior to a particular date and should always be borne in mind as a cause of finding no citations.

The general principles and rules of MEDLINE indexing are given in the *MEDLARS Indexing Manual Part 2 (1984)*. This is illustrated throughout with numerous examples of indexing policy for each category of *MeSH* headings and for the individual qualifiers.

Missing concepts

Although *MeSH* headings are available for the majority of concepts, it is sometimes necessary to use combinations of headings when the exact heading is not available, for example, DUODENAL DISEASES and TUBERCULOSIS, GASTROINTESTINAL for duodenal tuberculosis, or to use the next most general heading, for example MORAXELLA for the bacterium *Moraxella liquefaciens*. The specific bacterium can, of course, be retrieved by a combination of the *MeSH* heading MO-RAXELLA linked with the text word 'liquefaciens'.

Drugs and chemicals pose a particular problem in *MeSH* due to the sheer number of compounds appearing in the medical and pharmaceutical literature. A file maintained by the National Library of Medicine has entries for all drugs and biological factors that have appeared in the literature indexed for MEDLARS files, with indexing and automatic mapping instructions. A printed version is published and updated each year as *Medical Subject Headings — Supplementary Chemical Records*.

Searching MEDLINE

Before performing a search on any database one should do preparatory work and consider the kind of citations one is trying to retrieve and the best strategy for achieving this aim. Time spent in preparation can save wasted time and frustration at the CD-ROM or online terminal as well as missed references and unnecessary expense.

Both CD-ROM and online searching take place as an interactive dialogue between the searcher and the computer program. Command languages and the software facilities available for manipulating files differ between the various database hosts and between CD-ROM systems, but the basic principles of searching are similar in all systems. The Boolean operators 'AND', 'OR' and 'NOT' are used to link headings together. Brackets, including nested brackets, may be available to gather alternative headings or search statements together in groups. Word adjacency and word proximity operators may be available for finding the co-occurrence of textwords within sentences or paragraphs. Right-hand truncation of textwords or classification numbers is always available but left-hand truncation is not usually provided. An 'explode' facility may be provided to gather all the narrow headings under a broader heading within an hierarchical thesaurus like *MeSH*.

Microcomputer telecommunications software packages have been available for many years for personal computers which will dial up a database, run a prestored search profile and hold downloaded citations. 'Front-end' software called GRATEFUL MED has now been developed for automatic searching of MEDLINE and other NLM databases. This will run a search automatically for an untrained user by means of menus, but can also be used by skilled searchers in command mode. Using menus, the search formulation is constructed automatically from a typed-in sentence which is converted into groups of *MeSH* headings and truncated textwords. The software then dials up the NLM database through the telecommunications networks, logs in to the database and runs the search automatically. The retrieved citations are downloaded, and the system logs off from the network automatically. The citations resulting from the search can then be individually examined and evaluated off-line. The user's selection of relevant citations from those retrieved in the initial search is used to refine the search formulation which can then be re-run on the same file or a whole range of databases.

Online sources for MEDLINE

Online access to MEDLINE is provided by BLAISE-Link (which provides access from the UK and Eire to the NLM computer), BRS, Data-Star, Dialog, DIMDI, MIC-KIBIC, NLM, STN International and Télésystèmes-Questel. Most hosts now provide searching of the whole database as a single operation as well as partial searches on separate spans of years.

On BLAISE-Link and NLM the current file is updated weekly. The MESH VOCABULARY FILE and SDILINE, the latest month of MEDLINE, are also available as separate online files. *MeSH* Tree explosions can be performed using *MeSH* headings (rather than truncated Tree numbers which have to be used on other systems). Multiple file searches across different NLM databases are available, and records can be sorted and merged before being printed out. GRATEFUL MED is available from NLM within the USA and from BLAISE-Link within the UK and Eire.

Special features on BRS include the facility to read and print the full article text of citations from over 100 journals in COMPREHENSIVE CORE MEDICAL LIBRARY, and to link up and zoom in on the citations included within their lists of references.

Data-Star has the MESH VOCABULARY FILE for 1985 to date available online. DIMDI has the earliest records and provides 1964 to date as two files, whilst Dialog has the facility to merge records retrieved from a range of different databases and eliminate duplicate records before they are listed out.

CD-ROM sources for MEDLINE

Several different versions of MEDLINE are available on CD-ROM. COM-PACT CAMBRIDGE MEDLINE (Cambridge Scientific Abstracts) was the first version to be available and is widely used in UK medical libraries. Like most other versions it has menu-driven and command-driven modes of searching. The database is available on disc for 1966 onwards, with subscription options for spans of 25, 10 or 5 years, or for the current year alone, and it is updated monthly. An online linkage for BRS and GRATEFUL MED is included.

Dialog offers two versions of MEDLINE on compact disc. MEDLINE — CLINICAL COLLECTION CD Dialog Information Services covers *Abridged Index Medicus*, with some additional journal records, and provides the current year and two preceding years on a single disc, updated quarterly. DIALOG ONDISC MEDLINE CD provides the current year and up to five years of backfiles, and has menu and command searching modes. The command searching software uses the same commands as Dialog online, and a Dialog-Link facility provides access to all online databases on Dialog. CD-ROM searches can be run against MEDLINE online to obtain later citations not available on the current disc. From 1989 onwards each year's records take up two discs. The current year is updated monthly, and up to six years' backfiles are available.

CD PLUS/MEDLINE (formerly COMPACT MED-BASE) provides the complete MEDLINE files from 1966 onwards on seven discs. Used in conjunction with the CD Plus 200 workstation, which is available in an eight CD drive or three CD drive configuration, the system is claimed to be as fast as searching online. The workstation and software is designed for professional searchers, and has many useful and attractive features. For example, explosions of *MeSH* headings are performed rapidly, and pre-explosions of very heavily posted *MeSH* trees are stored on the system to increase the speed of retrieval. Networked and dial-up networked versions are available which allow up to eight simultaneous users. However, the price for the complete system of hardware and discs makes it uneconomic as an alternative to online for small and medium scale users of MEDLINE. A CD Plus 100 version with two CD drives is available for end users and smaller libraries. A fuller account of the features of CD-PLUS/MEDLINE is given by Whitsed (1990).

Ebsco offer two products: CORE MEDLINE Ebsco CD-ROM with records which correspond to two preceding years and the current year of *Abridged Index Medicus*, enhanced with records from additional journals, on a single disc and updated quarterly, and COMPREHENSIVE MEDLINE Ebsco CD-ROM. The latter version has a downloading facility to the British Library's ARTEL system for ordering inter-library loans.

MEDLINE ON SILVERPLATTER CD is a menu-driven system which can also be run on the MultiPlatter CD-ROM network package. A dial-in module is available which allows access from remote sites to the Multi-Platter network.

EMBASE (Excerpta Medica)

The computer database used in the production of the 44 abstract journals and two drug-related literature indexes of the Excerpta Medica Foundation is called EMBASE. Subject coverage includes the whole of biomedicine and basic clinical sciences but excludes nursing, psychology, dentistry, veterinary medicine and paramedical areas. Particular emphasis is given to covering the literature of drugs and pharmacology, including the biological effects of chemical compounds.

Coverage

Until recently, Excerpta Medica included items selectively from the journals it scanned and added 350 000 records each year. EMBASE now includes every item from 2900 biomedical journals and selected items from a further 600 journals. Approximately 400 000 citations per year are being added to the database and 60 per cent of the records have English abstracts. Abstracts are included on the basis of editorial judgement of the quality of the original articles. Books were included until 1980 but are no longer added. EMBASE includes a high proportion of European journals and selects and deselects titles for indexing far more frequently than MEDLINE. A *List of Journals Abstracted* is published annually, and a microfiche edition of the list is also available which gives cumulated details of journals indexed since 1977.

As well as original articles, EMBASE includes substantive editorials, conference proceedings and letters to the editor.

EMTREE

In 1988 a new classification system was introduced to replace EM-CLAS (the original Excerpta Medica CLASsification system used to organize the arrangement of the contents of the printed abstract journals and as one of the indexing systems of the database up until 1987). EM-TREE has 16 broad subject facets with up to four levels of hierarchical structure, and closely mirrors the subject organization of the *MeSH* tree structures: A — anatomical concepts, B — organisms, C — physical diseases, disorders and abnormalities, and so on. As in the *MeSH* Trees, each facet is divided into subgroups, for example, A1 — body regions, A2 — musculoskeletal system, and so forth, but at this level some differences in detail are apparent. EMTREE has 5300 codes with equivalent MALIMET (MAster LIst of MEdical Terms) headings.

Under the lowest level of the EMTREE codes is a large number of more specific MALIMET terms which are posted on to the EMTREE codes. The total number of MALIMET terms included within the structure is 23 500 and consists of the most frequently used indexing terms for EMBASE. A list of most of these headings has been published as Mini-MALIMET. The total structure thus contains almost one-and-a-half times the number of headings as *MeSH* but has shallower hierarchical arrangements.

MALIMET

The MAster LIst of MEdical Terms, MALIMET, is a controlled vocabulary of over 200 000 preferred headings, including more than 40 000 drugs and chemicals, and 250 000 synonyms. Synonyms are automatically converted into the preferred term by the MALIMET program. Since 1979 the subject indexing headings have been weighted to indicate major or minor concepts. On average, eight MALIMET terms are assigned to each article although up to 50 are permitted. A number of secondary indexing terms are also added without the use of a thesaurus, including trade and company names of drugs, and species of experimental animals.

EMTAGS

Concepts such as sex, age, type of study, common experimental animals and routes of drug administration are routinely recorded, and up to 25 EMTAG codes may be assigned to each article.

Searching EMBASE

Searches of EMBASE can be run using any combination of MALIMET terms, EMTREE codes, EMTAGS, and free text words, using the usual Boolean logical operators. EMTREE codes can be used to retrieve articles with all the subsidiary specific MALIMET indexing terms, similar to the explosion of *MeSH* Tree numbers in MEDLINE.

Unlike MEDLINE, EMBASE is not file-maintained for changes in descriptors so retrospective searches do need to be researched for changes in vocabulary. Some preprocessed search profiles are available on the

German host DIMDI which enable complicated searches to be performed with a single search term.

Sources for EMBASE

EMBASE is available online from BRS, Data-Star, Dialog and DIMDI and on compact disc as EXCERPTA MEDICA ABSTRACT JOURNALS ON CD-ROM SilverPlatter from 1984 to date. A current-awareness service on diskette, MEDICAL SCIENCE WEEKLY, covering over 1000 journals in the field of biomedicine from Excerpta Medica is also available.

BIOSIS/BIOSIS PREVIEWS

BIOSIS contains citations and abstracts from *Biological Abstracts* and *Biological Abstracts Reports, Reviews and Meetings*. The subject content is primarily biology and life sciences research but includes experimental human studies and some clinical medicine as well as pharmacology, biochemistry and other areas related to medicine. Citations are selected from over 9000 periodicals as well as monographs, reports and conference proceedings. BIOSIS is available online through BRS, Data-Star, Dialog, DIMDI, ESA-IRS and STN International. BIOLOGICAL ABSTRACTS ON COMPACT DISC (BA ON CD) SilverPlatter is also available.

Databases to specialized materials

Specialized medical databases devoted to records of books and monographs, audio-visual materials, and press cuttings are available, as well as a directory of health information providers.

AVLINE

AVLINE contains bibliographic records of all types of audio-visual materials in the field of medicine and health care, including dentistry and nursing in the collections of the National Library of Medicine. The file covers the period 1976 to date and contains over 21 000 records. Textwords and *MeSH* headings are available for subject searching, and the file can also be searched for type of media or specific running time. AVLINE is available online through BLAISE-Link and NLM.

BRITISH MEDICAL ASSOCIATION PRESS CUTTINGS

The BMA PRESS CUTTINGS file contains summaries of articles and items of medical interest from some 30 newspapers and UK radio broadcasts from 1984 onwards. The file is updated daily, and is available online through Data-Star.

CATLINE

The National Library of Medicine CATalogue onLINE (CATLINE) contains records of over 660 000 monographs, reports, and first issues of periodicals published since 1801. The file covers medicine, nursing and dentistry in all languages. Subject searching can be performed using *MeSH* headings, textwords or NLM class-marks. The file is updated weekly and can be accessed online through BLAISE-Link and NLM.

DIRLINE

The Directory of Information Resources online, DIRLINE contains 17 500 records to mainly U.S. professional societies, voluntary associations, government agencies, institutions, libraries, self-help/support groups, health information centres, poison control centres and other sources of help and information, but does include over 200 records for UK organizations. The file uses *MeSH* subject descriptors, and is available online through BLAISE-Link and NLM.

Databases to specialized subject areas

The acquired immunodeficiency syndrome, AIDS, has generated a spate of database activity. Among those available is the AIDS database produced by the Bureau of Hygiene and Tropical Diseases, which covers articles from over 1100 journals, as well as books and reports. The file contains 8000 records from 1984 onwards and is available online through BRS, Data-Star and DIMDI. A rather larger file is, AIDSLINE, is a subset of MEDLINE enhanced with records from CANCERLIT, HEALTH and other NLM databases, which contains over 40 000 records from 1980 onwards. AIDSLINE is available online through BLAISE-Link, Data-Star and NLM and on compact disc as AIDSLINE CD SilverPlatter. NLM also produces AIDSDRUGS, an online database giving details of nearly 100 agents which are currently being tested in clinical trials, and AIDSTRIALS a database of ongoing trials of treatments for AIDS. Both are available online through BLAISE-Link and NLM.

Ethical questions in medicine and health are the content of BIOETHICS produced by the Kennedy Institute of Ethics and the National Library of Medicine. The file contains nearly 31 000 graphical records from journals, monographs, newspaper articles and law reports from 1973 onwards. Records are indexed with terms from a specialized *Bioethics Thesaurus* related to *MeSH*. The file is available online through BLAISE-Link, DIMDI, NLM and Télésystèmes-Questel.

Cancer information is covered by a group of files. CANCERLIT, produced by the U.S. National Cancer Institute, covers all aspects of cancer from 3000 journals as well as books, conference proceedings and reports. CANCERLIT contains over 760 000 records from 1963 onwards. *MeSH* headings have been added to records of articles published from 1980 onwards, and all records contain abstracts.

CANCERLIT is available online through BLAISE-Link, BRS, DIMDI, Data-Star, Dialog and NLM, updated monthly, and on compact disc as CANCERLIT ON CD-ROM Cambridge Scientific Abstracts, covering the latest four years, updated quarterly.

CLINPROT contains summaries of almost 8000 clinical protocols using new anti-cancer drugs and treatments. Descriptions of the protocols and trials are supplied by the U.S. National Cancer Institute and cancer centres in the USA and elsewhere. The file is updated quarterly and is available online through BLAISE-Link, DIMDI and NLM.

PDQ (PHYSICIAN DATA QUERY), also produced by the National Cancer Institute, is a menu-driven service made up of three files and intended for use by doctors. The CANCER file contains updated information about the treatment and prognosis of 75 major types of cancer. The PROTOCOL file provides information on more than 1300 active clinical trials, 33 current and 6000 closed treatment protocols. The DIRECTORY file provides names, addresses and telephone numbers for 14 000 doctors and surgeons and 1600 organizations specializing in the care of cancer, mainly in the USA. The file is available online through BLAISE-Link, BRS and NLM and on compact disc as PDQ: PHYSICIAN DATA QUERY ON CD-ROM Cambridge Scientific Abstracts, updated quarterly.

DHSS-DATA is based on the abstracting and current awareness bulletins produced by the UK Department of Health Library. These cover the National Health Service, hospital administration, medical equipment and supplies, public health, primary care, occupational diseases, social services and social policy. Official reports, circulars and publications are covered as well as books and items from 1500 journals. The file covers 1983 onwards and is updated weekly. DHSS-DATA online is available on Data-Star and Scicon.

Information on non-clinical aspects of health care, health planning and management is provided by HEALTH (HEALTH PLANNING AND ADMINISTRATION). The file contains over 520 000 records from 1975 onwards compiled from MEDLINE with additional material selected from a further 750 journals. The file is produced by NLM in co-operation with the American Hospital Association and the Health Resources Administration, and has a structure similar to MEDLINE. HEALTH is available online through BLAISE-Link, BRS, Dialog, DIMDI and NLM, and on compact disc as CD-PLUS/HEALTH CD.

The history of medicine is covered by the HISTLINE (HISTory of medicine onLINE) file, source of the annual *Bibliography of the History of Medicine*. It comprises over 95 000 items from the CATLINE and MED-

LINE files from 1970 onwards, and is updated quarterly. HISTLINE is available online through BLAISE-Link and NLM.

MARTINDALE ONLINE is based on *Martindale: the extra pharmacopoeia*, and contains evaluated information on over 5000 drugs and medicines. Details of physical and pharmaceutical properties, dosage, adverse effects and interactions are included, as well as CAS Registry number, and alternative names. The information is gathered from many sources, and abstracts and citations to the literature are included in the records. MARTINDALE ONLINE is updated at six-monthly intervals and is available online through Data-Star and Dialog or in a CD-ROM version as MARTINDALE CD-ROM Micromedex. The CD-ROM version is also provided as part of the MICROMEDEX COMPUTERISED CLINICAL INFORMATION SYSTEM CD. This includes IDENTINDEX a complete emergency poison identification and management information system, IDENTIDEX, a capsule and tablet identification system, EMERGINDEX, an emergency medical care information system with literature abstracts, DRUGDEX, a referenced drug information system, and other drug-related information.

Occupational health and safety literature is provided by OSH-ROM CD SilverPlatter. This contains three databases NIOSHTIC from the TIS National Institute for Occupational Safety and Health, HSELINE from the UK Health and Safety Executive, and CISDOC from the International Occupational Safety and Health Information Centre of the International Labour Organization. HSELINE covers all the UK Health and Safety Commission publications, Health and Safety Executive publications, and items taken from journals, books, conference proceedings, reports and legislation. HSELINE is available online through Data-Star, ESA-IRS and Orbit.

Access to pharmaceutical literature is provided by a large number of databases. INTERNATIONAL PHARMACEUTICAL ABSTRACTS (IPA), corresponding to the American Society of Hospital Pharmacists publication of the same name, contains over 200 000 records from 1970 onwards on all aspects of pharmaceutical practice including drug testing, research, toxicity and adverse reactions, legislation, economics and ethics. Records contain descriptors from the *IPA Thesaurus*, Chemical Abstracts Service Registry numbers, FDA Adopted Names for drugs, and broad classification codes. INTERNATIONAL PHARMACEUTICAL ABSTRACTS is available online through BRS, Data-Star, Dialog and ESA-IRS, updated monthly, and on compact disc as INTERNATIONAL PHARMACEUTICAL ABSTRACTS ON CD-ROM Cambridge Scientific Abstracts, updated quarterly. A compilation which includes the American Society of Hospital Pharmacists *Drug Information Annual* and *Handbook on Injectable Drugs* as well as the complete INTERNATIONAL PHARMACEUTICAL ABSTRACTS database is also available on compact disc as the DRUG INFORMATION SOURCE CD Cambridge Scientific Abstracts.

The file for bibliographic information on population studies, family planning, fertility and contraception is POPLINE (POPulation information onLINE). The database is produced by NLM in co-operation with the Population Information Program of Johns Hopkins University and the Center for Population and Family Health of Columbia University. It includes information about family planning programmes and related legislation and policy issues. Journal and newspaper articles are covered as well as books, technical reports and grey literature. Most records have abstracts. The database contains over 175 000 records from 1970 onwards and is available online through BLAISE-Link and NLM.

Toxicology information is provided by the TOXLINE, TOXLIT and TOXNET databases. TOXLINE, with 861 000 records from 1981 onwards, and its backfile TOXLINE65, with 707 000 records spanning 1965 to 1980, contain seven subfiles of bibliographic data from different producers, which can be searched as a whole or as individual files. These include subfiles of toxicology information from MEDLINE (TOXBIB), BIOSIS, INTERNATIONAL PHARMACEUTICAL ABSTRACTS (IPA), and other sources. TOXLIT, with 857 000 records from 1981 onwards, and its backfile TOXLIT65, with 586 000 records from 1965 to 1980, contains complementary files of bibliographic information from the Chemical Abstracts Service which requires royalty payments for the use of records.

The TOXNET service is provided by NLM on a separate computer to the other NLM toxicology databases and gives access to 10 databases of toxicology data including HSDB (the Hazardous Substances Data Bank) with factual details of 4300 compounds, CCRIS (Chemical Carcinogenesis Research Information System) with nearly 2200 records, IRIS (Integrated Risk Information System) produced by the U.S. Environmental Protection Agency (EPA) containing factual health risk and EPA information on 400 chemicals, DART (Developmental and Reproductive Toxicology) a bibliographic database on chemical, physical and biological agents that may cause birth defects, with 5700 records, which continues ETICBAC (Environmental Teratology Information Center Backfile) with nearly 50 000 records, DBIR (the Directory of Biotechnology Information Resources) with over 1500 records, EMICBACK (Environmental Mutagen Information Center) backfile containing over 76 000 citations from 1950 onwards, TRI (the Toxic Chemical Release Inventory) as two files, TRI87 and TRI88, which contain information on the annual estimated releases of toxic chemicals to the environment in 1987 and 1988, and RTECS (the Registry of Toxic Effects of Chemical Substances) with over 105 000 records.

TOXLIT and TOXNET are available online through NLM and BLAISE-Link and TOXLINE through NLM, BLAISE-Link and Data-Star.

PSYCINFO is the database corresponding to *Psychological Abstracts* produced by the American Psychological Association. Over 1400 journals, as well as dissertations and technical reports are covered, and the database from 1980 onwards contains 20 per cent more references than the printed publication. The file covers 1967 onwards and contains over 670 000 records. It is available online through BRS, Data-Star, Dialog and DIMDI. A CD-ROM version is available as PSY-CLIT CD SilverPlatter covering 1974 to the present, with quarterly updates.

The NURSING & ALLIED HEALTH (CINAHL) database corresponds to the publication *Cumulative Index to Nursing & Allied Health Literature*. The file covers 1983 to date, contains over 100 000 records and is updated monthly. Nursing literature is the main subject area, but a significant amount of material on allied health disciplines is also included. Records are indexed with headings from a CINAHL *Subject Heading List* based on the *MeSH* model. NURSING & ALLIED HEALTH is available online through BRS, Data-Star and Dialog, and on CD-ROM as NURSING AND ALLIED HEALTH (CINAHL)-CD Silver Platter and CD PLUS/CINAHL CD.

Alternative medicine and allied health are the subject areas covered by the CATS/AMED (Current Awareness Topic Services Allied and Alternative Medicine) database produced by the British Library Medical Information Service, corresponding to the bibliographies *Complementary Medicine Index, Physiotherapy Index, Occupational Therapy Index, Rehabilitation Index*, and *Palliative Care Index*. 400 mainly English-language journals are covered as well as selected books, and records are indexed with a truncated and expanded version of *MeSH*. The database contains 40 000 records from 1985 onwards and is available online through MIC-KIBIC and Data-Star.

Major databases with overlap into medicine

Many databases contain some material of potential use to medicine. A number of major databases whose primary subject coverage is in other fields have areas of overlap with biomedicine and are mentioned below.

CA SEARCH the online database corresponding to *Chemical Abstracts* contains extensive bibliographic information from all areas of chemistry including biochemistry, pharmacology, analytical chemistry and pollution research covering a time span from 1967 to date. CA SEARCH is available through BRS, Dialog, Data-Star, ESA-IRS, Orbit, STN International and Télésystèmes Questel.

INSPEC 2, the online files of *Physics Abstracts, Electrical and*

Electronics Abstracts, and *Computer and Control Abstracts* contains material of interest to medicine, including the use of computers in biomedicine, electrophysiology, biomechanics, biophysics and the biomedical effects of radiation. INSPEC is available through BRS, Data-Star, Dialog, ESA-IRS, Orbit, and STN International.

LIFE SCIENCES COLLECTION covers 18 specialized abstracting journals in the area of biology from 1980 onwards. Of special interest are records provided on the biochemistry of proteins, nucleic acids and biological membranes, chemoreception, immunology, neurosciences and toxicology, as well as aspects of genetics, microbiology and virology. The database is available online through Dialog, and on compact disc as LIFE SCIENCES COLLECTION CD Cambridge Scientific Abstracts covering 1982 to date, updated quarterly.

SCISEARCH is a multidisciplinary file corresponding to the *Science Citation Index* with additional material from *Current Contents*, including *Current Contents, Clinical Medicine* and *Current Contents, Life Sciences*. The database gives a novel approach to literature searching, a citation index, which allows the retrieval of newly published articles which quote an existing citation as an authority. When a scientist quotes an earlier work in this way it implies a subject relationship between the content of the two papers. SCISEARCH allows one to use this inverted relationship to list all the papers in which the authority is currently quoted. As well as citation searching, the file also allows conventional subject retrieval. SCISEARCH is available online through Data-Star, Dialog and DIMDI. A compact disc version of SCIENCE CITATION INDEX CD Institute for Scientific Information is available from 1986 onwards. CURRENT CONTENTS ON DISKETTE current awareness services in six subject areas including CLINICAL MEDICINE and LIFE SCIENCES are also available from the Institute for Scientific Information. These provide weekly journal contents listings on floppy disc for use in personal computers which can be searched by keywords in titles and descriptors.

Material of relevance to medicine can, of course, be found in many other databases and this should not be taken as an exclusive list.

Ordering, file management, education and training

Online ordering of documents

Once an online search has been run and citations retrieved, the user will wish to read at least some of the cited documents. Several host systems provide online automatic document ordering facilities which can be used to obtain cited articles. These include BLAISE, Dialog and SDC Orbit.

Personal file management software

A personal collection of reprints, photocopies, books and journals resulting from searches and general reading rapidly builds up, and one soon needs an effective method of finding items amid the growing files of material. Card indexes and general database management systems for personal computers such as DBase or Cardbox can be used, but specialized bibliographic file management software makes the task much easier. Numerous software packages are available with the facility to import downloaded references from online and CD-ROM databases and incorporate them into a personal file system. A comparison of five different packages is given in Brantz and Galla (1988) and of nine packages by Herman (1991), including 'Reference Manager', whose features are described and reviewed by Lyon (1989), and 'Pro-Cite', described and reviewed by Hanson (1990).

Sources of education and training

Database producers and hosts are active in providing training in the use of their databases and services. Announcements of developments and changes in databases as well as information about dates and venues of courses are given in the house journals of the different hosts, for example, *BLAISE-Link Newsletter*, and *Chronolog* (Dialog). This information is collated and included in *Online Notes* a monthly newsletter published by the Aslib Information Resources Centre, which also includes information about CD-ROM developments, equipment for searching, books, manuals and user aids. A similar newsletter for CD-ROM products is *CD-ROM Newsletter* (Microinfo Ltd.).

Free or reduced-rate training databases are available online through the major hosts. MEDLEARN, available on BLAISE-Link and NLM, is a computer-assisted instruction program which teaches one how to perform simple searches on MEDLINE. ELHILL LEARN is a microcomputer-based training program for the NLM Elhill search and retrieval software. This is a precursor to other database-specific NLM microcomputer-based training programmes CHEMLEARN, TOX-LEARN and MEDTUTOR.

To keep up to date with developments, searchers have organized themselves into national and regional user groups. Online User Groups have regular meetings and frequently have speakers from database producers, vendors and online experts. They also provide a useful forum for the exchange of problems and experience. A list of UK online user groups is included as an appendix in *Going Online* (Aslib Information Resources Centre).

The *UK Online User Group Newsletter* summarizes the group's own and other major meetings and provides commentary on developments in the field of online information retrieval.

A CD-ROM (Biomedical) User Network has been formed within the UK Online User Group to provide a forum for the exchange of experience and information, and to act as a focus for liaison with CD-ROM producers and suppliers.

Database, Online, Online Review and *The Laserdisk Professional*, all published quarterly, are journals catering for online and CD-ROM searchers. They frequently contain articles about medical databases and news items about developments in products and services. Both *Database* and *Online* have a Caduceus column giving searching hints and commentary on the content and features of medical databases.

Future developments

Does the current trend towards CD-ROM signal the end of online as the main source of database information? Librarians on squeezed budgets have been enthusiastic about the fixed subscription cost of CD-ROM databases compared with the open-ended expense of online usage. Readers are enthusiastic about doing their own searching on CD-ROM databases rather than through an intermediary. The CD-ROM technology has improved dramatically, and is becoming as fast and convenient as online.

In the USA, GRATEFUL MED is being used by many thousands of doctors and researchers as a convenient way of gaining access to online information without having to leave their offices, laboratories or homes. The individual components of a fully integrated information system are already available. All that is required is for the individual components of search software, personal reference file, ADONIS and facsimile transmission to be joined together. Before too long perhaps we shall see a system which will run automatic searches from one's personal workstation, download the results, and then provide immediate delivery of any or all of the selected articles in facsimile, direct to the workstation from a central source.

References

Armstrong, C.J. and Large, J.A. (1990) *CD-ROM information products: an evaluative guide and directory*. Aldershot: Gower.

Brantz, M.H. and Galla, J. (1988) Is there an optimal bibliographic software package for end users? *Bulletin of the Medical Library Association*, **76**, 216-220.

Hanson, T. (1990) Pro-Cite: a review. *Health Libraries Review*, **7**, 237-239.

Herman, D. (1991) Downloading from MEDLINE: a comparison of personal database software. *Health Libraries Review*, **8**, 11-20.

Lyon, E. (1988) *Online medical databases 1989*. London: Aslib.

Lyon, E. (1989) 'Reference Manager' – a review. *Health Libraries Review*, **6**, 102-103.

Whitsed, N. (1990) Product review: CD-Plus MEDLINE. *Health Libraries Review*, **7**, 233-235.

CHAPTER SIX

Audio-visual materials

MARGARET C. STEWART

The importance of audio-visual (AV) aids in medicine has long been recognized — as Sir John McMichael, then Chairman of the Postgraduate Medical Federation, said in 1970:

> We have always been the first to demand any new advances which come along in illustrative techniques, to use them in medical education. Other sciences, even the physical sciences, lag well behind, and in fact the initiatives in developing audio-visual aids are stemming out from medicine ...

Although the absence of copyright libraries or legal deposit regulations for non-book materials has led to some difficulty in tracing and selecting suitable audio-visual aids, useful selection guides are available. This chapter concentrates on the situation in the UK, mentioning foreign materials only where they are of significant help to the British user.

History

Most historical information about the development and early use of audio-visual materials comes in the form of journal articles describing the development of particular audio-visual collections — e.g. Engel (1970a), Graves and Graves (1979) — and in the descriptive leaflets issued by such collections. However, Donald (1986) traces the subject back as far as ancient Egypt.

General surveys of how departments of medical illustration developed into audio-visual resource centres are given by Engel (1969,

1974) and Beard (1982). Townsend and Heath (1977) looked at the history of educational technology as applied to nursing. The report (Jones, 1965) of the working party chaired by Sir Brynmor Jones in 1963 not only described the history of audio-visual aids in scientific education, but also played a significant role in making it — although many of its recommendations have yet to be realized (Chessell, 1990).

One of the first specialist film libraries was that established by the British Medical Association (BMA) in 1946 (Engel 1970a,b) which took over 16-mm films formerly held by Kodak. This library was further developed between 1966 and 1989 under the auspices of the British Life Assurance Trust for Health Education (BLAT, later BLITHE) and is now once more in the care of the BMA Library. The Royal College of General Practitioners was the first in the medical field to set up, in 1957, a library of audiotapes and slides (Graves and Graves, 1970). It was not until 1970 that another of the royal colleges — the Royal College of Obstetricians and Gynaecologists established an audiotape/slide library (Roberts, 1970). The growing use of videotape in medicine is well documented by Paegle *et al.* (1980), Dranov *et al.* (1980), Van Son (1982) and Scroggie (1986). Holmes (1988) summarizes the development of videodiscs from the first experimental system in 1928.

From the earliest days of audio-visuals in medicine, users have formed themselves into societies and organizations to facilitate discussion of common problems. The Institute of Medical and Biological Illustration was founded in 1968 to bring together all those professionally engaged in audio-visual communication in the life sciences to stimulate the study and application of all aids to communication in medicine and biology. The predominant interest of many of its members was medicine and this was reflected in the 1989 name change to Institute of Medical Illustrators.

The Association of Programmed Learning and Educational Technology was developed in 1969 from the Association for Programmed Learning to reflect changing interests, and then in 1979 it became the Association for Educational and Training Technology. The Association's main aim is to promote communication amongst educational technologists and those of various disciplines who are interested in the subject.

The Scientific Film Association established a Medical Committee in 1944 to encourage the use of film for education, information and research, the publication of catalogues and of reviews of medical films, and the provision of advice to film-makers. The Committee disbanded in the early 1980s, as its work was being done by other more appropriate bodies. The Scientific Film Association amalgamated with the British Industrial Film Association in 1967 to become the British Industrial and Scientific Film Association (BISFA), and BISFA in turn merged with the UK arm of the International Television Association in 1988, becoming the International Visual Communications Association (IVCA), which is responsible for organizing prestigious festivals and awards schemes.

A fuller list of such organizations and their addresses (including organizations outside the UK) is given in each edition of the *International Yearbook Of Educational And Instructional Technology*, published for the Association of Educational and Training Technology by Kogan Page Ltd (Osborne, 1990) and in its American counterpart, the *Educational Media and Technology Yearbook* (Ely, 1988). But why use audio-visuals at all? One of the shortest and clearest arguments is an article written by McArthur (1982) for health professionals in developing countries. For lengthier explanations see Romiszowski (1988), Jones (1965), or almost any book on educational technology. Conclusively, A.H. Thompson (1986) quotes the statistics produced by the American Industrial audio-visual Association: 'We remember 10 per cent of what we read, 20 per cent of what we hear, 30 per cent of what we see and 50 per cent of what we both see and hear.'

Audio-visual formats

Very often the terms 'audiovisual' and 'non-book' are used synonymously. They are not synonyms. Indeed, Liebenow (1981) suggests that 'audiovisual' is to be seen as a 'sub-group within the area of non-books'. Writing on behalf of the International Federation of Library Associations (IFLA) Section of Statistics for the special audio-visual materials issue of the *IFLA Journal*, Liebenow continues

> It is assumed that criteria for audio-visual materials are that they need some sort of equipment for them to be made perceptible for the human being. For this reason, pictures, for example, regardless of whether they are paintings, graphics or photographs, should not necessarily be counted as being AV material, since they are directly perceivable to the naked human eye and are also present as pictures in books. Nevertheless, the opinions on this are divided.
>
> A very broad classification for AV materials is proposed, which nevertheless partially separates things which are closely related. This broad classification is based upon the human organ which perceives this material. Thus: auditory material, which reproduces only those things which are heard, visual material which is seen, and then the truly audio-visual material which is perceived by both the eye and the ear.

The first category covers records, tapes, audiocassettes and most compact discs; the second slides, transparencies and silent films; the third sound films, sound slide series, videocassettes, videodiscs, magnetic tapes with picture-tone records and picture records. Microforms however 'are not audio-visual material. They are nothing more than a reduced form of the printed book and are merely found in another form than is usual.' The use of computers as teaching aids is another grey area, especially computer simulations using sophisticated graphics packages. Almost by default — because they are not covered elsewhere — they are beginning to be included in the major audio-visual sources, where they fit logically alongside interactive video: videocassette or videodisc used in combination with a computer.

The above paragraph lists all the most common formats. Useful definitions of each and its respective advantages or disadvantages are given by McArthur (1982), Grills (1981), Casciero and Roney (1981), Pinion (1982), and Jones (1987).

Over the past few years, videocassette has become the most widely available format for medical users: Dranov *et al.* (1980), Van Son (1982), Hargie and Morrow (1986), Scroggie (1986). The drawback in the past was the mutual incompatibility of the formats most widely available but now, thanks largely to its success in the domestic market, VHS has emerged as the leader of the field. Only a few distributors make their programmes available in non-VHS format.

Some teachers/lecturers make use of different audio-visual media in one presentation, utilizing qualities special to each while the videodisc is claimed to have all the advantages of a multi-media presentation in one easy-to-use disc, The first videodiscs and their players went on sale in the UK during 1982, in direct competition with the prerecorded videocassette for home use. On the domestic scene they were not a success but for the professional user, two aspects of the videodisc have proved particularly valuable: its capacity for information storage (Grills, 1981; McArthur, 1982; Adrian, 1988); and its use with a computer to provide an interactive teaching/learning medium (Kwan, 1988; Bayard-White, 1991). Bryce and Stewart (1983a,b) and Holmes (1988) consider the wider applications of disc technology for medicine, and list projects already under way.

The potential of holography to ensure greater accuracy in radiotherapy and diagnostic radiology (White, 1987) and possibly in place of models for teaching is still being explored.

Contrary to opinions frequently expressed by proponents of the newer media the older, more simple, formats have not been superseded entirely. For example, the 35-mm slide is still very much in demand as a vehicle for medical illustrations as Gower Medical's ambitious project to produce a series of slide atlases indicates. Every atlas covers one particular medical topic (e.g. anatomy, ophthalmology, immunology) in several volumes, each containing hundreds of slides plus explanatory booklets and indexes. Meanwhile, a British Library-commissioned survey of slide collections (McKeown and Otter, 1989) identified nearly 700 non-commercial collections in the UK.

Storage and retrieval

Advice on storage varies between the user-orientated, with emphasis on ease of access to materials — Rydesky (1980), Pinion (1982), Weihs (1984) — and the highly technical, requiring careful control of temperature and humidity levels for archival conservation (FIAF/FIAT/IASA, 1989). Fothergill and Butchart (1990), Jones (1987) and Verny and Heider (for videotape only) (1982) consider aspects of storage, preservation and repair as part of the general maintenance of a collection. Drawing on her experience as Media Librarian at the Open University, Harrison (1987) discusses storage and long-term preservation for archival, reference and loan collections.

There is no one definitive guide on retrieval systems for medical slides. In 1982 Cockburn found, in a review of the literature, only seven accounts before he described the method he used. Since then many other authors have presented their own preferred systems: amongst the most interesting are Robertson (1985) and Nayler (1990).

Adrain (1988) points out that videodisc lends itself ideally as an archival storage medium for photographs, video frames, text and drawings. Over the last few years the Graves Educational Resource, formerly the Graves Medical Audiovisual Library (GMAL) has been amassing a collection of individual slides held by hospitals and universities throughout the UK, to form the National Medical Slide Bank. Now over 10 000 have been transferred on to a videodisc which purchasers can use for their own illustrative purposes. In 1990 the Wellcome Trust began to transfer the holdings of its museum archive on tropical medicine to videodisc, for eventual distribution to medical schools in the developed world and Third-World countries.

Selection

Producers and distributors

A substantial proportion of audio-visual materials for medicine have traditionally been produced in the audio-visual departments of large hospitals and medical schools, and kept for internal use. Gradually, as these departments have grown in size and importance, so the reputation of their products has spread, and other organizations have wanted to acquire them. In some cases, problems of copyright and the ethics of patient privacy have meant that the programmes have had to remain available to a restricted audience only. But some centres, like the University of Newcastle Regional Postgraduate Institute for Medicine and Dentistry and the University of London Audio-Visual Centre are able to sell or hire programmes they have produced. Others distribute materials through a commercial company.

As well as producing their own materials, large hospitals and medical schools hold collections of audio-visual aids produced elsewhere, e.g. the University of Southampton Department of Teaching Media and St. Bartholomew's Hospital Audio-Visual Teaching Department. Normally these are available only to their own staff and students, but a certain amount of interlending with other institutions takes place.

The full extent of audio-visual interlending was explored in British Library Research & Development Report 5526 (Pinion, 1980a) and a short account of its findings was published in *Interlending Review* (Pinion, 1980b). Following this, the National Committee on Regional Library Co-operation (NCLRC) established a working party to set up a pilot project for interlending audio-visual materials. Cornish (1989) reported on its activities to 1988, summing up that:

> The interlending of AV materials is not a large part of general interlibrary lending traffic and there is little sign of real growth, but whether this is because of the lack of a coherent system, of general awareness or of demand is not clear. Even in those areas which have a proper scheme there is little publicity for it and little growth.

The interlending situation with particular regard to health science materials is discussed by Cornish (1987),

Mention has already been made of the founding of the BMA Film and Video Library in 1946 (Engel,1970a,b) and the Graves Medical audio-visual Library (GMAL) in 1957 (Graves and Graves, 1979). Both act as distributors of audio-visual materials produced elsewhere, but whereas the BMA Film Library has encouraged film development by stringent testing of all titles submitted and by internationally recognized competitions, GMAL grew by commissioning and co-producing programmes to fill perceived needs. Other non-profit-making audio-visual distributors include the Open University, the Royal College of Obstetricians and Gynaecologists, the International Planned Parenthood Federation, the Scottish Central Film Library, and the Foundation for Teaching Aids at Low Cost — TALC, which specializes in slide sets and other teaching aids aimed at raising health-care standards in developing countries (Lunnon and King, 1986).

Foremost among the commercial distributors of medical audio-visual must be Oxford Educational Resources Ltd, which holds over 2000 titles in health and medicine, many originating from medical schools in the UK and overseas. Concord Video and Film Council, Edward Patterson Associates and the BBC also number important medical titles amongst their stock.

Pharmaceutical companies produce and distribute a not inconsiderable number of audio-visual materials, mostly videocassettes, for educational as well as promotional purposes. Notable amongst these are the MSD Foundation, which is sponsored by the pharmaceutical company Merck, Sharp and Dohme, and specializes in tape-slide and videocassettes for general practitioners, Bencard, ICI, Lipha and Rorer Pharmaceuticals.

Of the many significant audio-visual collections outside the UK, the largest must be the National Library of Medicine audio-visual Center, described in a history of the National Library of Medicine (Miles, 1982). The U.S. Army Academy of Health Sciences holds over 800 videotapes which are made available to recognized organizations submitting a blank tape for each programme required.

Some overseas collections have UK agents, e.g. the Sandoz Pharmaceutical Company (Switzerland) and the World Health Organization distribute their films through the BMA Film Library, and prints of films from the French Scientific Film Library are available through the Scottish Central Film and Video Library.

There are far too many audio-visual libraries and distributors to list in this short chapter. Appendix 2 lists the major directories of audio-visual suppliers in the UK and overseas.

Catalogues and directories: UK

The process of finding suitable audio-visual materials does not end with the identification of the major distributors and there are a number of guides to help the newcomer to the field to find the next step: Pinion (1982), Rydesky (1980) and Van Son (1982) have already been cited. The *International Yearbook of Educational and Instructional Technology* (Osborne, 1990) is invaluable, as is the *Educational Media and Technology Yearbook* (Ely, 1988).

Like book publishers, producers and distributors of materials print catalogues of items available. The British Universities Film and Video Council's encyclopedic guide *Distributors* (Grant and Sarmiento, 1990) describes the catalogues of more than 650 individual distributors in over 100 subject categories. The best of the catalogues are updated regularly and provide very full details of each programme author, running time, number of slides or frames where appropriate, date, intended audience and a brief synopsis of contents. The full catalogue of the Graves Educational Resources is an outstanding example. Because the catalogue is loose-leaf and is arranged by subject headings, GER can send just the relevant section to users with very specific subject interests. BBC Enterprises and the University of Newcastle Regional Postgraduate Institute for Medicine and Dentistry also produce extremely helpful catalogues. The European Multimedia Centre (EMC, 1991) publishes the *Interactive media courseware catalogue* which has claims to be the only such directory for ready-made interactive video teaching and resource discs on the British market. Oxford Educational Resources publishes a title list only but maintains full information on computer of all the programmes for which it is responsible: enquirers are encouraged to contact the company for a print-out of details of all materials of specific subject interest. Regrettably, some other audio-visual distributors provide only title lists without such a back-up.

Keeping track of the latest editions of each of these individual catalogues and remembering the subject coverage/audience level can be a nightmare. Geddes and Emery (1987) describe how, after abandoning a recording system based on 5 x 3 in. catalogue cards, they set up a computer database to handle their catalogue collection.

It is not surprising that the need has been felt for a *Medical books in print* of the audio-visual world. Perhaps the first British attempt was the catalogue published in 1948 by the Medical Committee of the Scientific Film Association and the Royal Society of Medicine, which gave details of some 200 films. The 1970 edition of this catalogue, *Medical films available in Great Britain*, produced with the assistance of the British Life Assurance Trust (Engel, 1970a), listed over 2100 titles. Since 1973 the BMA Film and Video Library has published, at regular intervals, an extensive catalogue to describe its own holdings (BMA/BLITHE, 1988) — now approximately 800 films — and all winners of the Certificate of Educational Commendation (see below). Contents are arranged under broad subject headings, supplemented by a title index.

For health education materials, the *Health education index* (1987) is unequalled. Aimed at schoolteachers, it describes books and audio-visual listed by health topic, and the directory of suppliers at the beginning is a useful guide to organizations working in the health-education field. The *Index* is fully revised every two to three years.

Materials on mental health topics from many distributors are pulled together into twelve subject directories by the Mental Health Media Council, providing a synopsis and full distribution details for each item.

In 1974 the Council for Educational Technology, assisted by the Department of Audio Visual Communication of the BMA and BLAT produced *HELPIS — medical* *, a directory of over 960 medical audio-visual materials (Council for Educational Technology, 1974) produced in institutions of higher education. Mostly films and videocassettes, the contents were arranged by Universal Decimal Classification (UDC) divisions with comprehensive subject and title indexes. This was an invaluable aid but is now extremely out of date. No new edition was ever produced because medical programmes began to be incorporated in the general *HELPIS* catalogue. *HELPIS*, one of several major multidisciplinary sources of information about audio-visual was first published in 1971 by the Council for Educational Technology and from 1976 by the British Universities Film and Video Council (BUFVC). Medicine was excluded from the early editions, when it was still unclear how much duplication there would be with the BMA/BLAT film catalogue. Another important directory published by the BUFVC was *Audiovisual materials for higher education*. The two directories were merged into one, the *BUFVC Catalogue* (on microfiche only) from 1984 when the distinction between audio-visual programmes produced *for* or *by* higher education no longer seemed as important as the need for easy retrieval of useful items, and BUFVC transformed *HELPIS* into an online database, accessible by subscribers. The last *BUFVC Catalogue* (Terris, 1990a) contained details of 7300 programmes, arranged by Universal Decimal Classification (UDC) and was a vital source of information about medical/health materials. It has now been replaced by the *BUFVC Handbook for film and television in education* (BUFVC, 1991) which includes feature articles and directories of sources. Full coverage of materials themselves is supplied by the AVANCE database described below. From time to time BUFVC also publishes, on paper, specialist subject listings of audio-visual materials.

As the BUFVC has so much experience in the provision of useful and up-to-date catalogues it is hardly surprising that they were among the bodies approached for help when the British Library decided to launch its own audio-visual directory, the *British catalogue of audio-visual materials* (British Library, 1979). Inspired by the British Library/ILEA** Learning Materials Recording Study (Ferris, 1981) the experimental edition, in 1979, was compiled from the collections held by the Reference Library of the ILEA's Central Library Resources Ser-

---

*   Higher Educational Learning Programmes Information Science
** Inner London Education Authority

vice, and the Higher Education Film Library and from selected publishers' catalogues. The catalogue used Dewey classification and provided title and subject indexes similar to those used by the BUFVC. Entries were rather brief and there was very little coverage of medical topics. The supplements, published in 1980 and 1983, drew additionally on information supplied by commercial and other distributors, and item entries were noticeably more detailed. This seemed to herald a significant advance in the bibliography of audio-visuals. Unfortunately, spending cuts within the British Library prevented further editions.

The nearest there is to a *British books in print* for all subjects is probably the *British national film and video catalogue* (Brown). Published quarterly by the British Film Institute (BFI), with annual cumulations, it aims to be a full listing of all films and videos released for non-theatric distribution in the UK. The introduction to the 1987 catalogue noted that in its first 25 years of existence it had listed over 60 000 programmes, of which 90 per cent were non-fiction — over a third of these were in applied sciences, medicine and technology. It does not claim to be completely comprehensive since there is no statutory obligation for distributors to inform the British Film Institute when they make a programme available, and the smaller distributors, in particular, may not be aware of the advantages of doing so. At the time of writing, the catalogue's future is in some doubt because of the funding cuts — its best hope may be to be absobed into the BUFVC. The British Film Institute also maintains an archive collection of 16-mm films and television programmes, and it published in 1980 a catalogue of its non-fiction holdings (BFI, 1980). This is disappointing as a record of medical titles.

It was the lack of any one definitive source of information that led to the compilation of the *International guide to locating audio-visual materials in the health sciences* (Jones, 1986). So many of the smaller organizations concerned with audio-visual materials in health have since merged or ceased to exist that it is now largely out of date but it may still serve to guide the newcomer to the field in the right direction.

Catalogues and directories: overseas

American directories of medical audio-visuals are dominated by the *National Library of Medicine Audio-visuals Catalog*, published quarterly since 1978, with an annual cumulation, to list and describe items held in the National Library of Medicine Audio-visual Center as well as relevant new materials. Prior to 1975 some audio-visuals had been included in the *National Library of Medicine Current Catalog*. In 1977 the Library published a separate volume, the *AVLINE Catalog* covering items catalogued in 1975 and 1976. The first *NLM Audio-visuals Catalog Annual Cumulation* was published for items new in 1977. Since 1978 the

NLM no longer includes any audio-visual materials except serial titles in the *NLM Current Catalog*. The *Audio-visuals Catalog* is arranged so that films, videocassettes and tape-slide programmes are easy to find under title or *MeSH* subject heading.

Apart from this there are numerous directories covering medicine as one of many educational topics. In 1981, Drolet was able to suggest 50 reference sources for answering enquiries on audiovisuals in any subject.

The *Educational Film/Video Locator* (1990) lists university rental sources for more than 50 000 films and videos, arranged by title, with additional indexes by subject and audience level.

The three *Videologs* (Business and technology; General interest and education; Health sciences) provide extensive coverage of U.S. videotape production. The *Health sciences videolog* (Videolog, 1981) lists over 7000 specialist videotapes and cassettes by title, cross-referenced in a index. The *Video Source Book* is an annual guide to available video material.

Audiocassettes may be located through a much more modest publication, the *Directory of spoken-word audio cassettes* (McKee, 1983).

An aid to finding medical and health education materials in any format is *Healthfinder: locating audio-visual materials* (National Health Information Clearing House, 1984). This lists directories of health-related audio-visuals, online databases and describes how to go about locating materials on specific health topics. Pemberton (1990) provides invaluable help to buyers by presenting in one volume the sales and preview policies of American suppliers of non-book materials and, significantly, incorporating a list of former names, subsidiaries and parent companies.

In Australia, the audio-visual Subcommittee of the Australian Council of Libraries and Information Services (ACLIS) produces *A directory of suppliers and lenders of audio-visual materials* — libraries and commercial suppliers — and *Audiovisual reference sources: an annotated list*, which is international in coverage. The Australian government also publishes a guide to finding sources (Rose and Dunlop, 1989).

Online services

The major online service for locating medical audio-visual materials is AVLINE, developed in 1973 as a component of MEDLARS and becoming operational in 1975. A full account of its background and development is given by Suter and Waddell (1982). The user's point of view is presented by Bridgman and Suter (1979). Access is through the MEDLARS online system or in microfiche catalogue form (i.e. *Health Sciences Audiovisuals* which is a quarterly cumulative print-out of everything on AVLINE). UK users have access to AVLINE and other MED-LARS services through the British Library BLAISE-Link service.

To complement its experimental printed edition, the *British catalogue of audio-visual materials*, the British Library introduced AVMARC, which now contains over 22 000 audio-visuals available in the UK. Entries follow the standard MARC format with additional information for physical description. This is accessible to users of BLAISE-Link. Unlike AVLINE, AVMARC is not restricted to medical topics.

In November 1989 the British Universities Film and Video Council installed a new in-house database AVANCE (Terris, 1990b). This incorporates the HELPIS database (previously maintained by the British Library on the BLAISE-Link system and the *BUFVC catalogue* plus new programmes added almost on a daily basis. In addition to information on audio-visual materials, including interactive videodisc and computer software, it holds details of books and periodical articles about the media and education. BUFVC staff are prepared to answer postal or telephone queries about the availability, production and use of audio-visual materials in higher education. For an annual subscription, users are entitled to free copies of various BUFVC publications, information during the year on new materials in specified subject areas, reduced prices at certain BUFVC events and use of the information service and reference library.

Probably the largest database of current and historical audio-visual materials is AV-ONLINE, maintained by NICEM, the National Information Center for Educational Media set up in 1966 at the University of Southern California to keep track of non-book materials. Containing some 400 000 items AV-ONLINE may be accessed via Dialog and is also available on compact disc through SilverPlatter Information Services.

FORMAT is a database of over 12 000 Canadian-produced audio-visual materials available online through the National Film Board of Canada (Bild, 1984).

For a description of the other online services listing audio-visuals on various aspects of health and medicine and instructions on how to use them, see the excellent manual *Searching online for health sciences audiovisuals* (University of Maryland, 1984).

Information services

Just as there are libraries prepared to compile bibliographies on specialist topics, so there are information centres which will provide resource lists (sometimes, lamentably, called 'mediagraphies') of audio-visual materials. These centres coexist with audio-visual libraries in institutions and societies which are able to provide services only to their own members.

The English National Board for Nursing, Midwifery and Health Visiting maintains the HEALTH CARE DATABASE (formerly AV-MINE in its precomputer days) from which it provides information to nurse teachers, health-care workers and educationalists on teaching/learning resources, research, organizations and career opportunities. Subjects covered relate to clinical aspects for all types of nursing, midwifery and health visiting; education; management; communication and health education. At present, searches can be requested by telephone, letter or electronic mail but it is hoped that online links will be established in the near future. Visitors can search the database for themselves. Searches are free to NHS staff: others pay a nominal fee. The HEALTH CARE DATABASE index gives full details of how to use the database, and the subject areas covered.

The Health Education Authority publishes, from time to time, lists of materials on different health topics, e.g. smoking, personal relationships. The BMA Film and Video Library offers an information and reference service on medical films and videos to members.

The Mental Health Media Council uses its database to assist enquirers looking for materials on specific topics. It also organizes 'preview days' around the country to give subscribers the opportunity to assess new materials for themselves.

Some organizations maintain reference centres where would-be purchasers can preview materials they may wish to use. The Audio-Visual Reference Centre at the BUFVC was established with financial assistance from the Nuffield Foundation as a preview and research facility for audio-visual materials produced in universities, polytechnics and other institutions of higher education. It now holds over 800 items. The International Visual Communications Association also maintains a large collection of award-winning programmes and viewing facilities for members in its London headquarters. The European Multimedia Centre houses a permanent exhibition of the latest hardware and software which may be demonstrated to members. The Scottish Council for Educational Technology offers preview facilities for SCET software and Open University videos.

Evaluation

Although reference centres such as those mentioned above exist and some distributors of materials offer preview facilities, it is frequently of help to the would-be purchaser/user to see a published review of the item, considering it in relation to its intended audience. Truett (1984) and Blake (1989) give advice on assessing the value of such reviews.

Journals

A number of journals devote space to listing and reviewing new materials, e.g. *Viewfinder* (British Universities Film and Video Council newsletter) and *Journal of Audiovisual Media in Medicine*. For comprehensive lists see the *International Yearbook of Educational and Instructional Technology* (Osborne, 1990), the *Audio-visual and microcomputer handbook* (Henderson and Humphreys, 1984), or the *Educational Media and Technology Yearbook* (Ely, 1988). A few major journals are listed in Appendix 3. The *Audio Video Review Digest* (Stetler, 1990) publishes compilations of reviews of any audio-visual media. Provan and Hunter (1985) performed the same function for exclusively health and medical programmes.

Assessment schemes

In 1970 the BMA Film Library undertook the critical assessment of all its holdings so that a new catalogue could be issued with sufficient information to help potential users in their selection (Engel, 1970a). At the same time the British Life Assurance Trust Certificate of Educational Commendation was instigated so that all films could be assessed by a special review panel made up of appropriate specialists according to the stated audience and purpose of the film. During the first 12 months, over 70 films were assessed, but fewer than 40 certificates could be awarded. This certification scheme is still in operation at the BMA and the certificates are highly valued by medical film producers. The BMA Film and Video Library also administers film and video competitions leading to various prizes for outstanding merit. Since 1991 it has also offered a medicine in the Media award for the best broadcast medical programme. Reviews of all award-winning films are published in the BMA catalogue *Health films and videos* (BMA/BLITHE Film Library, 1988). As new editions of this catalogue appear only infrequently, reviews are also printed as available in *Journal of audiovisual Media in Medicine*. The evaluation process was explained in a publication *Film in medical education* (CET/BLAT, 1973), produced by a special working party.

Films held in the French Scientific Film Library are reviewed by the BUFVC before being made available for hire: reviews are printed in the BUFVC's newsletter, *Viewfinder*.

Suter and Waddell (1982) explain how and why materials are reviewed before incorporation into AVLINE — the reviews may be seen both in the computer print-outs and the *National Library of Medicine Audio-visuals Catalog*.

Finally, Van Son (1982) includes a very helpful chapter on user-evaluation of videocassettes that could well be applied to other formats and the National Council for Educational Technology (1985) publishes an open learning guide on selecting media and how to evaluate them.

Equipment

Audio-visual equipment goes out of date even more rapidly than the contents of the films. Each user develops a fondness for particular makes or models, learns its 'foibles' and becomes an expert on its use and maintenance.

Newcomers to the field need unbiased advice on what to buy and how to look after it. Certain published guides have already established themselves as indispensable, for example the *USPECs* produced by the National Council for Educational Technology. *USPECs* (or User Specifications) are a series of regularly updated pamphlets intended as a means of providing information to educational users on the selection and operation of equipment for teaching and learning. USPECs published so far, free of charge, include *No. 28 — VHF Radio cassette recorders* (1983), *No. 30 — Sound systems* (1988), *No. 32 — Microcomputing* (2nd edn., 1988) and *No. 36 — Interactive video in education* (1989) and a new edition of *No. 15 — Video systems* is forthcoming. *USPEC information sheets* are also published to provide initial information about new equipment and technology of interest to education and training, Useful titles include: *No. 5 — Servicing equipment for use in educational technology* (1987) and *No. 8 — Batteries and their applications in A-V equipment* (1988).

The *Audiovisual Directory* (1991), from the publishers of the journal *Audiovisual* is the major UK annual guide to audio-visual equipment, dealers, programme production and production services and distributors.

Other serial publications that assist with equipment selection include: *Equipment Directory of Audio-visual, Computer and Video Products* (annual) which contains photographs, specifications and prices for every type and model of equipment offered by members of the International Communications Industries Association (formerly National Audio Visual Association); *AV market place* (1991) which lists more than 6000 suppliers of equipment or services; *Audio-visual and microcomputer handbook* (Henderson and Humphreys, 1984) which advises on choosing and hiring equipment; and *International Yearbook of Educational and Instructional Technology* (Osborne, 1990) which carries a list of manufacturers of particular categories of hardware.

Fothergill and Butchart (1990) describe how different kinds of equipment work and what could go wrong: Crowe (1984) gives guidance on selection and evaluation which is invaluable to a wider audience than the school media centres for whom she is writing. Schroeder and Lare (1979, 1990) explain repairs and maintenance.

Conclusion

Finally, what happens next for audio-visual aids in medicine? We still await the introduction of legal deposit and the publication of the definitive information source. There may be hope: the British Library is reported to have asked the Office of Arts and Libraries to carry out an inquiry into the extension of legal deposit to cover audio-visuals (Cullen and Pinion, 1990).

Publishers and university audio-visual departments continue to explore the possibilities of interactive video as a teaching device and the full potential of holography in medical education has yet to be realized.

On the negative side, audio-visual is still seen in some circles as an optional adjunct to teaching, and audio-visual departments are amongst the first to be hit as financial cuts in higher education bite (Evans, 1990). Chessell (1989), writing after the death of Sir Brynmor Jones, comments that his seminal report (Jones, 1965) was 24 years before its time: it may be the time now for educators to go back to that report and push for implementation of its recommendations.

References

ACLIS AV Subcommittee (ed.) *A directory of suppliers and lenders of audiovisual materials* and *Audiovisual reference sources: an annotated list*. Queensland: Australian Council of Libraries and Information Services AV Subcommittee.

Adrain, R.S. *et al.* (1988) Laser video disk archival storage. *Journal of audiovisual Media in Medicine*, **11**, 129-138.

Audiovisual directory (1991) Croydon: EMAP Vision.

AV market place (1991) Ann Arbor, MI: Bowker.

Bayard-White, C. (1991) *Interactive video handbook and directory*. London: European Multimedia Centre.

Beard, L.F.H. (1982) Aids to medical education. *Media in Education and Development*, **15**, 28-30.

BFI (1980) *National film archive catalogue. Vol. 1.: Non-fiction films*. London: BFI.

Bild, D. *et al.* (1984) Computerized information system operates for AV materials. *Canadian Library Journal*, **41**, 323-330.

Blake, V.L.P. (1989) The role of reviews and reviewing media in the selection process: an examination of the research record. *Collection Management*, **11**, 1-40.

Bridgman, C.F. and Suter, E. (1979) Searching AVLINE for curriculum-related audiovisual instructional materials. *Journal of Medical Education*, **54**, 236-237.

BMA/BLITHE Film Library (1988) *Health films and videos*. London: BMA/BLITHE.

British Library (1979) *British catalogue of audiovisual materials, 1st experimental edition*. Also *1st supplement* (1980); *2nd Supplement* (1983). London: British Library Bibliographic Services Division.

Brown, M. *British National Film and Video Catalogue*. (Quarterly, with annual cumulations) London: British Film Institute.

Bryce, C.F.A. and Stewart, A. (1983a) How to use videodiscs in medical education. Part 1. *Medical Teacher*, **5**, 6-9.

Bryce, C.F.A. and Stewart, A. (1983b) Videodiscs in medical education. Part 2. *Medical Teacher*, **5**, 57.

BUFVC (1991) *BUFVC handbook for film and television in education* 1991-1992. London: BUFVC.

Casciero, A.J. and Roney, R.G. (1981) *Introduction to AV for technical assistants*. Littleton, CO: Libraries Unlimited Inc.

CET/BLAT (1973) *Film in medical education — production and use*. London: Council for Educational Technology/BLAT.

Chessell, G. (1990) Audiovisual resources for learning — a brave new world unrealized? *Journal of Audiovisual Media in Medicine*, **13**, 17-19.

Cockburn, N. (1982) Slide retrieval systems — a pharmaceutical industry approach. *Journal of Audiovisual Media in Medicine*, **5**, 27-29.

Cornish, G. (1987) Interlending of audio-visual materials: a neglected national resource for medical and health libraries. *Health Libraries Review*, **4**, 164-171.

Cornish, G. (1989) Report: National Committee on Regional Library Co-operation. *Audiovisual Librarian*, **15**, 103-106.

Council for Educational Technology (1974) *HELPIS — medical, 1st edn. A catalogue of audiovisual and other educational materials in medicine and allied fields produced by institutions of higher education in the UK*. London: Councils and Education Press Ltd.

Crowe, V.M. (1984) Choosing technologies for school library media centres: hardware selection. *Drexel Library Quarterly*, **20**, 51-63.

Cullen, P. and Pinion, C. (1990) Seen and heard: news. *Audiovisual Librarian*, **16**, 56.

Donald, G. (1986) The history of medical illustration. *Journal of Audiovisual Media in Medicine*, **9**, 44-49.

Dranov, P. *et al.* (1980) *Video in the 80s: emerging uses for television in business, education, medicine and government.* White Plains, NY: Knowledge Industry Publications Inc.

Drolet, L.L., Jr. (1981) Reference readiness for AV questions. *American Libraries*, **12**, 154-155.

Educational film/video locator (1990) ...of the consortium of College and University Media Centres and R.R. Bowker, 5th edn. Ann Arbour, MI: Bowker.

Ely, D.P. *et al.* (eds.) (1988) *Educational media and technology yearbook.* Littleton, CO: Libraries Unlimited Inc.

EMC (1991) Interactive media courseware catalogue. London European Multimedia Centre.

Engel, C.E.E. (1969) Some trends in medical education through audio-visual aids. *British Journal of Hospital Medicine*, November Equipment Supplement, 17-19.

Engel, C.E.E. (1970a) Films and the BMA. *Update*, May, 620, 647-648.

Engel, C.E.E. (1970b) Some innovations and investigations in medical education. In *Aspects of educational technology, vol IV*, ed. A.J. Bajpai and J.F. Leedham, pp. 26-33, London: Pitman.

Engel, C.E.E. (1974) Medical illustration in the new Health Service — 4. Broadening the base. *Medical and Biological Illustration*, **24**, 174-176.

Equipment directory of audio-visual, computer and video products (Formerly *AV equipment directory*) (annual). Fairfax, VA: International Communications Industries Association.

Evans, T. (1990) Making media work. *AV User*, No. 25, 22-24.

Ferris, D.J. (1981) *Learning materials recording study: report of a study funded by the British Library.* London: Council for Educational Technology.

FIAF/FIAT/IASA (1989) *Archiving and audiovisual heritage.* Papers from 1987 Joint FIAF/FIAT/IASA Technical Symposium. Berlin: Stiftung Deutsche Kinemathik.

Fothergill, R. and Butchart, I. (1990) *Non-book materials in libraries: a practical guide*, 3rd edn. London: Clive Bingley.

Geddes, G. and Emery, L. (1987) A computer index to AV publishers' catalogues. *Audiovisual Librarian*, **13**, 217-219.

Grant, C. and Sarmiento, M. (eds) (1990) *Distributors: the guide to video and film sources for education and training.* London: BUFVC.

Graves, J. and Graves, V. (1970) *3rd Conference on the use of Audiotape in Medical Teaching, 14th October 1970*, p. 2. Chelmsford: Medical Recording Service Foundation.

Graves, J. and Graves, V. (1979) The changing use of a tape-slide library. *Journal of Audiovisual Media in Medicine*, **2**, 95-101.

Grills, C.M. (1981) Training, researching and learning with videodisc. *Videodisc/Teletext*, **1**, 14-17.

Hargie, O.D.W. and Morrow, N. (1986) Analytical and practical considerations of illustrative model video-tapes. *Journal of Audiovisual Media in Medicine*, **6**, 65-68.

Harrison, H.P. (1987) Conservation and audiovisual materials. *Audiovisual Librarian*, **13**, 154-162.

Health Education Index (1987) 9th edn. London: Edsall.

Health Sciences Audiovisuals (quarterly) Bethesda, MD: National Library of Medicine. [Each issue some 80 microfiche.]

Henderson, J. and Humphreys, F. (eds) (1984) *Audio-visual and microcomputer handbook*, 4th edn. London: Kogan Page.

Holmes, R. (1988) Laser disc technology: the implications for medicine and medical information. *Audiovisual Librarian*, **14**, 210-210.

Jones, B. (Chairman) (1965) *Audio-visual aids in higher scientific education*. Report of the committee appointed by the University Grants Committee, the Department of Education and Science and the Scottish Education Department in February 1963. London: HMSO.

Jones, M.C. (1987) *Non-book teaching materials in the health sciences*. Aldershot: Gower.

Kwan, R.M.F. *et al.* (1988) Use of interactive video in teaching history-taking to medical students: a pilot project. *Journal of Audiovisual Media in Medicine*, **11**, 121-124.

Liebenow, P.K. (1981) From the Section on Statistics. [IFLA and audiovisual materials] *IFLA Journal*, **7**, 335-336.

Lunnon, R. and King, F.S. (1986) Teaching aids at low cost. *Journal of Audiovisual Media in Medicine*, **9**, 105-107.

McArthur, J.R. (1982) Conventional and high-technology teaching methods for educating health professionals in developing nations. *Journal of Audiovisual Media in Medicine*, **5**, 21-26.

McKee, G. (ed.) (1983) *Directory of spoken-word audiocassettes*, 3rd edn. New York: Jeffery Norton.

McKeown, R. and Otter, M.E. (1989) *National survey of slide collections*. (BL Research Paper No. 67). London, British Library.

McMichael, J. (1970) Have we proved the effectiveness of tape? In *3rd Conference on the use of audiotape in medical teaching, 14th October 1970*, ed. J. Graves and V. Graves. p. 54, Chelmsford: Medical Recording Service Foundation.

Miles, W.D. (1982) *A history of the National Library of Medicine*, Chapter XXIV. Washington DC: U.S. Government Printing Office.

National Council for Educational Technology (1985) *How to find and adapt materials and select media* (Open Learning Guide 8). London: NCET.

National Health Information Clearinghouse (1984) *Healthfinder: locating audiovisual materials*. Washington DC: NHIC.

National Library of Medicine Audio-visuals Catalog (quarterly, with the

4th issue being the annual cumulation). Bethesda, MD: National Library of Medicine.

Nayler, J. (1990) The CPHA's ICD-9. CM as a coding source for medical slide filing. *Journal of Audiovisual Media in Medicine*, **13**, 55-60.

Osborne, C.W. (ed.) (1990) *International yearbook of educational and instructional technology*. London: Kogan Page.

Paegle, R.D. *et al.* (1980) Videotaped vs traditional lectures for medical students. *Medical Education*, **14**, 389-393.

Pemberton, J.M. (1990) *Policies of audiovisual producers and distributors: a handbook for acquisition personnel*, 2nd rev. edn. Metuchen, NJ and London: Scarecrow.

Pinion, C.F. (1980a) *The interlending and availability of audiovisual materials in the UK: Report of a survey conducted in 1979* (BLR&D Report 5526). Boston Spa: British Library.

Pinion, C.F. (1980b) The interlending and availability of audiovisual materials in the United Kingdom: report of a survey conducted in 1979. *Interlending Review*, **8**, 55.

Pinion, C.F. (1982) Audiovisual materials. In *Handbook of special librarianship*, ed. L.J. Anthony, 5th edn., p. 28. London: Aslib.

Provan, J.B. and Hunter, J. (eds) (1985) *Health media review index: a guide to reviews and descriptions of commercially available non-print-material for the medical, mental, allied health, human service and related counselling professions*. Metuchen, NJ: Scarecrow.

Roberts, D.W. (1970) The Royal College of Obstetricians — audiovisual aids — present position and plans for the future. In *3rd Conference on the use of audiotape in medical teaching, 14th October 1970*, p. 18, ed. J. Graves and V. Graves. Chelmsford: Medical Recording Service Foundation.

Robertson, S.J. (1985) 'Cardbox' as an ideal programme for clinical filing. *Journal of Audiovisual Media in Medicine*, **8**, 19-21.

Romiszowski, A.J. (1988) *The selection and use of instructional media: a systems approach*, 2nd edn. London: Kogan Page.

Rose, M. and Dunlop, P. eds. (1989) *Finding and keeping: a researcher's guide to audiovisual resources in Australia*. Canberra: Australian Government Publishing Service.

Rydesky, M.M. (1980) Audiovisual media: special library asset or bane? In *Special librarianship: a new reader*, ed. E.B. Jackson, pp. 521-529. London: Scarecrow.

Schroeder, D. and Lare, G. (1979) *Audiovisual equipment and materials: a basic repair and maintenance manual,* Vol. 1. Metuchen, NJ: Scarecrow.

Schroeder, D. and Lare, G. (1990) *Audiovisual equipment and materials: a basic repair and maintenance manual,* Vol. 1. Metuchen, NJ: Scarecrow.

Scroggie, I.P. (1986) Videorecording and high-definition television systems for the late 1980s: a review. *Journal of Audiovisual Media in Medicine,* **6,** 91-94.

Stetler, S.L. (ed.) (1990) *Audio video review digest 1989.* Gale Research.

Suter, E. and Waddell, W.H. (1982) AVLINE: a database and critical review system of audiovisual materials for the education of health professionals. *Journal of Medical Education,* **57,** 139-155.

Terris, O. (1990a) *BUFVC catalogue.* London: BUFVC [7 microfiches with 48-page booklet listing distributors.]

Terris, O. (1990b) AVANCE: a multimedia database. *Audiovisual Librarian,* **16,** 112-115.

Thompson, A.H. (1986) Knowledge or format — which comes first? *Audiovisual Librarian,* **12,** 184-188. Quotation from O. Patterson (ed.) (1962) *Special tools for communication.* Chicago Industrial Audiovisual Association.

Townsend, I. and Heath, J. (1977) Is educational technology infectious? In *Aspects of educational technology, vol. XI. The spread of educational technology,* ed. P. Hills and J. Gilbert, pp. 189-195. London: Kogan Page.

Truett, C. (1984) Evaluating software reviews: a review of the reviews. *Library Software Review,* **3,** 371-378.

University of Maryland (1984) *Searching online for health sciences audiovisuals* Baltimore, MD: Southeastern/Atlantic Regional Medical Library Services (University of Maryland).

USPECS and *USPEC information sheets.* London: National Council for Educational Technology.

Van Son, L.G. (ed.) (1982) *Video in health.* White Plains, NY: Knowledge Industry Publications Inc.

Verny, R.G. and Heider, M. (1982) Selecting and using video programs. In *Video in health,* ed. L.G. Van Son, pp. 97-124. White Plains, NY: Knowledge Industry Publications Inc.

Video Source Book (annual) New York: National Video Clearing House Inc.

Videolog (1981) *The health sciences videolog,* 2nd edn. New York: Video-Forum.

Weihs, J. (1984) *Accessible storage of nonbook materials.* Phoenix, AZ: Oryx Press.

White, N. (1987) Holography — the clear plate syndrome. *Journal of Audiovisual Media in Medicine,* **10,** 135-137.

APPENDIX 1 Addresses of organizations

Association for Educational and Training Technology, c/o The Centre for Continuing Education, The City University, Northampton Square, London EC1V 0HB.

Australian Council of Libraries and Information Services AV Subcommittee. Secretary: Gulcin Cribb, The Audiovisual Library, The University of Queensland, St Lucia, Queensland, A4072 Australia.

Bencard Film Library, Promotional Services Dept, Bencard, Great West Road, Brentford, Middlesex TW8 9BD.

BBC Education and Training Sales, BBC Enterprises Ltd, Woodlands, 80 Wood Lane, London W12 0TT

British Film Institute, 21 Stephen Street, London W1P 1PL.

BLAISE Information Services, The British Library National Bibliographic Service, 2 Sheraton Street, London W1V 4BH.

BMA Film and Video Library, The Nuffield Library, BMA House, Tavistock Square, London WC1H 9JP.

British Universities Film and Video Council, 55 Greek Street, London W1V 5LR.

Concord Video and Film Council Ltd, 201 Felixstowe Road, Ipswich IP3 9BJ.

Edward Patterson Associates, Treetops, Cannongate Road, Hythe, Kent CT21 5PT.

English National Board for Nursing, Midwifery and Health Visiting, Resource and Careers Services, Woodseats House, 764a Chesterfield Road, Sheffield S8 0SE. For HEALTH CARE DATABASE *index* and further *Update indexes* contact the Publications Department at the same address.

European Multimedia Centre, 24 Stephenson Way, London NW1 2HD.

Foundation for Teaching Aids at Low Cost, PO Box 49, St Albans, Herts AL1 4AX.

Gower Medical Publishing Ltd, Middlesex House, 34-42 Cleveland Street, London W1P 5FB.

Graves Educational Resources, Holly House, 220 New London Road, Chelmsford, Essex CM2 9BJ.

Health Education Authority, Hamilton House, Mabledon Place, London WC1H 9TX.

ICI Pharmaceuticals Division, Alderley Park, Macclesfield, Cheshire SK10 4TF.

Institute of Medical Illustrators, 27 Craven Street, London WC2N 5NX.

International Planned Parenthood Federation, Regent's College, Inner Circle, Regent's Park, London NW1 4NS.

International Visual Communications Association, 5–6 Clipstone Street, London W1P 7EB.

Lipha Pharmaceuticals Ltd, Harrier House, High Street, Yiewsley, West Drayton, Middlesex UB7 7QG.

University of London Audio-Visual Centre, North Wing Studios, Senate House, Malet Street, London WCIE 7JZ.

Mental Health Media Council, 380 Harrow Road, London W9 2HU

MSD Foundation, Tavistock House, Tavistock Square, London WC1H 9LG.

National Council for Educational Technology, Sir William Lyons Road, Science Park, Coventry CV4 7EZ.

NICEM, Access Innovations, PO Box 40130, Albuquerque, NM 87196, USA.

National Library of Medicine Audiovisual Center, 8600 Rockville Pike, Bethesda, MD 20209, USA.

University of Newcastle Regional Postgraduate Institute for Medicine and Dentistry, University of Newcastle upon Tyne, 11 Framlington Place, Newcastle upon Tyne NE2 4AB.

Open University Educational Enterprises Ltd, 12 Cofferidge Close, Stony Stratford, Milton Keynes MK11 1BY.

Oxford Educational Resources Ltd, Academic House, Oakfields, Eynsham, Oxford OX8 1TH.

Rorer Pharmaceuticals Ltd, St Leonards House, St Leonards Road, Eastbourne, East Sussex BN21 3YG.

Royal College of Obstetricians and Gynaecologists, 27 Sussex Place, Regent's Park, London NW1 4RG.

St Bartholomew's Hospital Audio Visual Teaching Department, The Robin Brook Centre for Medical Education, West Smithfield, London EC1A 7BE.

Scottish Council for Educational Technology Information Resource Centre, 74 Victoria Cresent Road, Glasgow G12 9JN.

Scottish Central Film and Video Library, 74 Victoria Crescent, Glasgow G12 9JN.

SilverPlatter Information Services, 10 Barleymow Passage, London W4 4PH.

University of Southampton AV Resources Unit, Department of Teaching Media, South Academic Block, Southampton General Hospital, Southampton SO9 4XY.

U.S. Army Academy of Health Sciences, Attn: HSA-SMD, Fort Sam Houston, TX 78234, USA.

The Wellcome Trust Tropical Diseases Videodisc Project, 183 Euston Road, London NWI 2BN.

APPENDIX 2 Directories listing producers/distributors of audio-visual aids

ACLIS AV Subcommittee (ed.) *A directory of suppliers and lenders of audiovisual materials.* Queensland: Australian Council of Libraries and Information Services AV Subcommittee.

Audiovisual directory (1991) Croydon: EMAP Vision.

AV market place (1991) Ann Arbor, MI: Bowker.

AV source directory: a subject guide to health science AV producer/distributor catalogs. Chicago, IL: Greater Midwest Regional Medical Library Network.

Dyke, R. (ed.) (1979) *Audio-visual centres in institutions of higher education in Europe.* Warwick: University of Warwick/UNESCO.

Ely, D.P. *et al.* (eds) (1988) *Educational media and technology yearbook.* Littleton: Libraries Unlimited Inc.

European Multimedia Yearbook 1992 (1991) London European Multimedia Centre.

Geddes, G. and MacKechnie, J. (1981) *AVSCOT checklist of UK audio visual software producers.* Glasgow: AVSCOT.

Grant, C. and Sarmiento, M. (eds) *(1990) Distributors: the guide to video and film sources for education and training.* London: BUFVC.

Henderson, J. and Humphreys, F. (eds) (1984) *Audio-visual and microcomputer handbook,* 4th edn. London: Kogan Page.

Jones, M.C. (1986) *International guide to locating audio-visual materials in the health sciences.* Aldershot: Gower.

McKeown, R. (1989) *National directory of slide collections.* (British Library Information Guide No. 12). London: British Library.

NICEM (1989) *Index to AV producers and distributors.* 7th edn. Medford, NJ: NICEM/Plexus Publishing.

Oliver, E. (ed.) (1989) *Researcher's guide to film and television collections,* 3rd edn. London: BUFVC.

Osborne, C. W. (ed.) *(1990) International Yearbook of Educational and Instructional Technology.* London: Kogan Page.

Pemberton, J.M. (1990) *Policies of audiovisual producers and distributors: a handbook for acquisition personnel,* 2nd rev. edn. Metuchen, NJ and London: Scarecrow.

Terris, O. (1990) *BUFVC Catalogue.* London: [BUFVC. 7 microfiches with 48-page booklet listing distributors.]

APPENDIX 3 A select list of journals concerned with audio-visual aids in medicine.

Those marked * carry reviews of new materials
Biomedical Communications
Health Libraries Review
*Health Service Journal**
*Journal of Audiovisual Media in Medicine**
Journal of Family Practice
Public Health Reports

The following, although not specifically concerned with medicine, frequently carry items of interest to medical readers. For lists of other journals on the use of audio-visual aids generally and on audio-visual equipment, see sources cited in the text.

Audio Visual
Audiovisual Librarian
AV User
European Multimedia Bulletin
Interactive Update
Screen Digest
Videodisc Newsletter (BUFVC)
Viewfinder (BUFVC)

CHAPTER SEVEN

Anatomy and physiology

R.J. MOORE

The long-established anatomical and physiological sciences, dealing with biological structure and function, can be seen as precursors of many of today's biomedical sciences, having given birth to biochemistry, cell and molecular biology (via 'physiological' chemistry), developmental biology, embryology, and the great upsurge in the neurosciences and biophysics. They have contributed to the development of many other fields through technical innovations in microscopy, measurement, monitoring and control.

These factors have obviously influenced the literature and resulted in anatomical and physiological information being spread over a wide area of information sources. This chapter will aim to cover this wide spectrum both in terms of subject area and information sources such as monographs, journals, indexing and abstracting services, data books, reviews etc.The sources given are not intended to be exhaustive but to highlight the main areas of importance. In some cases older works are given, as well as recent publications: these can still be of considerable value in indicating the development of the disciplines and also placing current work in historical perspective.

Primary sources of information

Journals

Original work appears principally in periodicals but other forms of publication must be kept in mind, such as symposia, conferences, research reports, and theses. Means of locating this material is covered in the sections on abstracting and indexing services. Many papers relevant to anatomy and physiology appear in journals of general scientific or medical interest, e.g. *Nature, Science, Proceedings of the Royal Society of London, Proceedings of the National Academy of Sciences (USA), British Medical Journal, The Lancet, Journal of Experimental Medicine*, etc. Specialist medical journals which often contain papers bearing on the normal subject are many, e.g. *Gut, Thorax, Gastroenterology, etc.* It is clear that many periodicals are needed in research in these two major basic medical sciences. The position is clear on examining the *List of Journals Indexed in Index Medicus* which is published each year with the January issue of *Index Medicus* (see p. 52), it includes subject and geographical listings. A check of the headings Anatomy (which includes morphology), Cytology (which includes microscopy), Embryology (which includes developmental biology and teratology), Histocytochemistry and Physiology, shows that almost 300 other journals are likely to be relevant. Even then, these headings do not include still more specialized journals, e.g. *Circulation Research*. Incidentally, the subject and geographical sections of the *List* enable one to ascertain quickly the titles of journals in any particular field or country, so that it is not necessary to give here more than a representative selection of the most important titles in these basic sciences. Each country has its leading journals — in the UK the *Journal of Anatomy* and the *Journal of Physiology*, in the USA the *American Journal of Anatomy* and the *American Journal of Physiology*. Clearly these four cannot publish the leading work in every field (despite the increase in the size of all four) and some journals have gained equal repute in their more circumscribed spheres, e.g. *Journal of Applied Physiology, Journal of Neurobiology*.

The following list is confined to the more important journals published in English; those in other languages may be traced through the subject and country listings in the *List of Journals Indexed in Index Medicus*.

ANATOMY

Acta Anatomica
American Journal of Anatomy
Anatomical Record

Anatomy and Embryology
Journal of Anatomy

CELL BIOLOGY

Cell
Cell and Tissue Research
European Journal of Cell Biology

Journal of Cell Science
Journal of Histochemistry and Cytochemistry

Experimental Cell Research
Journal of Cell Biology

Journal of Structural Biology
Tissue and Cell

DEVELOPMENTAL BIOLOGY

Development
Developmental Biology
Journal of Developmental Physiology

PHYSIOLOGY

Acta Physiologica Scandinavica
American Journal of Physiology
Comparative Biochemistry and Physiology
Experimental Physiology
Journal of Applied Physiology

Journal of Cellular Physiology
Journal of General Physiology
Journal of Physiology
Pflüger's Archiv: European Journal of Physiology
Quarterly Journal of Experimental Physiology

CARDIOLOGY

Cardiovascular Research
Circulation Research
Respiration Physiology

ENDOCRINOLOGY

Endocrinology
Journal of Endocrinology
Journal of Reproduction and Fertility

NEUROSCIENCES

Brain Research
Developmental Neuroscience
International Journal of Developmental Neuroscience
Experimental Brain Research
Experimental Eye Research
Hearing Research
Journal of the Autonomic Nervous System

Journal of Comparative Neurology
Journal of Neurocytology
Journal of Neurophysiology
Journal of Neuroscience
Neuroscience
Neuroscience Letters
Vision Research
Pain

For those who wish to keep up to date with the latest developments there is the choice of either regularly scanning new issues of journals in a good library or using a current-awareness service (either printed or computer-based). In practice, most people use both methods. *Current Contents: Life Sciences*, which reproduces the contents pages of over

1200 biomedical journals, appears weekly; it is also provided on a diskette for use on a personal computer.

Abstracting services

Abstracting services are discussed in Chapter 3, but some account of those serving these basic medical sciences is necessary here. Currently there are two main sources for extensive informative abstracts, *Excerpta Medica* and *Biological Abstracts*; however, it must be remembered that MEDLINE (the computer-based version of *Index Medicus*) provides abstracts of approximately 70 per cent of papers included.

Excerpta Medica has, since 1968, provided a keyword subject index in each issue, and the annual indexes appear soon after the completion of the volume; the abstracts are reasonably informative. The relevant sections are (parts per annum are in parentheses):

1. Anatomy, anthropology, embryology and histology (10 parts)
2. Physiology (24 parts)
3. Endocrinology (24 parts)
8. Neurology and neurosurgery (32 parts)
21. Developmental biology and teratology (8 parts)
27. Biophysics, bio-engineering and medical instrumentation (10 parts)

Excerpta Medica is also available online and as CD-ROM.

Biological Abstracts vies with *Chemical Abstracts* in its sophisticated structure and extensive coverage, dealing with 9000 primary journals and monographs, and serving all the life sciences. Each semimonthly issue has a classified arrangement with author, taxonomic, subject and organism indexes. It is also available online and as CD-ROM.

Examples of other relevant abstracting services confined to specific fields include the following:

Calcified Tissue Abstracts (quarterly, classified, author and subject indexes)

Chemoreception Abstracts (quarterly, author and subject indexes)

Nutrition Abstracts and Reviews; Series A — Human and Experimental Neuroscience Abstracts (monthly, author and subject indexes)

Other abstracting journals: *Berichte über die gesamte Physiologie* and *Physiological Abstracts* should not be overlooked.

Indexing services

For most anatomists and physiologists the printed *Index Medicus* (also available online, see Chapter 5) is indispensable. New users should study the introduction (printed in each issue) and the annual list of subject headings *(MeSH)* — this contains an alphabetical list of all headings used together with a categorized list.

The development in 1967 of *BioResearch Index*, now *Biological Abstracts RMM (Reports, Reviews, Meetings)* as an adjunct to *Biological Abstracts* has greatly assisted in tracing research reports, reviews, books, and papers at meetings. Each year this index reports 250 000 research papers in addition to and different from the more than 275 000 reports in *Biological Abstracts*. The *Index* appears semi-monthly and includes a complete list of publications covered and the same types of author and subject indexes as its parent publication. Other sources of information on symposia and meetings are: *Index of Conference Proceedings* which does not actually list the contents of such proceedings; these are covered by the *Index to Scientific and Technical Proceedings*, published by the Institute for Scientific Information (ISI), which includes biomedical material (this is available online).

In addition to these general indexes, there are a number which serve limited areas. An example is the *Bibliography of Reproduction*, begun in 1963; it is a classified monthly index to books and periodical articles on all aspects of reproduction in vertebrates, including man. Approximately 300 000 items have been recorded and a bibliographical service, both manual and computer-based, is run by the producing body, Reproduction Research Information Service, Cambridge. Each monthly issue has an author index; half-yearly subject indexes are available. Separate printed bibliographies on specific topics can be obtained.

Other bibliographies which have now ceased publication, probably because of the easier availability of specialized bibliographies via computer-accessible databases, include: *Bibliographia Histochemica, Index of Tissue Culture, Bibliographia Neuroendocrinologica* and *Electroencephalography and Clinical Neurophysiology — Index to Current Literature*.

A wide variety of specialized current-awareness bulletins are produced. Two examples of suppliers are: The Medical Information Service of the British Library at Boston Spa, Wetherby, W. Yorkshire, LS23 7BQ and The Biomedical Information Service at the University of Sheffield, Sheffield, S10 2JF.

Retrospective bibliographies

Over the years many specialized printed bibliographies have been compiled; these are dated now and not quite so useful and have been replaced to a certain extent by on-demand computer-searchable databases used in conjunction with earlier reviews. However, some of the older bibliographies still have value and examples are:

Bibliography of electroencephalography, 1875-1948 compiled by M. Brazier (Suppl. 1 to the journal *Electroencephalography and Clinical Neurophysiology*, 1950)

Bibliography of research in tissue culture, 1884-1950 edited by M.R. Murray and G. Kopech (Academic Press, 1950)

Bibliography of hearing by S.S. Stevens *et al.* (Harvard University Press, 1950)

Bibliography on the sense of taste, 1566-1966 compiled by R.M. Pangborn and I.M. Trabue (appended to *The chemical senses and nutrition* edited by M.R. Kare and O. Maller, Johns Hopkins, 1967)

Bibliography on muscle receptors, their morphology, pathology and physiology by E. Eldred *et al.* (Supplement 3 to *Experimental Neurology*, 1967)

Secondary sources

While it may be convenient to speak of primary and secondary sources, one cannot forget that journals contain material that is not necessarily original, while new information may first appear in a symposium or some other non-periodical publication. There are also journals which are in any case secondary source material since they are confined to the review type of article.

The following section deals with those forms of literature which present an ordered statement of knowledge on a given subject, though of varying scope and depth, i.e. handbooks, treatises, textbooks, monographs and symposia. As an intermediate step, however, consideration must first be given to reviews, mostly collected in serial publications, though occasionally found in isolated surveys of progress. Authorship may be collective, and some symposia offer the best exposition on certain topics. Other methods of presenting facts may be pictorial (atlases), documentary (data handbooks) or simply explanatory (dictionaries, terminology) and these are treated in succeeding sections.

The ever-changing approach to the study and teaching of the medical sciences has resulted in a new literature. Some of these works concern individual subjects and are mentioned in those contexts, but some publications of a general interdisciplinary nature may be cited here.

The first is *A companion to medical studies* edited by R. Passmore and J.S. Robson (3 vols, Blackwell Scientific Publications, 1974, 1980, 1986). The first two volumes cover the preclinical sciences, structure and function being co-ordinated (Volume 1, *Anatomy, biochemistry, physiology and related subjects*, 3rd edn., 1986; Volume 2, *Pharmacology, microbiology, general pathology and related subjects*, 2nd edn., 1980). The other two publications are shorter but also based on a wider approach to the study of human structure and function: *Introduction to the study of man* by J.Z. Young (2nd edn., Oxford University Press, 1974) and *Human biology; an introduction to human evolution, variation, growth, and adaptability* edited by G.A. Harrison *et al.* (3rd edn., Oxford University Press, 1988).

Reviews

The value of this type of secondary source material is perhaps best underlined by the existence of the *Bibliography of Medical Reviews* as a prominent feature of *Index Medicus*. While the majority of such articles are contained in serials entirely devoted to this form of literature, there are still many reviews to be found in journals intended primarily for original papers; in addition, reports of the review type may be found in the annual volumes of symposia of various societies, e.g. the Society for Experimental Biology. Discovering such articles is facilitated by the *Bibliography of Medical Reviews*.

The following list may be of use in searching for reviews in the fields concerned:

*Advances in Anatomy, Embryology
    and Cell Biology*
Advances in Biophysics
Advances in Cell Culture
Annual Review of Biophysics
Annual Review of Cell Biology
Annual Review of Neuroscience
Annual Review of Nutrition
Annual Review of Physiology
Biological Reviews
Brain Research Reviews (a section of
    the journal *Brain Research*)
British Medical Bulletin
*Cold Spring Harbor Symposia on
    Quantitative Biology*
*Current Topics in Developmental
    Biology*
Endocrine Reviews
Harvey Lectures
*International Review of Connective
    Tissue Research*
International Review of Cytology
International Review of Neurobiology

News in Physiological Sciences
Nutrition Abstracts and Reviews
Physiological Reviews
Progress in Biophysics and Molecular
    Biology
Progress in Brain Research
Progress in Histochemistry and
    Cytochemistry
Progress in Neurobiology
Progress in Sensory Physiology
Quarterly Review of Biology
Quarterly Reviews of Biophysics
Reviews of Physiology, Biochemistry
    and Pharmacology
Symposia of the Society for
    Developmental Biology
Symposia of the Society for
    Experimental Biology
Trends in Neurosciences

Systematic works, textbooks, monographs

Anatomy, histology, embryology

The old anatomical handbooks in this field have become dated and with changes in terminology often difficult to use: Bardeleben's *Handbuch der Anatomie des Menschen* (8 vols in 19, Jena, 1896-1934) and Quain's *Elements of anatomy* (11th edn., 4 vols in 8, Longmans, 1908–1929) are without successors. For general works with the most detail there is still *Gray's anatomy* by P.L. Williams and R. Warwick (37th edn., Churchill Livingstone, 1989) and *Cunningham's textbook of anatomy* by G.J. Romanes (12th edn., Oxford University Press, 1981), both of which successfully resist the passage of time. For students there are Grant's *Method of anatomy* by J.V. Basmajian (11th edn., Williams and Wilkins, 1989), *Clinically orientated anatomy* by K.L. Moore (2nd edn., Williams and Wilkins, 1985) and *Anatomy as a basis for clinical medicine* by E.C.B. Hall-Craggs (2nd edn., Urban and Schwarzenberg, 1990). The regional approach is used in *Anatomy, regional and applied* by R.J. Last (7th edn., Churchill Livingstone, 1984), and in *Anatomy: a regional study of human structure* by E. Gardner (5th edn., Saunders, 1986). For guides in dissecting there are *Cunningham's manual of practical anatomy* (15th edn., 3 vols, Oxford University Press, 1986) and the *Manual of human anatomy* by J.T. Aitken *et al.* (3rd edn., 3 vols, 1975). Of particular use in the dissecting room is *Human dissection* by C.C. Chumbley (Wolfe, 1988)

Histology is one subject still comprehensively covered by one of the great German treatises: the *Handbuch der mikroskopischen Anatomie des Menschen* founded by W. von Möllendorf and now edited by A. Oksche and L. Vollrath (7 Bände in 43 parts to date, Springer, 1927-) There is no lack of textbooks of histology, of which the most important include those by D.W. Fawcett and W. Bloom, *Textbook of histology* (11th edn., Saunders, 1986), *Cell and tissue biology; a textbook of histology* by L. Weiss (6th edn., Urban and Schwarzenberg, 1988), *Basic histology*, by L.C. Junqueira (5th edn., Lange, 1986), and P.R. Wheater *et al.*, *Functional histology*, 2nd edn., Churchill Livingstone, 1987). Researches on ultrastructure have led to more specialized works: *Cell and molecular biology* by E.D. De Robertis (8th edn., Lea and Febiger, 1987), *Ultrastructure of the mammalian cell* by R.V. Krstic (Springer, 1979), *Histology and human neuroanatomy* by H. Elias *et al.* (4th edn., Wiley, 1978), *Molecular biology of the cell* by B. Albertis *et al.* (2nd edn., Garland, 1989) and *Introduction to biological membranes* by M.K. Jain and R.C. Wagner (2nd edn., Wiley, 1988). There are also numerous works on techniques, e.g. H.M. Carleton's *Histological technique* (5th edn., Oxford University Press, 1980), *Theory and practice of histological techniques* by J.D. Bancroft and A. Stevens (3rd edn., Churchill Livingstone, 1990), *Cellular pathology technique* by C.F. Culling (4th edn., Butterworths, 1985), *Biological stains* by H.J. Conn (9th edn., Williams and Wilkins, 1977), *A colour atlas of histology* by M.B.L. Craigmyle (2nd edn., Wolfe, 1986). Histochemical methods are ever-growing in number: guides to their use include *Histochemistry; an explanatory outline of histochemical and biophysical staining* by R.W. Horobin (Butterworths, 1982) and *Histochemistry, theoretical and applied* by A.G.E. Pearse (4th edn., 2 vols, Churchill Livingstone, 1980, 1985).

In the field of embryology useful textbooks for medical studies are *Langman's medical embryology* by T.W. Sadler (6th edn., Williams and Wilkins, 1990), and *The developing human* by K.L. Moore (4th edn., Saunders, 1988). For the scientific worker the following will be useful: *An introduction to embryology* by B.I. Balinsky (5th edn., Saunders, 1981), *Introduction to concepts in developmental biology* by A. Monroy and A.A. Moscona (University of Chicago Press, 1980), *Introduction to molecular embryology* by J. Brachet and H. Alexandre (2nd edn., Springer, 1986), *Patten's foundations of embryology* by B.M. Carlson (5th edn., McGraw-Hill, 1988), *Developmental biology; a comprehensive synthesis* edited by L.W. Browder, Plenum, 1985-). Experimental methods may be found in *Manipulating the mouse embryo* by B.L.M. Hogan (Cold Spring Harbor, 1986), *Culture of animal cells* by R.I. Freshney (2nd edn., Liss, 1987), *An atlas for staging mammalian and chick embryos* by H. Butler and B.H.J. Juurlink (CRC Press, 1987) and *The house mouse* by K.Theiler (Springer, 1989).

Among works of reference for embryologists are the 'normal tables', containing descriptions of embryos at successive stages of development; at best not only external details are given, but also an account of the various organs. The existence of these standard descriptions obviates the need for repeating them and also assists identification of which stage another author is discussing, if this should be in doubt. The basic series of these works was the *Normentafeln zur Entwicklungsgeschichte der Wirbeltiere* edited by F. Keibel (16 vols, G. Fischer, 1897-1938). Many others have since been published, and a detailed list is given in Bellairs' *Developmental processes in higher vertebrates* (Logos Press, 1971).

The culture of cells and tissues has applications in other branches of medical research, and the bibliographies already indicate what may be relevant here. A basic text on the subject is *Cell and tissue culture* by J. Paul (6th edn., Churchill Livingstone, 1989, while *Cells and tissues in culture* edited by E.N. Willmer (3 vols, Academic Press, 1966), is an older, but very extensive, treatise.

Physiology

The *Handbook of physiology* (Oxford University Press) is the creation of the American Physiological Society, with contributions by physiologists from many other countries. Its aim is 'the comprehensive but critical presentation of the state of knowledge in the various fields of functional biology'. The sections cover the physiological sciences in their entirety and will be systematically revised. The arrangement of Sections, most consisting of a number of volumes is:

Section 1. The nervous system
Section 2. The cardiovascular system
Section 3. The respiratory system
Section 4. Adaptation to the environment
Section 6. The gastrointestinal system
Section 7. Endocrinology
Section 8. Renal physiology
Section 9. Reactions to environmental agents
Section 10. Skeletal muscle

One other work which should be cited, since it is to some extent complementary, is the *Handbook of sensory physiology* with various editors (Springer 1971-1979). The series is updated by *Progress in Sensory Physiology*.

General physiology has produced some notable textbooks, now a little dated, e.g. Bayliss' *Principles of general physiology* (5th edn., 2 vols, Longmans, 1959-1960 and H. Davson's *Textbook of general physiology* (4th edn., 2 vols, Churchill, 1970). Established texts in human physiology are *Physiology of the human body* by A.C. Guyton (6th edn., Saunders, 1984), *An introduction to human physiology* by J.H. Green (4th edn., Oxford University Press, 1976), *Physiology and biophysics* edited by T.C. Ruch and H.D. Patton (1973-1982), *Introduction to physiology* by H. Davson and M.B. Segal (5 vols, Academic Press, 1975-1980), *Textbook of physiology* by D. Emslie-Smith *et al.* (11th edn., Churchill Livingstone, 1988), *Physiology* by E.E. Selkurt (5th edn., Little, Brown, 1984).

Medically-slanted texts are *The physiological basis of medical practice* by C.H. Best and N.B. Taylor (11th edn., Williams and Wilkins, 1985), *Samson Wright's Applied physiology* by C.A. Keele and E. Neil (13th edn., Oxford University Press, 1982) and *Textbook of medical physiology* by A.C. Guyton (7th edn., Saunders, 1986), among others. More specialized works include; *Experiments in physiology* by G.D. Tharp (5th edn., Burgess, 1986) for students. For the research worker there is *Methods in cell biology* (Academic Press, 1964-). Recent developments in neurophysiological techniques are reported in *Journal of Neuroscience Methods* and surveyed by the review journals such as *Annual Review of Physiology*. The role of computers is well covered by *Microcomputers in physiology; a practical approach* edited by P.J. Fraser (IRL Press, 1988).

Systems of the body

The nervous system more than any other has seen a widespread increase in all forms of the relevant literature; at the same time older material may still be needed, such as *Histologie du système nerveuse de l'homme et des vertébrés* by S. Ramón y Cajal (2 vols, Paris, 1909-1911; reprint Madrid, Instituto Ramón y Cajal (1952-1955). Also, some forms are confused, e.g. *Progress in Brain Research* (1-, Elsevier, 1963), the scope of which is wider than the title indicates, and which includes symposia, monographs and reviews of progress; work of basic importance may be found in *Publications of the Association for Research in Nervous and Mental Diseases* (vol 1-, Williams and Wilkins, 1920-).The integrated approach to the study of the nervous system is found in *Medical neurobiology* by W.D. Willis and R.G. Grossman (3rd edn., Mosby, 1981) and *Neurological anatomy in relation to clinical medicine* by A. Brodal (3rd edn., Oxford University Press, 1981). Useful textbooks include *Neuroanatomy* by D.E. Haines (2nd edn., Urban and Schwarzenberg, 1987) and *Human neuroanatomy* by M.B. Carpenter and J. Sutin (8th edn., Williams and Wilkins, 1983).

The embryology and histology of the nervous system are treated in various works: *Developmental neurobiology of the autonomic nervous system* by P.M. Gootman (Humana, 1986), from the research angle, and *Developmental neurobiology*, a monograph by M. Jacobson (2nd edn., Plenum, 1978). Textbooks on neurophysiology are *Neurophysiology* by R.H.S, Carpenter (2nd edn., Arnold 1990), and *Fundamentals of neurophysiology* by R.F. Schmidt (3rd edn., Springer, 1985).

Monographs and other works on special topics of importance are so numerous that any attempted listing would be both selective and misleading. Up-to-date information on important classical works can be easily obtained from review papers or the more general treatises. The almost overwhelming flow of new books is best monitored using the standard bibliographical tools together with routine examination of the book review sections of the general and specialized journals.

The literature on the brain has grown to such a volume that it has its own history, *The human brain and spinal cord: a historical study ... from antiquity to the twentieth century* by E. Clarke and C.D. O'Malley (University of California Press, 1968). It is not possible here to cover all aspects of research on the structure and function of the brain: some current studies still refer to classic works such as *Histological studies on the localisation of cerebral function* by A.W. Campbell (Cambridge University Press, 1905), *The integrative action of the nervous system* by C.S. Sherrington (Yale University Press, 1906) and *The cytoarchitectonics of the human cerebral cortex* by C. von Economo (Oxford University Press, 1929). Many have since worked in this field, and the following is a select list in chronological order of some other major works still in use:

Brain mechanisms and intelligence by K.S. Lashley (Chicago University Press, 1929; Dover, 1963); *The primate thalamus* by A.E. Walker (Chicago University Press, 1938); *The hypothalamus* by W.E. Le Gros Clark *et al.* (Oliver and Boyd, 1938); *The cerebral cortex of man* by W. Penfield and T. Rasmussen (Macmillan, 1930).

Three modern classics are: *Principles of neural science* edited by E.R. Kandel and J.H. Schwartz (2nd edn., Elsevier, 1985); *From neuron to brain* by S.W. Kuffler *et al.* (2nd edn., Sinauer, 1984); *Programs of the brain* by J.Z. Young (Oxford University Press, 1978).

The series *Progress in Brain Research*, already cited, reports on the various aspects of current research. The special sense organs are treated in the *Handbook of sensory physiology* mentioned above. Two introductions to the subject are *Fundamentals of sensory physiology* by R.F. Schmidt (3rd edn., Springer, 1986) and *The senses* by H.B. Barlow and J.D. Mollon (Cambridge University Press, 1982). For individual organs the following works are important:

1. Vision: the two works by S. Polyak, *The retina* (Chicago University Press, 1941) and The *vertebrate visual system*

(Chicago University Press, 1957) together with the encyclopaedic *Vision and visual dysfunction* edited by J. Cronly-Dillon (17 vols, Macmillan, 1990); and also *The eye* edited by H. Davson (2nd edn., 6 vols, Academic Press, 1967-1974). Vision by D. Marr (Freeman, 1982) and *Physiology of the retina and visual pathway* by G.S. Brindley (2nd edn., Arnold, 1970).

2. Hearing: *An introduction to the anatomy and physiology of speech and hearing* by J.F. Jarvis (Jauta, 1978) and *An introduction to the physiology of hearing* by J.O. Pickles (2nd edn., Academic Press, 1988)

3. Taste and smell: *Neurobiology of taste and smell* by T.E. Finger and W.L. Silver (Wiley, 1987)

4. Touch: *Mechanisms of cutaneous sensation* by D. Sinclair (Oxford University Press, 1981)

With respect to other systems of the body, the secondary literature is smaller and sometimes out of date. Where no recent treatise or monograph exists, reference should be made to the appropriate section of the *Handbook of physiology* or to one of the larger general textbooks. For physiology the valuable monograph series of the Physiological Society should be remembered: this began in 1953, and was originally published by Arnold and, more recently, by Cambridge University Press and Academic Press; recent volumes include *Energetic aspects of muscle contraction* and *Atrial receptors*. The following list indicates titles likely to be of use for other systems:

1. Locomotor system: *Biochemistry and physiology of bone* edited by G.H. Bourne (2nd edn., vols 1-4, Academic Press, 1972-77); *Physiology and pathophysiology of the skin* edited by A. Jarrett (9 vols, Academic Press, 1973-86); *Biochemistry and physiology of the skin* edited by L.A. Goldsmith (2 vols, Oxford University Press, 1983); *Muscle* by J. Squire (Benjamin, 1986).

2. Circulatory system: *Circulatory physiology* by J.J. Smith (3rd edn., Williams and Wilkins, 1990); *Cardiovascular dynamics* by R.F. Rushmer (4th edn., Saunders, 1976) and *The human cardiovascular system* by J. T. Shepherd and P.M. Vanhoutte (Raven Press, 1979); and *Introduction to cardiovascular physiology* by J.R. Levick (Butterworths, 1990).

3. Respiratory system: *Physiology of respiration* by J.T. Comroe (3rd edn., Year Book Medical Publishers, 1987) and *Regulation of breathing* by R. Hornbein (2 vols, Dekker, 1981).

4. Digestive system: *Physiology of the digestive tract* by H.W.

Davenport (5th edn., Year Book Medical Publishers, 1982); *Digestive system physiology* by F.A. Sanford (Arnold, 1982) and, for a short introduction, *A digest of digestion* by H.W. Davenport (3rd edn., Year Book Medical Publishers, 1988).

5. Urinary system: *The kidney* by B.M. Brenner and F.C. Rector (3rd edn., 2 vols, Saunders, 1986) and *Principles of renal physiology* by C.J. Lote (2nd edn., Croom Helm, 1987).

6. Lymphatic system, body fluids: *Lymphoid cells* edited by J.I. Gallin (Raven, 1983) and *Physiology and pathophysiology of the cerebrospinal fluid* by H. Davson (Churchill, 1987).

7. Endocrine system: *Textbook of endocrine physiology* edited by J. E. Griff in and S. R. Ojeda (Oxford University Press,1988); *Endocrine physiology* by C.R. Martin (Oxford University Press, 1985); *Endocrinology* by L.J. Degroot *et al.* (3 vols, Grune and Stratton, 1979); *Essential endocrinology* by J. Laycock and P. Wise (2nd edn., Oxford University Press, 1983).

8. Reproductive system: F.H.A. Marshall's *Physiology of reproduction*, edited by G.E. Lamming (4th edn., 2 vols, Churchill Livingstone, 1990); *Essential reproduction* by M.H. Johnson and B. Everitt (3rd edn., Blackwell, 1988); *Human reproduction and developmental biology* by D.J. Begley *et al.* (Macmillan, 1980); The ovary, edited by S. Zuckerman (2nd edn., 3 vols, Academic Press, 1977-78); Lactation: a comprehensive treatise, edited by B.L. Larson and V.R. Smith (4 vols, Academic Press, 1974-78).

9. Nutrition: *Davidson's human nutrition and dietetics* by R. Passmore and M.A. Eastwood (8th edn., Churchill Livingstone, 1986); *Human nutrition: a comprehensive treatise*, edited by R.B. Alfin-Slater and D. Kritchevsky (3 vols in 4, Plenum, 1979-80).

Atlases

While the older type of anatomical atlas continues, newer works resulting from the use of the electron microscope and of the stereotaxic instrument are multiplying. J.C.B. Grant's *Atlas of anatomy* (8th edn., Williams and Wilkins, 1983), R.M.H. McMinn and R.T. Hutchings' *A colour atlas of human anatomy* (2nd edn., Wolfe Medical Publications, 1988) and *Wolf-Heidegger's atlas of human anatomy* by H. Frank *et al.* (4th edn., Karger, 1990), *Sobotta atlas of human anatomy* (Urban and Schwarzenberg, 1990) are all popular; the first two also include descriptive text. To microscopic anatomy is added ultrastructure: atlases of micrographs with accompanying descriptions are *Atlas of descriptive histology* by E.J. Reith and M.H. Ross (3rd edn., Harper and Row, 1977), *Ultrastructural pathology of the cell and matrix* by F.N. Ghadially (3rd edn., Butterworths, 1988) and *Fine structure of cells and tissues* by K.R. Porter and M.A. Bonneville (4th edn., Lea and Febiger, 1974).

For the study of embryology there are W.W. Matthew's *Atlas of descriptive embryology* (3rd edn., Macmillan, 1986), and the three volumes of H. Tuchmann-Duplessis *et al.*, *Illustrated human embryology* (Chapman and Hall, 1972-1974). Of those atlases with more specialized objectives, the following are available: for general studies on the brain, *A colour atlas of the brain and spinal cord* by M.A. England and J. Wakely (Wolfe, 1990), while, for dissecting, *Human brain* by N. Gluhbegovic and T.H. Williams (Harper and Row, 1980) is valuable; for dental studies there are *A colour atlas and textbook of oral anatomy* by B.K.B. Berkovitz *et al.* (Wolfe Medical Publications, 1978) and *A colour atlas of the head and neck* by R.M.H. McMinn *et al.* (Wolfe Medical Publications, 1981). In the field of comparative anatomy, there are the *Atlas of cat anatomy* by H.E. Field and M.E. Taylor (2nd edn., Chicago University Press, 1969), and — with atlases incorporated in the text — *The anatomy of the dog* by M.E. Miller *et al.* (Saunders, 1964) and *The anatomy of the rat* by E.C. Greene (1935, reprinted, Hafner, 1968).

The stereotaxic instrument for the three-dimensional investigation of the brain was invented by R.H. Clarke some years before World War I. However, it is only in the last few decades that it has been widely used and atlases of the deep structures of the brain of man and of various animal species published as a result: *Stereotaxy of the human brain* by G. Schaltenbrand and A.E. Walker. (2nd edn., Thieme, 1982), *Atlas for stereotaxy of the human brain* by G. Schaltenbrand and W. Wahren (2nd edn., Thieme, 1977).

Stereotaxic atlas of the human thalamus and adjacent structures by J. Andrew and E.S. Watkins (Williams and Wilkins, 1969), relates to man. For comparative studies the following stereotaxic atlases may be noted:

> Baboon: R. Davies and R.D. Huffman (University of Texas Press, 1968)
> Chimpanzee: M.R. DeLucchi *et al.* (University of California Press, 1966)
> Rhesus monkey, *Macaca mulatta*: R.S. Snider and J.C. Lee (Chicago University Press, 1961)
> Java monkey, *Macaca irus*: T.R. Shantha *et al.* (Karger, 1968)
> Cebus monkey: S.L. Manocha *et al.* (Clarendon, 1968)

Squirrel monkey, *Saimiri sciureus*: R. Emmers and K. Akert (University of Wisconsin Press, 1963)
Cat: R.S. Snider and W.T. Niemer (Chicago University Press, 1961)
Brain stem — A.L. Berman (University of Wisconsin Press, 1982)
Diencephalon — H.H. Jasper and C. Ajmone-Marson (National Research Council of Canada, 1954)
Hypothalamus — R. Bleir (Johns Hopkins Press, 1961)
Dog:
S. Dua-Sharma *et al.* (MIT Press, 1970)
R.K.S. Lim *et al.* (C.C. Thomas, 1960)
Rat:
R.J. and J.R. Olds (Wolfe Medical Publications, 1977); L.J. Pellegrino *et al.* (2nd edn., Plenum, 1979); G. Paxinos and C. Watson (2nd edn., Academic Press, 1986)
Developing brain — N.M. Sherwood and P.S. Timiras (University of California Press, 1970)
Diencephalon — D. Albe-Fessard *et al.* (CNRS, Paris, 1971)
Forebrain and lower brain stem — J.F.R. Konig and R.A. Klippel (Williams and Wilkins, 1963)

Reference books

Data handbooks

The great volume of data established in anatomical and physiological research has been digested and made available in several publications. Probably the biggest compilation of this kind is the series *Tabulae biologicae* (22 vols, W. Junk, 1925-1963); the last four volumes are Vol. 19 *The Cell* (1939-1951), Vol. 20 *Growth of man* (1941), Vol. 21 *Digestion* (1954) and Vol. 22 *The Eye* (1947-1963). This work contains a mass of fully documented data not always accessible elsewhere.

More recently, an excellent series edited by P.L. Altman and D.S. Dittmer for the Federation of American Societies for Experimental Biology, entitled the *FASEB biological handbooks*, has appeared. So far the following volumes have been issued: *Blood and other body fluids* (1961, reissued 1971), *Growth, including reproduction and morphological development* (1962), *Environmental biology* (2nd edn., 1983), *Metabolism* (1968), *Respiration and circulation* (1971), *Biology data book* (2nd edn., 3 vols, 1983), *Cell biology* (1976), *Human health and disease* (1977), and *Inbred and genetically defined strains of laboratory animals* (2 vols, 1979).

The application of mathematics and physics to preclinical medical sciences may involve both theory and practice. *Medical physics* by A.C. Damask (3 vols, Academic Press, 1978-1984) will be of use in the physical and mathematical aspects of biomedical research. *Biomathematics; the principles of mathematics for students of biological and general science* by C.A.B. Smith (4th edn., 2 vols, Griffin, 1966-1969), is still very useful: it can be supplemented by a series of monographs, *Biomathematics*, edited by S.E. Levin (Springer, Jan 1973-). Methodology is covered by *Statistical methods for research workers* by R.A. Fisher (15th edn., Hafner, 1973), and *Armitage's statistical methods in medical research* edited by G. Berry (2nd edn., Blackwell, 1987) and data by the *Statistical tables for biological, agricultural and medical research* by R.A. Fisher and F. Yates (6th edn., Longman, 1974). For the student there are *Statistical exercises in medical research* by J.F. Osborn (Blackwell, 1979), and *Statistics at square one* by T.D.V. Swinscow (7th edn., British Medical Association, 1980).

Dictionaries

The major medical and biomedical dictionaries are covered in Chapter 4. However a useful specialized dictionary is *Henderson's dictionary of biological terms*, which has now reached its 10th edition (Longmans, 1990.

Anatomical nomenclature

Modern anatomical nomenclature is based on the *Basle Nomina anatomica* (BNA) of 1895, which was revised in the UK, in 1933, by the Anatomical Society at Birmingham (BR) and in Germany, in 1933, by the German Anatomical Society at Jena (JNA or INA). The Fifth International Congress of Anatomists at Oxford in 1950 agreed to produce a new standard revision, which was ready for the Paris Congress in 1955 (PNA). The current authority is found in the *Nomina anatomica* (6th edn., Churchill Livingstone, 1989), which was approved by the 12th International Congress of Anatomists, London, 1985, and includes *Nomina histologica* (3rd edn.) and *Nomina embryologica* (3rd edn.). A comparative study of the three systems — BNA, JNA and PNA — has been made by T. Donath in his *Anatomical dictionary* (Pergamon, 1969), which presents them — with an explanatory dictionary and a list of authors named in eponyms, with biographical data. For a straightforward equation of PNA and BR nomenclature, the Appendix to *Butterworths Medical dictionary* edited by MacDonald Critchley (2nd edn., Butterworths, 1978) is very useful. A guide for students is *Anatomical terms; their origin and derivation* by E.J. Field and R.J. Harrison (3rd edn., Heffer, 1968).

Historical sources

Anatomy

Charles Singer's *Evolution of anatomy* (Paul Kegan, 1925), an invaluable reference work, was reprinted as *A short history of anatomy from the Greeks to Harvey* (Dover, 1957). Two other useful works are G.W. Corner's *Anatomy* (Hoeber, 1930) and R.H. Hunter's *A short history of anatomy* (2nd edn., Bale, 1931). J.L. Choulant traced the evolution of anatomical illustration in *Geschichte und Bibliographie der anatomischen Abbildung* (Weigel, 1852); an English translation was published in 1920 by Chicago University Press and reprinted with additional material in 1945. Jessie Dobson's *Anatomical eponyms* (2nd edn., Livingstone, 1962) is a biographical dictionary of anatomists whose names are perpetuated in the nomenclature; it includes definitions of the structures, eponyms and references to the works in which they are described.

Embryology

Joseph Needham's *History of embryology* (2nd edn., Cambridge University Press, 1934) is an exhaustive account with good illustrations and a valuable bibliography. *The rise of embryology* by A.W. Meyer (California University Press, 1939) includes a good bibliography, and Vols 2-5 of H.B. Adelmann's *Marcello Malpighi and the evolution of embryology* (Cornell University Press, 1966) provides an extensive account of the development of embryology. Other useful sources are *A history of embryology* by T.J. Horder *et al.* (Cambridge University Press, 1985) and *Essays on the history of embryology and biology* by J.M. Oppenheimer (Massachusetts Institute of Technology, 1967).

Physiology

J.F. Fulton's *Selected readings in the history of physiology* (2nd edn., C.C. Thomas, 1966) is an excellent introduction to the subject. The readings extend from Aristotle to twentieth-century writers and give access to many classical accounts otherwise difficult to come by. Other languages are translated into English. Michael Foster's *Lectures on the history of physiology* (Cambridge University Press, 1901; reprinted 1924), although lacking in modern material is worth reading. K.J. Franklin's *Short history of physiology* (2nd edn., Staples, 1949) and Fulton's *Physiology* (Hoeber, 1931) though small, are useful. The best systematic account is probably K.E. Rothschuh's *Geschichte der Physiologie* (Springer, 1953) of which there is a revised and expanded English translation by G.B. Risse (Krieger, 1973); this includes a new English bibliography. A more recent account of the development of physiology is to be found in *The pursuit of nature; informal essays on the history of physiology*, edited by A.L. Hodgkin *et al*. (Cambridge University Press, 1977.) A valuable recent work is *Founders of British physiology; a biographical dictionary, 1820-1885; 1885-1914*, by W.J. O'Connor (Manchester University Press, 1988, 1991). Two works on the neurophysiology have been produced by M.A.B. Brazier — *A history of neurophysiology in the 17th and 18th centuries* (Raven Press, 1984) and *A history of neurophysiology in the 19th century* (Raven Press, 1987). Finally, an opportunity to obtain insight into the reality of physiological research is given by the prefatory chapter in each volume of the *Annual Review of Physiology*. These are written by leading international physiologists and give a detailed account of their scientific lives.

CHAPTER EIGHT

Biochemistry, biophysics and molecular biology

J.F.B. ROWLAND

Biochemistry is the study of the molecular changes that occur within living tissues. Biophysics is the study of living organisms by the techniques and concepts of physics. Out of the two subjects has grown molecular biology, which has so greatly enhanced man's understanding of the fundamental processes of life. The boundaries between these three disciplines are arbitrary. Biochemistry has traditionally concerned itself with the elucidation of metabolic reaction pathways, the study of the enzymes that catalyse the steps in those pathways and the mechanisms of control of the pathways. Molecular biology is taken to mean the study of the processes whereby an organism reproduces itself: the replication of DNA, the synthesis of RNA, the synthesis of protein and the relationships between the structure and the function of nucleic acids and of proteins. Biophysics has concentrated on the study of systems, such as membranes, biological fluids and muscle, where physical models are most applicable.

The field covered by these three subjects is itself interdisciplinary. They draw most heavily upon the fundamental concepts of chemistry, physics and mathematics — which may explain their relative unpopularity among medical students! Basic biological knowledge is necessary for the biochemist (this word, here and later, is taken to encompass the biophysicist and the molecular biologist), and this becomes the more true the closer to the molecular level the biological knowledge draws. So cell biology, physiology and microbiology are disciplines closely related to biochemistry. Pharmacy, medicinal chemistry and agricultural chemistry are sciences where biochemical knowledge is extensively used. As is conventional, 'the chemistry of natural products' has been omitted from the definition of biochemistry. This area — the study, by purely chemical methods, of materials of organic origin, without any intention of elucidating the reactions that occur *in vivo* — is normally considered part of organic chemistry. However, chemical or physical studies of model systems are included in the subject matter of this chapter; an example might be the physical study of a model membrane.

There is a tendency for scientists to read, and to contribute to, the literature of the subject in which they originally trained. As biochemical techniques and concepts have achieved wider and wider usage, this has meant that essentially biochemical work has been reported in the literature of adjoining disciplines, because the authors regard themselves as 'chemists', say, or 'pharmacists', rather than 'biochemists'.

One other important point must be borne in mind about biochemistry. It is an essentially bipartite profession. On the one hand, the research biochemist has a general responsibility to broaden human knowledge and is therefore a very heavy user of the literature, and a prolific contributor to it. He or she may well work in a medical research laboratory, but has no responsibility, directly or indirectly, to specific patients. Clinical biochemists, on the other hand, belong to one of the professions ancillary to medicine. They are primarily practitioners rather than researchers and are responsible to physicians and through them to patients. Their responsibility is to assist the diagnosis and treatment by the application of biochemical techniques and so they write rather less in the literature, and probably read it rather less, than research biochemists. Further, there is a separate literature of clinical biochemistry in which they write and read. When one reads of the spectacular growth of biochemistry and its literature over recent decades, it is mainly research biochemistry that is meant. Clinical biochemistry has grown in both volume and importance, and is an essential department in every hospital, but its growth has not been of such a spectacular kind.

That all of science has grown at a remarkable rate in recent years is well known. But biochemistry has grown even faster than most sciences. A measure of this is the biochemical sections of *Chemical Abstracts*. As is discussed later, there are some biochemical papers in other sections of *Chemical Abstracts*, but the biochemical sections do give an indication of the size and growth of the subject. A third of the abstracts in *Chemical Abstracts* are now in the biochemical sections, in spite of the youth of biochemistry compared with other branches of chemistry.

The actual numbers of papers in the biochemical sections at five-year intervals from 1969 to 1989 are given in Table 8.1, which shows that the proportion levelled out at 34–35 per cent in the 1980s.

Table 8.1. Number of abstracts appearing in the biochemical sections of *Chemical Abstracts* **1969–1989**

Year[*]	Number of abstracts in biochemical sections	Total number of abstracts in *Chemical Abstracts*	Biochemical sections as percentage of whole
1969	70 472	252 320	27.9
1974	103 228	333 624	31.0
1979	150 975	436 887	34.6
1984	161 600	460 569	35.1
1989	167 207	489 191	34.2

[*]The figures for 1969 were provided by Dr J.T. Dickman, Chemical Abstracts Service; those for 1974–1989 were calculated by the author.

The very rapid growth of biochemical research in the 1960s and 1970s is thought, by some biochemists, to stem from new laboratory techniques. It is certainly true that biochemical research has always faced formidable difficulties of practical technique attempting as it does to elucidate the chemical changes that occur within living cells. The major sources of this difficulty are:

1. The chemical changes involve very small quantities of reactants.

2. The biological samples under investigation are, by chemical standards, very complex mixtures.

3. It is desirable to study the reactions while the cell continues to live.

It is also certainly true that certain modern techniques have rapidly become the standard methods of the biochemical research laboratory. Among these, the various chromatographic and electrophoretic separation methods are of primary importance: gas–liquid, thin-layer, paper, ion-exchange and molecular-sieve chromatography, and paper, thin-layer and gel electrophoresis are examples of the many different techniques now in use. Another important technique is the use of radioactively and other isotopically labelled compounds; these assist in solving both the problem of small quantities and the problem of studies *in vivo*; radioautography is especially useful with the latter problem. Thus, the literature of methods and techniques is of high importance to the biochemist; with the usual indexes it is often harder to track down a method that one needs than to find a general discussion of results in an area of the subject.

Primary journals

Research biochemists are rather more likely than some other types of scientist (chemists, for example) to work in universities, colleges, medical schools, medical research institutes or hospitals, and rather less likely to work in commercial or industrial employment. This is another factor that contributes to their very large production of literature; their work is not so likely to be written in the form of confidential internal reports. Patent literature is also of correspondingly more limited importance in pure biochemistry — a contrast to its very great importance in the literature of the adjoining field of pharmaceutical chemistry. Furthermore, the very rapid development of techniques, concepts and factual knowledge in biochemistry means that the delays inherent in book publication are not often tolerable to the research biochemist. Consequently, publication in the scientific journals is of the highest importance. There is a large and increasing number of major journals covering the whole breadth of biochemistry, biophysics or both. The most important of these (with year of foundation and country of publication) are:

Journal of Biological Chemistry (1905) (USA) is a journal of very high standards, well respected in the field; it is produced by the American Society for Biochemistry and Molecular Biology.

Biochemistry (1962) (USA) is published by the American Chemical Society and carries the biochemical papers that previously would have appeared in *Journal of the American Chemical Society*; as this origin suggests, it has a slight stress on the more chemical side of biochemistry. It is a journal of very high standards.

Biochemical Journal (1906) (UK) is the oldest established UK journal in the field, and is published by the Biochemical Society. It is the preferred channel of publication for UK biochemists, but also carries a considerable amount of overseas matter; its standards are high, although it is sometimes criticized for its stress on the more classical areas of the subject; more modern material tends to find its way into the *Journal of Molecular Biology*. Papers delivered at meetings of the Society, formerly carried at the back of the journal in a Proceedings section, are now published in a separate journal called *Biochemical Society Transactions* (1973).

Biochimica et Biophysica Acta (1947) (Netherlands) accepts papers in English, French or German and is, perhaps, the journal of choice for most continental biochemists. It is also the most voluminous of the leading biochemical journals and appears in several simultaneous volumes, divided by subject matter (Lipids and Lipid Metabolism; Nucleic Acids and Protein Synthesis; Biomembranes; Gene Structure and Expression; Protein Structure and Molecular Enzymology; Molecular Cell Research; Bioenergetics; General Subjects). Review volumes are now also included, among them Reviews on Cancer, Reviews on Biomembranes, and Reviews on Bioenergetics.

Journal of Biochemistry (1922) (Japan) is published in English, and is the preferred journal of Japanese authors. Biochemically based industries, especially those based on fermentation processes for chemical and pharmaceutical production, are prominent in Japan and consequently much biochemical research of a high calibre is performed there.

Biokhimiya (1936) (USSR) is the leading Russian journal in this field. The Soviet Union was less renowned for life sciences than for engineering and physical sciences; however, the life sciences have been catching up in recent years. A cover-to-cover translation of *Biokhimiya*, entitled *Biochemistry: Biokhimiya*, is published in the USA.

Biological Chemistry Hoppe-Seyler was, as *Hoppe-Seylers Zeitschrift für physiologische Chemie* (1877) (Germany), the first journal devoted to the biochemical field. but, with the relative decline of Germany from its former position as the predominant scientific nation, it is less pre-eminent than it once was. Like most major German journals it is now published almost entirely in English.

Biochemische Zeitschrift (1906) (Germany) was a similar publication to *Hoppe-Seyler*; however, when in 1967 the Federation of European Biochemical Societies started to publish the new *European Journal of Biochemistry* (1967) (Germany), it replaced the *Zeitschrift*, which had been entirely in German. The new *European Journal* accepts papers in English, French or German, but English predominates.

Journal of Molecular Biology (1959) (UK) has rapidly established itself as one of the most respected scientific journals in the world. It is edited from the Laboratory of Molecular Biology in Cambridge, a laboratory of exceptional renown, and its subject field is the most rapidly developing and exciting part of the whole biochemical area. These factors combine to make publication in this journal unusually prestigious, and consequently its editorial standards are particularly high.

Biochemical and Biophysical Research Communications (1959) (USA) is a fast-publication organ. Urgent papers are published very quickly by photographic reproduction of the author's original typescript.

FEBS Letters (1968) (Germany) is a similar fast publication journal produced by the Federation of European Biochemical Societies.

The European Molecular Biology Organization (EMBO) at Heidelberg now has a similar journal, the *EMBO Journal*, published since 1982 from the UK.

Archives of Biochemistry and Biophysics (1942) (USA), *International Journal of Biochemistry* (1970) (UK) and *Bioscience Reports* (Short Papers and Reviews *in Molecular and Cellular Biology*) (1981) (UK) complete the list of the major journals that tend to contain papers from a variety of countries.

In addition to the above, there are an increasing number of essentially 'national' biochemical journals, and some of these are:

Acta Biochimica et Biophysica Hungarica (1966) (Hungary)

Acta Biochimica Polonica (1954) (Poland)

Biochimica e Biologia Sperimentale (1961) (Italy)

Canadian Journal of Biochemistry and Cell Biology (1923) (Canada)

Indian Journal of Biochemistry and Biophysics (1964) (India)

Physiological Chemistry and Physics and Medical NMR (1969) (USA)

Studii si Cercetari de Biochimie (1959) (Romania)

In addition to these, there are also several purely biophysical journals, of which the best known is *Biophysical Journal* (1960) (USA). Others are:

Biofizika (1956) (USSR)

Bulletin of Mathematical Biophysics (1939) (USA)

Radiation and Environmental Biophysics (1963) (Germany)

Studia Biophysica (1966) (Germany)

As one might expect in an interdisciplinary field that is growing rapidly, biochemistry has spilled out of its own journals and a large proportion of the important papers appear in more general periodicals. A large amount of literature on biochemistry, biophysics and molecular biology appears in *Nature* (1868) (UK), for example.

The *Proceedings of the National Academy of Sciences of the United States of America* (1915) has been the journal chosen for the announcement of many major biochemical discoveries, and doubtless will continue to be so in the future. Other general journals that regularly carry biochemical papers are:

Annals of the New York Academy of Sciences (1823) (USA)

Comptes Rendus des Séances de L'Académie des Sciences, Série C: Sciences Chimiques et Série D: Sciences Naturelles (1835) (France)

Doklady Akademii Nauk SSSR (1828) (USSR)

Endeavour (1942) (UK)

Experientia (1945) (Switzerland)
Life Sciences (1962) (UK)
Naturwissenschaften (1913) (Germany)
Proceedings of the Royal Society, Series B (1800) (UK)
Proceedings of the Society for Experimental Biology and Medicine (1903) (USA)
Science (1883) (USA)

In recent years, the growth in biochemistry and the increasing specialization of biochemists have led to the appearance of a number of journals covering specific areas of biochemistry. These include:

Biochemical Genetics (1967) (USA)
Biochemical Pharmacology (1951) (UK)
Biochemical Systematics and Ecology (1973) (UK)
Biopolymers (1963) (USA)
Biorheology (1962) (UK)
Carbohydrate Research (1965) (Netherlands)
Cereal Chemistry (1924) (USA)
Chemistry and Physics of Lipids (1966) (Ireland)
Comparative Biochemistry and Physiology (1960) (USA)
Enzyme (1961) (Switzerland)
Histochemical Journal (1968) (UK)
Histochemistry (1958) (Germany)
Insect Biochemistry and Journal of Insect Physiology (1971) (UK)
Journal of Bioenergetics and Biomembranes (1970) (USA)
Journal of Cellular Biochemistry (1972) (USA)
Journal of Histochemistry and Cytochemistry (1953) (USA)
Journal of Lipid Research (1959) (USA)
Journal of Neurochemistry (1957) (USA)
Journal of Steroid Biochemistry (1969) (UK)
Lipids (1966) (USA)
Journal of Nutritional Science and Vitaminology (1954) (Japan)
Lipids (1966) (USA)
Molecular and Cellular Biochemistry (1973) (Netherlands)
Molecular and Cellular Biology (1981) (USA)
Molecular Immunology (1964) (UK)
Molecular Pharmacology (1965) (USA)
Nucleic Acids Research (1974) (UK)
Photochemistry and Photobiology (1962) (UK)
Phytochemistry (1961) (UK)
Process Biochemistry (1966) (UK)
Soil Biology and Biochemistry (1969) (UK)
Steroids (1963) (USA)

A great deal of biochemical research is reported in the journals of adjoining fields of science. It is clearly not possible to mention all of these, and many are covered in other chapters of this book. Some of the more important that often contain biochemical work are listed below:

CHEMISTRY

Acta Chemica Scandinavica (1947) (Denmark)
Journal of the American Chemical Society (1879) (USA)
Journal of the Chemical Society (various sections) (1849) (UK)

PHYSIOLOGY

American Journal of Physiology (1898) (USA)
Journal of Cell Physiology (1932) (USA)
Journal of General Physiology (1918) (USA)
Journal of Physiology (1878) (UK)
Pflügers Archiv: European Journal of Physiology (1868) (Germany)

PHARMACY AND PHARMACOLOGY

British Journal of Pharmacology (1947) (UK)
Journal of Pharmacology and Experimental Therapeutics (1909) (USA)
Journal of Pharmacy and Pharmacology (1919) (UK)
Journal of Pharmaceutical Sciences (1911) (USA)

MEDICINAL CHEMISTRY AND BIOCHEMISTRY

Arzneimittelforschung (1951) (Germany)
Biochemical Medicine (1967) (USA)
Journal of Experimental Medicine (1896) (USA)
Journal of Medicinal Chemistry (1959) (USA)

MICROBIOLOGY

Archives of Microbiology (1930) (Germany)
Journal of Applied Bacteriology (1945) (UK)
Journal of Bacteriology (1916) (USA)
Journal of General Microbiology (1947) (UK)
Journal of General Virology (1967) (UK)
Microbiology and Immunology (1957) (Japan)

AGRICULTURAL AND FOOD CHEMISTRY

Journal of the Agricultural Chemical Society of Japan (1924) (Japan)
Journal of Agricultural and Food Chemistry (1950) (USA)
Journal of Food Science (1936) (USA)
Journal of the Science of Food and Agriculture (1953) (UK)

MEDICAL PHYSICS

Physics in Medicine and Biology (1956) (UK)

CANCER RESEARCH

British Journal of Cancer (1947) (UK)
Cancer (1948) (USA)
Cancer Research (1944)
European Journal of Cancer and Clinical Oncology (1965) (UK)
International Journal of Cancer (USA)
Japanese Journal of Cancer Research: Gann (1907) (Japan)
Journal of the National Cancer Institute (1940) (USA)

NUTRITION

British Journal of Nutrition (1947) (UK)
Journal of Nutrition (1928) (USA)

BIOENGINEERING

Biotechnology and Bioengineering (1962) (USA)
Journal of Medical Engineering and Technology (1977) (UK)
Medical and Biological Engineering and Computing (1963) (UK)

CELL SCIENCE

Journal of Cell Biology (1955) (USA)
Journal of Cell Science (1966) (UK)

In addition to these, there are the specialized journals for the clinical biochemist, such as:

Clinica Chimica Acta (1956) (Netherlands)
Clinical Chemistry (1955) (USA)
Clinical and Experimental Pharmacology and Physiology (1974)
Clinical Pharmacology and Therapeutics (1960) (USA)
Clinical Science (1933) (UK)
European Journal of Clinical Pharmacology (1968) (Germany)
Journal of Clinical Pathology (1947) (UK)
Journal of Laboratory and Clinical Medicine (1915) (USA)
Laboratory Investigation (1952) (USA)
Medical Laboratory Sciences (1944) (UK)
Metabolism Clinical and Experimental (1952) (USA)
Scandinavian Journal of Clinical Laboratory Investigation (1949) (Norway)

And also there are the very useful journals devoted to techniques, of which the most significant are:

Chromatographia (1968) (Germany)

Journal of Chromatographic Science (1969) (USA)

Journal of Chromatography (1958) (Netherlands)

Journal of Electron Microscopy (1953) (Japan)

Journal of Labelled Compounds (1969) (Belgium)

Laboratory Practice (1952) (UK)

Medical Laboratory Sciences (1915) (USA)

Organic Mass Spectrometry (1968) (UK)

Science Tools — The LKB Instrument Journal (1953) (Sweden)

Separation Science (1966) (USA)

And, most important of all the methodological journals, there is *Analytical Biochemistry* (1960) (USA).

As the amount of biochemical research undertaken and the number of practising biochemists have increased, so the pressure on space in the established journals has caused them to increase in size, and has brought new ones into being. Further, the rapid development of the subject has brought impatience with the slow and gentlemanly publishing methods that once prevailed. The 'Letter to *Nature*' has long been popular with authors as a vehicle for brief and urgent communications of important discoveries; work can appear in print within a month of being written. The popularity of this method of publication led to the establishment of *Biochemical and Biophysical Research Communications*, which photographically reproduces the author's typescript to achieve very rapid publication of short reports. *FEBS Letters*, produced by the Federation of European Biochemical Societies, now provides a European counterpart. Established journals carrying full-length papers now often contain a section of short communications, receiving accelerated treatment: *Biochimica et Biophysica Acta* and *Biochemical Journal* now both do this. None of these fast-publishing media, however, dispenses with strict editorial control of the quality of the papers; the short papers, like full-length papers in all the reputable primary journals, are published only after being approved by acknowledged scientific experts acting as editors and referees. It was intended that these fast-publishing media should carry preliminary reports of work that would ultimately appear as a full-length archival paper, and consequently the editing of the short papers is less stringent than that of full-length ones. Unfortunately it often happens that the fuller paper never appears, and the short communication remains the only report in the literature of that particular piece of work. Another recently launched rapid-publication journal for short papers is *Bioscience Reports*.

The Elsevier–North Holland group of publishers has also launched a series of rapid publication journals called *Trends in ...*, in newspaper format. *Trends in Biochemical Sciences*, known as *TIBS*, is probably the most successful of these chatty news journals; it was founded in 1976. It has been joined by *Trends in Pharmacological Science* (*TIPS*), founded in 1980, and *Trends in Genetics* (1985). All three are edited from Elsevier's Cambridge (UK) offices.

Abstracts, title-lists and indexes

It is impossible for a hard-working research scientist to look at all the journals that might contain articles of interest, and for many years scientists have depended on abstracting journals. The first twenty sections of *Chemical Abstracts* cover biochemistry very fully. These sections are listed in Table 8.2; they appear fortnightly in the odd-numbered issues. Certain biochemical papers — notably those on biochemical macromolecules — can appear in other sections of *Chemical Abstracts*. The biochemical sections can be purchased as a separate publication if required, though such a purchase does not include any volume indexes. *Chemical Abstracts* covers conference proceedings, books and patents as well as journal articles. *Biological Abstracts* also covers this field in its sections entitled 'Biochemistry', 'Metabolism', 'Enzymes' and 'Biophysics'. Biochemical papers in other sections (such as 'Chemotherapy',

Table 8.2. Biochemical sections of *Chemical Abstracts*, 1990

Section number	Section title
1	Pharmacology
2	Hormones (mammalian)
3	Biochemical genetics
4	Toxicology
5	Agrochemicals
6	General biochemistry
7	Enzymes
8	Radiation biochemistry
9	Biochemical methods
10	Microbial biochemistry
11	Plant biochemistry
12	Non-mammalian biochemistry
13	Mammalian biochemistry
14	Mammalian pathological biochemistry
15	Immunochemistry
16	Fermentations and bioindustrial chemistry
17	Food and feed chemistry
18	Animal nutrition
19	Fertilizers, soils, and plant nutrition
20	History, education and documentation

'Medical and Clinical Microbiology', 'Muscle', 'Immunology' or 'Plant Physiology, Biochemistry and Biophysics' can be traced by use of the CROSS index. The publishers of Biological Abstracts also publish BioResearch Index, a Keyword-in-Context (KWIC) index of papers and conference proceedings that are *not* included in *Biological Abstracts*. Another abstracts journal in this field is *Excerpta Medica*; Section 29: 'Biochemistry', contains relevant abstracts in this field, but Section 3: 'Endocrinology', Section 4: 'Microbiology' and Section 26: 'Immunology, Serology and Transplantation' may contain items of biochemical interest as well. The biochemical sections of two famous general abstracting journals — the French *PASCAL* and the Russian *Referativnyi Zhurnal* — are also very valuable, especially for their coverage of foreign-language material.

Each of these journals gives full bibliographical references to papers, a summary of their contents, and author and subject indexes. A somewhat different type of abstract is provided by *Current Abstracts of Chemistry and Index Chemicus*. Here the abstracts are mostly in the form of structural diagrams of chemical compounds, with little text; however, it is a rather specialized abstracts journal covering organic and pharmaceutical chemistry, and biochemistry is rather on the fringe of its coverage. Numerous other specialized abstracts journals exist; a relevant title worth mentioning here is *Analytical Abstracts*, useful for methodological information. The British company Information Retrieval Ltd. has now sold its abstracts journals, including *Genetics Abstracts, Virology and AIDS Abstracts, CSA Biochemistry Abstracts* and *Microbiology Abstracts* to Cambridge Scientific Abstracts of Bethesda, Maryland.

Clinical biochemistry has, since 1969, had its own abstracts journal, entitled *Clinical Biochemistry*. There is another named *Current Clinical Chemistry* (Pergamon, 1974–).

There are other journals which give only the titles and bibliographic references of papers, without any abstract. The most widely used of these is *Current Contents*, which consists of photographic reproductions of the contents pages of the original journals. There are several editions in different subject areas, each appearing weekly; *Current Contents: Life Sciences* covers biochemistry and chemistry. It also contains an author index to the title pages. Another title-list journal is the computer-produced *Chemical Titles*; the main body of the journal consists of a KWIC index of the titles; each index entry gives an abstract number, and this refers to a list of the full bibliographic citations in the back of the issue. Biochemistry is towards the margin of the coverage of *Chemical Titles*, however, *Index Medicus* is another title-list journal; in this case the entries are given under index headings, chosen from a standard list of terms (Medical Subject Headings). Many of the more medical biochemical papers appear in it (see Chapter 3).

Reviews

While the abstracts and the title-list journals help the scientist to keep up with the flood of new papers appearing, they do not offer any critical appraisal of the research. In most fields of science, there are now regular series of publications entitled *Annual Review of ..., Advances in ..., Progress in ...,* or some similar title. In these volumes, which are usually annual and in hard covers, acknowledged authorities review the year's progress in various fields, sifting the work and criticizing it, and providing bibliographies. Usually the book contains a number of such review articles, so as to cover the whole range of the subject given in the book's title. These volumes are of great value to research workers, especially, perhaps, in keeping up to date in fields a little way removed from their central interest. Numerous such series exist in biochemistry and biophysics, of which the most important is probably *Annual Review of Biochemistry*, published by Annual Reviews Inc., founded in 1932.

Other more specialized publications are:

Advances in Carbohydrate Chemistry and Biochemistry (Academic Press)

Advances in Comparative Physiology and Biochemistry (Academic Press)

Advances in Enzyme Regulation (Pergamon Press)

Advances in Enzymology (Wiley Interscience)

Advances in Lipid Research (Academic Press)

Advances in Microbial Physiology (Academic Press)

Advances in Prostaglandin, Thromboxane and Leukotriene Research (Raven)

Advances in Protein Chemistry (Academic Press)

Advances in Second Messenger and Phosphoprotein Research (Raven)

Advances in Steroid Biochemistry and Pharmacology (Academic Press)

Progress in Biochemical Pharmacology (Karger)

Progress in Nucleic Acid Research and Molecular Biology (Academic Press)

Progress in Phytochemistry (Interscience)

Recent Progress in Hormone Research (Academic Press)

Subcellular Biochemistry (Plenum)

For the biophysicist there is also *Advances in Biophysics* (Japan Scientific Societies Press/Elsevier), and for the clinical biochemist there are *Advances in Clinical Chemistry* (Academic Press), *Progress in Clinical Pathology* (Grune and Stratton), *Year Book of Pathology and Clinical Pathology* (Year Book Medical Publishers) and *Recent Advances in Clinical Biochemistry* (Churchill Livingstone).

Series in adjoining fields often contain reviews relevant to biochemists; among these are:

Advances in Applied Microbiology (Academic Press)

Advances in Biomedical Engineering (Academic Press)

Advances in Cancer Research (Academic Press)

Advances in Drug Research (Academic Press)

Advances in Immunology (Academic Press)

Advances in Metabolic Disorders (Academic Press)

Advances in Pharmaceutical Sciences (Academic Press)

Advances in Pharmacology and Chemotherapy (Academic Press)

Annual Reports on the Progress of Chemistry (The Royal Society of Chemistry)

Annual Review of Microbiology (Annual Reviews Inc.)

Annual Review of Pharmacology and Toxicology (Annual Reviews Inc.)

Annual Review of Physiology (Annual Reviews Inc.)

Annual Review of Plant Physiology (Annual Reviews Inc.)

Current Topics in Membranes and Transport (Academic Press)

Progress in Industrial Microbiology (Churchill Livingstone)

Progress in Medical Genetics (Grune and Stratton)

Progress in Medicinal Chemistry (North-Holland)

Progress in Medicinal Chemistry (Butterworths)

Year Book of Cancer (Year Book Medical Publishers)

All these series are annual and in hard covers. There are also review journals that appear more frequently, commonly quarterly, in soft covers; they do not attempt to cover the whole of their field in each issue. No such journal exists in biochemistry, but in biophysics there are *Quarterly Review of Biophysics* and *Progress in Biophysics and Molecular Biology* — the latter was formerly one of the annual volumes, but has been converted into a review journal. In adjoining fields there are:

Bacteriological Reviews

Biological Reviews

British Medical Bulletin

Chemical Reviews

Royal Society of Chemistry Reviews (a merger of *Quarterly Reviews of the Chemical Society* and *Royal Institute of Chemistry Reviews*)

Physiological Reviews

In biochemistry there exists also *Essays in Biochemistry*; this appears annually in soft covers and contains a number of specialized reviews, but not a comprehensive coverage every year. The value of this publication is that it is aimed at undergraduates reading biochemistry, and therefore assumes rather less prior knowledge than most scientific journals. It is published by Academic Press for the Biochemical Society. The same idea has now been extended to clinical biochemistry. The Biochemical Society and the Association of Clinical Biochemists jointly publish *Essays in Medical Biochemistry*, the first issue of which appeared in 1975. In a similar context, mention should be made of *Scientific American*; articles in this journal often give excellent coverage of a topic for a newcomer.

Some journals mostly concerned with primary scientific papers include review articles from time to time. Among journals that do this are *Journal of Lipid Research* and *Physics in Medicine and Biology*. The journal *Progress in Histochemistry and Cytochemistry* (Gustav Fischer Verlag) appears in soft covers and consists of just one review per issue. Recently, the *Biochemical Journal* has started to carry reviews, and for readers' convenience these are republished at the end of the year bound together in an extra issue entitled *BJ Reviews*.

Finally, among these various types of review, come the less frequent type of review series that attempt to take a longer term view of progress, no easy task in such a rapidly evolving subject, but one that needs to be undertaken by some leading researchers if the subject is to have a sense of direction. Unfortunately, the three main series that exist have all been allowed to fall seriously behind events; it is to be hoped that at least one of them will appear again in a new edition. They are:

Currents in Biochemical Research, edited by D. E. Green (3rd edn., Wiley Interscience, 1968)

Progress in biochemistry since 1949, edited by F. Haurowitz (5th edn., Wiley Interscience, 1959)

Recent advances in biochemistry, edited by T.W. Goodwin (4th edn., Churchill, 1960)

To assist in keeping track of the review literature, a third tier of 'indexes to reviews' now exists. Relevant to the problem in biochemistry are:

Bibliographic Index, edited by M. Frank (Wilson, 1958–)

Index to Reviews, Symposia, Volumes and Monographs in Organic Chemistry (Pergamon, 1962–)

Each of these is a continuing series, updated annually.

Conferences and symposia

Another source of information that is extensively used in many fast-progressing areas of science is the scientific meeting, conference or symposium. These can be divided into two types: the regular general meetings of scientific societies, and specialized meetings to discuss a particular topic, though there are, of course, borderline cases. The general meetings — international, or more local — provide opportunities for scientists to deliver a large number of short papers describing their current work. The information that emerges from them is therefore up to date, but it is usually subject to far less quality control than is applied to journal articles. Some of the work subsequently appears in such articles, in a fuller form; other pieces of work do not reach a conclusive enough state for publication and are never heard of again. In the biochemical field the most important such meetings are the International Congresses of Biochemistry, of which a number have now been held. The publication of their proceedings has taken rather variable forms; for example, the fourth congress (Vienna, 1958) ran to 15 volumes because full texts of all the papers were given, whereas the sixth (New York, 1964) appeared in only two volumes. In the latter case, only abstracts of the ordinary papers were issued, and they occupied one volume; the plenary lectures, which are of a more review-like nature, were given in full in the other volume.

The meetings of the Federation of European Biochemical Societies are of similar importance; their proceedings are, however, published as a regular series, Proceedings of the Federation of European Biochemical Societies. In the USA a number of societies publish their proceedings in a joint journal called *Federation Proceedings*, the joint body being called the Federation of American Societies for Experimental Biology. Closer to home, the papers given at the regular meetings of the (UK) Biochemical Society are published as *Biochemical Society Transactions*; again, however, it must be stressed that they are not subject to the editorial control that is applied to the *Biochemical Journal*. The Biochemical Society also holds more specialized symposia from time to time, and these are published as a separate series entitled *Biochemical Society Symposia*.

The information value of the large general meetings is, however, probably greater for those who attend the meetings than for those who read the proceedings afterwards. The specialized symposia, on the other hand, often provide, in their published proceedings, reviews of specialized topics that remain authoritative and valuable for years. Important series of symposia regularly covering biochemical topics are:

Biochemical Society Symposia
Brookhaven Symposia in Biology
Ciba Foundation Symposia
Cold Spring Harbor Symposia on Quantitative Biology
Colloquia on Protides of the Biological Fluids
Federation Proceedings, Symposia
Symposia of the International Society for Cell Biology
Symposia of the Society for Experimental Biology
Symposia of the Society for General Microbiology

Each of these series is published regularly, on a different topic on each occasion, in book form except for the last mentioned. If a recent volume in one of these series covers a topic of interest, it will be of great value.

There are, of course, also many 'one-off' symposia and ones in lesser series, whose proceedings subsequently appear. These can be difficult to track down, though they are covered by *Chemical Abstracts*. Some examples are:

Regulation of macromolecular synthesis by low molecular weight mediators, edited by G. Koch and D. Richter (Academic Press, 1979)

Nonsense mutations and tRNA suppressors, edited by J. E. Celis and D. Smith (Academic Press, 1979)

Natural sulfur compounds, edited by D. Cavallini, G. E. Gaull and V. Zappia (Plenum, 1980)

Biomolecular structure and function, edited by P. Agris (Academic Press, 1978)

Various lists of forthcoming and past conferences exist to help a searcher to locate an appropriate volume of proceedings. Probably the most useful is *Interdok — Directory of Published Proceedings* (Interdok Corp.). This appears monthly and gives a list of conferences, arranged chronologically by the date of the conference, each entry giving the title, editor, publisher and price of the proceedings. At the back there are indexes of subjects, sponsors, and editors of the proceedings. A similar service is provided by the *Index to Conference Proceedings* published by the British Library Document Supply Centre (Boston Spa, West Yorkshire, UK).

There are also series of invited lectures, whose published texts subsequently serve as reviews of the field. Among those that appear as independent publications are:

Ciba Lectures in Microbial Chemistry
The Harvey Lectures
E. R. Squibb Lectures on the Chemistry of Microbial Products

Other similar lectures are given in response to the award of a medal or prize to a distinguished scientist by a scientific society, and are subsequently published in the society's journal. Journals which contain such lectures from time to time include the *Biochemical Journal*, *Journal of General Microbiology* and *European Journal of Biochemistry*.

Metabolic maps

A form of 'review' which is peculiar to biochemistry is the metabolic map. This is a chart showing diagrammatically the metabolic pathways that have been demonstrated to exist. These are often supplied by the manufacturers or distributors of biochemical laboratory materials. Koch-Light Laboratories, for example, distribute a large chart entitled

Metabolic pathways by D. E. Nicholson, which is updated annually. It is in four colours and covers all the main areas of metabolism. It is accompanied by an explanatory booklet containing an index and notes on the reactions. The same author, with S. Dagley, has also produced a more detailed book entitled *An introduction to metabolic pathways* (Blackwell, 1970), in which the evidence for the pathways is presented. Two other manufacturers who produce charts are Boehringer (*Biochemical pathways*, two charts, 1965) and Gilson Medical Electronics (*Intermediary metabolism* by H. J. Sallech and R. W. McGilvery, four charts, 1963). The famous biochemist W. W. Umbreit produced a set of charts bound into book form, entitled *Metabolic maps* (two volumes, Burgess, 1952–1960), but this publication is now out of date. The textbook *Introduction to modern biochemistry* by P. Karlson (4th edn., Academic Press, 1974) contains several large pull-out charts of metabolic pathways. Another book, *Graphic biochemistry: metabolism of biological molecules* by T. B. Bennett (Macmillan, 1968), contains many reactions laid out in diagrammatic form.

Any of the large charts can be used very profitably as a rapid *aide mémoire*; it is a good idea to have one of them up on the laboratory wall so that one can consult it to refresh one's memory when reading something else.

Books

It is more true in biochemistry than in most subjects that a book is bound to be out of date before it is published, but this does not deter biochemists from writing and reading them. The books may be classified into several types:

1. Large multi-volume treatises covering an area of the subject in great depth.
2. Monographs covering a very specialized area — these may be published as part of a monograph series, of which *Methuen's Monographs on Biochemical Subjects* is probably the best known, or as an isolated event.
3. Textbooks for students at various levels.
4. Encyclopaedias and dictionaries.
5. Handbooks and other compilations of data.

The leading multi-volume treatises are:

Comparative biochemistry, edited by M. Florkin and H. S. Mason (7 vols, Academic Press, 1960–1964)

The enzymes, edited by P. D. Boyer (13 vols, 3rd edn., Academic Press, 1970–)

The carbohydrates by W. Pigman and D. Horton (3 vols, 2nd edn., Academic Press, 1972)

The proteins, edited by H. Neurath (5 vols, 3rd edn., Academic Press, 1977)

The hormones, edited by G. Pincus, K. V. Thimann and E. B. Astwood (5 vols, Academic Press, 1948–1964)

The vitamins, edited by W. W. Sebrell and R. S. Harris (vols 1–5) and P. Gyorgy and W.N. Pearson (vols 6–7) (7 vols, 2nd edn., Academic Press, 1967–)

Enzymes and metabolic inhibitors, edited by J. L. Webb (5 vols, Academic Press, 1963–)

Metabolic pathways, edited by D. M. Greenberg (6 vols, 3rd edn., Academic Press, 1965–1972)

Biochemistry of animal development, edited by R. Weber (2 vols, Academic Press, 1965–1967)

Handbuch der Pflanzenphysiologie, edited by W. Ruhland (18 vols, Springer, 1955–)

Mammalian protein metabolism, edited by H. N. Munro and J. B. Allison (4 vols, Academic Press, 1964–1970)

Molecular biology of human proteins, with special reference to plasma proteins by H.E. Schultze and J. F. Heremans (Elsevier, 1966–)

Molecular genetics, edited by J.H. Taylor (Academic Press, 1963–)

Chemistry of the amino acids by J. B. Greenstein and M. Winitz (3 vols, Wiley, 1961)

Biochemistry of the amino acids by A. Meister (2 vols, 2nd edn., Academic Press, 1965)

The amino sugars, edited by R.W. Jeanloz and E. A. Balazs (Academic Press, 1965–)

Metabolic inhibitors: a comprehensive treatise, edited by R. M. Hochester, M. Kates and J. H. Quastel (3 vols, Academic Press, 1972)

Bio-organic chemistry by E. E. van Tamelen (4 vols, Academic Press, 1978)

Isozymes: genetics and evolution by C. L. Markert (4 vols, Academic Press, 1975)

The most ambitious of these publications, however, is *Comprehensive biochemistry*, edited by M. Florkin and E. H. Stotz (36 vols, Elsevier, 1961–). This treatise covers the entire subject, each volume being devoted to a specialized area. One drawback of these treatises, especially the larger ones, is the fact that the different volumes are always out of date to different extents at any one time. Recently, a series entitled *New comprehensive biochemistry* has started to appear; it is edited by A. Neuberger and K. Brocklehurst and published by Elsevier, and the first volume on *Hydrolytic enzymes* appeared in 1987.

Monographs appear in large numbers every year. In addition to the Methuen series already mentioned, there are also three relevant series from Academic Press (*Molecular Biology, Advanced Biochemistry*, and *Medicinal Chemistry*), and also Elsevier's '*BBA Library*' (linked with the journal *Biochimica et Biophysica Acta*). Springer-Verlag produces a series called *Molecular biology, biochemistry and biophysics*. In Butterworths *MTP International review of science* there is a Biochemistry Series. Any list of recent significant titles will soon be overtaken by time, but some recent monographs are nevertheless mentioned:

Molecular biology of RNA: New perspectives by M. Inouye and B.S. Dudock (Academic Press, 1987)

Liposomes — a practical approach by R.R.C. New (IRL Press, 1990)

Eicosanides and the gastrointestinal tract, by K. Hillier (MTP Press, 1988)

Supramolecular enzyme organization by P. Friedrich (Pergamon, 1984)

Molecular biology of the gene by J.D. Watson, N.H. Hopkins, J.W. Roberts, J.A. Steitz and A.M. Weiner (4th edn., Benjamin Cummings, 1987)

Molecular mechanisms of transmembrane signalling by P. Cohen and M.D. Houslay (Elsevier, 1985)

Over the years many leading biochemists have set out to produce textbooks of the subject for students at various levels. Many of the ones now in use are of U.S. origin, and have been written in response to the trend in the USA for basic college courses in biology to have a considerable biochemical emphasis. Others are larger works, intended to cover the whole of the subject for the student specializing in it. They rarely succeed, since an undergraduate specializing in biochemistry will, by the time the latter part of the course is reached, need to be more up to date than a textbook can be. Nonetheless, every student needs to have one of the large texts within easy reach for continual reference, and these can be of similar use to non-students. Not all the major textbooks have been regularly up-dated, and the appended list includes only those that have appeared in a new edition relatively recently:

Biochemistry, by F.B. Armstrong (2nd edn., Oxford University Press, USA, 1983)

Introduction to physiological and pathological chemistry, by L.E. Arnow (9th edn., Mosby, 1976)

The biochemistry of the tissues, by W. Bartley and L.M. Birt (2nd edn., Received, Wiley, 1976)

Biochemistry: a comprehensive review, by N.V. Bhagavan (2nd edn., Lippincott, 1978)

Biochemistry illustrated, by P.N. Campbell and A.D. Smith (Churchill Livingstone, 1988)

Lecture notes on biochemistry, by J.K. Candlish (Blackwell Scientific, 1984)

Outlines of biochemistry, by E.E. Conn, P.K. Stumpf, G. Bruening and R.H. Doi (5th edn., Wiley, 1987)

Biochemistry, by S.P. Datta and J.H. Ottaway (3rd edn., Baillière Tindall, 1976)

Review of physiological chemistry, by H.A. Harper (21st edn., Lange Medical, 1988) (now entitled *Harper's Biochemistry*)

Principles of biochemistry, by A.L. Lehninger (2nd edn., Worth Publishers Inc., 1982)

Biochemistry — a case-oriented approach, by R. Montgomery, K.L. Dryer, T.W. Conway and A.A. Spector (3rd edn., Mosby, 1980)

Human biochemistry, by J.H. Ottaway and D.K. Apps (4th edn., Baillière Tindall, 1984)

The chemistry of life, by S. Rose (2nd edn., Pelican, 1979)

Biochemistry, by L. Stryer (3rd edn., Freeman, 1988)

Principles of biochemistry, E.L. Smith, R.L. Hill, I.R. Lehman, R.J. Lefkowitz, P. Handler and A. White (7th edn., McGraw-Hill, 1983)

Comprehensible biochemistry, by M. Yudkin and R. Offord (Longmans, 1973)

Biochemistry, by G. Zubay (2nd edn., Macmillan, USA, 1988)

Textbooks on the clinical side are *Textbook of clinical chemistry*, by N.W. Tietz (10th edn., Saunders, 1986), *Clinical chemical pathology*, by C.H. Gray, P.J.N. Howorth and M.G. Rinster (10th edn., Edward Arnold, 1985), *A new short textbook of chemical pathology*, by D.N. Baron, J.T. Whicker and K.E. Lee (5th edn., Edward Arnold, 1989) and *Varley's practical clinical chemistry*, edited by Alan H. Gowenlock (8th edn., Heinemann, 1988).

A recent development is the appearance of programmed texts for biochemistry students. Unlike more orthodox textbooks, these cannot be used as reference books, but only as learning aids. As such, therefore, they are perhaps of less interest to the average reader of this book; a few are, however, mentioned, in case the reader should happen to be a complete newcomer to biochemistry:

Guide to cellular energetics, by L.C. Carter (W.H. Freeman, 1973)

Multiple choice questions in biochemistry, H. Hassall, A.J. Turner and E.J. Wood (Churchill Livingstone, 1985)

Life's basis: macromolecules, by G.E. Parker and T.B. Mertens (Wiley, 1973)

Biochemistry — a functional approach, by R.W. McGilvery (3rd edn., Saunders, 1983)

Also aimed at the student reader are books of quantitative problems for use as exercises, such as *Quantitative problems in biochemistry*, by E.A. Dawes (6th edn., Longmans, 1980) and *Quantitative problems in biochemical science* by R. Montgomery and C.A. Swenson (2nd edn., Freeman, 1976).

There have been very few attempts to produce alphabetically arranged dictionaries or encyclopaedias in this field, possibly because of the frequent updatings that would be necessary. An attempt is *The encyclopaedia of biochemistry*, edited by R.J. Williams and E.M. Lansford, Jr (Van Nostrand Reinhold, 1967), which is very useful as a quick reference tool for information outside one's own special area of knowledge. Another is *Concise encyclopedia of biochemistry*, by M. Brewer and T. Scott (de Gruyter, 1983), a translation of *Brockhaus ABC Biochemie*, Leipzig).

The Merck Index of chemicals and drugs (11th edn., 1989), though confined to information about individual compounds, is another very useful tool. Two other alphabetical books, both edited by P. Gray, that are also of value in the biochemical field are *Encyclopaedia of biological sciences* (2nd edn., Van Nostrand Reinhold, 1969) and *Dictionary of the biological sciences* (1967), Further alphabetical dictionaries have also appeared: *Dictionary of biochemistry* by J. Stenesh (Wiley-Interscience, 1975), *Glossary of molecular biology* by A. Evans (Butterworths, 1974) and, on the clinical side, *Glossary of clinical chemical terms* by P. Haisman and B. Muller (Butterworths, 1974), and *A–Z of clinical chemistry* by W. Hood (MTP Press, 1980).

A number of handbooks exist for use when one needs not so much a full discussion or a definition, but more a single piece of reliable data. The 'Rubber Bible', *Handbook of chemistry and physics* (71st edn.,

1990), is as indispensable to biochemists or biophysicists as it is to their non-biological colleagues. The same publishers (Chemical Rubber Publishing Co.) have now also produced other handbooks more specifically for biochemists: *Handbook of biochemistry and molecular biology* (3rd edn., 1976) and *Practical handbook of biochemistry and molecular biology* (1989). Apart from these, the most important purely biochemical handbook is probably *Data for biochemical research*, edited by R.M.C. Dawson, D.C. Elliot, W.H. Elliot and K.M. Jones (3rd edn., 1986); it is designed specifically to be useful in the laboratory and has therefore been kept compact. For more exhaustive coverage, one might turn to *The biochemist's handbook* edited by C. Long (1961), which contains over 300 tables of data on all aspects of biochemistry — for example, enzymes, chemical composition of biological tissues, nutritional data and metabolic pathways. It is now out of date and a new edition would be welcome. Another compilation that, like the *Merck Index*, concentrates on compound data is *Specifications and criteria of biochemical compounds* (Committee on Biological Chemistry and Chemical Technology, U.S. National Academy of Sciences); this is loose-leaf so that supplements can be added to it. It first appeared in 1960 and supplements have appeared since. It gives full information on each compound: structure, sources, method of preparation, physical criteria (melting point, specific rotation, chromatographic mobilities and extinction coefficients), methods of assay, stability, and methods of storage. Another handbook of considerable value is *Biochemisches Taschenbuch* edited by H. M. Rauen (2 vols, 2nd edn., 1964), and another is *Handbook of biochemistry and biophysics*, edited by H. C. Ramm (1966). Several handbooks that cover parts of the subject exist; these include *The enzyme handbook* edited by T. E. Barman (1969, 2 vols; Supplement I, 1974) and *The Pfizer handbook of microbial metabolites. Atlas of protein structure and sequence*, edited by M. O. Dayhoff, attempts to give the amino acid sequence of every protein for which the sequence has been determined, and by 1978 had reached the third supplementary volume to volume 5. A competitor to Dayhoff is *Handbook of protein sequence analysis* by L. R. Croft (2nd edn., Wiley, 1980), and an equivalent volume in a specialized area of protein chemistry is *Variable regions of immunoglobulin chains* by E. A. Kabat, T. T. Wu and H. Bilofsky (National Institutes of Health, 1976). New computer-based databanks of sequences have now largely replaced these printed works, and are discussed in the last section of this chapter. An indispensable volume for the serious biochemist is *Enzyme nomenclature: recommendations 1978 of the International Union of Pure and Applied Chemistry and the International Union of Biochemistry* (Academic Press, 1979); this gives not only the rules for the classification and nomenclature of enzymes, but also coverage of enzyme kinetics; it also contains 3859 references and is thus an important bibliography of enzymology.

There are also two handbooks designed for the clinical biochemist. The older one is another of the Chemical Rubber Publishing's publications, *Handbook of clinical laboratory data* (2nd edn., 1968), and the newer is *Biochemical values in clinical medicine* by R. D. Eastham (7th edn., John Wright, 1985).

Methods and techniques

The importance of technical information has already been stressed and some specifically 'methods' journals have been mentioned. However, many of the most important techniques were originally described in the 'experimental' section of a paper in a general biochemical journal. The most celebrated example is a paper by O. H. Lowry (*Journal of Biological Chemistry*, vol. 193, page 265, 1951). This paper describes the standard method of measuring the concentration of protein in a solution and is reckoned to be the most frequently cited reference in the whole of science. How would one find a similar, but less famous, reference to a method, if one did not know where to look?

There fortunately exist numerous handbooks of laboratory methods for biochemists. Some of these appear as serial publications, often annually:

Methods of biochemical analysis, edited by D. Glick (Interscience, 1954–). Volumes appear annually, and both chemical and biological assays of materials of biochemical importance are described in full laboratory detail.

Biochemical preparations (Wiley, 1949–) appears less frequently (about once every 1–2 years) and gives details of methods for the preparation or isolation of compounds and enzymes, independently checked.

Methods in medical research (Year Book Medical Publishers, 1955–) is more general but usually includes methods of interest to the biochemist.

Chromatography reviews, edited by M. Lederer (Elsevier, 1959–), which covers electrophoretic as well as chromatographic methods, is an important aid to the biochemist, these separation methods being so central in biochemical research.

Advances in tracer methodology, edited by S. Rothschild (Plenum, 1962–), covers this important area of isotopic tracer methods.

Methods in enzymology, previously edited by S. P. Colowick and N. O. Kaplan, but now with various editors (Academic Press,

1955–), was originally a multi-volume treatise, but since 1966 has been converted into a serial publication, volumes appearing two or three times a year. It is probably the most authoritative of these series, the scope of the work being far broader than the title suggests. Methods for the preparation and for the assay of a large number of enzymes are indeed given, but so are the preparation of enzyme substrates, methods for the handling of biological materials, protein purification techniques, metabolic studies and isotopic methods. Sufficient detail is given for the methods to be used without further reading. Volume 183 (1990), entitled *Molecular evolution — Computer analysis of protein and nucleic acid sequences*, edited by R.F. Doolittle, covers a field which is considered in more detail later in this chapter.

Advances in Chromatography is edited by J.C. Giddings and R.A. Keller (Arnold, 1966–).

Laboratory techniques in biochemistry and molecular biology, originally edited by T. S. Work and E. Work (North-Holland, 1969) is one of the major series of this type; it had reached volume 19 by 1988, by which time R.H. Burdon and P.H. van Klippenberg had become series editors.

Methods in molecular biology, edited by J.A. Last and A.I. Laskin (Marcel Dekker, 1972–) covers the important molecular biological area.

Clinical biochemistry is also served by one of the series, *Standard methods of clinical chemistry*, edited by D. Seligson (Academic Press, 1953–).

Several large treatises exist on the methodological side of biochemistry. Amongst these are:

Methods in hormone research, edited by R.I. Dorfmann (2nd edn., Academic Press, 1968–)

Physical techniques in biological research, edited by G. Oster and A. W. Pollister (6 vols, 2nd edn., Academic Press, 1968)

Techniques in protein biosynthesis, edited by P. N. Campbell and J. R. Sargent (3 vols, Academic Press, 1967–1973)

Newer methods of nutritional biochemistry, by A. A. Albanese (Academic Press, 1964–)

Methods in carbohydrate chemistry, edited by R. L. Whistler and M. L. Wolfrom (5 vols, Academic Press, 1962–1965)

Moderne Methoden der Pflanzenanalyse, edited by K. Paech and M. V. Tracey (vols 1–4), H. F. Liskens and M. V. Tracey (vols 5–) (Springer, 1956–). This book is mostly in English

Experimental biochemistry, by J. M. Clark and R. L. Switzer (Freeman, 1977)

Electron microscopy of enzymes, edited by M. A. Hayat (4 vols, Van Nostrand Reinhold, 1975)

A laboratory manual of analytical methods in protein chemistry, edited by P. Alexander and R. J. Block (5 vols to date, Pergamon, 1960–)

Monographs on methods are legion, but some are in such constant use in biochemical laboratories that they must be singled out. I. Smith's *Chromatographic and electrophoretic techniques* (vol. 1: *Chromatography*; vol. 2: *Electrophoresis*) (4th edn., Heinemann, 1976) is an essential book of this kind. Other important works on separation methods are:

Separation methods in biochemistry, by C.J.O.R. Morris and P. Morris (Pitman, 1964)

New biochemical separations, by A. T. James and L. J. Morris (Van Nostrand, 1963)

Separation techniques in chemistry and biochemistry, by R. A. Keller (Dekker, 1967)

Laboratory handbook of chromatographic methods, edited by O. Mikes (Van Nostrand, 1966)

Separation methods in organic chemistry and biochemistry, by F. J. Wolf (Academic Press, 1969)

There are also numerous more specialized works on different separation methods. A representative selection is given:

Thin-layer chromatography: a laboratory handbook, by J. S. Kirshner (Interscience, 1967)

Quantitative paper and thin-layer chromatography, edited by E. J. Shellard (Academic Press, 1968)

Techniques of thin-layer chromatography in amino acid and peptide chemistry, by G. Pataki (2nd edn., Ann Arbor Science Publishers, 1968)

The practice of gas chromatography, by L. S. Ettre and A. Zlatkis (Interscience, 1967)

A programmed introduction to gas chromatography, by J. B. Pattison (Heyden, 1969)

Gas-phase chromatography of steroids, by K. B. Eik-Nes and E. C. Horning (Springer, 1968)

Quantitative gas–liquid chromatography of amino acids in proteins and biological substances, by C. W. Gehrke (Analytical Biochemistry Laboratories, 1969)

Gas chromatography, by H. Determan (Springer, 1968)

Electrophoresis, by D. J. Shaw (Academic Press, 1969)

Electrophoresis and immunoelectrophoresis, by L. Cawley (Little, Brown, 1969)

Methods in zone electrophoresis, by J. R. Sargent (BDH Publication, 1969)

Gel electrophoresis of nucleic acids: a practical approach, by D. Rickwood and B. D. (Hames, IRL Press, 1982)

As mentioned earlier, the use of radioactive tracers in elucidating biological reactions has been very great and, not surprisingly, large numbers of books on these techniques have also appeared. Some of these are mentioned below:

Principles of radioisotope methodology, by G. D. Chase and J. L. Rabinowitz (2nd edn., Burgess, 1966)

Radiotracer techniques in biological sciences, by C. H. Wang and D. L. Willis (Prentice-Hall, 1965)

Tritium-labelled molecules in biology and medicine, by L. E. Feinendegen (Academic Press, 1967)

Isotopes in biology, by G. Wolf (Academic Press, 1964)

Radioactive isotopes in biochemistry, by E. Broda (Elsevier, 1960)

Labelled nucleotides in biochemistry, by R. Monks, K. G. Oldham and K. C. Tovey
(Radiochemical Centre, 1971)

The spectroscopic techniques that have revolutionized organic chemistry in recent years have, with the exception of ultraviolet spectroscopy, been rather slower to be adopted in the biochemical laboratory. This is probably because the complexity of the chemical systems within living organisms makes the spectra very hard to interpret. Nevertheless, most of these methods have now come into use in the biochemical laboratory, often with the aid of the computer for interpretation. Books describing the particular application of these methods to biological systems are listed; there are, of course, also large numbers of books describing the techniques themselves without special reference to biological use:

Nuclear magnetic resonance in biochemistry, by T. L. James (Academic Press, 1975)

Interpretation of the ultraviolet spectra of natural products, by A. I. Scott (Pergamon, 1964)

Structure elucidation of natural products by mass spectrometry, by H. Budzikiewicz, C. Djerassi and D. H. Williams (2 vols, Holden–Day, 1964)

Magnetic resonance in biological systems, edited by A. Ehrenberg, B. G. Malstrom and T. Vanngard (Pergamon, 1967)

The biological and biochemical applications of electron spin resonance, by D. J. E. Ingram (Hilger, 1969)

Fluorescence assay in biology and medicine by S. Udenfreund (1st vol., 3rd printing, Academic Press, 1965; 2nd vol., Academic Press, 1969)

One technique very specific to biochemistry is ultracentrifugation, for the separation of sub-cellular particles and biological macromolecules, and the measurement of their molecular weights. The authoritative work on this technique is *The ultracentrifuge in biochemistry* by H. K. Schachman (Academic Press, 1959), and a very useful book for the newcomer to the subject is *An introduction to ultracentrifugation* by T. J. Bowen (Wiley, 1970). Other works on the subject are:

Mathematical theory of sedimentation analysis, by H. Fujita (Academic Press, 1962)

Ultracentrifugal analysis in theory and experiment, edited by J. W. Williams (Academic Press, 1963)

Ultracentrifugation, by J. S. McCall and B. J. Potter (Baillière Tindall, 1973)

Some of the less modern, but still important, classic methods are provided with major works that are essentials of the biochemical laboratory. One of these is H. U. Bergmeyer's *Methods of enzymatic analysis* (Verlag-Chemie and Academic Press, 1963), which describes the use of enzymes as analytical tools, often for the assay of other enzymes — a technique which has been responsible for many of the most elegant determinations of metabolic pathways, and one that also finds use in clinical biochemistry. H. U. Bergmeyer has now produced a more up-to-date book entitled *Principles of enzymatic analysis* (Verlag-Chemie, 1978). Another classic is *Manometric techniques* by W. W. Umbreit, R. H. Burris and J. F. Stauffer (Burgess, 1963). Manometric techniques were one of the earliest major tools of the biochemist, and are still very useful today in the study of any enzymic reaction that involves the evolution or absorption of a gas. The book is much more general than the title suggests and could, indeed, serve as an introductory text to practical biochemistry in general.

In the specialized but important area of protein chemistry, *Techniques in protein chemistry* by J. Leggett Bailey (2nd edn., Elsevier, 1969) was the authoritative work; it described all the major methods used in elucidating the amino acid sequence of proteins. However, this area has now been thoroughly automated (see later in this chapter) and the book is obsolete. A number of other recent books on methods in particular areas of the subject are also mentioned herein, although, as with monographs in biochemistry generally, the list given is only a selection of recent publications from an enormous number:

Biochemistry and methodology of lipids, edited by A. R. Johnson and J. B. Davenport (Wiley-Interscience, 1971)

Amino acid determination — Methods and techniques, by S. Blackburn (Arnold, 1968)

Procedures in nucleic acid research, edited by G. L. Cantoni and D. R. Davies (Harper and Row, 1967)

Protein sequence determination, edited by S. B. Needleman (Chapman and Hall, and Springer, 1970)

An introduction to isozyme techniques, by G. J. Brewer and C. F. Sing (Academic Press, 1970)

Analysis of triglycerides, by C. Litchfield (Academic Press, 1972)

A flexible system of enzymatic analysis, by O. H. Lowry and J. V. Passoneau (Academic Press, 1972)

Handbook of micromethods for the biological sciences, by G. Keleti and W. H. Lederer (Van Nostrand Reinhold, 1974)

Introduction to protein sequence analysis, by L. R. Croft (Wiley, 1980)

And, on the clinical side, there are *Clinical chemistry and automation: a study in laboratory proficiency* by R. Robinson (Griffin, 1972) and *Automation of a biochemistry laboratory* by G. E. Sims (Butterworths, 1972).

History of biochemistry

The serious student of biochemistry ought to spend at least a little time learning about the history and development of the subject; indeed, the historical method of approach improves one's understanding of some of the more complex areas of the subject, such as molecular biology. One follows the train of thought of the pioneers and thus better appreciates the reasons why currently held theories have evolved.

No journals are devoted specifically to the history of biochemistry, but papers on the history of biochemistry can be found in the more general *Journal of the History of Medicine and Allied Sciences* (1946–) (USA), *Medical History* (1957–) (UK), *Koroth* (1953–) (Israel), *Isis* (USA), *Sudhoffs Archiv* (Germany), etc. Papers in *Perspectives in Biology and Medicine* (1957–) are often written in a more personal and biographical style than those in most journals. A valuable source for biographical data is *Selected bibliography of biographical data for the history of biochemistry since 1800* by J. S. Fruton (2nd edn., American Philosophical Society, 1977).

The treatise *Comprehensive biochemistry* edited by Florkin and Stotz, mentioned earlier, devotes vols 30 to 36 to the history of the subject. The most recent editions of these volumes date from 1986. Other important works on the subject are:

The biochemical approach to life, by F. R. Jevons (2nd edn., Allen and Unwin, 1968)

Reflections on biochemistry, edited by A. Kornberg, B. L. Horecker, L. Cornudella and J. Oro (Pergamon, 1977)

From medical chemistry to biochemistry, by R.E. Kohler (CUP, 1972)

Search and discovery, edited by B. Kaminer (Academic Press, 1970)

Molecules and life, edited by J. S. Fruton (Wiley-Interscience, 1972)

Development of biochemical concepts from ancient to modern times, by H.M. Leicester (Harvard University Press, 1974)

Wanderings of a biochemist, by F. Lipmann (Wiley-Interscience, 1971)

Machina carnis: the biochemistry of muscular contraction and its historical development, by D.M. Needham (CUP, 1971)

And perhaps the most famous book yet written describing biochemical history in the making is *The double helix* by James Watson (Weidenfeld and Nicolson, 1968).

Current awareness: aid from mechanized services

A large proportion of biochemists — especially those in academic institutions — obtain help in keeping up to date from an 'invisible college' of associates, former colleagues and friends working in different laboratories around the world. The members of such informal groups correspond with one another, visit one another's laboratories, and meet at various international congresses, meetings, symposia and like events. In considering the flow of information in any science, it is important to remember the 'invisible college' and to consider both its merits and its drawbacks. Its greatest merit is its timeliness; its second is probably the ease with which one can keep up to date by this method —

indeed, research scientists tend to mingle their personal and working lives to such an extent that it may become virtually a leisure activity. Perhaps because of this, its drawbacks tend to be overlooked. First, this form of communication is rather exclusive; information reaches only those who belong to the 'college', and this tends both to intensify specialization and to undervalue work done by outsiders or written in an unfamiliar language. Secondly, the information that passes is informal, and thus research workers' enthusiasm for their current project may lead them to describe it in a biased way; also, verbal communications are unlikely to be filed properly for future reference, and the recipients of the information have to depend on their fallible memory of what was said. The 'invisible college' is probably most important at the frontiers of knowledge, where only a small number of groups of high-powered specialists are working on the same problem. Modern technology has now arrived in the invisible college; the use of the academic telecommunications networks (JANET in the UK, BitNet in the USA, etc.), themselves now interlinked, and electronic mail, bulletin board and computer conference software has now become widespread among academic biochemists. Once the number of interested parties becomes large, then the formal communication system has to be used. Biochemistry, biophysics and, especially, molecular biology are rapidly-developing subjects and thus a fair proportion of their practitioners are working on the frontiers. However, one must not forget the large groups of workers who do not belong to the international 'jet-set' of scientists — the university teachers in the lesser research schools with a large teaching load; the research workers in industrial laboratories; the practising physicians; the students. Their need for keeping up to date is for a quick method of sorting through the large weekly output of papers to establish the few that they need to read.

Many maintain that it is sufficient to scan a few leading journals — typically 15 to 20 — and that 'everything important' is in these. Many studies have demonstrated that this argument is false, relevant papers in almost any specialization being scattered over a surprisingly large number of journals. Further, this attitude tends to devalue any work not published in English. A wiser approach is regularly to scan *Current Contents* or (less effectively for biochemistry) *Chemical Titles* or *Index Medicus* for relevant-looking titles. A fair number of scientists, however, use *Chemical Abstracts*, *Biological Abstracts* or *Excerpta Medica* directly for their current awareness, despite the large number of abstracts that each now includes and the consequent tedium of scanning them.

The magnitude of the task of keeping up to date with the flood of literature has produced its own specialists, the information scientists. To date they have been more active in industrial than in academic laboratories, possibly because industry is more ready to direct the way in which research workers should use their precious time. Thus, biochemistry being an essentially academic subject, biochemists were until recently less aware than, say, chemists of recent activities in tie field of information handling.

Computer-based 'selective-dissemination-of-information' services are now publicly available in a number of disciplines. These result as by-products from the computerized typesetting now used by the major abstracts journals. The magnetic tapes used for the typesetting are themselves sold by the abstracts journals' publishers, and these can be searched by computer for topics of interest to the individual user. Large industrial concerns buy the tapes and search them in-house for their own scientists. But services are available publicly as well.

The magnetic-tape version of *Science Citation Index* (p. 54, 105) is made available by the tape's producers, the Institute for Scientific Information, whose UK office is in Uxbridge, Middlesex; and the machine-readable versions of *Chemical Abstracts* and *Biological Abstracts* are both searched by the Royal Society of Chemistry at Cambridge. One can also do current-awareness searches on the interactive online search systems mentioned below.

Each of these services searches regular issues of the tapes for the user's interests, and sends a print-out of the relevant references. It is important to realize, however, that the potential users must be prepared to put some work initially into compiling their search formulation; the computer looks only for those words it is told to look for, and thus a poorly thought-out search formulation gives poor results.

The subject area in which scientists need to keep absolutely up to date is probably fairly specific. They will, however, need to keep more generally abreast of developments in a wider area. The scientific news magazines, such as *New Scientist* and *Nature*, are helpful here. But for more regular, if less frequent, background coverage, the *Annual Reviews*, *Advances* and *Progress* series described earlier are probably paramount. Though a few months out of date when they appear, they do give authoritative descriptions of the previous year's progress in their specific fields. As the sheer quantity of scientific research increases, these reviews are likely to become more and more important — provided always that sufficiently eminent scientists are prepared to write them.

Exhaustive retrospective searches

There are a number of occasions when an exhaustive search of the past literature of a subject is needed; for example, when a completely new research project is due to commence. This is commonly when a new research student is starting work, when an industrial researcher is required to change to a new topic, or when an academic researcher moves to a different establishment with a different research emphasis. Another occasion is when some unexpected result alters the course of research, and reveals that the research team lacks knowledge of the new area. Again, results may suggest a new hypothesis, and this has to be tested by checking on past work that might refute or confirm the new theory. In all these cases one wants to find every publication that has ever had a bearing on the subject.

Such a search is usually an iterative process; the area of information required is first defined, and a first search reveals too much informtion or (less likely) too little. The area is then redefined and the search continued.

Probably the place to start in such a search is in the indexes of the appropriate review serials, or the *Interdok* index of conferences. This leads to reviews of different ages that are relevant to the topic and yield some references to the primary literature. For the period since the latest relevant review, one needs to resort to the indexes of the appropriate abstracts journal. *Chemical Abstracts* is probably the first choice. It has decennial or (more recently) quinquennial indexes; for the period since the last quinquennial index, one has to use the volume (six-month) indexes. All of these indexes can be used to search for topics or for authors, but if the subject indexes are used, it must be remembered that one is confined to the index headings which the indexer thought appropriate for the paper; titles, as such, are not indexed. For the period since the last six-month index, the KWIC index of the titles that appears at the back of each weekly issue must be used. If this last procedure seems too tedious, one could try looking through the reproduced contents pages in the recent issues of *Current Contents* instead.

Another method of covering the recent literature is to use the *Science Citation Index*, a description of which is included in Chapter 3.

Online information retrieval services

Chapter 5 of this book covers the use of online information retrieval services in the medical sciences generally, and details of accessing *Medline*, *Excerpta Medica*, etc., online will not be repeated here. However, as was mentioned above in the discussion of printed abstracts journals, the most important database for biochemists is undoubtedly *Chemical Abstracts*, which Chapter 5 does not cover. Online searching of chemical databases in general and of *Chemical Abstracts* (CA) in particular are covered in depth in Chapter 6 of the companion volume

Information sources in the chemical sciences (4th edn., 1992) entitled 'Online searching for chemical information' and written by G.G. Vander Stouw of Chemical Abstracts Service. For those without access to that volume a brief description is provided here.

Chemical Abstracts has been published since 1907 but in general only data from 1967 onwards are available in machine-readable form. The available data include the abstracts, bibliographical details and keywords, and the index entries for each paper which are used to produce the semi-annual Volume Indexes and quinquennial Collective Indexes of CA. The data are arranged in different ways by the different online hosts, whose services are as follows.

BRS	file named CHEM covers 1977 to date
CAN/OLE (Canada)	covers 1977 to date
Data-Star	file named CHEM covers 1967 to date
Dialog	file named CA Search covers 1967 to date
ESA/IRS	file named CHEMABS covers 1967 to date
Orbit	separate files cover each Collective Index period and are named from the first year of their coverage: CAS67, CAS72, CAS77, CAS82, etc.
Télésystèmes-Questel	similar to Orbit, but named EUCAS67, etc.

Each vendor has arranged each file internally to suit its own software system and command language. However, the vendor STN International, which is part-owned by Chemical Abstracts Service (CAS), has a more complete database owing to CAS's controversial policy of not releasing all of its data to other hosts. In particular, the CAS Registry System, which is a file of almost 10 million chemical substances and contains in most cases their structures in the form of connection tables, is available to STN, but not to other hosts, with the exception of Télésystèmes-Questel.

CAS Online, on STN, therefore provides (in addition to all the bibliographical, abstracts and indexes information available through the other hosts) access to the files through chemical structure and substructure searching; the user draws a structural fragment on his terminal screen and the search provides those compounds that contain the fragment. There are also services for searching for particular types of reaction (CASReact) and for searching the kind of generalized structures often found in patents (MarPat). Compounds retrieved by means of a structure search can be carried across to a bibliographical search in order to find papers referring to the compounds in question.

In general, biochemists will perhaps be slightly less interested than pure chemists in these structure search facilities, and may therefore decide to avoid the additional costs of CAS Online and utilize the other vendors listed above. One major consideration in choosing a host will be the range of other databases available with the same host; STN, in general, leans towards the physical rather than the biomedical sciences in its choice of databases. Dialog and the European host Data-Star cover the medical sciences more widely. Chemical databases are not, in general, available from BLAISE-Link or the NLM.

Databanks in molecular biology

In the rapidly advancing field of molecular biology, computerized information retrieval is becoming an integral part of the research activity itself, rather than a separate part of the scientist's work. Since the elucidation of the genetic code by Watson and Crick in 1953, research in molecular biology has concentrated on discovering the structures of nucleic acids and proteins and the relationship between their structure and function. This has resulted in the accumulation of much data on the sequences of these macromolecules (amino acid sequences of proteins and nucleotide sequences of nucleic acids) and smaller quantities of three-dimensional structure data based on X-ray crystallographic investigation. In the early period, such research was very time-consuming and the number of structures known increased only slowly. Recently, however, computerized sequencing methods have become widespread and the number of protein and nucleic acid sequences known has therefore risen rapidly, moving into the tens of thousands. Three-dimensional structures have accumulated much more slowly and the known ones are still numbered only in the hundreds; methods of predicting three-dimensional structure from one-dimensional sequence algorithmically form a very active area of current research.

Although workers in this field have published conventionally in the journal literature, printed publication is an inefficient and uneconomic way of disseminating large numbers of sequences or of crystallographical coordinates. Since in all cases today such data will have arisen from computerized laboratory equipment and therefore exist in machine-readable form from the outset, logic suggests their storage and retrieval in the same form. Furthermore, the computer–based databanks themselves form a research tool in sequencing further samples, since the databanks can be searched for near-matches of new incomplete sequences with known sequences.

Sequencing of nucleic acids is easier than sequencing proteins, largely because there are only four different nucleotide types in nucleic acids and 20 different amino acids in proteins. Nowadays, therefore, the normal procedure is to sequence a nucleic acid and then, knowing the genetic code, to predict the sequence of the protein for which the nucleic acid codes; software exists also for this translation.

This area of research has come into great prominence lately as a result of the U.S. government's decision to fund an effort to find the sequence of the entire human genome over the next 15 years. This project brings biomedical science into the arena of 'Big Science' alongside nuclear physics and astrophysics, for the first time. The project is headed by James Watson who, with Francis Crick, discovered the genetic code almost 40 years ago.

The Human Genome project will incorporate within its infrastructure a major element of computerized databank services. These will be based on existing collections of sequences and three-dimensional structures, which will, however, have to be expanded greatly and be provided with improved hardware and software accordingly. There will have to be improved co-ordination between the different services under the overall umbrella of the Human Genome project; as will be seen, this co-ordination has begun.

Volume 183 of *Methods in Enzymology*, edited by R. F. Doolittle and published in February 1990, covers the whole area of databases, databanks and computer software used in support of the molecular biology research enterprise very fully, and is recommended as further reading in this important area.

The major existing sequence collections are listed below. In general these are not accessed via the usual commercial hosts such as Dialog, STN, Data-Star, etc., but over the academic networks such as BitNet which (as mentioned above) are also increasingly used as the preferred channel of communication for informal contacts between academic scientists in the advanced countries. In addition, copies of the databanks are often held in-house at the major molecular biological research establishments, in order that they can be used as research tools in day-to-day work in the laboratory. They are distributed on floppy disks, magnetic tape, or in some cases compact disk-read only memory (CD-ROM), with regular updates.

> GenBank (Los Alamos National Laboratory, USA) — over 9000 nucleic acid sequences
>
> EMBL Data Library (European Molecular Biology Laboratory, Germany) — over 7000 nucleic acid sequences
>
> Protein Identification Resource (National Biomedical Research Foundation, USA) — over 7000 partial or complete protein sequences and over 2000 nucleic acid sequences
>
> PRF SEQDB (Protein Research Foundation Japan) — over 12 000 protein and peptide sequences

DNA Data Bank of Japan (Ministry of Education, Science and Welfare, Japan) — nucleic acid sequences

MIPS (Martinsried Institute for Protein Sequences, Germany) — protein sequences

These and some other smaller organizations are now collaborating and seeking to make their collections compatible with the National Biomedical Research Foundation in Washington, DC, which is taking the lead in managing the co-operation.

Another databank that is so far unique is the Complex Carbohydrate Structure Database, administered by the U.S. Department of Energy (DoE). While molecular-biological interest has centred on nucleic acids and proteins, many polysaccharides of biological origin have also been studied; since a proportion of proteins are glycoproteins, and the sugar moiety is often of functional significance to the protein, there is in fact a connection with the major area of interest. Only in 1986, however, was an initiative taken by the DoE to set up a databank of known polysaccharide structures; this contained 2000 entries by 1989 and is expected to contain 5000 by 1991. The file is distributed on floppy disks from the University of Georgia.

In addition to the sequence databanks mentioned above, the much smaller collection of three–dimensional structures is available in the form of the Protein Data Bank (PDB) from the Brookhaven Laboratory in the USA. This contains about 400 sets of atomic co-ordinates, although the number of proteins that have been investigated at sufficient resolution to allow the construction of an atomic model is a little higher, perhaps 500. The number of biological macromolecules that have been crystallized in pure form is about 1200, so there is a considerable backlog of work in this area. The PDB is distributed on magnetic tape. Recently a program was written which can co-ordinate searches of the PDB with those of the main sequence databanks (GenBank, etc.), as a step towards the eventual goal of predicting three-dimensional structures from sequences. If a protein of known sequence is not in the PDB (as is likely, with 14 000 sequences known and only 400 three-dimensional structures in the PDB), the program will attempt to find nearest matches amongst sequences to one whose structure is known in three dimensions. It is called Integrated Sequences Integrated Structures (ISIS).

It can be seen, therefore, that information work in the biochemical sciences has progressed from being a merely ancillary service to the research effort, to being nowadays an integral part of that effort and a major contributor to the must exciting biochemical research project ever conceived, the Human Genome project.

Acknowledgements

I am grateful to Dr J. M. Turner, author of the corresponding chapter in the companion volume on *Information sources in the biological sciences* in this series, for assisting in the compilation of lists of publications in this chapter. I also acknowledge pre-publication access to the chapter by Dr Gerald G. Vander Stouw on online chemical information in *Information sources in chemistry*, which provided information for the new section on *Chemical Abstracts* online. I thank Dr Maria Sillince, who allowed me to use information from her thesis at Loughborough University on 'Databases for the Molecular Sciences', which provided much of the new information on protein and nucleic acid structure databanks; in the same connection I thank Dr Bruce W. Birren of California Institute of Technology, especially for drawing my attention to volume 183 of *Methods in enzymology* before it was available in the UK. The opinions expressed and any errors or omissions are, however, entirely my own.

CHAPTER NINE

Public health

B. FURNER and GAYNOR MESSENGER

According to Holland *et al.* (1984)

> Public health is concerned with defining the problems facing communities in the prevention of illness and thus studies of disease aetiology and promotion of health. It covers the investigation, promotion, and evaluation of optimal health services to communities and is concerned with the wider aspects of health within the general context of health and the environment. Other terms in common use such as community medicine, preventive medicine, social medicine and population medicine have acquired different meaning according to the country or setting.

So wrote the editors of a major textbook in this subject and it is quoted to show how all-encompassing this subject is potentially – and as a consequence how difficult it is to treat in a work such as the one of which this chapter forms a part. This chapter concerns itself only with those information sources on the health of populations as a whole, and the delivery of health-care services to populations – i.e. public health in general. It encompasses the related disciplines of epidemiology and vital statistics which are the bases of all health programmes. Subjects which could be regarded traditionally as component parts of public health such as child health, geriatrics, maternity services, family planning and demography, food hygiene, water supply and sanitation, environmental hygiene and pollution are not covered explicitly though many are dealt with in the bibliographical resources listed. An exception is occupational health, as this is not dealt with elsewhere in this book and selected major, current reference sources have been included here. An attempt is made merely to guide the reader to some of the more important sources of information in selected areas. The approach is by form and then by subject: first, primary sources — textbooks, journals and official publications (including statistical sources); second, abstracting and indexing services and other bibliographies. Important organizations and libraries in the field are included at the end.

Major reference works, textbooks and monographs

Though called a textbook the *Oxford textbook of public health* (3 vols; 2nd edn., edited by W.W. Holland, R. Detels and G. Knox, Oxford, OUP, 1991) is much more an encyclopaedia of the subject. Volume 1 leads the reader through the historical determinants of health to the overall scope and strategies of public health. Major determinants of health and disease are described, with a broad outline of factors concerned with the development of disease. Methods and strategies by governments to control health hazards are discussed. Volume 2 deals with the processes of health promotion, ranging from scientific and regulatory processes used to control the physical environment and the spread of infectious diseases to the involvement of governments and international organizations. Volume 3 is concerned with the investigative methods used in public health. Major disease groups, systems of the body, and special care groups are treated systematically to review the public health issues they raise.

The American equivalent, a larger work in one volume, is the mammoth *Maxcy-Rosenau-Last public health and preventive medicine* (13th edn., edited by J. M. Last, Norwalk, CN: Appleton-Century-Crofts, 1992). This contains 75 chapters by 167 contributors arranged in sections covering public health methods; communicable diseases; environmental health; behavioural factors affecting health; non-communicable and chronic disabling conditions; and health-care planning organization and evaluation. It is an invaluable resource, particularly of statistical information and epidemiological data pertaining to specific conditions and diseases, and replete with references. One important sourcebook is the *Handbook of health, health care and the health professions*, edited by David Mechanic (Free Press, 1983). It presents issues of health and health care in broad historical and socio-cultural dimensions, examines major health risks and epidemiological studies, health-care delivery systems, and health occupations.

Many of the texts referred to in the equivalent chapter of the previous edition of this book have not in fact been superseded by new editions and the reader is referred to them: however, though they serve as valuable background reading, their date of publication renders them unsuitable for inclusion here. Four texts that can be mentioned are *Es-*

sential community medicine (including relevant social services) by R. N. and L. J. Donaldson (MTP Press, 1983); *Health, society and medicine: an introduction to community medicine* by R. M. Acheson and S. Hagard (Blackwell Scientific Publications, 1984); and, both American, *Handbook of community health* by M. Grant (4th edn., Lea & Febiger 1987) and *Community health* by L. W. Green and C. L. Anderson (5th edn. Times Mirror/Mosby, 1986).

There is a review series, of which the latest is *Recent advances in community medicine – 3*, edited by A. Smith (Churchill Livingstone, 1985). Two very useful works emanating from the Open University Press that would grace the shelves of any medical library (or interested layman) are *Health and disease: a reader*, by Nick Black and others (1984), and *The health of nations* prepared by the U205 Course Team (Book III, 1985), an explanation of national and international patterns of disease. Two monographs which offer a non-developed-country perspective on public health are *Epidemiology and the community control of disease in warm climate countries*, edited by Derek Robson (2nd edn., Churchill Livingstone, 1985) and *Strategies for primary health care: technologies appropriate for the control of disease in the developing world*, edited by J.A. Walsh and K. S. Warren (University of Chicago Press, 1986).

Organization of health services

UNITED KINGDOM

The publication of the Government White Paper *Working for patents* has set in motion a period of radical change throughout the hospital and family practitioner services sectors in the UK. An overview of the new structure and organization of the NHS resulting from this is given Chris Ham's *The new National Health Service: organization and management* (Radcliffe Medical Press, 1991). Audrey Leathard's *Health care provision: past present and future* (Chapman & Hall, 1990) summaries the development of health services in England and Wales from 1900 to 1990 and looks at the major implications of the White Paper. A brief introduction to the overall organization of the NHS is given in the National Association of Health Authorities and Trusts' *NHS handbook* (7th edn. Macmillan, 1991) edited by Barbara Connah and Ruth Pearson. This contains much useful information on many aspects of the NHS, and includes a reference section. A more in-depth account is given in Ruth Levitt and Andrew Wall's *The reorganised National Health Service* (3rd edn. Chapman & Hall, 1984). This also includes a chapter covering the different arrangements in Scotland, Wales and Northerh Ireland. However, this predates *Working for patients*.

A brief introduction to the overall organization of the NHS is given in the National Association of Health Authorities *NHS handbook* (4th edn., Macmillan, 1989) edited by Barbara Connah and Susan Lancaster. This contains much useful information on many aspects of the NHS, and includes a reference section.

The fourth edition was written before the publication of *Working for patients* but a preliminary section has been included which outlines the major proposal for reform, and summarizes the first eight working papers published immediately following the White Paper. A more in-depth account is given in Ruth Levitt and Andrew Wall's *The reorganized National Health Service* (3rd edn., Chapman & Hall, 1984). This also includes a chapter covering the different arrangements in Scotland, Wales and Northern Ireland. However, this entirely predates *Working for patients*.

Trends in policy within the NHS are analysed by a number of health service research institutes, such as the Centre for Health Economics (University of York), King's Fund Institute (King Edward's Hospital Fund for London) and Nuffield Institute for Health Service Studies (University of Leeds). Publications from these centres are a good source of current information on health services policies.

The *Hospitals and Health Services Yearbook*, edited by N. W. Chaplin and published annually by the Institute of Health Services Management is another principal source of information. It includes a listing of statutory instruments and circulars, and summarizes recent reports on the health service as well as providing a directory of addresses of a wide range of health and health-related organizations. A selected bibliography of health service literature is another valuable inclusion.

OVERSEAS

Comparative information on the structure and organization of health systems in other countries is extensive. A useful recent publication is *The international handbook of health-care systems* edited by Richard B. Saltman (Greenwood Press, 1988). This surveys 21 countries, including the UK, the USA and several Eastern European countries. A slightly older study is *Comparative health systems: descriptive analyses of fourteen national health systems* (Pennsylvania State University Press, 1984), edited by Marshall W. Raffel. *Hospital management international* (International Hospital Federation, 1989–) formerly the International Hospital Federation *Official yearbook* is a useful annual text on trends in health services internationally, and is a compilation of short papers on many health service issues.

Though not a textbook, this seems the appropriate place to refer the reader to a vital set of publications, the World Health Organization's

Seventh report on the world health situation: evaluation of the strategy for health for all by the year 2000 (WHO, 1986–87). There are 7 volumes, one for each of WHO's six regions and one giving a global review. Each regional volume gives, in varying degrees, much valuable background and statistical data concerning the health status and health systems for each country.

Current publications covering the health systems of the countries in Europe are harder to trace. The World Health Organization's *Health services in Europe* (3rd edn., WHO, 1981) is in two volumes. Volume 1 illustrates the social, political, economic and geographic factors which shape the health services in Europe, while volume 2 gives statistical information which is directly comparable for each country. The *Eurohealth handbook* (Robert S. First Inc., 1982) includes reviews of the health-care systems, morbidity, mortality, etc. of 18 European countries, and it also provides a section on 'sources of information' for statistics and government agencies in each country.

Financing of health services

UNITED KINGDOM

The reforms proposed in *Working for patients* have included major changes in health service financial arrangements. The *Introductory guide to NHS finance* (Healthcare Financial Management Association, 1991) gives a brief outline of the new arrangements, effective from April 1991. Brief outlines of the pre-White Paper financial arrangements are given in Levitt and Wall, mentioned above. An important in-depth study is Tom Jones and Malcolm Prowle's *Health service finance: an introduction* (3rd edn. Certified Accountant Educational Trust, 1987). It includes chapters on alternative sources of finance; improving efficiency; and the use of information technology in financial management.

OVERSEAS

A discussion and comparison of various methods of financing health services in the major developed countries is to be found in William A. Glaser's *Paying the hospital: the organization, dynamics and effects of differing financial arrangements* (Jossey-Bass, 1987). It covers France, Germany, England, Holland, Switzerland, Canada and the USA, and is arranged by topic rather than by country. The advantages and disadvantages of particular methods are summarized.

Two other useful publications which provide comparative analyses of health-care expenditure and systems, mainly in Europe are: *Financing and delivering health care: a comparative analysis of OECD countries* (OECD, 1987) and *Health care systems in transition: the search for efficiency* (OECD, 1990). The latter also includes a compendium of statistics on health-care expenditure and other data, which is an update of tables first published in *Measuring health care 1960–1983: expenditure, costs and performance* (OECD, 1985).

Health data and information

The six reports of the Steering Group on Health Services Information, chaired by Edith Körner (1982) outline the minimum data sets for health service information required at national and local level. The reports cover hospital services, patient transport services, manpower information, radiotherapy, paramedical services, maternity and family planning services, community services, and financial information. Phil Windsor's *Introducing Körner: a critical guide to the work and recommendations of the Steering Group on Health Services Information* (British Journal of Healthcare Computing, 1986) provides an excellent shortened guide to the six reports. A practical guide to the use and interpretation of health service statistical data in general is Christopher Day's *From figures to facts* (King's Fund on behalf of the NHS/DHSS Health Services Information Steering Group, 1985). This is aimed primarily at Health Authority members, and is useful for the general reader with no prior knowledge of statistics. It covers measures of waiting lists, bed use, planning norms, and manpower statistics, and includes case studies in the use of these measures.

Health Service indicators (or performance indicators) which allow individual health authorities to compare their own performance against that of other districts have been available since 1983. The main package is available as a set of computer discs to run on a microcomputer. In book form, *Comparing health authorities: Health Service indicators 1983–1986* (Department of Health and Social Security, 1988) covers a selection of key indicators and gives guidance on their use. Christopher Day's *Taking action with indicators* (HMSO, 1989) outlines the background to Health Service indicators and describes how they may be used to provide information in a number of different situations.

Occupational health and medicine

The International Labour Office has published the mammoth *Encyclopaedia of occupational health and safety* (2 vols; 3rd edn., 1983 reprinted with modifications 1989). It is intended for those responsible for managing workers' health and safety, especially in developing countries, as well as for those who have technical responsibilities in this field but do not have access to adequate library facilities. It contains over 1100 articles from over 1000 authors, and some 6000 bibliographical references are given. Three major British textbooks are: *Textbook of occupational medicine*, edited by J. Keir Howard and F. H. Tyrer (Churchill Livingstone, 1987); *Occupational health practice*, by H. A. Waldron (3rd edn., Butterworth, 1989); and the classic, *Hunter's Diseases of occupations* — under Hunter's authorship this work reached six editions — it is now edited by P.A.B. Raffle and others (1987, Hodder & Stoughton). Two useful quick reference books are: *Pocket consultant: occupational health* by J. M. Harrington and F. S. Gill (2nd edn., Blackwell Scientific Publications, 1987) and *A synopsis of occupational medicine* by F.H. Tyrer and K. Lee (2nd edn., Wright, 1985).

American works in this field include *Occupational medicine: principles and practical applications* by Carl Zenz (2nd edn., Year Book Medical Publishers, 1988, and *Patty's industrial hygiene and toxicology*, now edited by G. D. and F. E. Clayton (3rd edn. in 4 vols, Wiley, 1978–81).

There are two review series: *Recent advances in occupational health – 3*, edited by J. M. Harrington (Churchill Livingstone, 1987) and *Current approaches to occupational health – 3*, edited by A. Ward Gardner (Wright, 1987).

Epidemiology

There is an extensive literature on epidemiology and only major works can be listed here. An excellent sourcebook, originally produced for epidemiologists and public health workers in developing countries, is *The challenge of epidemiology: issues and selected readings*; compiled by Carol Buck and others (PAHO, 1988. *PAHO Scientific Publication No. 505*). Still a comprehensive and useful book is *Foundations of epidemiology* by A.M. and D.E. Lilienfeld (2nd edn., OUP, 1980). Three important textbooks of epidemiological theory and techniques are: *Epidemiology in medicine* by C.H. Hennekens and J.E. Buring (Little, Brown, 1987); K.J. Rothman's *Modern epidemiology* (Little, Brown, 1986); and *Mausner & Bahr Epidemiology — an introductory text*, by J. J. Mausner and S. Kramer (2nd edn., Saunders, 1985).

Those seeking information on the epidemiology of diseases in general may find these works of interest: *A world geography of human disease*, edited by G.M. Hoare (Academic Press, 1977); *The epidemiology of diseases*, by D.L. Miller and R.D.T. Farmer (Blackwell, 1982); *Epidemiology of common diseases* by H. Pedeh and R.F. Heller (Heinemann, 1984); and *The geography of non-infectious disease* by M.S.R. Hutt and D.P. Burkett (OUP, 1986).

Though beyond the scope of this chapter, demography and population studies is a field of interest to epidemiologists. The *International encyclopaedia of population*, edited by J.A. Ross (2 vols, Free Press,

1982) contains valuable information on mortality and morbidity trends, globally, regionally and nationally. A useful dictionary should be noted here — *A dictionary of epidemiology* edited by J.M. Last for the International Epidemiological Association (2nd edn., OUP, 1988).

Journals

Any bibliography of papers on public health and epidemiological topics will show that many of these are published in the standard general medical journals, such as the *British Medical Journal* or the *New England Journal of Medicine*; and these therefore should be borne in mind. Summarized below are the major specialized journals of public health and related disciplines.

Public health

Important public health journals include the *American Journal of Public Health* (Washington DC); *Journal of Public Health Medicine* (Oxford) (formerly *Community Medicine*); *Preventive Medicine* (New York), *Public Health* (London), *Public Health Reports* (Washington, DC). There is also the excellent *Annual Review of Public Health* (New York). The *Journal of Infectious Diseases* is a major primary source of information on the clinical, microbiological, epidemiological and public health aspects of the subject. There are numerous public health journals relating to specific geographical regions, including, the *Asia-Pacific Journal of Public Health* (Honolulu); both the *Boletín de la Oficina Sanitaria Panamericana* (Washington, DC) and *Bulletin of the Pan American Health Organization* (Washington DC) covering Central and South America; and the *Scandinavian Journal of Social Medicine* (Stockholm). The late 1980s has seen attention being drawn to the public health problems of Eastern Europe: the *Journal of Hygiene, Epidemiology, and Immunology* (Prague/Basle) contains papers in English from research workers in that region.

There are national journals of public health which are of more than local interest – examples include the *Canadian Journal of Public Health* (Ottawa); *Indian Journal of Public Health* (Calcutta); and *Salud Pública de México* (Mexico, DF). For further titles, readers should consult the *List of Journals Indexed in Index Medicus* under the country or area concerned.

Epidemiology

The important epidemiological journals of interest to public health specialists are: *American Journal of Epidemiology* (Baltimore);

Epidemiology and Infection (Cambridge); *European Journal of Epidemiology* (Rome); *International Journal of Epidemiology* (Oxford); *Journal of Clinical Epidemiology* (Oxford) (formerly the *Journal of Chronic Diseases*); and the *Journal of Epidemiology and Community Health* (London). There is an important annual review — *Epidemiologic Reviews* (Baltimore). Those readers seeking information on the epidemiology of specific diseases or groups of diseases should consult the specialist journals in those areas.

Health services

A great many journals are available in this field (see Cook, 1987). The following is a very selective list from those available. The *Health Service Journal* (London) is a weekly publication covering topical issues in health services, primarily in the UK. *Health Services Management* (London) formerly *Hospital and Health Services Review* – the official journal of the Institute of Health Services Management – is also useful for short articles on current issues. The *International Journal of Health Planning and Management* (Chichester) is international and multidisciplinary in scope and covers 'major issues in health planning, and management systems and practices'. *Medical Care* (Philadelphia) also covers all aspects of health services planning, provision and evaluation but focuses primarily, though not exclusively, on the USA. *Journal of Management in Medicine* (London) covers the growing need of clinical professionals for information on health services delivery. The *International Journal of Health Services* (Amityville, NY) is broadly devoted to health and social policy, political economy and sociology, history and philosophy, and ethics and law as they relate to public health. *Health Policy and Planning* (Oxford) is concerned with health policy issues in the developing world.

The fields of health-service finance and health economics are covered by the *Journal of Health Economics* (Amsterdam) and *Health Care Financing Review* (Baltimore), though the latter covers primarily issues related to the UK.

The Health Education Authority publishes *Health Education Journal* (London) which deals mainly with issues in the UK. *Health Promotion International* (Oxford), formerly *Health Promotion*, covers health promotion and health education issues throughout the world. Research in health education and health promotion is covered by *Health Education Research: Theory and Practice* (Oxford).

In the field of social medicine, *Social Science and Medicine* (Oxford) is of major importance, covering health economics, health policy, medical anthropology, medical ethics, medical psychology and medical sociology. The *Journal of Health and Social Behavior* (Washington,

DC) publishes articles that apply sociological concepts and methods to the understanding of health, illness and medicine in their social context. More social-science-orientated but relevant journals are *Social Biology* (Madison), *Social Psychiatry* (Berlin) and *Social Policy and Administration* (Oxford). *The Milbank Memorial Fund Quarterly* (New York) publishes symposia, many of which deal with various aspects of medical care.

Two specific medico-social, public-health issues should be mentioned — addiction and AIDS. *Alcoholism* (New York), *British Journal of Addiction* (London), *International Journal of Drug Policy* (Liverpool) and *Bulletin on Narcotics* (Geneva) are major publications. While general medical journals carry major papers on AIDS and related issues, several new specialist journals have arisen in this field. Among those covering the public health and social issues are *AIDS and Public Policy Journal* (Frederick, MD); *AIDS: Education and Prevention* (New York); and *AIDS Care* (London). *AIDS* (London) and *Journal of Acquired Immune Deficiency Syndromes* (New York) contain epidemiological studies. In 1987 an important annual review series began – *Current Topics in AIDS* (Wiley, Chichester).

Occupational and environmental health

In the fields of environmental health, occupational health and medicine the following are among the leading English-language journals: *Archives of Environmental Health* (Washington, DC); *British Journal of Industrial Medicine* (London); *Environmental Health Perspectives* (Washington, DC); *International Archives of Occupational and Environmental Health* (Berlin); *Journal of Occupational Accidents* (Amsterdam); and *Scandinavian Journal of Work, Environment and Health* (Helsinki). A useful review publication is *Occupational Medicine: State of the Art Reviews* (Philadelphia). Published quarterly, as a hardback, each volume is devoted to a special topic and each volume lists the themes of previous and forthcoming volumes.

Official publications of international agencies, government departments and other organizations including statistical sources

The publications of the World Health Organization — both emanating from its headquarters in Geneva and from its six Regional Offices around the world — are of enormous value. Many of these appear in its various series, which are all indexed by author, title, series and subject in WHO *Publications Catalogue*. At the time of going to press the most recent covered 1948–1989, but updated supplements are regularly issued. Of particular relevance to public health workers is the series *Public Health Papers* (Geneva) and *Public Health in Europe* (Copenhagen), but relevant publications also appear as *Technical Reports, Euro Reports and Studies* and *Offset Publications*. WHO produces much vital epidemiological and statistical data: the *Weekly Epidemiological Record* and *WHO Statistics Quarterly* contain detailed analyses of selected health topics of current epidemiological interest. The *World Health Statistics Annual* gives vital statistics and life tables, and causes of death, by sex and age, for member countries for stated years that differ from country to country. In addition each issue contains a global overview of selected aspects of the world health situation, and a special section on a particular topic of public-health interest – recent editions have covered information on health personnel (1988) and monitoring cardiovascular diseases (1989). From time to time WHO publishes a *Report on the world health situation* of which the seventh is the most recent. Entitled *Evaluation of the strategy for health for all by the year 2000*, the report is in seven volumes: the first is a global review and each subsequent volume covers a specific WHO region.

Epidemiological information, vital statistics and information on the health status of a particular region and countries can be hard to trace – it may be necessary to search an indexing publication such as *Tropical Diseases Bulletin* by country for a recent paper giving such information or scan regional medical journals (e.g. *West African Medical Journal*). Three useful regional statistical sources are: *CAREC Surveillance Report* (Port of Spain) a monthly bulletin of epidemiological information covering 19 member countries of CAREC, the Caribbean Epidemiological Centre; *SEAMIC Health Statistics* (South East Asia Medical Information Centre, Tokyo), a yearbook of health statistics covering countries of South East Asia (Brunei, Indonesia, Japan, Malaysia, Philippines, Singapore, Thailand); and the annual *Health Statistics in Nordic Countries* (Copenhagen) contains useful vital and health statistics for Denmark, Finland, Iceland, Norway and Sweden, published by the Nordic Statistical Secretariat.

Each country will differ in its ability to collect and disseminate its vital and health statistics: for many countries these can only be discerned in summary from the annual government medical reports (if available) or from census reports. Others make available a wide range of statistical information. A very useful guide to such statistics is given on pages 138–49 of Michael Alderson's *Mortality, morbidity and health statistics* (Macmillan, 1988) — an invaluable source in this field, with guides to a variety of morbidity statistics and statistics on specific diseases, and containing a superb 50-page bibliography. Britsh statistical sources are outlined in the next section. American statistics are well documented. The *Morbidity and Mortality Weekly Report* is published by the Centers for Disease Control, Atlanta, and lists cases of specified notifiable diseases by state, as well as publishing accounts on current public health interest, with occasional supplements on specific issues. The final part of each year (issued much later) is an annual *Summary of Notifiable Diseases, United States*. The Secretary of Health and Human Services produces an annual report on the health status of the nation: *Health, United States* (USPHS) which is full of valuable statistical information. The National Center for Health Statistics (3700 East-West Highway, MD 20782) produces a number of valuable documents of interest to public-health workers, including the *Monthly Vital Statistics Report* and the associated *Vital and Health Statistics* which is published in a variety of sections: series 5 covers comparative international vital and health statistics on selected topics. A guide to US health statistics is *Health statistics: a guide to information sources* by F. O. Weise (Gale, 1980); though it is now out of date, it is as a useful guide to publications at that date.

Organization and financing of health services in Britain

A range of publications is available giving statistical information on the staffing, financing and activity of the British health services. *Health and Personal Social Services Statistics for England* (HMSO) is an annual publication from the Department of Health giving summarized information mainly at Regional level on finance; manpower; and activity of hospital, family practitioner, community health and personal social services. A useful companion to this is the Office of Health Economics' *Compendium of Health Statistics* (7th edn., OHE, 1989) published irregularly. This covers similar material to *Health and Personal Social Services Statistics*, but also includes discussion of the data, and illustrative figures and charts. Health service statistics for Wales, Scotland and Northern Ireland are published separately as *Health and Personal Social Services Statistics for Wales* (HMSO); *Scottish Health Statistics* (Common Services Agency); and *Health and Personal Social Services Statistics for Northern Ireland* (Belfast, DHSS). Statistical information given in these sources may not be directly comparable. Information in the OHE *Compendium* usually covers Britain as a whole.

Quite detailed information on hospital in-patient or day-case activity (based on a 1 in 10 sample of patients in hospitals in England) is available in the *Hospital In-patient Enquiry* (HMSO, 1987) published by the DHSS and Office of Population Censuses and Surveys (OPCS). However, the most recent information available covers 1985 with a volume summarizing the years 1979–1985. The recommendations of the Körner inquiry necessitated a change in data collected, and information is now based on consultant episodes, rather than discharges and deaths. By late 1990, there had been no replacement publication.

Financial information on the average hotel and staffing costs of providing in-patient and day-case treatment in hospitals is available in the DoH and Welsh Office's *Health Services Costing Returns* (National Health Service). Summarized accounts for the NHS as a whole are also available: *Summarised Accounts of Health Authorities and Family Practitioner Committees in England and Wales ... (HMSO)*. The former Department of Health and Social Security published a summary of the statistics which are collected: *A guide to health and social services statistics* (DHSS, 1987) with a list of DHSS contact points and a bibliography. No account is taken of the Körner proposals, however, and though it is arranged as a broad subject index, more detailed indexing would be helpful. Complaints about the NHS and their investigation are summarized in the *Annual Report of the Health Service Commissioner* (HMSO).

For information on the vital statistics and health status of individual countries comprising the UK, census reports and the annual medical reports provide detail not available elsewhere. For England and Wales the OPCS publishes an annual reference series, including the following subjects: family statistics; death, morbidity, population estimates and projections, abortions, etc. This is supplemented by a series of *OPCS Monitors* designed for the quick release of selected information. For example, Series WR is the *Registrar General's Weekly Returns*, listing notifications of births, deaths and infectious diseases for England and Wales. Comparable statistics for Scotland and Northern Ireland appear in the annual reports from the Registrar General for those countries. There are also the annual reports of the Chief Medical Officer of the Department of Health *On the State of the Public Health*, and equivalent reports of the Welsh Office and the Scottish Home and Health Department.

Communicable disease statistics are published in the Public Health Laboratory Service's *CDR – Communicable Disease Report* covering England, Wales and Ireland. Data for Scotland are given in the weekly *Communicable Diseases Scotland.*

Health Trends (London) is a quarterly journal published by the Department of Health, aimed at disseminating 'information bearing on the [health] service and not otherwise readily available to the professions working in it' (Godber, 1969). Another irregular publication aiming to disseminate information quickly is the Department of Health's *Statistical Bulletin* (London). This releases information on various NHS hospital activities, e.g. waiting list reports, prescriptions dispensed, NHS hospital activity statistics. The Departments of Health and Social Security, the Scottish Home and Health Department, and the Welsh Office also publish reports on special topics. Recent reports have covered nursing skills mix; ENT services in Scotland, and Community Health Councils in Wales. Other occasional reports on aspects of health services delivery are published by the National Audit Office. Recent studies range from financial management in the NHS, to hospital building in England, to the provision of maternity services.

The Health and Safety Executive produces a series entitled *Health and Safety Statistics: 1981–82* (HMSO, 1985), *1983* (HMSO, 1986), *1984–85* (HMSO, 1987) and *1985–86* (HMSO, 1988). Though apparently an annual publication, each volume covers a longer period than is implied by its title and the volumes need to be consulted together.

Abstracts, indexes and other bibliographies

Public health

Public health is bibliographically scattered. Catalogues of libraries collecting in this field are an obvious source, and here the various series of the National Library of Medicine's catalogues and its *Current Catalog* are of prime importance.

A.J. Bunch's *Health care administration: an information sourcebook* (Capital Planning Administration, 1979) is a useful guide to mainly British publications and sources, although a new edition is needed. A valuable selected bibliography is *Health service literature: a bibliography* by A.J. Bunch and J. Payne in *Hospitals and Health Services Yearbook* (edited by N.W. Chaplin, Institute of Health Services Management. 1991). The bibliography, a regular inclusion in the yearbook, is intended as a guide to the most important recent publications in the field.

Ray Elling's *Cross-national study of health systems* (Gale, 1980) is a valuable bibliography. It is published in two volumes, one covering countries, world regions and special problems; the other covers concepts, methods and data sources. For those interested in primary health care in developing countries, the Evaluation and Planning Centre (now the Health Policy Unit) at the London School of Hygiene and Tropical Medicine has published an excellent series of reviews and annotated bibliographies in the field. Among subjects covered so far have been: primary health care approach in developing countries (1981); medical anthropology and primary health care (1990); and national policies on community health workers (1988). *SALUS: low-cost rural health care and health manpower training* (International Development Research Centre, Canada, 1975–84) is an important series of 15 volumes providing annotated bibliographies with a special emphasis on developing countries.

There are three major abstracting journals in the field of public health. *Abstracts on Hygiene and Communicable Disease* selectively abstracts that literature which reports advances in knowledge or provides 'state of the art' reviews. *Excerpta Medica* has two sections of interest to public health workers: Section 17 covers public health, social medicine and epidemiology, while Section 46 covers environmental health and pollution control.

The new major public-health problem, AIDS, is now supported by several abstracting journals. *Current AIDS Literature* (London) is a comprehensive monthly abstracting journal published by the Bureau of Hygiene and Tropical Diseases, which also produces (in collaboration with WHO) *WHO AIDS Technical Bulletin*, aimed particularly at developing countries. *Excerpta Medica* introduced Section 54, devoted to AIDS, in 1989.

Public Health News (Bureau of Hygiene and Tropical Diseases), launched following the rise of public interest in Britain in the late 1980s in public health issues, is a useful monthly digest of reports on public health issues culled from the popular and scientific press. It is international in scope but is biased towards Britain in its coverage of news. *Healthcare Parliamentary Monitor*, published fortnightly while Parliament sits, is a digest reporting all proceedings in Parliament concerned with health matters.

For the older literature on public health, it is necessary to use published library catalogues including the *Index-Catalogue of the Surgeon General's Library*. The *Dictionary Catalogue of the London School of Hygiene and Tropical Medicine* (7 vols, G.K. Hall, 1965, and *Supplement*, 1970) forms a wide-ranging bibliography of the literature of preventive and tropical medicine. The *John Crerar Library (Chicago) Classified Subject Catalog* vols 18 and 19, (G.K. Hall, 1967) shows the holdings in hygiene and public health of a great scientific library.

Health services finance, planning and management

A major work is the *International bibliography of health economics* (2 vols, by C.A. Blades *et al.*, Wheatsheaf, 1986). It is a comprehensive, annotated guide to English-language sources since 1914. Three major serial publications are available covering information on planning, management and financing of health services in general, and of hospitals and health care units of all kinds. *Excerpta Medica. Section 36: Health Policy, Economics and Management* covers international literature. *Health Service Abstracts* (1985–) previously entitled *Hospital Abstracts* (1961–1984) is published by the libraries of the UK Departments of

Health and Social Security. It indexes UK government reports and circulars within the field, and also other books and reports in addition to the journal literature. *Hospital Literature Index* (1945–) published by the American Hospital Association is more extensive in its scope and coverage of the journal literature, but with index entries only. Neither publication attempts to cover material on clinical aspects of patient care.

A useful source of information on management issues in nursing and allied health fields is the *Cumulated Index of Nursing and Allied Health Literature* (Glendale Adventist Medical Center, 1956–). This indexes most English-language nursing journals, together with many other allied health, biomedical and health-related journals. From 1984, all new nursing and allied health books from major health-care publishers have also been indexed.

Health education and personal health

For consumer health information, the reader should refer to Chapter 23. The library of the Health Education Authority produces a monthly current-awareness publication, *Journal Articles of Interest to Health Educators* (Health Education Authority). The *Consumer Health and Nutrition Index* (1985–) edited by Alan M. Rees may also provide useful material. In addition, *Health Service Abstracts* (1985–) has a subsection devoted to preventive medicine and health education. The *Health Education Index* (Edstall Professional Services, irregular) does not index journal literature, but is a good source for audiovisual materials in health education, and does provide a list of books, booklets and leaflets in the field.

Occupational health

A detailed listing of important historical sources on occupational health can be obtained by reference to the appropriate section in the previous edition of this work, and to *Occupational health: a guide to sources of information* by S. Gauvain (Heinemann Medical, 1974) which was at the time a comprehensive review of all types of information sources then available. An excellent review of current knowledge is the *Encyclopaedia of occupational health and safety* (ILO, Geneva, 3rd edn., 1983 – reprinted with modifications, 1989). The *Barbour health and safety library* is a microfiche compilation, regularly updated, of all relevant literature and codes of practice. *Excerpta Medica* continues to abstract important world literature on occupational health and hygiene in *Section 35: Occupational Health and Industrial Medicine*.

Vital statistics and epidemiology

Bibliographies of health and disease statistics can save much research. Good examples are *Reviews of United Kingdom statistical sources. Vol. IX. Health surveys and related studies* by M. Alderson and R. Dowie (Pergamon, 1979), together with other volumes in this series, of which the general editor is W. F. Maunder; *A guide to health and social services statistics* (Department of Health and Social Security, 1974); and *Health statistics: a guide to information sources* by F. O. Weise (Gale, 1980). The US National Center for Health Statistics publishes a useful *Catalog of Publications*, one covering 1962–1979 (US Public Health Service, 1980) and 1980–86 (USPHS, 1987). Two valuable compendia of information, both by Michael Alderson, are *International mortality statistics* (Macmillan, 1981), and *Mortality, morbidity and health statistics* (Macmillan, 1988). The US National Center for Health Statistics produces the *International health data reference guide, 1989* (USPHS, 1990). An excellent pathfinder through the maze of British official statistics in this field is B. Benjamin's *Population statistics: a review of UK sources* (Gower, 1989).

Bibliographies of diseases are too numerous to mention here but should not be ignored. Collective works of value which are basic tools for any chronological epidemiological study are, among others, *Handbook of geographical and historical pathology* by A. Hirsch, translated from the second German edition by C. Creighton (New Sydenham Society, London 1883–1886), *Welt-Seuchen-Atlas ... World atlas of epidemic diseases* by E. Rodenwaldt (Hamburg 1952–1957); and G. M. Howe's *National atlas of disease mortality in the United Kingdom* (2nd edn. Nelson, 1970). Histories of diseases and of epidemiology are also useful sources.

The study of population growth and control is of increasing significance in vital statistics. The United Nations publishes much valuable work in the field of demography and this can be traced through its *Documents Index*. The *Population Index* (Princeton, 1935–) is a quarterly abstracting periodical and includes morbidity and mortality.

Lastly, mention should be made of *Current Bibliography of Epidemiology* (1969–1977). Derived from the MEDLARS tapes, it covered epidemiology and preventive medicine and was indexed in more depth than *Index Medicus*.

Online databases and CD-ROM

Public health specialists will find the general medical databases MEDLINE and EXCERPTA MEDICA of use. Of particular interest to them will be PUBLIC HEALTH AND TROPICAL MEDICINE (PHTM), available online through the German host DIMDI. PHTM contains the entire bibliographical database of the Bureau of Hygiene and Tropical Diseases and is in effect the online version of *Abstracts on Hygiene and Communicable Disease, Tropical Diseases Bulletin* and *Current AIDS Research.* LILACS, the Latin American and Caribbean Health Sciences Literature database, is available on CD-ROM, produced by the Pan American Health Organization. It also contains REPIDISCA, the Pan American Information and Documentation Network on sanitary engineering and environmental sciences. POPLINE, available both online and in CD-ROM, is a valuable tool for the public health specialist. It contains over 200 000 citations with abstracts (including those listed in *Population Index*) in the fields of demography, family planning, vital statistics, maternal and child health, AIDS in developing countries, and general health, law and policy issues; and it goes back as far as 1827.

The major public health problem of AIDS is covered by *Compact AIDS Library*, a CD-ROM published by Maxwell Communications. It contains the AIDS Knowledge Base from San Francisco General Hospital, full text of recent AIDS-related articles from standard medical journals such as the *New England Journal of Medicine* and *Journal of Infectious Diseases*, AIDS-related citations from MEDLINE and the Bureau of Hygiene and Tropical Diseases, and of the American Foundations for AIDS Research's *AIDS/HIV Experimental Treatment Directory.*

Health services planning, organization and management

The two major online databases in the field are the equivalents of *Health Service Abstracts* and *Hospital Literature Index.* Covering mainly UK material, though with some European and North American literature, is DHSS DATA (1983—), the catalogue of the libraries of the Departments of Health and Social Security. Included on this database are UK government reports in the health and social services field, circulars and press releases. HEALTH PLANNING & ADMINISTRATION (1975–) is produced by the American Hospital Association in conjunction with the National Library of Medicine. It consists of some MEDLINE records, together with additional documents supplied by the AHA. It includes some European and UK journals but does not cover UK official reports or circulars. It is also available on CD-ROM as HealthPLAN-CD. CINAHL also has its online equivalent — NAHL: NURSING AND ALLIED HEALTH LITERATURE (1983–) and is available on CD-ROM.

OSH-ROM is a collection on CD-ROM of occupational health and safety information containing the bibliographic databases of the U.S. National Institute for Occupational Safety and Health; ILO's International Occupational Safety and Health Information Centre; and the British Health and Safety Executive's Major Hazards Incidents Data Service. TOXLINE available both online and in CD-ROM, contains citations to published material and research in progress in, among others, the fields of adverse drug reactions, chemical carcinogenesis, drug toxicity, food contamination, occupational and environmental hazards, and water treatment.

History of public health

The origins and development of the public health movement are succinctly described by S.P.W. Chave in the first chapter of the *Oxford textbook of medicine: volume 1* (edited by W. W. Holland *et al.*, Oxford University Press, 1984). C. F. Brockington's *A short history of public health* (2nd edn., Churchill, 1966), G. Rosen's *A history of public health* (MD Publications, 1958), and W. M. Frazer's *A history of English public health 1834—1939* (Baillière Tindall, 1950) provide modern accounts. Sir John Simon's *English sanitary institutions* (Castle, 1890) is a contemporaneous account of the development of public health in nineteenth-century England. A modern account is A.S. Wohl's *Endangered lives: public health in Victorian Britain* (Dent, 1983). A highly readable account of one aspect of 'state medicine' is *Recalling the Medical Officer of Health; writings of Sydney Chave*, edited by M. Warren and H. Francis (King Edward's Hospital Fund for London, 1987). Of specialist interest is *The social history of occupational health* edited by P. Weindling (Croom Helm, 1985).

Historical accounts of the creation of the British National Health Service are to be found in B. Abel-Smith's *The National Health Service: the first thirty years* (HMSO, 1978), John E. Pater *The making of the National Health Service* (King Edward's Hospital Fund for London, 1981) and Frank Honigsbaum's *Health, happiness and security: the creation of the National Health Service* (Routledge, 1989). An extremely detailed account of the NHS from its inception to more recent times is in process of publication; to date volume 1 has appeared of Charles Webster's *The health service since the war* entitled *Problems of health care: the National Health Service before 1957* (HMSO, 1988).

A systematic account of international health work from its beginning to modern times is N. M. Goodman's *International health organizations and their work* (2nd edn., Churchill Livingstone, 1971). The World Health Organization publishes studies on various aspects of international public health in its series *History of International Public Health*, of which No. 6, *Smallpox and its eradication* (by F. Fenner *et al.*, Geneva, 1988) is a monumental account (in 1460 pages) of the international battle to eradicate this infectious disease from the world, culminating in success in 1980.

Finally, the journal *Social History of Medicine* (Oxford, 1988–) publishes articles which will be of interest to the public health historian.

Useful organizations

The library of the London School of Hygiene and Tropical Medicine (Keppel Street, London WC1E 7HT; Tel: 071-927 2283) is a large collection specializing in preventive and tropical medicine and allied disciplines. Though the library of a postgraduate medical school it is open to visitors who wish to consult its specialized holdings. Its catalogue was published in 1965, with a supplement in 1970 (*see above*). Since January 1991 its holdings of material from 1980 onwards have been available online as part of the library catalogue held on the LIBERTAS system of University College London. This can be accessed through JANET, the British Joint Academic Network, address A 000005112800. The library at the King's Fund Centre for Health Services Development (126 Albert Street, London NW1 7NF. Tel: 071-267 6111) is a specialist collection covering health services management, planning and organization. It is open for reference to all who wish to consult the collections.

Other useful organizations to approach for material on health services management are:

Nuffield Institute for Health Service Studies (University of Leeds, 71-75 Clarendon Road, Leeds LS2 9PL. Tel: 0532-459034)

Health Services Management Centre (University of Birmingham, Park House, 40 Edgbaston Park Road, Birmingham B15 2RT. Tel: 021-455 7511)

Scottish Health Service Centre (Scottish Health Service Management Development Group, Crewe Road South, Edinburgh EH4 2LF. Tel: 031-332 2335)

For health education and health promotion material a useful source is the Health Promotion Information Centre at the Health Education Authority (Hamilton House, Mabledon Place, London WC1X 9TX. Tel: 071-383 3833). For information relating to occupational health and safety, a valuable resource is the library of the Health and Safety Executive (Broad Lane, Sheffield S3 7HG. Tel: 0742 76814).

References

Cook, S. (1987) A core list of periodicals for health-care management libraries. *Health Libraries Review*, **4**, 14.

Godber, G. (1969) Introduction. *Health Trends*, **1**, 1.

CHAPTER TEN

Pharmacology and therapeutics

D.H. CALAM

The information sources considered in this chapter have been selected to cover not only the fields of pharmacology and therapeutics in the strict sense, but also areas of pharmaceutical science concerned particularly with drugs, their development and control. This broader selection is deliberate because the pharmaceutical field is not examined specifically elsewhere in the book. The range of medicines available continues to develop and change with scientific and technical advances. In the past few years, genetic engineering techniques have given access to protein drugs that were previously unavailable, and so to new areas of therapy and prophylaxis. Advances in chemical synthesis and separation science, together with increased awareness of the structural specificity of biological action, have heightened interest in drugs that are single stereoisomers and not mixtures. Yet other advances in pharmaceutical technology are leading to the introduction of new delivery systems for established drugs. With increased sensitivity and specificity of analytical methods has come increased knowledge of pharmacodynamics and pharmacokinetics both in animals and man. These and other developments have been accompanied by greater legislative control over marketing of medicines and greater interest on the part of patients receiving them.

As the pace of change shows no sign of slackening, information sources play a crucial role in meeting the challenge of maintaining awareness of these developments. Rapid progress in the field of communications and computers is having a marked influence on these sources and the use that is made of them. The volume and diversity of information and its origins can present formidable problems to someone searching on a given topic and the solution is increasingly to gain access to printed sources through a database system. The potential to do so electronically and online is being realized not only from libraries but from individual offices through personal computers and computer networks. An important gain that has come from such developments has been the reduction in time between publication of data and their general accessibility. Publication times themselves may also shorten, for example, through the acceptance of submitted papers on computer disks. Data in a compendium like *Martindale* can now be studied online (including CD-ROM) as they are updated and the time cannot be far off when pharmacopoeial requirements can be examined in the same way.

Information retrieval

Chapters 3 and 5 deal in detail with indexes, abstracts and retrieval systems. This section only summarizes the main sources of information for the subject matter of this chapter. The great increase in availability and use of personal and other computer systems and familiarity with them, together with the growth of electronic data transmission, has caused a significant alteration in the balance from use of hard-copy indexing and abstracting sources towards use of databases on- and offline.

Current Contents in its various editions is one of the most timely indexing systems, sometimes including titles before the publication appears. It is readily available in printed form and on diskette, and can also be consulted through the database files SCISCAN and SCISEARCH. The more specialized listings such as *Index Medicus* and *Index Chemicus* are not so up to the minute but have the advantage of sorting titles under subject headings which facilitates more efficient searching. The hard-copy versions provide a solid base for screening the literature for a lead into abstracting sources. In the case of INDEX MEDICUS, the database version contains more extensive entries than the hard copy.

A manual search of recent literature can be carried out efficiently using the *Science Citation Index* (*SCI*) (see Chapter 3). Given a key article or review, *SCI* permits direct entry to the literature in which such an item has been cited and enables the construction of citation trees from which the major contributors to a field can be identified and a fresh search developed. *Chemical Abstracts* provide an alerting service every two weeks of abstracts on selected topics from the main database. These *CASelects* include blood coagulation, drug delivery systems and dosage forms, drug interactions and structure–activity relationships.

Many databases are now available. They are updated weekly or less frequently and their coverage is slowly extending backwards to older literature. Online database services, such as the Radio Suisse Data-Star, provide a convenient route to many of them through a common entry point. In this way, ready access can be obtained to a range of approximately 50 biological/medical sources including CHEMICAL ABSTRACTS, CURRENT BIOTECHNOLOGY ABSTRACTS, EXCERPTA MEDICA, INTERNATIONAL PHARMACEUTICAL ABSTRACTS, MARTINDALE ONLINE, MEDLINE, PHARMAPROJECTS, SIDE EFFECTS OF DRUGS and TOXLINE. The use of some is facilitated by availability of free training files. The enhanced value of searching abstracts by database arises from the opportunities offered to search free text and not just keywords and to refine a search online in order to reduce the number of items to a manageable figure. This is a particular advantage bearing in mind that MEDLINE and EXCERPTA MEDICA, each drawn from about 3000 journals, are increasing at about 250 000 abstracts annually. As well as online retrieval, offline prints can be made. Specific, personalized searches can be run on a regular basis and provided as an offline copy. Because of the growth in size, coverage and diversity of database sources, their use should be considered for any extensive literature search or one in an unfamiliar field.

Databases also offer opportunities to access other information. PHARMACEUTICAL AND HEALTHCARE INDUSTRY NEWS contains a file from 1982 of *Scrip*, the international newsletter on the pharmaceutical industry; DIOGENES consists of selected unpublished U.S. Food and Drug Administration (FDA) documents obtained under the Freedom of Information Act, full-text FDA publications on drug regulation and pharmaceutical newsletters; BIOCOMMERCE DATA includes a directory of information about organizations involved in biotechnology.

Primary sources

Over the years it has become more and more difficult to read widely and in depth in any discipline because of the steady increase in size and number of journals. The individual reader must decide which are the core journals of prime interest and which are of less importance. This is probably done most easily by studying issues of *Current Contents* in the *Life Sciences* or *Clinical Medicine* editions (Institute for Scientific Information) over a period of several weeks. The contents pages, taken as a whole, of journals published frequently (at least monthly) provide an excellent insight to the subject matter and degree of specialization of the journal. Review publications produced quarterly or annually can be located by reference to the cumulated journal index, which appears tri-annually, and to the biannual lists of journal coverage.

The following list, arranged broadly by discipline, is a selection of primary journals intended to provide sources for original literature, in some cases (indicated with an asterisk) with brief review articles and annotations. The classification of some titles is arbitrary since they cover several fields.

Pharmacology and therapeutics

Agents and Action*
Archives Internationales de
    Pharmacodynamie et de Thérapie
Archives of Toxicology
Biochemical Pharmacology
British Journal of Pharmacology
Drug Metabolism and Drug
    Interactions
European Journal of Pharmacology
Farmakologiya i Toksikologiya
General Pharmacology
Immunopharmacology and
    Immunotoxicology
Journal of Pharmacokinetics and
    Biopharmaceutics

Journal of Pharmacology and
    Experimental Therapeutics
Molecular Pharmacology
Naunyn-Schmiedeberg's Archives of
    Pharmacology
Neuropharmacology
Pharmacological Research
    Communications*
Pharmacology
Pharmacology and Therapeutics
Pharmacology and Toxicology
Teratology
Toxicology and Applied
    Pharmacology

Clinical pharmacology

British Journal of Clinical
    Pharmacology
Clinical Pharmacology and
    Therapeutics
Drugs
European Journal of Clinical
    Pharmacology
International Journal of Clinical
    Pharmacology
Therapy and Toxicology
Thérapie

together with core medical journals, e.g. *The Lancet, British Medical Journal, Journal of the American Medical Association, New England Journal of Medicine.*

Pharmaceutical and chemical sciences

Acta Pharmaceutica Suecica
Annales Pharmaceutiques Françaises
Antimicrobial Agents and
    Chemotherapy

Archiv der Pharmazie
Arzneimittel-Forschung
Chemical and Pharmaceutical
    Bulletin

Chemico-Biological Interactions
Chirality
Drugs of the Future
European Journal of Medicinal
Chemistry
Il Farmaco Edizione Scientifica
Journal of Antibiotics
Journal of Antimicrobial
*Chemotherapy**

Journal of Medicinal Chemistry
Journal of Pharmaceutical and
Biomedical Analysis
*Journal of Pharmaceutical Sciences**
Journal of Pharmacy and
*Pharmacology**
Khimiko-Farmatseuticheskii Zhurnal
Pharmaceutica Acta Helvetiae
Die Pharmazie

Some primary information on the development of drugs appears in core chemical journals, such as *Helvetica Chimica Acta, Journal of the American Chemical Society, Journal of the Chemical Society (Perkin Transactions), Bulletin de la Société Chimique de France, Chemische Berichte.*

Reviews

In addition to the brief reviews in some journals listed above, indicated by an asterisk, similar reports may also be found in periodicals such as *Pharmaceutical Journal, Deutsche Medizinische Wochenschrift* and *Schweizerische Medizinische Wochenschrift*, and longer articles in those such as *Pharmacological Reviews*. The annual review issue of *Analytical Chemistry* includes a literature review on pharmaceutical chemistry. The *British Medical Journal* frequently contains short reviews on topics such as 'New Drugs' and 'Today's Treatment' and these are cumulated from time to time in separate publications. A valuable source for general awareness is *Trends in the Pharmacological Sciences*. The *British Medical Bulletin* is a quarterly with each issue reviewing a specific topic under guest editor(s). Volume 46, No.1 (1990) is an excellent critical overview of use of drugs in the elderly.

There are, of course, several series publications of the 'Advances' type. Among the more important of these are *Annual Review of Pharmacology* and ... *of Medicine* (Annual Reviews Inc.), *Advances in Drug Research* (Academic Press, published since 1964, which consists of long articles on specific topics; *Advances in Pharmacology and Chemotherapy* (Academic Press), published from 1969 as a continuation of the two previously separate series; *Progress in Drug Research*, edited by E. Jucker and U.A. Meyer (Birkhauser Verlag), provides survey articles of pharmaceutical research; *Progress in Medicinal Chemistry* (Elsevier) contains reviews by specialists in different disciplines concerned with development and study of new drugs; *Annual Reports in Medicinal Chemistry* (Academic Press) has similar aims. *Drug Metabo-*

lism Reviews, edited by F.J. Di Carlo (Dekker), beginning in 1973, and *Progress in Drug Metabolism* edited by J.W. Bridges and L.F. Chasseaud (Taylor and Francis), a series commencing in 1976, review this area of activity. Finally, *Recent Advances in Clinical Pharmacology and Toxicology*, edited by P. Turner and A.N. Volans (Churchill Livingstone) covers a further field of interest.

Three other periodicals which contain short articles rather than reviews and which attempt to provide unbiased and critical information should be mentioned. All are produced by non-profit organizations. The first is the *Drug and Therapeutics Bulletin*, edited by A. Herxheimer and J. Collier and published by the Consumers Association (London). It consists of four pages every fortnight and contains general articles, as well as others that reassess old drugs and critically discuss new ones, particularly in comparison with existing methods of treatment. The second of this type is the *Adverse Drug Reaction Bulletin*, edited by D.M. Davies, published every two months by Meditext (Weybridge). It has the same four-page format the as *Drug and Therapeutics Bulletin* and is similar in style. The third short-article periodical is a U.S. counterpart: the *Medical Letter on Drugs and Therapeutics* (editorial chairman, H. Aaron), published fortnightly by The Medical Letter Inc. (New York). This has similar aims and format to the others and was formerly known as *Drugs and Therapeutic Information*.

Adverse reactions to drugs and drug interactions are a very important factor in therapy and themselves are responsible for significant numbers of hospital admissions. There are several excellent sources of information about adverse reactions and side-effects. The most recent information can be tracked through *Adverse Reaction Titles* (Excerpta Medica International Abstracting Service), a monthly bibliography from more than 3000 biomedical journals. In addition to indexes and monographs, *Side Effects of Drugs Annual* (Excerpta Medica) edited by M.N.G. Dukes and L. Beeley provides a critical and timely account of new information on adverse drug reactions and interactions. One valuable feature is the 'special review', a brief (one to two pages) critical assessment of older findings and ideas in the light of new knowledge. These reviews are printed in italics in appropriate chapters throughout the volume. *Meyler's Side effects of drugs*, edited by M.N.G. Dukes (11th edn., Excerpta Medica, 1989) is a comprehensive and authoritative guide.

Information on topics of current importance to practitioners is also circulated from official sources. In the UK, the Committee on Safety of Medicines produces, as an occasional series, *Current Problems*, which draws attention to problems giving rise to concern and seeks reports from doctors. The *FDA Bulletin* is a similar U.S. publication.

Monographs

The selection of significant books and monographs is a difficult task because few are read from cover to cover, and in any rapidly changing field they have an inherent tendency to date rather quickly. This short list is not exhaustive.

Goodman and Gilman's The pharmacological basis of therapeutics, edited by A.G. Gilman, T.W. Rall, A.S. Nies and P. Taylor (8th., Macmillan, 1990), is a classic work which provides a bridge between basic medical science and clinical usage of drugs. The 70 chapters, in 17 main sections, have been prepared by many distinguished contributors. A minor disadvantage is the emphasis on U.S. trade names. Other major reference monographs include the Springer-Verlag *Handbooks of experimental pharmacology*, for example volume 99 (*Pharmacology of peptic ulcer disease*, edited by M.J. Cullen and S.J. Benjamin, 1991); the constituent volumes of the *International encyclopedia of pharmacology and therapeutics* (Pergamon), many of which have been published as supplements to the review journal *Pharmacology and Therapeutics*. *Remingtons's pharmaceutical sciences* edited by A.R. Gennaro (18th edn., Mack Publishing, 1990) is a massive 'treatise on theory and practice of pharmaceutical sciences and essential information about pharmaceutical and medicinal agents'. The reader should judge how far this intention is met.

The range of textbooks on pharmacology and therapeutics includes the *Oxford Textbook of clinical pharmacology and drug therapy* by D.G. Graham Smith and J.K. Aronson (Oxford, 1984), *Principles of drug action: the basis of pharmacology* by W.B. Pratt and P. Taylor (3rd edn., Churchill Livingstone, 1990), *Clinical pharmacology* by P. Turner and A. Richens (5th edn., Churchill Livingstone, 1986) and *Clinical Pharmacology* by D.R. Lawrence (6th edn., Churchill Livingstone, 1987). A more specialist area is covered by *Poisoning diagnosis and treatment*, edited by J.A. Vale and T.J. Meredith (Update Books, 1981).

The *Merck Manual of diagnosis and treatment*, editor-in-chief R. Berkow (15th edn., 1987) is an established U.S. handbook for physicians. It provides information about the aetiology, investigation and treatment of a wide range of conditions. Drug names and trade names reflect the book's origin. There is increasing interest in the specificity of pharmacological, toxicological and other biological actions of individual stereochemical forms of drugs, many of which were first used as isomeric mixtures and a good source for information on this topic is *Chirality and biological activity*, edited by B. Holmstedt, H. Frank and B. Testa (Wiley-Liss, 1989).

Among books dealing with the field of adverse drug reactions and interactions may be mentioned a *Manual of adverse drug interactions* by J.P. Griffin *et al.* (4th edn., Wright, 1988), *Textbook of adverse drug reactions* by D.M. Davies (3rd edn., Oxford University Press, 1991), *Drug interactions* by I.H. Stockley (2nd edn., Blackwell, 1991) and *Adverse reactions to drug formulation agents* by M. Weiner and I.L. Bernstein (Dekker, 1989).

Pharmacopoeias

The object of a pharmacopoeia is to lay down specifications for the quality of important and widely used drugs. These specifications are 'official' and are intended to ensure that all marketed versions of such drugs are of high quality. This activity long pre-dates, and is complementary to, control of quality through national licensing systems where information is confidential to the producer and the licensing authority. Further, pharmacopoeial requirements apply throughout the life of a product and may differ from those applied at the time of manufacture. Many countries produce their own pharmacopoeias which are revised periodically by committees of experts. The escalating cost of developing new drugs means that a world market is sought for their sale and one consequence is an increasing tendency to apply uniform criteria of drug quality through multinational use and production of pharmacopoeias.

The duty to publish a *British Pharmacopoeia* (*BP*) was laid upon the General Medical Council by the Medical Act 1858, and the first edition was published six years later. In recent times, revisions have appeared at regular intervals with addenda to the main volume in between. Under the provisions of the Medicines Act 1968, responsibility for the *BP* was transferred to the Health Ministers, who authorize publication after the edition has been prepared on behalf of the Medicines Commission. The 1973 edition was the first to appear under these arrangements. The *BP*, like others, declares a date from which its contents become 'official' and supersede those of previous volumes. The current *BP 1988* is in two volumes, the first of which contains monographs on drug substances, including definitions, descriptions, tests for identity, purity and properties, assays, information about action and use and labelling. It also includes a collection of infra-red reference spectra. The second volume consists of specifications for preparations (such as tablets and injections), blood and immunological products, and some surgical materials, together with a series of appendices with information about reagents, procedures and general requirements. At present the *BP* is the only pharmacopoeia to provide a compilation of infra-red reference spectra for identification, instead of reference materials with which analysts prepare their own spectra. Unlike certain other pharmacopoeias (for example, the French), the tests are advisory not mandatory, but in the event of dispute there is an obligation to justify any departure from them. Edited monographs from the *European Pharmacopoeia* are included and indicated by a five-pointed star.

Addenda containing new and revised material are published, usually annually, between the main editions and now have consecutive pagination. The index is cumulative and so the one in the latest *Addendum* provides direct access to all references in the main volumes and *Addenda*. The *Addendum* is likely to be the last before the next full edition. The requirements of the *British Pharmacopoeia* are enforced in many Commonwealth and other countries. Medicines specifically for veterinary use feature in a separate volume with a similar format, the *British Pharmacopoeia (Veterinary) 1985* with an *Addendum* 1988. One additional feature is a section on action and use and usual dosage range for a variety of animal species.

The *European Pharmacopoeia (EP)* is prepared in two official languages, English and French, under the auspices of the Council of Europe by the terms of a Convention of 1964. The events leading to this and subsequent developments are described in the slim *European Pharmacopoeia: A review of its history and functions* by H.S. Grainger, its first Secretary (Maisonneuve, 1981). The eight founder countries (Belgium, France, Italy, Luxembourg, The Netherlands, UK, West Germany and Switzerland) have increased to 20 by accession of the remaining members of the European Community and some other countries. The *EP* is drafted by groups of experts, not necessarily drawn from all the countries, and the draft is approved by a main Commission representative of the national authorities. Thus, the requirements of the *EP* represent the agreed views of most countries in western Europe. Publication of the second edition commenced in 1980 in a loose-leaf format. The reasons for adopting this, and the system for publication, are explained in the preface. In essence, advances in methods and the complexity of drug substances demand frequent revision of monographs. The loose-leaf presentation should facilitate replacement of sections and of monographs in the correct sequences as they are revised. New material is issued in annual fascicules. Because of national variations in prescribing and the large range of excipients that may be incorporated in drug dosage forms, the monographs of the *European Pharmacopoeia* are almost exclusively for parent substances. The few exceptions concern complex biological products.

Under the terms of the Convention, it is agreed that the monographs should become official in each country from a specified date and that they are included in and supersede existing monographs in the national pharmacopoeias. There is no obligation to include a particular monograph, but if included it must not be changed and no alternative is permitted. *EP* monographs currently represent about 40 per cent of those for bulk substances in the *BP* and about one quarter of the whole. Translations into other languages, for example German and Spanish, are official only if authorized or if the monographs appear as part of the national pharmacopoeia of a country signatory to the Convention. Because the various national pharmacopoeias are used in other countries, the influence of the *EP* extends beyond Europe, particularly to the countries of Latin America and the former colonies of the UK and France. This influence will grow through the interest of Eastern European countries in joining the Council of Europe and the impact of the single market in the European Community in 1993 on pharmaceutical suppliers to the region.

In 1987, publication commenced of *Pharmeuropa*, a periodical intended to provide information about the work of the European Pharmacopoeia Commission and to permit feedback from users of the *EP*. It contains draft monographs, articles and letters.

Before the *EP* Convention was signed, the Scandinavian countries had reached a similar agreement concerning a *Nordic Pharmacopoeia*, produced in several languages. The main volumes that appeared in 1963 have been updated by means of loose-leaf addenda. Further development of the *Nordic Pharmacopoeia* has been overtaken by accession to the *EP* Convention of the countries involved.

Following a precedent set by the League of Nations, the World Health Organization produces the *International Pharmacopoeia*. The third edition is in the course of publication. Unlike earlier editions which employed material from some national pharmacopoeias, this edition is intended to meet the specific needs of developing countries. Volume 1, published in 1979, contains general methods of analysis, and volumes 2 and 3 (1981 and 1988) contain quality specifications. The aim is to provide specifications for the drugs appearing on the 'essential' list recommended by WHO, together with common excipients and dosage forms, at a level to ensure their safety and efficacy without recourse to complex methods or imposing unduly stringent criteria. A further aim is to provide general methods which can form the basis for control of other products. The *International Pharmacopoeia*, which is produced by an international group of experts and has no legal force in itself, is available for official adoption by any member state of WHO.

Main editions of the *United States Pharmacopeia (USP)* (XXIInd edn., 1990) appear every five years. Although produced by the U.S. Pharmacopeial Convention, independent of government, the *USP* has official status. Each edition has a preface describing the history of the *USP* and the changes since the previous edition. A second book of drug standards, the *National Formulary (NF)*, was merged with the *USP* in 1975 and is now bound into the *USP* as a separate section. Following reorganization of their contents, the *USP* section concerns drug substances and dosage forms while the *NF* deals with pharmaceutical ingredients. Supplements to the *USP* are published every six months. They have continuous pagination and a cumulative index. An insight into pharmacopoeial revision is provided by *Pharmacopeial Forum*, published every two months. This gives details of in-process revision of monographs for the *USP* with discussion and explanation, and proposes policy changes; comments are sought. Each issue contains a cumulative index.

Although the pharmacopoeias described above are the most important for English readers, a number of others are interesting for comparison of their approach and content. The *Pharmacopoeia Helvetica* (7th edn., 1987), is published in loose-leaf form and in three languages (French, German, Italian). The monographs are similar to those of the *BP*, but include cautions (e.g. incompatibility) and guidance on possible changes such as sensitivity to light.

The *Pharmacopée Française* (10th edn.) has a loose-leaf presentation. The monographs of the *EP* are included and identified as such; the other monographs are prepared in the same format. One feature is an appendix on drug interactions arranged by therapeutic classification. Supplements are prepared annually and the changes in them are highlighted on green paper. A separate volume of recommended dosages has been published (1988). Reflecting national differences in medical practice, monographs for homoeopathic mother tinctures are included in the 6th *Supplement* (1989). Both France and Germany produce homoeopathic pharmacopoeias. The *Formulaire National* is a complementary volume containing details of preparations such as ointments and tablets.

The *Deutsches Arzneibuch (DAB)* (9th edn.) for West Germany was published in 1986 with later supplements. It includes a statement permitting the use of non-pharmacopoeial methods if they give the same result as the official one — in accord with the policy of the *BP*. A *Kommentar* (commentary) on the previous edition (*DAB8*), was prepared by H. Bohme and K. Hartke and gave descriptive and explanatory notes. East Germany also produced a *Deutsches Arzneibuch* and in due course some merger of the contents of the two may be anticipated. The *Deutscher Arzneimittel Codex 1986* is a separate publication covering additional but supplementary materials. The Italian pharmacopoeia (*Farmacopea Ufficiale*, 1985 and 1st supplement, 1988) contains tables of usual dosages and legal information of concern to pharmacists on classification of drugs, and equipment that should be available in a pharmacy. Certain foreign pharmacopoeias are published in English translation and are therefore more readily accessible than might appear at first sight, for example, the *10th Japanese Pharmacopoeia* (1986) and the *Pharmacopoeia of India* (3rd edn., 1985).

Volume 1 of a *British Herbal Pharmacopoeia 1990* (British Herbal Medical Association) has been published and further volumes are in preparation. It contains monographs for botanical drugs with references to the *EP* and *BP* and a brief indication of action. A companion *British Herbal Compendium* giving therapeutic and other information is also in preparation.

Drug indexes and compendia

Reference volumes in which are collected details of all drugs currently available fall into two groups: those that merely provide details of proprietary preparations and their manufacturers, and those that provide greater detail about the individual active substances, their indications and adverse reactions, and the preparations containing them. The former group are, of course, essential to pharmacists and are produced in many countries, usually annually. The library of the Royal Pharmaceutical Society of Great Britain, in London, holds a wide range of them. The *Monthly Index of Medical Specialities (MIMS)* is widely circulated to general practitioners and doctors free and to others with a professional interest. Each issue contains details of new products in the form of a data sheet, discontinued products, lists of drugs in a pharmacological classification with presentation, composition and contraindications, together with a therapeutic index and a combined alphabetical and nonproprietary name index. The *Pharmaceutical Journal* also provides regular information about new products and product changes. The *Chemist and Druggist Directory* (Benn Brothers) is an annual trade directory and buyers' guide. It contains information about products, tabulated details of drug interactions, a tablet and capsule guide, a résumé of the Medicines Acts and a section providing information about companies with interests in pharmacy and pharmaceuticals.

An analogous American volume is the *Drug Topics Red Book* (Medical Economics Co.), an annual which provides product information not only about proprietaries, but also other drug store merchandise, such as cameras, as well as a colour guide for product identification and a section on drug interactions. An interesting feature of the drug entries is the National Drug Code system. This consists of a four- or five-figure code allotted to each manufacturer by the Food and Drugs Administration. Each product is then further coded with a four-figure code and finally a two-character package code. The identity and package size of each product is thus uniquely defined. There are other similar American publications such as the *American Drug Index* (Lippincott), which gives details of composition, presentation and use of products in alphabetical order with cross-indexing for generic, brand, chemical and *USP/NF* names. Thus, it is relatively simple to find a drug or combiniation even if only one major constituent is known. There is also a manufacturer/distributor index. Another American book, the *Merck Index* (11th edn., 1989, Merck), is rather more an organic or pharmaceutical chemistry reference work. It includes details of about 10 000 substances with a strong medical bias. Each entry contains a definition with references to the original literature or reviews and very brief details of therapeutic use where appropriate. There is an extensive cross-index of names as well as indexes for therapeutic categories, formulae and *Chemical Abstracts* registry number.

The indexes for other countries are prepared on similar lines to those described above. The German *Rote Liste* (Editio Cantor, Aulendorf/ Wüttenburg) is an annual similar to the *American Drug Index*. It is a collection of product information and includes pharmacological and pharmacokinetic data and recommendations for treating overdoses. It is now available on disc for IBM-PC. The French *Dictionnaire Vidal* (*OVP*) is also an annual, but is brought up to date 10 times during the year by the *Cahiers de Bibliographie Thérapeutique Française*. The *Dictionnaire* consists mainly of a listing providing details of therapeutic products covering composition, properties, indications, dosage and presentation, with a similar section on dietary and other products. It also includes a compound name index with trade/product name, a pharmacological classification giving trade names in each group and a listing of manufacturers and producers with their products.

L'Informatore Farmaceutico (Organizzazione Editoriale Medico-Farmaceutica, Milan), the Italian directory of drugs and manufacturers, is in two volumes with a separate index. Volume 1 lists all products by trade name with composition, presentation and code, together with over-the-counter preparations (e.g. baby products, diabetic foods). Volume 2 includes a list of drug substances, a therapeutic classification, a list of medicinal plants and information about manufacturers and concessionaires. The whole is kept up to date by the *Notiziario Medico Farmaceutico*.

Among many other such indexes, the following are given to provide some indication of geographical coverage: *Prescription Products Guide* (Australia and New Zealand); *Indice de Especialidades Farmaceuticas* (Spain); *Felleskaterlog* (Norway); *Israel Drug Compendium*; *Indian Pharmaceutical Guide* and the regional editions of *MIMS*.

The Royal Pharmaceutical Society library holds a comprehensive proprietary drug index on cards listed by trade name with details of composition, action and use, manufacturer and country. This has been compiled from data such as new product indexes and also from the literature. It includes drugs which have not been marketed commercially as well as proprietaries. Many of the entries have been compiled from the journal *Unlisted Drugs* (Pharmaco-Medical Documentation Inc.,

Box 429, Chatham, New Jersey). This is issued monthly and provides current-awareness coverage of all newly reported drugs which are not yet listed by name, composition and manufacturer in a basic drug compendium such as *Martindale* (see below). It also contains reviews of new books on drugs and certain other data. Information about each drug is given under the following headings: name, composition, equivalent preparation, manufacturer, pharmacological or clinical activity, reference. Information may also be provided by a structural diagram, dosage, synonyms and any earlier references in the journal. An interim index of numbers and names appears in July and an annual index after December. There is also a cumulative index. A valuable service is provided in the alternative supply of the data on cards each month. An index Guide is produced at irregular intervals. The journal *Drugs of the Future* contains similar snapshots of products under development.

The second group of drug compendia comprises those which provide more descriptive information than the group dealt with above. Some of these are annual volumes but many appear less frequently. Foremost among the English volumes is *Martindale's Extra pharmacopoeia*, edited by J.E.F. Reynolds (29th edn., Pharmaceutical Press, 1989). The aim of this is to provide practising physicians and pharmacists with up-to-date information on all substances in current use, whether official, unofficial or proprietary. It is compiled from the literature and draws on many pharmacopoeias and national formularies. Large numbers of references and abstracts are included. Part 1, which forms the bulk of the book, contains almost 4000 monographs grouped into chapters reflecting current therapeutic practice. Each chapter opens with an introduction of background information, often with a classification and description of classes of drugs within the group, followed by monographs on individual substances. Each monograph includes some or all of the following information: name of the drug together with official name and synonyms; molecular formula and molecular weight; list of foreign pharmacopoeias in which the drug may be found; dose, including information as to division and time, and paediatric dose; description and brief details of physical and pharmaceutical properties; dependence; adverse effects; antidotes; precautions, absorption and fate; uses. Brief abstracts may be provided under these headings, compiled from the literature. Finally, details are given of official preparations and of proprietary preparations available in the UK and proprietary names in use elsewhere. There is extensive cross-referencing. Part 2 contains short monographs on about 800 (new, obsolescent) drugs and ancillary substances and Part 3 is a selective list of 670 proprietary medicines available over the counter and which may be advertised to the public.

Martindale, which was first published in 1883 and has appeared at intervals since, is probably the key book for the bookshelf of anyone whose main interest is covered by the subject matter of this chapter. Certainly it should be readily available. It contains a mass of detailed information and provides direct access to original literature. The individual 'chapters', read as a whole, provide a succinct review of current therapeutics and clearly indicate those areas in which more effective and specific drugs are needed. Like all the best reference books, once opened it tempts one to digress into other pages. This edition has been compiled from a computer-based databank and the entries, which are now updated continuously, can be accessed online. Not surprisingly, *Martindale* is often used as the yardstick by which similar volumes are measured in reviews. Few measure up to it.

The *British National Formulary* (*BNF*) (British Medical Association and the Pharmaceutical Press) is revised and published every six months. Its aim is to promote effective prescribing and it is prepared for the benefit of professional staff in the National Health Service. The main section consists of chapters dealing with the drugs and preparations used for treatment of diseases of particular body systems, such as the respiratory system, or for a particular purpose, such as vaccines. Guidance is given about costs, and the preference of the panel of experts who compile the *Formulary* for particular preparations is indicated. In addition, there is a section on drug interactions, advice on prescribing in renal impairment and other special situations and an extensive index. Although the current policy of the *BNF* has been subjected to some criticism, the widespread distribution of the book to doctors, pharmacists and students completing their courses for these professions ensures that its opinions and recommendations have considerable impact. In an era of cost-consciousness, local formularies are also produced by some hospitals and health authorities in order to rationalize prescribing in their areas.

A U.S. view of available treatments is provided in the *Year book of drug therapy* (Year Book Medical Publishers). One of the American volumes similar to *Martindale* is *AMA drug evaluations* (American Medical Association). This provides details of pharmaceutical preparations for those prescribing, dispensing and administering drugs. The chapters are arranged in groups by therapeutic use, with a short introductory section. Each drug has a monograph which includes dose, route of administration and proprietary names. Although there are similarities with *Martindale*, the coverage is in some respects narrower. One area in which confusion may arise is with regard to proprietary names. Those given here are largely confined to those of North America, whereas *Martindale* provides names used in many countries. Although this may be considered a minor point, the immediate relevance of some of the information in the AMA volume is lost as a result.

The growing demand for information about products to be available in a defined style for physicians and for patients, has resulted in publication of compendia in several countries. The Medicines Act 1968 (see p. 231) requires that data sheets for medicinal products, to a format prescribed by regulation, be circulated to practitioners by the manufacturer. To simplify the system, the Association of the British Pharmaceutical Industry produces the *ABPI Data Sheet Compendium*. This combines data sheets from most companies, listed in alphabetical order, together with a product (trade mark) index, an index of non-proprietary names and a list of participating companies. Each sheet contains entries under the headings: presentation, uses, dosage and administration, contra-indications, etc., pharmaceutical precautions, legal category, package quantities, further information and product licence number.

The British Medical Association guide to medicines and drugs, edited by J. Henry (British Medical Association, 1988), is — despite its cumbersome title — an authoritative attempt to provide patients with basic information on more than 200 widely used drugs. Extensive use is made of graphical presentation of data and there is background information about therapeutic classification. A different approach is made in *A consumer's guide to prescription medicines* by B. Copper and L. Gerlis (Hamlyn, 1990) which is a straightforward alphabetical listing under trade and non-proprietary names providing details of the nature and use of each product with extensive cross-references. Since it is intended to reinforce the information about prescribed drugs given to the patient by the physician, no injectable preparations are included. Consumer interest in medicines means that many other guides of varying quality and coverage are published.

USP dispensing information, which has expanded from information previously included in the *National Formulary*, now consists of three volumes. Volume I, in two parts, is for the 'health care professional' and contains data similar to the ABPI compendium. Each entry comprises official name, dose form, category, pharmacology, precautions, side and adverse effects, patient consultation, dosages and storage. Volume II is particularly interesting being intended for use by the patient and for display in a pharmacy or hospital. The entries are written in less technical language and consist of name, explanation of use, information about proper use, precautions and side effects. It is suggested that copies of the relevant entries are made for the patient to take home. Volume III, which was first included in the 1989 edition, is entitled 'Approved Drugs and Legal Requirements'. Its purpose is to provide information about use of drugs, administration, dosage and commercial production as well as legal requirements governing them. The *Physicians' desk reference* (Medical Economics) is another U.S. annual, which has latterly included information about non-prescription drugs. It contains data sheets edited into a standard format with indexes for manufacturers' and product names, and products by category and generic name. There is a product identification colour guide and information is grouped by manufacturer. An uncommon feature is the section on diagnostic products. *Drug facts and comparisons* (Lippincott) is a similar loose-leaf compilation of product package literature also in a standard format arranged in sections by broad therapeutic classification.

Other similar compendia include the *MIMS Annual*, for Australia, which incorporates the Australian Drug Compendium and has entries in the data sheet format; the *Repertorio Terapeutico*, from the publishers of *L'Informatore Terapeutico*, which contains entries for about 5000 drugs and mixtures in both Italian and English; *FASS* (Farmaceutiska Specialiteter i Sverige), and the new *Japan Pharmaceutical Reference* (1st edn., 1989) containing data sheets for Japanese products and an appendix of new active substances approved in Japan since 1980.

The *Compendium Suisse des medicaments* (Documed, 1989) is similar to the *USP dispensing information* and consists of two volumes of product information for the medical professions; a separate volume containing a non-proprietary name index, therapeutic classification and manufacturers' lists; and a fourth volume with information intended for the patient, for example, when to take the product.

One problem associated with the study of drugs in current use, and that soon emerges, is the plethora of names which may be used for one substance in several countries. There are three reference volumes which are of importance with regard to the assignment of officially accepted names for drugs. International non-proprietary names (INN) are established by WHO for drugs in international use. A guide to the system is to be found in *WHO Chronicle*, 1981, **35**, 172-175. Lists are published regularly in *WHO Drug Information* and a cumulative list appears at intervals. The latest, *International non-proprietary names for pharmaceutical substances no. 7* (WHO, 1988), is a computer print-out of INN in Latin, English, French, Russian and Spanish. It includes national names where these differ significantly from the INN. Chemical names and graphic formulae are not included and must be found in the separate published lists. *British approved names 1990* (HMSO, 1990) is the most recent complete list of official names prepared by the British Pharmacopoeia Commission. The entries give official and chemical names, trade names, *Chemical Abstracts* registry number, manufacturer(s), code numbers and a therapeutic classification based on that in the *BNF* (p. 227). The existence of pharmacopoeial monographs is indicated. Guiding principles for selection of names are given, together with guidance on systematic chemical nomenclature of some groups of compounds, and a proprietary name/approved name cross-index.

The authorized list of names for use in the USA appears regularly as *USAN and the USP dictionary of drug names* (United States Pharmacopeial Convention, 1991). U.S. Adopted Names (USAN) are chosen usually when a drug is under development and so may never reach the market. The main listing is of USAN and names used in the USP/NF. Full entries include the name, chemical synonyms, empirical and structural formulae, *Chemical Abstracts* registry number, use, trade names and manufacturers. There is extensive cross-indexing. For convenience, INN for drugs not in use in the USA are given in one appendix and miscellaneous other non-proprietary names, for example for obsolete preparations, in another. Indexes of registry numbers and formulae are included.

Valuable compilations of synonyms are available: the most extensive is probably *Organic-chemical drugs and their synonyms* by M. Negwer in three volumes (6th edn., Akademie-Verlag, 1987). This lists over 9000 drugs and more that 80 000 synonyms. Entries are included by incremental molecular formulae. The following are given for each drug: structural and empirical formulae; *Chemical Abstracts* registry number; systematic names; salts which may be in use; synonyms, including official names; and therapeutic use. Volume 3 contains a group index for identification of drugs related chemically or pharmacologically.

The *Index Nominum 1987* (Société Suisse de Pharmacie, 1987) is the 13th edition of a volume revised at regular intervals. The main language is French, with instructions for use in English and German as well. It is a compilation of synonyms for therapeutic substances on an international basis and consists of an alphabetical list of drug names, including extensive cross-references. The key entries take the International Nonproprietary Name or another national approved name and give the chemical name, structural formula, therapeutic class, trade names and sources, and monograph titles in internationally important pharmacopoeias. If one name for a drug is known, any others can be traced very easily.

Legal requirements

At a time when statutory controls are imposed widely on medicinal products for both prescription and non-prescription use, legal requirements deserve a brief mention.

WHO drug information provides an overview of topics concerning drug development and regulation, relating this to therapeutic practice. It contains reports on individual substances, advisory notices, regulatory matters and discussion of policy issues involving drugs. A slim guide *Medicines and ethics* is produced every six months with the *Pharmaceutical Journal* and provides pharmacists with details of the law covering sale, supply and classification of medicines, together with information on labelling and other matters. Cumulated amendments appear monthly in the *Pharmaceutical Journal*.

A major piece of legislation in this country is the Medicines Act 1968, which exerts control over all aspects of manufacture, wholesaling, retailing and import of 'medicinal products', a class of substance which is defined very widely. This Act has had far-reaching effects on the pattern of drug development and use, and amplified earlier controls, which were much less extensive. It is implemented by a series of Statutory Instruments. Editorials on and a survey of the first ten years of the Act are in *British Journal of Clinical Pharmacology*, 1981, **12**, 447-463. The annual reports of the Medicines Commission and of the major committees established under the Act are published collectively by HMSO and provide details of their various activities and terms of reference. The Department of Health (Medicines Control Agency) issues *MAIL: Medicines Act Information Letter* several times per year. Although intended primarily for holders of licences issued under the Act, the contents are often of more general interest. The Agency also issues booklets giving notes for guidance on various aspects of application of the Medicines Act.

The accelerating influence of European Community requirements on national legislation continues to have an impact in the pharmaceutical field, as in others. EC Directives are published in the *Official Journal of the European Communities*, both when first proposed and when adopted. They are reprinted in the *Pharmaceutical Journal*. These Directives provide the framework for moves towards the single market from 1993 and have far-reaching consequences. As well as setting the criteria by which applications for marketing should be assessed, procedures are in place and being extended to facilitate centralized assessment of many applications. The Commission of the European Communities has published information, legal requirements and guidance in a set of five volumes of *Rules governing medicinal products in the European Community*. These contain texts of Directives relating to human and veterinary medicines, information for applicants, notes for guidance and details of good manufacturing practice. The 1989 edition of the *UK guidance notes on applications for product licences MAL 2* (Medicines Control Agency) explains the background to the change from national to Community requirements.

The major statutory control in America is exercised under the Federal Food, Drug and Cosmetic Act 1938 as subsequently amended. One particularly significant group of amendments (the Kefauver-Harris amendments) was enacted in 1962.

Similar legislation is in force or being introduced in many other countries, and is one field included in the quarterly *International Digest of Health Legislation*, collated and published by WHO. With a greater awareness of the risks as well as the benefits of drug treatment, it is inevitable that such legislation will increase rather than diminish.

History

Although historical sources are considered in Chapter 24 the reader's attention is drawn to a few sources of particular relevance. Early works are annotated in L.T. Morton's *Medical bibliography* (5th edn., Gower, 1991), which includes original publications up to about 1960 (for example, the original descriptions of the isolation of antibiotics) together with later histories. A special supplement to the *Journal of Pharmacy and Pharmacology* in April 1976 entitled 'Frontiers in Pharmacology', a collection of papers to mark the 50th anniversary of the founding of the pharmacological laboratories of the (Royal) Pharmaceutical Society of Great Britain, includes several entertaining accounts of the early activities of those laboratories. A further source of historical information is the lectures given on the occasion of award of the Nobel Prizes. These appear in *Science* within a few months of delivery and are published elsewhere.

Many standard textbooks acquire historical value over the years because, apart from their rarity, they provide an insight into the scientific development of a field. R.T. Williams' *Detoxication mechanisms* (1st edn., Chapman and Hall, 1947) is an example from the area of metabolism. The acquisition and study of such books can be an interesting and enlightening pastime.

CHAPTER ELEVEN

Tropical medicine

CATHERINE M. DEERING

Tropical medicine can no longer be considered an exotic or unusual branch of the profession; nor is it now of interest simply because of an increase in rare diseases made possible by increased air travel. Today tropical medicine is a multidisciplinary subject with a large and growing body of literature. In addition to preventing the spread of communicable diseases, the discipline encompasses a wide diversity of health problems in 'developing' countries: refugees, disasters, poverty, the provision of appropriate health care, appropriate technology, community participation, and many other issues. Topics such as AIDS, which has special relevance in the tropical context, have meant that every medical undergraduate must now acquire some knowledge of the specialty.

Journals

General tropical medicine

There are several major periodicals in the English language devoted largely or entirely to general tropical medicine, and to associated subjects, such as parasitology and entomology. The *Annals of Tropical Medicine and Parasitology* has been published since 1907 by the Liverpool School of Tropical Medicine, covering all aspects of tropical medicine and related sciences; its particular strength is the inclusion of papers from researchers in every part of the world. The *American Journal of Tropical Medicine and Hygiene*, the official organ of the

American Society of Tropical Medicine and Hygiene, Baltimore, has been published since 1952.

Also of great importance in this field are the *Transactions of the Royal Society of Tropical Medicine and Hygiene*, the official journal of that Society, and the *Journal of Tropical Medicine and Hygiene*, which emanates from the London School of Hygiene and Tropical Medicine. All the above publish the results of original research initiatives, often of a highly technical nature; all are published in English. *Tropical Doctor* continues to address the practical needs of medical workers in remote areas, with shorter papers and advice on the conditions and difficulties they are likely to meet.

To these important general journals must be added the vital serial publications of national medical associations and other regional bodies. The *Southeast Asian Journal of Tropical Medicine and Public Health* is the official publication of the Southeast Asian Ministers of Education Organization (SEAMEO) Regional Tropical Medicine and Public Health Project, which has given rise to many very important initiatives. This project was established in 1967 to help improve the health of the region by pooling manpower resources to upgrade existing research and training facilities. Other national and regional journals include the *African Journal of Medicine and Medical Sciences*, the *Central African Journal of Medicine*, the *East African Medical Journal*, the *Indian Journal of Medical Research*, the *Journal of the Kuwait Medical Association*, the *Journal of the Nepal Medical Association*, the *Journal of the Pakistan Medical Association*, the *Medical Journal of Malaysia*, the *Medical Journal of Zambia*, the *Papua New Guinea Medical Journal*, the *Saudi Medical Journal* and the *West Indian Medical Journal*.

Several European nations besides the UK have extensive interests in tropical medicine, and this is reflected in their periodical publications. From France, and from Francophone Africa, the following publish many significant papers annually: the *Bulletin de la Société Exotique et de ses Filiales* (Paris), *Cardiologie Tropicale* (Abidjan), *Dakar Médical (Dakar)*, *Médecine d'Afrique Noire* (Dakar), *Médecine Tropicale* (Marseilles), and *Revue d'Élevage et de Médecine Vétérinaire des Pays Tropicaux* (Paris). The Belgian Society of Tropical Medicine publishes the *Annales de la Société Belge de Médecine Tropicale* (Brussels). *Acta Tropica* is published by Elsevier in Holland in association with the Swiss Tropical Institute in Basel.

Parasitology

The study of parasites is vitally important in tropical medicine, and there has been a sharp increase in the past few years in the number of journals devoted to the subject. *Parasitology*, which originated in 1908, remains a leading journal in the field, which includes *Journal of Parasitology*, the journal of the American Society of Parasitologists, *Journal of Helminthology*, *Experimental Parasitology*, *International Journal for Parasitology*, *Molecular and Biochemical Parasitology*, *Parasite Immunology*, *Veterinary Parasitology* and *Parasitology Today*. The last title, publication of which begun in 1985, has quickly established itself as a popular forum for original articles and the exchange of newsworthy information, in a readable format which is rather more relaxed than the traditional journal. *Folia Parasitologica*, which emanates from the Czechoslovak Academy of Sciences, publishes the work of scholars from all parts of Europe, and *Parasitology Research*, which was founded as *Zeitschrift für Parasitenkunde*, is the organ of the German Society for Parasitology (Deutsche Gessellschaft für Parasitologie).

In other languages, *Angewandte Parasitologie* was published by the Parasitological Society of the former DDR (Parasitologische Gessellschafte der DDR); most of its papers are in German. The *Korean Journal of Parasitology* publishes some of its papers, and abstracts of many more, in English. Also of note are *Parassitologia*, a quarterly journal from Rome (Istituto di Parassitologia), and *Annales de Parasitologie Humaine et Comparée* appears in French, although some papers recently have been in English.

Entomology

A great deal of pertinent research now takes place in the field of medical entomology, and the following are the most important journals: the *Bulletin of Entomological Research*, published by the Commonwealth Agricultural Bureaux, *Canadian Entomologist*, the *Memoirs of the Entomological Society of Canada*, *Insect Science and its Application*, *Journal of Economic Entomology*, *Journal of Insect Physiology*, the *Journal of the American Mosquito Control Association*, *Journal of Medical Entomology*, *Mosquito News* and the journals of the Royal Entomological Society of London: *Ecological Entomology*, *Physiological Entomology*, *Systematic Entomology* and *Medical and Veterinary Entomology*.

Beiträge zur Entomologie publishes the work of European scholars in English, French and German; it emanates from the former Akademie der Landwirtschaftswissenschaften der DDR in Berlin.

Child health

A number of very interesting journals are devoted to the study of children in the tropics. *Annals of Tropical Paediatrics* is published by the Department of Tropical Paediatrics and International Child Health of the Liverpool School of Tropical Medicine. The British Paediatric Association publishes the *Archives of Disease in Childhood* in London. *Children in the Tropics* is the review of the International Children's Centre in Paris. This Centre was created by the French government in 1949, with the purpose of furnishing international agencies dealing with child care, with training facilities, and educational tools in the field of child health and development. The Paediatric Association of Nigeria produces the *Nigerian Journal of Paediatrics*, which, in particular, gives useful information on work and research being undertaken in various teaching hospitals in Nigeria. Similarly, the Indian Academy of Paediatrics in New Delhi publishes *Indian Paediatrics*; every article is screened for clinical relevance, and the proceedings of symposia are included.

Abstracting and indexing services

The abstracting service central to the discipline is *Tropical Diseases Bulletin*, produced by the Bureau of Hygiene and Tropical Diseases in London. This was started in 1908 as an intergovernmental information service under the titles of *Sleeping Sickness Bureau Bulletin* and *Kala-Azar Bulletin*. Now in its 87th volume, it continues its strong tradition of only abstracting papers which describe advances in knowledge or treatment of tropical disease. Each year the *Bulletin* includes a number of review articles on various major topics which are generally held to be among the best of the state-of-the-art surveys available. A major feature of the *Bulletin* is the excellence of the indexing; annual author, subject and geographical indexes are provided. The complementary *Abstracts on Hygiene and Communicable Diseases* focuses on communicable disease in countries outside the tropics. A valuable new initiative is the inclusion of *Public Health News*, which contains items on public health from the major newspapers and other sources scanned by the Bureau's staff. This is also available separately with its own annual index.

The CAB (Commonwealth Agricultural Bureaux) International Information Services at Wallingford, Oxon, produce and maintain a very important database for agriculture, land management and public health, among other subjects, and some of their hard-copy publications are directly relevant to the study of various aspects of parasitology and entomology. The most important are *Review of Medical and Veterinary Entomology, Biocontrol News and Information, Protozoological Abstracts, Helminthological Abstracts* and *Veterinary Bulletin*.

Part of *Excerpta Medica* (Amsterdam, Elsevier), section 17, is also concerned with public health, social medicine and epidemiology and *Current Contents: Life Sciences* can also be useful, although the reader will need to be selective. All the above are searchable through online hosts and on compact disk, and any reader interested in this approach to the literature should consult the relevant chapter.

Some other abstracting services focus on specific diseases. *Schisto Update*, from the Edna McConnell Clark Foundation of New York, is produced in co-operation with the National Library of Medicine MED-LARS service. This reproduces the abstracts relevant to the study of schistosomiasis from *Index Medicus*, and is distributed free of charge to interested individuals and institutions. The Tsetse and Trypanosomiasis Information and News Service at the Overseas Development Natural Resources Institute, Chatham, Kent, disseminates information on tsetse and trypanosomiasis control to scientists involved in the problems of African trypanosomiasis, in the *Tsetse and Trypanosomiasis Information Quarterly*. The Service is sponsored by the World Health Organization, the Food and Agriculture Organization of the United Nations, and the Overseas Development Natural Resources Institute, among others, and produces the *Quarterly* in both French and English editions. Non-commercial recipients in Africa may be entitled to receive it free of charge. *Courrier: Revue Médico-Sociale de l'Enfance* is published by the International Children's Centre in Paris in both French and English, and is devoted to the field of paediatrics, though it is not exclusively tropical.

The Southeast Asian Medical Information Centre (SEAMIC) and the International Medical Foundation of Japan in Tokyo are at present working on a SEAMIC *Index Medicus*, the early stages of which look extremely promising. They have already published BIBLIOMED-SM (Singapore and Malaysia): 1974–1979, published in 1982, the *Philippine Index Medicus* 1975–1979, published in 1985, the *Indonesian Index Medicus* 1975–1979, published in 1987, and the *Thai Index Medicus* 1975–1979, published in 1988. The 1980–1984 edition should be forthcoming within the next few years; the various parts are planned in one volume.

Bibliographies

A major contribution to the bibliography of primary health care and related disciplines began in 1975, when the International Development Research Centre in Ottawa initiated the series, *Salus: low cost rural health care and health manpower training: an annotated bibliography with special emphasis on developing countries* (IDRC, 1975-) This aimed to gather information on non-traditional health-care delivery systems in remote regions of the world, and was designed to be of use in the planning, operation and evaluation of systems providing rural health-care services. A particular effort was made to include unpublished grey literature. Ten volumes have been published at irregular intervals.

The IDRC has also supported the Museum and Reference Centre of the TROPMED National Centre of Thailand, Faculty of Tropical Medicine, Mahidol University, in its efforts to exchange information on major mosquito-borne diseases. The *Annotated bibliography on mosquito-borne diseases in Asia* was first published in 1983, covering dengue and dengue fever, Japanese B encephalitis, filariasis, malaria and mosquitoes. Further editions have been produced, covering 1984 and 1985.

Official publications of international agencies

The publications of the World Health Organization, both serial and monographic, are a crucial resource for the whole spectrum of tropical medicine. The *Public Health Papers* addresses such topics as health manpower, policy and planning, health systems support, management, etc. The *Technical Report* series continues a strong record of publication of the work of various Expert Committees on specific diseases, biological standardization, drug dependence, food additives, vectors and pests, etc. The status of most of the major diseases has been reviewed thoroughly in the 1980s.

The WHO has initiated an AIDS series, giving guidelines on the development of national AIDS prevention and control programmes. The 'Health for All' series contributes to, and monitors the progress of, the Organization's aspiration of 'Health for all by the year 2000', laid down at the Alma-Ata conference in 1978.

Various regional offices of the WHO – European, South-East Asia, Africa, the Western Pacific – maintain their own published series for topics of particular relevance to the region. Of particular prominence is the Pan American Health Organization. It has produced an official *Boletín* since 1922, with articles mainly in Spanish. It also distributes *Disaster Preparedness in the Americas*, an *Epidemiological Bulletin*, and the *EPI (Expanded Programme on Immunization) Newsletter*. The *WHO Publications Catalogue 1948–1989*, published in 1989, is the most concise and convenient guide to available material.

Other very valuable periodicals from the WHO are the *Weekly Epidemiological Record*, which provides up-to-date information on the incidence and distribution of important diseases; the *World Health Statistics Quarterly*, the *World Health Statistics Annual*, the *International Digest of Health Legislation*, *World Health Forum* and the *Bulletin of the World Health Organization*. *WHODOC: List of Recent WHO Publications and Documents* is issued every two months, covering all publications and a selection of documents of interest to health administrators and personnel.

The Southeast Asian Medical Information Centre (SEAMIC) regularly publishes the proceedings of its workshops and seminars on tropical disease and other health problems in the SEAMIC Publications Series. Recently the scope of this series has widened to include urbanization, primary health care and microcomputers for health planning.

Monographs and major textbooks

The standard textbook on tropical medicine in the English language is still '*Manson*', which was first published in 1898. *Manson's Tropical diseases* (Baillière Tindall, 1987), edited by P. E. C. Manson-Bahr and D. R. Bell, is now in its 19th edition. There is extensive coverage of all tropical diseases and the editors have aimed at a manual with relevance to both the clinician in the tropics and the doctor faced with the wider responsibilities of the district medical officer. With this very practical end in view, all the main clinical sections of the book have been written by practising physicians. The substantial appendices remain a notable feature of the book; lengthy sections on medical protozoology, medical helminthology, medical entomology and the laboratory diagnosis of tropical disease obviate the need for purchasers to acquire a separate textbook of parasitology.

A much shorter, but still very valuable, guide to the spectrum of diseases is *Lecture notes on tropical medicine* by D.R. Bell (Blackwell Scientific Publications, 3rd edn., 1990). This is a very practical book, giving a concise account of conditions and including case presentations and self-assessment questions. A chapter on AIDS has been included.

Another standard volume, that known as *Adams and Maegraith*, i.e. *Clinical tropical diseases* (Blackwell Scientific Publications, 9th edn., 1989) was edited by Brian Maegraith shortly before his death in 1989. Here the chapters are presented in alphabetical order of disease; there is increased coverage of viruses to include AIDS and Kaposi's sarcoma, and the chapter on malaria has been revised to include details of recent advances in the treatment of drug-resistant parasites. *Tropical and geographical medicine* (McGraw Hill, 2nd edn., 1990) by Kenneth S. Warren and Adel A.F. Mahmoud is clinical in emphasis, but contains a series of appendices on defining clinical syndromes, the geographic distribution of major infectious diseases and therapeutic approaches.

The standard U.S. book on the subject, *Hunter's Tropical medicine* (Saunders, 6th edn., 1984) is edited by G. Thomas Strickland. The latest edition has been almost completely rewritten; the majority of the contributors are American, but there are substantial sections by UK contributors and from doctors working in tropical countries.

Also American is A.S. Benenson's *Control of communicable diseases in man* (American Public Health Association, 14th edn., 1985). This does not aim to be a standard textbook; instead it is a manual presenting basic information on how to recognize a disease, how to manage patients and limit the spread of infection. It considers communicable diseases globally, and although many of the conditions described are not specifically tropical, a great deal of space is devoted to 'exotic' diseases. Smallpox is still covered, although now eradicated, on the grounds that an appropriate source of information is necessary, should its reappearance be suspected.

Leprosy

Jopling's *Handbook of leprosy* (Heinemann, 4th edn., 1988) now has two authors, W.H. Jopling and A.C. McDougal. The handbook covers much new ground in multidrug therapy, and reaffirms the importance of the role of paramedicals, or auxiliaries, in controlling the disease. There is a concise and useful glossary especially provided for readers in this capacity.

In 1988 the World Health Organization published the second edition of *Guide to leprosy control* (Geneva, 1988). This is based in part on work done in the 1980s by various Study Groups, whose deliberations have been published in the Technical Report series. This *Guide* aims to provide all background information necessary for planning and implementing successful control programmes. *Leprosy*, edited by Robert C. Hastings (Churchill Livingstone, 1985) is a textbook which also considers the large amount of new research information available on the disease since the publication of *Leprosy in theory and practice* by R.G. Cochrane and T.F. Davey (Wright, 1964).

Cholera

There is still no major work bringing together advances in research and practical help in patient care for cholera, although a great deal is being published on this and other diarrhoeal diseases. *Dialogue on diarrhoea* is a readable and informative source of information on the topic; it is distributed free to developing countries. The International Centre for Diarrhoeal Diseases Research, Dhaka, Bangladesh, produces the *Journal of Diarrhoeal Diseases Research*, a forum for original research articles, and a thorough, annotated bibliography on the subject.

Smallpox

The world's last naturally occurring case of smallpox was in Somalia, in 1977. In 1966 the World Health Assembly decided to establish an Intensified Smallpox Eradication Programme, with an annual allocation of $2.4 million. Its goal was the complete elimination of the disease within ten years. On 8 May 1980, the Thirty-Third World Health Assembly adopted a resolution declaring that smallpox had been eradicated globally; it also recommended that this extraordinary feat should be fully recorded. *Smallpox and its eradication* (WHO, 1988), by F. Fenner, D.A. Henderson *et al.* takes the Intensified Programme as its main focus and describes the many different activities it embraced. A full account of the clinical and epidemiological features of the disease is included, a history of smallpox vaccination, and a consideration of immunological and virological aspects of the now extinct disease.

Malaria

L.J. Bruce-Chwatt's *Essential malariology* (Heinemann Medical, 1955) which went into its second edition in 1985, is now a classic. The most important recent publication has been *Malaria: principles and practice of malariology* (Churchill Livingstone, 1988), edited by W.H. Wernsdorfer and Sir Ian McGregor. Almost 40 years after Boyd's *Malariology* (Saunders, 1949) this interdisciplinary study presents a comprehensive survey of all aspects of the subject. It is orientated principally to malaria as a human disease, but substantial coverage of experimental studies of animal malarias is included where this is informative in describing the dynamics of infection. The large and thorough bibliography draws on the usual sources, and also provides information on the material on the disease in unpublished documents of the World Health Organization Malaria Action Programme and the Division of Vector Biology Control, from whose directors copies can usually be obtained.

W. Peters' *Chemotherapy and drug resistance in malaria* (Academic Press, 2nd edn., 1987), also gives a wide-ranging survey of the last two decades' literature, providing a concise account of recent work on both the malaria parasites themselves and the continuing search for new antimalarial compounds.

Trypanosomiasis

The African trypanosomiases (Allen and Unwin, 1970), by H.W. Mulligan, although an old textbook now by medical standards, is still worth consulting for the breadth of its consideration of the subject and its large bibliography. Similarly, *The trypanosomes of mammals*, by C.A. Hoare

(Blackwell Scientific Publications, 1972) was a milestone in the subject and remains an excellent example of the zoological approach to the disease. These texts can be brought up to date by reading Anthony M. Jordan's *Trypanosomiasis control and African rural development* (Longman, 1986), which addresses itself to disease control mechanisms, and vector control in particular, and gives lucid examples of control campaigns. There is also in-depth consideration of the ecological background to the sleeping sickness problem. Although there is a long bibliography, Jordan has not attempted an exhaustive review of existing literature; he has, however, tried to emphasize the less widely disseminated views of recent workers.

In *The biology of Trypanosoma and Leishmania: parasites of men and domestic animals* (Taylor and Francis, 1983), D.H. Molyneux and R.W. Ashford have attempted to present a summary of knowledge of the biology of what they call the 'haemoflagellates' and their vectors, at such a level that it can be read by the non-specialist. They explain how an understanding of various characteristics of these parasites could lead to elucidation of wider biological problems. Selected texts for further reading are given at the end.

For the veterinary side of the subject, *Trypanosomiasis: a veterinary perspective* (Pergamon, 1986), by Lorne E. Stephen tries to fill the gap Hoare identified in this aspect of the disease. This is a discursive and conversational book in some respects, but it is rigorous in its examination of the different species of *Trypanosoma* and their effects on economically important animals. Diagnostic procedures, chemotherapy and zoonotic aspects are also covered. Its long bibliography is well researched and thorough.

Schistosomiasis

Over 200 million people are believed to be infected with schistosomiasis, or bilharziasis, and the disease seems to be spreading through irrigation schemes and dams, the building of which creates new snail habitats. Two publications of the 1980s have brought together the work of many distinguished researchers on both the clinical and public-health significance of the disease. In 1987 Baillière Tindall devoted a volume of its series, *Clinical Tropical Medicine and Communicable Diseases: International Practice and Research*, to this topic, edited by A.A.F. Mahmoud. This includes descriptions of the clinical syndromes and diagnostic methods developed by doctors and scientists; it also covers the management of control strategies and the possibility of creating vaccines. *The biology of schistosomes: from genes to latrines* (Academic Press, 1977), edited by David Rollinson and Andrew J.G. Simpson, as its title suggests, integrates studies on all major aspects of the biology of schistosomes, from basic facets of the organisms to molecular analyses. The chapters contain well-balanced lists of references, but its citation of articles and books is nevertheless selective, as the editors wish to concentrate on presenting the significant concepts.

In 1985, Cambridge University Press published an account of a single project which investigated the advantages and disadvantages of various control methods in a particular geographic location, the island of St. Lucia. *Schistosomiasis: the St. Lucia project* (CUP, 1985), by Peter Jordan, describes in detail the project which has become widely known in all circles interested in parasitic research. It is essential reading for all involved in designing control strategies, whether at administrative or laboratory level.

Child health

On present trends, it has been estimated that more than 100 million children will die from illness and malnutrition in the 1990s; 50 million of these deaths will be from diseases which can be inexpensively treated or prevented. This frightening statistic is provided in *The state of the world's children 1990* (OUP, Unicef, 1990), edited by James P. Grant, Executive Director of the United Nations Children's Fund. This annual report, which began publication in 1980, very usefully summarizes the position of the very young and helpless in the world's poorest countries. It provides authoritative information on the progress of immunization, breast feeding, child spacing, literacy, life expectancy and school enrolment, and very useful tables of figures on basic indicators, nutrition, health, education, demographic and economic indicators and the rate of progress. *Diseases of children in the tropics and subtropics* (Edward Arnold, 4th edn., 1990), edited by D.B. Jelliffe and J.P. Stanfield, has become something of a classic.

The *Nelson Textbook of paediatrics* (13th edn., Saunders, 1987) is not exclusively tropical, but contains much information relevant to the care of children in tropical countries. This edition was edited by R.E. Behrman and V.C. Vaughan. In the same category is *Textbook of paediatrics* (Churchill Livingstone, 3rd edn., 1984), edited by J.O Forfar and G.C. Arneil.

Primary health care

The World Health Organization published the declaration of Alma-Ata in 1978, calling on the governments of the world to strive for 'Health for all by the year 2000', launching one of the great public-health movements of modern times. Many important works have been published recently, contributing to and monitoring the progress of this aspiration. The WHO's seventh report on the world health situation, *Evaluation of the strategy for health for all by the year 2000* (WHO, 1987) was derived principally from contributions of member states on their own evaluation of national strategies for the attainment of the goal. Further WHO publications of note are *From Alma-Ata to the year 2000: reflections at the midpoint* (WHO, 1988), which brings together various papers and comments on the declaration arising from the Forty-First World Health Assembly at Riga in 1988 and a number of short publications dealing with health indicators, managerial techniques, and programme evaluation principles have been published in the 'Health for All' series. There were ten publications in this series in 1989.

Health services management

Since the Alma-Ata declaration it has been generally acknowledged that major constraints in achieving 'Health for all by the year 2000' are lack of skills in health management in the developing countries, and poor management support infrastructures, in areas such as transport, health information and drug provision. The Seventy-Third Session of the WHO Executive Board, which convened in Geneva in 1984, urgently advised the strengthening of managerial capacity. Much general management literature, found in a variety of sources, is of use in studying this area, but three publications specifically about health management are of note. The African Medical and Research Foundation of Kenya has produced a two-volume *Health service management* (Nairobi: AMREF, 1988), edited by S. Kanani, J. Maneno and P. Schlutter; volume I contains learning materials developed for workshops on problem solving and health management, and volume II the materials on health planning and the proceedings of a practical workshop. *Management training strategies for developing countries* (Boulder: Lynne Rienner, 1987), by J. E. Kerrigan and J. S. Luke, assesses the state of management training in the Third World, examines the strengths and weaknesses of different training approaches currently utilized, and provides practical recommendations for more effective training initiatives. Finally, although not targeted directly at developing world problems, *Managing health professionals* (Chapman and Hall, 1989) addresses the main personnel management elements where health professionals are concerned.

General parasitolology

Monographs abound on every detail of the rapidly growing discipline of parasitology. The publication of Craig and Faust's *Clinical parasitology* (Lea and Febiger, 9th edn., 1984) under the authorship of Paul C. Beaver, R.C. Jung and E.W. Cupp originally appeared in 1970. This continues the original intention of providing a handbook source of essential facts for physicians, and for graduate and postgraduate students. It also gives approved methods of diagnosis, treatment and control of parasitic diseases. The number of zoonotic species described has been expanded. *Modern parasitology* (Blackwell, 1982), edited by F.E.G. Cox, does not try to duplicate any such information: instead it tries to isolate and stress less usual aspects, such as chemotherapy, nutrition, epidemiology, immunity and prospects for vaccination. A complete chapter is devoted to the literature, providing a useful and concise summary of approaches to the subject.

Another large textbook, *General parasitology* (Academic, 2nd edn., 1986), by Thomas C. Cheng, presents the 'classical', basic information fully and lucidly, and particular attention is paid to taxonomy. This work is aimed primarily at biologists, rather than doctors and medical students, but this second edition does devote more space than the first to species of medical importance. Extensive references are provided at the end of each chapter.

A book specifically written as an introductory text is *Medical parasitology* (Gower, 1990) by Ralph Muller and John R. Baker. A notable feature of this book is the excellence of the illustrations, all of which are in colour. New techniques in molecular biology, such as infraspecific variation, and immunodiagnosis, are described, and the reading list, though short, is up to date and well chosen to reflect the most modern scholarship. *Parasites and human disease* (Arnold, 1985), by W. Crewe and R.D. Haddock, addresses the question of parasitic infections which occur outside the tropics, and which would therefore constitute a public-health problem, rather than a localized matter of concern for the infected individual. The book emphasizes the biology and transmission of parasites, on laboratory and clinical diagnosis, and on therapy. It also serves as a concise introductory text for individuals intending to work in warm climates.

Immunity to parasites: how animals control parasitic infections (Arnold, 1984), by Derek Wakelin, is concerned with the field of immunoparasitology. It concentrates on selected host–parasite relationships where immunologically-orientated research has been important.

The field of veterinary parasitology is also expanding. Two very helpful points of reference are: G.M. Urquhart *et al.*, *Veterinary parasitology* (Longman, 1987), a book aimed at veterinarians involved in the diagnosis, treatment and control of diseases in domestic animals. Here details of classification are kept to a minimum, as they are of limited value to the veterinarian, and taxonomic information is presented only at generic level. Secondly, the Commonwealth Agricultural Bureaux International and the Institut d'Élevage et de Médecine Vétérinaire des Pays Chauds, France, have now produced a *Manual of tropical veterinary parasitology* (Wallingford: CAB, 1989). The objective of the manual is to provide technical livestock service personnel and producers with information on helminths which they may have to identify and deal with. For practical reasons, the descriptions of parasitic diseases is based on autopsy techniques, i.e. focusing on the organ. Diagnostic methods are dealt with fully, and there is a section on currently available anthelmintics.

General entomology

A concise and useful introduction to the subject can be found in M.W. Service's *Lecture notes on medical entomology* (Blackwell, 1986) which presents the basics of insect-borne diseases and insect parasites for students of medicine, hygiene, public health and parasitology. The book is very clearly illustrated, facilitating identification of the insects described. Anyone requiring further detail should consult *Comprehensive insect physiology, biochemistry and pharmacology* (Pergamon, 1985), edited by G.A. Kerkut and L.I. Gilbert, an exhaustive work of 12 volumes, in which the literature reviews should save researchers a great deal of time.

History

H.H. Scott's *A History of tropical medicine* (Arnold, 1939) is an exhaustive study of the subject. Parasitology is well covered by W.D. Foster's *History of parasitology* (Livingstone, 1965), and R.T. Leiper's paper 'Landmarks in medical helminthology' in the *Journal of Helminthology*, 1929, 7, 101-110, is a useful contribution. W.H.S. Jones's *Malaria and Greek society* (Manchester University Press, 1909) is a classic in its field. A more recent study has been published by L.J. Bruce-Chwatt and J. de Zulueta: *The rise and fall of malaria in Europe: an historico-epidemiological study* (OUP, 1980). Two works on leprosy worthy of note are D.A. Zamabaco's *La Lèpre à travers les sièecles et les contrées* (Masson, 1914) and A. Weymouth's *Through the leper squint: a study of leprosy from pre-Christian times to the present day* (Selwyn and Blount, 1938). *A history of bubonic plague in the British Isles* by J.F.D. Shrewsbury (Cambridge University Press, 1970) is an extensive study with 76 pages of references and 27 page bibliography. *Health in tropical Africa during the colonial period* edited by E.E. Sabben-Clare *et al.* (Oxford University press, 1980) is based on the proceedings of a symposium held in Oxford in 1977.

Tropical medicine and parasitology: classic investigations compiled by B.H. Kean *et al.* (2 vols, Cornell University Press, 1978), provides a valuable collection of texts not easily available otherwise. Finally, not a history but a perspective of strategies for the future is found in the proceedings of a 1977 conference, *Tropical medicine from romance to reality* edited by C. Wood (Academic Press, 1979).

CHAPTER TWELVE

Pathology, clinical and experimental

ANNE COLLINS

with contibutions on Cancer from M.K. Gallico and on AIDS from Suzanne Bates.

Pathology is the scientific study of disease processes. It includes observation of the structural and functional changes throughout the course of a disease. In its widest sense the subject covers all aspects of the cause and effect of abnormalities of function or structure resulting from any agent that has damaging effects on the body whether it be a genetically caused inherited disease or one caused by chemical or biological agents. Involved in the full understanding of the subject are the disciplines of morbid anatomy, histology and cytology, immunology, biochemistry, haematology, microbiology, physiology and clinical medicine. For this reason this chapter cannot attempt to be comprehensive but simply to act as a guide to the literature of a very wide-ranging subject. For the same reason, some topics are not dealt with here, the reader being directed to the specific chapter concerned with that subject.

Indexes and abstract journals

Indexes, abstracts, bibliographies and reviews are dealt with in detail in Chapter 3. *Index Medicus* and its forerunners and *Excerpta Medica* will provide most of the information required by the pathologist for retrospective searching and this can be supplemented for current awareness by *Current Contents: Life Sciences*.

Index Medicus is an extremely comprehensive index to the medical sciences. The list of journals indexed includes some 66 titles under the heading of 'Pathology' alone while several hundreds of titles are listed under related headings for, as we have already seen, almost every aspect of medicine can have its pathological significance.

Excerpta Medica is published in a number of sections, those most use to pathologists being Section 5, General Pathology and Pathological Anatomy; Section 21, Developmental Biology and Teratology; and Section 26, Immunology, Serology and Transplantation.

Databases

Online and CD-ROM sources of information retrieval are dealt with in detail in Chapter 5 but, again, we should mention here that databases such as MEDLINE, CANCERLINE, EMBASE provide access to bibliographic information (and abstracts). References can be retrieved in these systems using indexing terms combined together with Boolean operators. The resulting list of references will accurately reflect the subject of the search.

The development of optical disc technology (CD-ROM – Compact Disc-Read-Only-Memory) has brought automated literature retrieval within reach of the enquirer himself. The financial constraints imposed by telecommunication and connect time costs as well as less-than-friendly software has tended to keep online searching within the province of the librarian or the information officer who has acted as an intermediary, interpreting the enquiry into computer terms. CD-ROM, which runs on a personal computer and has software designed with the inexperienced searcher in mind, has brought about a revolution in information retrieval. The biomedical area has been well served and MEDLINE was one of the first bibliographic databases to become available. CANCERLIT, PDQ, COMPACT LIBRARY: AIDS and AIDS KNOWLEDGE BASE are all relevant sources which are described in more detail later in the chapter under the appropriate subject headings. EMBASE has recently entered the market with a version of the database containing the abstracts published between 1984–87; more recent material is being split by subject in a similar way to the printed version although at present only a limited number of subject areas is being covered. EXCERPTA MEDICA CD: PATHOLOGY and IMMUNOLOGY AND AIDS are probably of interest.

Current-awareness services on floppy disc are also increasingly relevant. Services such as CURRENT CONTENTS, REFERENCE UPDATE and MEDICAL SCIENCE WEEKLY contain up-to-the-minute bibliographic information, much of which will be of interest to the pathologist.

General textbooks and atlases

There are numerous excellent general textbooks of pathology. Many of them are long established and are updated at frequent intervals. The selection of a general textbook depends to some extent upon personal taste, or the currently fashionable choice, but some of those that are most popular are:

Anderson's Pathology, edited by J.M. Kissane (2 vols, 9th edn., Mosby, 1990)

Boyd's Textbook of pathology, by A.C. Ritchie (9th edn., Lea and Febiger, 1990)

General pathology, by J.B. Walter and M.S. Israel (6th edn., Churchill Livingstone, 1987)

Introduction to general pathology, by W.G. Spector (3rd edn., Churchill Livingstone, 1989)

Muir's Textbook of pathology, edited by J.R. Anderson (12th edn., Edward Arnold, 1985)

Pathology: the mechanisms of disease, by R.A. Cawson (2nd edn., Mosby, 1989)

Pathology illustrated, by A.D.T. Govan, P.S. MacFarlane and R. Callander (2nd edn., Churchill Livingstone, 1989)

Robbins Pathologic basis of disease, edited by R.S. Cotran, V. Kumar and S.L. Robbins (4th edn., Saunders, 1989)

Books on surgical pathology include:

Ackerman's Surgical pathology, edited by J. Rosai (2 vols, 7th edn., Mosby, 1989)

Diagnostic surgical pathology, edited by S.S. Sternberg *et al.* (2 vols, Raven Press, 1989)

Pathology in surgical practice, edited by G.J. Hadfield, M. Hobsley and B.C. Morson (Edward Arnold, 1985)

Principles and practice of surgical pathology, by S.G. Silverberg (2 vols, 2nd edn., Churchill Livingstone, 1988)

Surgical pathology, by W. Coulson (2 vols, 2nd edn., Lippincott, 1988)

Atlases have long been a popular medium since so much of the information is essentially visual in nature. The earliest atlas, by Julius Vogel, *Icones histologiae pathologicae* appeared in 1843 and a second, by Hermann Lebert, *Physiologie pathologique ou recherches cliniques, experimentales et microscopiques* in 1845. Of more recent works, the *CIBA Collection of medical illustrations* edited by Frank H. Netter and published in eight volumes (CIBA Pharmaceutical Co., 1985–1986) is an important example. Others include: *Basic histopathology: a colour atlas and text*, by P. Wheater *et al.* (Churchill Livingstone, 1985); *Colour atlas of histopathology,* by R.C. Curran (3rd rev. edn., Oxford University Press, 1985); *Colour atlas of surgical pathology*, by W. Guthrie and R. Fawkes (Wolfe Medical, 1982).

Slide sets

A natural extension of the colour atlas is the slide set because of the visual character of the subject. Several of the publishers of atlases also publish slide sets, either to accompany an atlas or as separate entities. A very short selection includes:

Blood under the microscope, by G.F. Riedler and V. Graswinckel (Wolfe Medical) [214 slides with a textbook of 180 pages]

Disease entities by W. Siegenthaler and W. Ostermayer (Wolfe Medical) [310 colour slides with a booklet containing brief comments on each slide]

Blood and bone marrow cell recognition and interpretation, by V. Minnich *et al.* (Raven Press/American Society of Clinical Pathologists Press, 1982) [A series of ten slide presentations each accompanied by a cassette and a short monograph]

Journals

Many of the clinical medical journals publish papers that are relevant to the pathologist so material is often to be found there as well as in the specialist journals of pathology. Modern pathology is usually considered to date from the publication by Rudolph Virchow of his famous book *Die Cellularpathologie in ihrer Begründung auf physiologische und pathologische Gewebelehre* (Hirschwald, 1858). Some specialist journals of pathology, still in publication, precede this book, as does Virchow's own *Virchow's Archiv für pathologische Anatomie und Physiologie.* By the end of the century, *Zentralblatt für allgemeine Pathologie und pathologische Anatomie* (1892) and the *Journal of Pathology and Bacteriology* (1892) were in publication and still continue, the latter, since 1969, being renamed the *Journal of Pathology.* Amongst those that are of interest are: *American Journal of Pathology, American Journal of Clinical Pathology, American Journal of Surgical Pathology, Archives of Pathology and Laboratory Medicine, Experimental and Molecular Pathology*, and *Human Pathology*, all from the USA; *British Journal of Experimental Pathology* which became known as *Journal of Experimental Pathology* in 1990, and *Histopathology* from the UK, and *Pathology* from Australia. From Asia there are the *Indian Journal of Pathology and Microbiology* and the *Malaysian Journal of Pathology*.

Very specialized titles also exist such as *Veterinary Pathology* and *Journal of Invertebrate Pathology* which have a more limited readership. Other specialist journals are listed in the relevant sections on succeeding pages.

Review publications

A number of journals publish review articles and some concentrate entirely on this type of paper. They can often be identified by titles such as *Annual Review of ...*, *Recent Advances in ...*, *Year Book of ...*, and titles of particular interest to pathologists include:

Advances in Pathology, edited by C.M. Fenoglio-Preiser (Year Book Medical, 1988–)

Current Topics in Pathology, edited by C.L. Berry and E. Grundmann (Springer-Verlag)

International Review of Experimental Pathology, edited by G.W. Richter and M.A. Epstein (Academic Press, 1962–)

Pathology, edited by A.D. Fayemi (9th edn., Elsevier, 1988)

Pathology Annual, edited by S.C. Sommers, P.P. Rosen and R.E. Fechner (Appleton-Century-Crofts, 1966–)

Methods

As we saw at the beginning, the study and practice of pathology involves a wide range of disciplines and methods. They all have their own literature and, although the following sections cannot attempt to be comprehensive they will give an indication of the very wide area upon which the pathologist must draw for his information.

Autopsy

The post-mortem examination of the patient carried out with the intention of finding out the cause of death, the extent of the disease or the injuries that caused the death, and also the effect of any therapeutic intervention or any conditions that were unrecognized before death but may have affected the course of the disease is an important part of pathology. The development of techniques such as needle biopsy, endoscopy, and a variety of scanning and imaging techniques has had an effect on the use of autopsy in that much information can be obtained during life. While, in the past, many diagnoses were made at the postmortem examination it now has a role in revealing changes in the patterns of many diseases, the unexpected and unwanted effects of many drugs and other therapeutic procedures, and in demonstrating the natural history of a disease process.

Two books dealing with autopsy are *The coroner's autopsy: a guide to non-criminal autopsies for the general pathologist* by B. Knight (Churchill Livingstone, 1983) and *Post-mortem procedures: an illustrated textbook*, by G.A. Gresham and A.F. Turner (Year Book Medical Publishers, 1979). A useful atlas is *An atlas of gross pathology*, by C.D.M. Fletcher and P.H. McKee (Edward Arnold, 1987).

Histological methods

Histological methods are used to study the tissues removed from patients in surgical procedures. Histopathology is the study of the structural changes in diseased tissues by the examination of tissue sections or smears using the naked eye, light or electron microscopy. These studies involve a knowledge of cytology, which is the branch of biology concerned with the study of cells, and histology which involves the treatment of tissue and cells with special chemicals which make the structures more clearly visible in microscopic examination.

Journals devoted to histological methods include the *Journal of Histochemistry and Cytochemistry*, which is the official journal of the Histochemical Society, *Histopathology*, the journal of the British Division of the International Academy of Pathology and *Histochemical Journal*. Some recent books on histological techniques including the use of dyes and stains and histochemistry are as follows.

HISTOLOGICAL TECHNIQUES

Theory and practice of histological techniques, edited by J.D. Bancroft and A. Stevens (3rd edn., Churchill Livingstone, 1990)

DYES AND STAINS

Conn's Biological stains, edited by R.D. Lillie (9th edn., Williams and Wilkins, 1977)

Staining procedures, edited by G. Clark (4th edn., published for the Biological Stain Commission by Williams and Wilkins, 1981)

Synthetic dyes in biology, medicine and chemistry, by E. Gurr (Academic Press, 1971)

Colour atlas of histological staining techniques, by A. Smith and J.W. Bruton (Wolfe Medical, 1977)

HISTOCHEMISTRY

Histochemistry, theoretical and applied, by A.G.E. Pearse (2 vols, 4th edn., Churchill Livingstone, 1980-85)

Histopathological technic and practical histochemistry, by R.D. Lillie and H.M. Fulmer (4th edn., McGraw Hill, 1976)

Microscopy

Microscopy is the examination of tissue and cell structure with the aid of an enlarging instrument. This may be an optical microscope or an electron microscope. There are many microscopic techniques including: stereoscopic microscopy in which a pair of low-power microscopes are used giving a large depth of focus; polarized light microscopy which uses light which is vibrating in a single plane; electron microscopy, which uses a beam of light to visualize particles too small to be resolved by a light microscope. It permits details of tissue to be seen clearly at magnifications of 100 000–150 000 times. This development had an enormous effect in pathological research because of the detail it revealed. In routine pathology, however, it has been less important partly because of the expense of the equipment but also because the processing, section cutting and subsequent examination of the material is too time consuming.

There are journals specifically concerned with microscopy, for example *Journal of Microscopy*, published in Oxford, which was known as the *Journal of the Royal Microscopical Society* until 1969. It was first published in 1878. *Scanning Microscopy* and *Ultrastructural Pathology* are also of interest.

Numerous books have been published about the use of the microscope. A useful series of pamphlets published jointly by the Royal Microscopical Society and Oxford University Press and known as *Microscopy handbooks* began in 1984 and now includes some 22 volumes. Many of them are relevant and titles include *An introduction to the optical microscope*, by S. Bradbury (Microscopy Handbooks, No. 1 rev. edn., Oxford University Press, 1989) and *The operation of the transmission electron microscope*, by D. Chescoe and P. J. Goodhew (Microscopy Handbooks No. 2, Oxford University Press, 1984). Other books include *Fundamentals of light microscopy*, by M. Spencer (Cambridge University Press, 1982), *The microscope and how to use it*, by P.B. Carona (Gulf Publications, 1970) and *Microscope technique*, by W. Burrells (Halstead Press, 1977).

Electron microscopy is covered by books such as *Introduction to electron microscopy*, by C.E. Hall (2nd edn., McGraw-Hill, 1966), *Practical methods in electron microscopy*, edited by A.M. Glauert (10 vols, North-Holland 1972–1985), *Diagnostic electron microscopy*, by J.V. Johannessen and M. Sobrinho-Simoes (Hemisphere Publishing Corporation, 1982), *Introduction to diagnostic electron microscopy*, by B. MacKay (Appleton-Century-Crofts, 1981), *Electron microscopy in human medicine*, edited by J.V. Johannessen (11 vols, McGraw-Hill, 1979–1985) and *Principles and practice of electron microscopy*, by I.M. Watt (Cambridge University Press, 1985).

Photomicrography also has specialized texts including *An introduction to photomicrography*, by D.J. Thomson and S. Bradbury (Oxford University Press, 1987).

Experimental animals

The use of experimental animals is a controversial matter and there is much strong opposition to the practice. There can be no doubt, however, that their use has permitted considerable advances in the understanding of many processes. Among the journals dealing with the subject are *Laboratory Animals*, *Laboratory Animal Science* and the *Journal of the Institute of Animal Technicians*.

A vital text for any laboratory using animals is *UFAW Handbook on the care and management of laboratory animals*, edited by T.B. Poole (6th edn., Longman Scientific, 1987). There are many other books about the care and handling of laboratory animals, such as *Handbook for the animal licence holder*, edited by H.V. Wyatt (Institute of Biology, 1980), while publications also exist which provide information about the holdings of species and strains. Among these are *International index of laboratory animals giving sources of animals throughout the world*, edited by M.F.W. Festing (5th edn., Laboratory Animals, 1987), 'Standardized nomenclature for inbred strains of mice: eighth listing for the International Committee on Standardized Genetic Nomenclature for Mice', by J. Staats (*Cancer Research*, 1985, **45**, 945-977). Between publication of the listings, additions and deletions to strain holdings appear in *Mouse News Letter* and *Inbred Strains of Mice*.

The use of laboratory animals in research is covered by books such as *Methods of animal experimentation*, edited by W.I. Gay (7 vols, Academic Press, 1965–1989), while books dealing specifically with pathology include *Pathology of laboratory animals*, edited by K. Benischke *et al.* (2 vols., Springer-Verlag, 1978), *The pathology of laboratory animals*, by W.E. Ribelin and J.R. McCoy (2nd printing, C. C. Thomas, 1971) and *Pathology of laboratory mice and rats*, edited by

P.L. Altman (Pergamon Press, co-publishers with the Federation of American Societies for Experimental Biology, 1985).

There are also many specialized texts dealing with a particular type of laboratory animal. Examples are:

Colour atlas of the rat: a dissection guide, by R.J. Olds (Wolfe Medical, 1979)

Experimental and surgical technique in the rat, by H.B. Waynforth (Academic Press, 1980)

Laboratory rat, Vol. 1, Biology and diseases; Vol. 2, Research applications, edited by H.J. Baker *et al.* (Academic Press, 1979 and 1980)

Pathology of the Fischer rat: reference and atlas, edited G.A. Boorman *et al.* (Academic Press, 1990)

Biology of the laboratory mouse, by the staff of the Jackson Laboratory and edited by E.L. Green (2nd edn., McGraw-Hill, 1966; reprinted, Dover, 1975)

The nude mouse in experimental and clinical research, edited by J. Foch and B.C. Giovanella (Academic Press, 1978)

The biology of the guinea pig, edited by J.E. Wagner and P.J. Manning (Academic Press, 1976)

The biology of the laboratory rabbit, edited by S.H. Weisbroth *et al.* (Academic Press, 1974)

The pig as a laboratory animal, by L.E. Mount and D.L. Ingram (Academic Press, 1971)

Controls and checks on the use of animals for experimental purposes do exist and a statistical report produced under the provisions of the Cruelty to Animals Act 1876 is *Statistics of experiments on living animals: Great Britain*, by the Home Office (HMSO, annual). Another official publication is *House of Commons Papers: Code of practice for the housing and care of animals used in scientific procedures*. Great Britain, Home Office, House of Commons Paper 107, 1989 (HMSO).

Opposition to animal experiments has led to a search for alternatives and a recent report on the subject is *Alternatives to animal use in research, testing and education*, by the United States Congress, Office of Technology Assessment (Dekker, 1988). Also on the emotive subject, a book which covers legislation in the UK, Europe and the USA descriptions of the major activities involving experimental animals, and ethical issues is *Animals in research: new perspectives in animal experimentation*, edited by D. Sperlinger (John Wiley, 1981).

Systemic pathology

In this section we will consider the special pathology of the more important diseases of particular organs or systems. It is impossible to provide an exhaustive coverage and in many cases only one or two recent sources will be cited. Some sections will, however, be treated in greater depth.

Systemic pathology, edited by W.St C. Symmers (6 vols, 2nd edn., 1976–80, 7 vols to date, 3rd edn., Churchill Livingstone, 1986-) is a multivolume work, now entering its third edition, and attempts to deal with systemic pathology in one work. First published in two volumes in 1966, the second edition required six volumes, and the third edition, the work of 19 specialist editors, will require 15 volumes, each dealing with only one or part of one system.

Ageing

The biology of the ageing process is the study of the causes and mechanisms underlying the gradual deterioration of structure and function that is characteristic of ageing. A multidisciplinary journal that publishes original research, theoretical and review articles dealing with the fundamental mechanisms underlying the ageing process, including man, is *Mechanisms of Ageing and Development* (Limerick). Cellular ageing is dealt with in *Time, cells, and ageing*, by B.L. Strehler (2nd edn., Academic Press, 1977). Many of the books dealing with gerontology include the biological aspects of the ageing process together with the clinical patient-orientated considerations and the social aspects of old age. Useful material is to be found in *The biology of aging*, by J.W. Brookbank (Harper and Row, 1990), *The biomedical basis of gerontology*, by D.A. Hall (Wright-PSG, 1984) and *Textbook of geriatric medicine and gerontology*, edited by J.C. Brocklehurst (3rd edn., Churchill Livingstone, 1985).

AIDS (Acquired Immunodeficiency Syndrome)

A number of specialist journals are currently published in this area. *AIDS Research and Human Retroviruses* features papers discussing basic research into HIV. The social aspects of AIDS, public policy issues, HIV education and counselling initiatives are covered by the American *AIDS Patient Care, AIDS Education and Prevention* and the European orientated *AIDS Care. AIDS, Journal of Acquired Immune Deficiency Syndromes* and the more broad-based *International Journal of STD and AIDS* feature a cross-section of research, clinical, epidemiological and social items.

A variety of abstracting and indexing services is available by which to monitor the ever-increasing volume of journal literature on HIV and AIDS. Two such monthly current-awareness bulletins published in Britain are *AIDS Information* (Leeds University Press) and *Current AIDS Literature* (Bureau of Hygiene and Tropical Diseases); a US publication in the same vein is *ATIN — AIDS Targeted Information Newsletter* (Williams and Wilkins). *AIDS Index* (City of London Polytechnic) concentrates more on the social aspects of HIV and AIDS and indexes articles primarily from non-scientific journals, along with books, pamphlets and audio-visual materials. The *AIDS Resource List* (Health Education Authority) details the availability of materials on all aspects of HIV and AIDS for different age, social and occupational groups.

Specialist databases for material on HIV and AIDS include AIDS (Bureau of Hygiene and Tropical Diseases) compiled from literature abstracted and annotated in house; AIDSLINE (National Library of Medicine), a compilation of the HIV and AIDS-related information from their MEDLINE, CANCERLIT, and CATLINE databases; HEALTH PLANNING AND ADMINISTRATION file, and abstracts from papers presented at the international conferences on AIDS in 1989 and 1990; AIDSTRIALS (NLM), which provides data on the status of clinical trials of drugs and vaccines and the criteria for selection of participants; AIDSDRUGS (NLM) which gives information on the agents being tested in these clinical trials, and the AIDS KNOWLEDGE BASE FROM SAN FRANCISCO GENERAL HOSPITAL (Massachusetts Medical Society/Medical Publishing Group) which is an electronic textbook written by experts from the Hospital with information on the pathogenesis, diagnosis and epidemiology of AIDS, management and prevention strategies, and social and public health information.

A further source of AIDS information, somewhere between the current-awareness bulletin and the online database is the COMPACT LIBRARY: AIDS (Massachusetts Medical Society/Medical Publishing Group). The CD-ROM, which is updated quarterly, holds HIV and AIDS-related citations from MEDLINE, AIDSLINE, AIDSTRIALS, AIDSDRUGS, and the Bureau of Hygiene's AIDS database, text from the American Foundation for AIDS Research experimental treatment directory, and the AIDS KNOWLEDGE BASE along with full text from nine biomedical journals.

Owing to the rate at which new research findings on HIV and AIDS are published, textbooks in this subject area may contain outdated facts and figures almost from their date of publication. A valuable source of information, however, is *AIDS: etiology, diagnosis, treatment and prevention*, edited by V.T. DeVita, S. Hellman and S.A. Rosenberg (2nd edn., Lippincott, 1988) which discusses a variety of basic research as well as clinical and public health issues. A more concise, though still very comprehensive publication is *AIDS: pocket book of diagnosis and management*, edited by A. Mindel (Edward Arnold, 1990). Once again the subject is covered by colour atlases in *A colour atlas of AIDS and HIV disease*, by C.F. Farthing, S.E. Brown and R.C.D. Staughton (2nd edn., Wolfe Medical, 1988).

A resource which overcomes the problem of currency of information is the UK published *National AIDS Manual* (NAM Publications) which is produced in loose-leaf format and regularly updated. It provides information on a cross-section of issues including safe sex, counselling, treatment, research, and living with AIDS, and contains lists of addresses of helplines, HIV/AIDS agencies, needle exchange schemes and sexually-transmitted disease clinics.

Statistics of AIDS cases in the UK are collated by the Public Health Laboratory Service/Communicable Diseases Surveillance Centre and their figures published in *Answer* (Communicable Diseases (Scotland) Unit). Statistics for the USA are reported weekly by state in the *Morbidity and Mortality Weekly Report* (Centers for Disease Control). Data on AIDS cases worldwide is compiled by the World Health Organization and published in a quarterly list by continent and country in the *Weekly Epidemiological Record*.

Bone and bone marrow

Texts include:

Atlas of bone marrow pathology, by B. Frisch and R. Bartle (Kluwer Academic, 1990)

Biopsy pathology of bone and bone marrow, by B. Frisch *et al.* (Biopsy Pathology Series) (Chapman and Hall, 1985) 'Bone pathology' (*Journal of Applied Pathology*, 1987, **5**(3)), edited by E. Bonocci (S. Karger, 1987)

Bone tumors: clinical, radiologic, and pathologic correlations, edited by J.M. Mirra *et al.* (2 vols, Lea and Febiger, 1989)

Pathology of bone, by P.A. Revell (Springer-Verlag, 1985)

Pathology of the bone marrow, edited by K. Lennert and K. Hubner (Gustav Fischer Verlag, 1984)

Breast

Texts include:

Atlas of breast pathology, by F. Linell and O. Ljungberg (Munksgaard, 1984)

Atlas of breast pathology, by R.R. Millis (Current Histopathology series, Vol. 7) (MTP Press, 1984)

Benign breast disease, by J.A. Smallwood and I. Taylor (Edward Arnold, 1990)

Biopsy pathology of the breast, by J.P. Sloan (Chapman and Hall, 1985)

International histological classification of tumours, No. 2, Histological typing of breast tumours (2nd edn., World Health Organization, 1981)

Cancer

The literature of oncology, the study of tumours, dominates that of any other discipline: In 1989 12.8 per cent of all references in MEDLINE were indexed by a term from the 'Neoplasms' tree of *MeSH*, representing 44 625 papers compared with 30 192 (11.4 per cent) in 1979. The National Cancer Act of 1971 in the USA, which substantially enlarged the role of the National Cancer Institute (NCI) and which launched the US National Cancer Program, and governmental emphasis in the UK at the same time which led to increased attention to cancer, underlie much of the growth within the subject. Control of the literature, the rapid development of knowledge and developing technology all pose considerable challenges for information retrieval.

The number of journals devoted to oncology rises yearly, but there are a number of long-standing titles that undoubtedly carry most importance: virtually all are associated in some way with the major organizations involved in cancer research. Equally balanced between clinical and research papers is the *British Journal of Cancer* and *International Journal of Cancer*. The recently renamed *European Journal of Cancer* and the American *Cancer* and *Journal of Clinical Oncology* are the major clinical titles, whilst, also from the USA, *Cancer Research* is predominantly centred on experimental research. In addition, all sub-divisions of oncology, medical, paediatric, radiation, and surgical, have their own specialist journals, whilst much cancer material is published in the journals of every specialty and of course in the standard non-specialist titles.

In the field of general textbooks certain titles have established themselves as standard works, e.g. *Cancer: principles and practice of oncology* by V.T. DeVita *et at.* (2 vols, 3rd edn., Lippincott, 1989). This is probably the pre-eminent single title which covers both biological and clinical aspects. Good introductions to the subject for the newcomer are: *Manual of clinical oncology* edited by C.D. Sherman *et al.* (4th edn., Springer-Verlag for the International Union Against Cancer, 1987) and *Lecture notes on clinical oncology* by B.W. Hancock and J.D. Bradshaw (2nd edn., Blackwell Scientific Publications, 1986).

By contrast, reviews of both uncommon histological types of tumour and unusual presentations by site of familiar types are provided by *Textbook of uncommon cancer* edited by C.J. Williams *et al.* (Wiley, 1988).

Three important monograph series which publish both experimental and clinical volumes are *Recent results in cancer research* (Springer-Verlag), *Developments in oncology* (Nijhoff) and *IARC scientific publications* (Oxford University Press for the International Agency for Research on Cancer), whilst a very useful annual review is *Cancer Chemotherapy and Biological Response Modifiers Annual* (formerly *Cancer Chemotherapy Annual*) (Elsevier) which summarizes systemic therapy by both compound and by tumour site. In the field of annuals *Yearbook of Cancer*, (Year Book Medical) reports major papers from the previous year with extended abstracts and editorial comment.

Much effort has been put into the development of classification schemes for universal application, represented by the *International classification of diseases for oncology (ICD-O)* (World Health Organization, 1976) which is used internationally for the coding and exchange of registration data. Universal histological criteria are laid down in the 26 volumes of *International histological classification of tumours* (World Health Organization, 1967-81) and *Atlas of tumor pathology* (2nd series, Armed Forces Institute of Pathology, Washington, DC, 1966-), both of which treat tumours of separate body sites or organs in individual volumes. The anatomical extent of cancer within a single patient (the 'staging') has been the subject of other international schemes, published in standard form in *TNM classification of malignant tumours*, edited by P. Hermanek and L.H. Sobin (4th edn., Springer-Verlag for the UICC, 1987) and its companion: *TNM atlas: illustrated guide to the TNM/pTNM - classification of malignant tumours*, edited by B. Spiessl *et al.* (3rd edn., Springer-Verlag for the UICC, 1989). North American experience is represented by the *Manual for staging of cancer*, American Joint Committee on Cancer (3rd edn., Lippincott, 1988).

Further reference sources of value are the *International directory of specialized cancer research and treatment establishments (UICC technical report series)* 5th edn., 1990, which cites statistics, the major research interests and the senior personnel of each centre; similar in approach, although listing individual projects, is the annual *Directory of On-going Research in Cancer Epidemiology* (IARC scientific publications).

English and Welsh statistics for cancer are found in two OPCS series: *MB1, Cancer statistics: registrations*, for cases registered in any one year, is presented by age, occupation, and region for each site or type, and includes the occasional *Cancer statistics: survival* with data for the one-, three- and five-year survival rate. Series *DH2, Mortality statistics*, gives a breakdown of cases by tumour type and age group.

Both series are published at least three years in arrears. For Scotland these data can be found in *Scottish health statistics* (Common Services Agency). Also from the IARC is the continuing series *IARC monographs on the evaluation of carcinogenic risk of chemicals to man* which evaluates evidence of carcinogenic effect for an increasing number of compounds.

Control of the primary literature is clearly important, given its size, and several printed bibliographic services attempt it. Intended for the laboratory scientist is *Current Advances in Cancer Research* (Pergamon Press), a monthly cross-referenced listing derived from the CABS database. The NCI publishes *Cancergrams*, a monthly series of some 60 bulletins on both clinical and research topics citing, with several months' delay and with the authors' abstracts, papers deemed by the editors to be significant publications. In the UK, *Oncology Information* (Oncology Information Service, Leeds University) is a purely clinical current-awareness series of 19 bulletins with a strong emphasis on speed and comprehensiveness of citation.

Retrospective literature searching (apart from *Index Medicus*) is available online in CANCERLIT, the NCI's database which since 1980 has been indexed using *MeSH* and which now contains over 841 000 items. The oncology content of MEDLINE is now loaded into CANCERLIT, which is augmented with grey literature, theses and conference proceedings, although the value of this extra, hard-to-obtain, material is doubtful. CANCERLIT was briefly published as *Oncology Abstracts* (Cambridge Scientific Abstracts 1986–88). In searching either MEDLINE or CANCERLIT it should be remembered that there exists a regularly revised supplement to the MEDLARS indexing instructions, the *Tumor key* which is a subordinate thesaurus of histological types (latest edition, 1989). Two other NCI-produced online databases are centred on North American experience: CANCERPROJ describes about 6000 currently active research projects registered at the NCI whilst CLINPROT provides summaries of over 2000 clinical trials in progress with their protocols, again largely in the USA. Finally, in both printed form and on diskette for PCs is *Current Opinion in Oncology* (Current Science). The printed version reviews annually all aspects of clinical oncology in rotation, supplemented with retrospective and annotated bibliographies. The reference listings are available on diskette with bimonthly updates.

An innovative database is PHYSICIAN DATA QUERY (PDQ) which has been widely described by its creators (see, for example, Hubbard *et al.*, 1987). PDQ is a full-text state-of-the-art source of consensus information on the staging and treatment of cancer, updated monthly by an editorial board. Menu-driven, it is intended to allow end users to 'keep abreast of advances in treatment, to identify appropriate clinical research trials ... and to retrieve information on specialists for consultation or referral'.

The cancer information file is the core of the system, providing data on the therapy and prognosis of each stage of every tumour type with some recent references; it is possible to transfer to CLINPROT from within PDQ to identify protocols for the selected tumour or stage and PDQ also contains a listing of over 12 000 clinicians and 1400 organizations, mostly North American. In the longer term the creators intend that PDQ should include access to CANCERLIT. Despite considerable publicity there is little evidence of its overall acceptability although a recent report (Angier *et al.*, 1990) found it well received in a small trial. European users may not find the protocol and clinician sections of much use, nor may they agree with some of the consensus statements.

New applications of CD-ROM in oncology appear regularly and PDQ and CANCERLIT are both available in this format. The journal *Cancer* is also available in a full-text CD-ROM version of the 1988 and 1989 volumes and other journals will surely follow. More interesting are some of the products which combine sources. *Oncodisc* (Lippincott) provides the last three years' data from CANCERLIT, the full version of PDQ and the full text of DeVita *et al.*, *Cancer*, the AJCC *Manual for staging*, recent volumes of Lippincott's own yearbook, *Important advances in oncology* and, it is planned, the full text of original papers. The intention is an integrated personal reference source and an early appraisal has been published by Schipma (1988). A purely bibliographic CD-ROM from SilverPlatter, CANCER-CD, combines the data from three sources, CANCERLIT, EMBASE and *Year Book of Cancer*. Where each source duplicates a reference, these have been merged whilst retaining unique information from each file; all items carry an abstract but there are differences in indexing practice and record structure. Finally, and in acknowledgement of the models in which so much progress has been researched, animal tumours are discussed in *Pathology of tumours in laboratory animals*, with specific volumes on rat and mouse models (IARC scientific publications, 1990).

Cytology

Cytology is that branch of biology which is concerned with the study of cells, including their anatomy, chemistry, pathology and physiology. Advances in techniques such as fibreoptic technology, fine needle aspiration and stereotactic biopsy have meant that cytologic specimens can be obtained from most body sites with a minimum of trauma while new methods of analysis such as DNA probes, immunocytochemistry and flow cytometry can be used with the specimens. Cytopathology has therefore become a major diagnostic technique in the clinical setting, allowing clinicians to make immediate decisions about treatment and management.

Amongst the journals concerned with cytology are *Acta Cytologica, Analytical and Quantitative Cytology and Histology, Cell, Cell and Tissue Kinetics* (which became *Cell Proliferation* in 1990), *Cytopathology*, a new journal in 1990 and the official journal of the British Society for Clinical Cytology and also of the cytological societies of Australia, Belgium, Denmark, Holland and Greece, which will publish articles about those aspects of cytology that will increase knowledge and understanding of the aetiology, diagnosis and management of diseases in man, and *Diagnostic Cytopathology*.

There are several extremely popular books on the cell including *The cell*, by D.W. Fawcett (2nd edn., Saunders, 1981), *Molecular biology of the cell*, by B. Alberts *et al.* (2nd edn., Garland Publishing, 1989) and *Molecular cell biology*, by J. Darnell, H. Lodish and D. Baltimore (2nd edn., Scientific American Books, 1990).

A practical text and atlas written for community pathologists and others providing a pathology service is *Practical cytopathology*, edited by R. W. Astarita (Churchill Livingstone, 1990).

A book written specifically for medical laboratory scientific officers which concentrates on practical work but also covers many aspects of the laboratory environment, such as health and safety, and computers, and also includes a chapter on information collection and use and guidelines on the presentation of dissertations and lectures, is Basic histology and cytology for medical laboratory scientists, by A.W. Currie (Churchill Livingstone, 1988).

Not surprisingly there are numerous atlases covering both general and specialized aspects of cytology including *Atlas of general cytology* by O.A.N. Husain (MTP, 1982), *Atlas of diagnostic cytopathology*, by C. Gompel (Wiley, 1978), *Colour atlas of gynaecological cytology*, by O.A.N. Husain and E.B. Butler (Wolfe Medical, 1989) and *Cytology of body cavity fluids: a colour atlas*, by E.B. Butler and C.M. Stanbridge (Chapman and Hall, 1986).

Ear

Texts include:

A colour atlas of ear disease, by R.A. Chole (Wolfe Medical 1982)

Diseases of the ear: clinical and pathologic aspects, by M. Hawke and A.F. Jahn (Lea and Febiger, 1987)

Pathology of the ear, by H.F. Schuknecht (Harvard University Press, 1974)

Pathology of the ear, by I. Friedmann (Blackwell, 1974).

Endocrine pathology

A new discipline that has made substantial progress in recent years concerns the abnormalities of endocrine glands and the hormone-producing cells. A new journal dealing with the subject is: *Endocrine Pathology* and among the books are *Diagnosis and pathology of endocrine diseases*, by G. Mendelsohn (Lippincott, 1988) and *Functional endocrine pathology*, by K. Kovacs and S. Asa (Blackwell Scientific Publications, 1989).

Eye

Texts include *A colour atlas of ocular tumours*, by M.A. Bedford (Wolfe Medical, 1979), *Greer's Ocular pathology*, by D.R. Lucas (4th edn., Blackwell Scientific Publications, 1989), *International histological classification of tumours, No. 24, Tumours of the eye and its adnexa* (World Health Organization, 1980) and *Ocular pathology: a text and atlas*, by M. Yanoff and B.S. Fine (3rd edn., Lippincott, 1989).

Forensic pathology

The journals that deal with forensic pathology are the *American Journal of Forensic Medicine and Pathology* and the *Journal of Forensic Sciences*.

General forensic texts include *Essentials of forensic medicine*, by C.J. Polson, D.J. Gee and B. Knight (4th edn., Pergamon Press, 1985), *Simpson's Forensic medicine* by B. Knight (10th edn., Edward Arnold, 1991), *Forensic medicine: a study in trauma and environmental hazards*, by C.G. Tedeschi *et al.* (3 vols, Saunders, 1977) and *Forensic medicine: a guide to principles*, by I. Gordon, H.A. Shapiro and S.D. Berson (3rd edn., Churchill Livingstone, 1988).

More specialized books include *Closed head injury: its pathology and legal medicine*, by R. Crompton (Edward Arnold, 1985), *Forensic histopathology*, by W. Janssen, translated by S. Foster (Springer-Verlag, 1984), *Forensic pathology*, by D.J. DiMaio and V.J. Dimaio (*Practical aspects of criminal and forensic investigations* series) (Elsevier, 1989) *Practical forensic pathology*, by C.V. Wetli (Igaku Shoin, 1988).

This aspect of pathology also has its atlases, among them *Colour atlas of forensic pathology*, by G.A. Gresham (Wolfe Medical, 1975, 3rd impression 1984), *Colour atlas of forensic dentistry*, by D.K. Whittaker and M.G. MacDonald (Wolfe Medical, 1989) and *Colour atlas of trauma pathology*, by H. Fischer, C.J. Kirkpatrick and M.E. Aronson (Wolfe Medical, 1991).

Gastrointestinal tract

Gastrointestinal pathology, by B.C. Morson and I.M.P. Dawson (3rd edn., Blackwell Scientific Publications, 1990) is a comprehensive account of the pathology of the gastrointestinal tract which sets out to give the subject a clinical perspective. By the same first author is *Colour atlas of gastrointestinal pathology*, by B.C. Morson (Oxford University Press, 1988) and *Gastrointestinal and oesophageal pathology*, edited by R. Whitehead (Churchill Livingstone, 1989) covers the normal structure of the gastrointestinal tract together with the kinetics of its maintenance, function and motility in the first section of the book. The remaining sections consider pathological states arranged under the broad headings of pathological processes.

The World Health Organization's *International histological classification of tumours* has three sections covering this subject: *No.4, Histological typing of oral and oropharyngeal tumours* by H. Watanabe et al., 2nd edn., Springer-Verlag, 1990; *No. 18, Gastric and oesophageal tumours (1977)*; *Histological typing of intestinal tumours* by J.R. Jass and L.H. Sobia (2nd edn., Springer-Verlag, 1989).

Biopsy is covered by *Atlas of gastrointestinal biopsy pathology*, by I.M.P. Dawson (MTP Press, 1983), *Biopsy diagnosis of the digestive tract*, by H. Rotterdam and S.C. Sommers (Raven Press, 1981), *Biopsy pathology of the oesophagus, stomach and duodenum*, by D.W. Day (Chapman and Hall, 1986) and *Biopsy pathology of the small intestine*, by F.D. Lee and P.G. Toner (Chapman and Hall, 1980).

Atlases include *Atlas of gastrointestinal pathology*, by F.A. Mitros (Gower Medical, 1988) and *Colour atlas of the digestive system*, by R.E. Pounder, M.C. Allison and A.P. Dhillon (Wolfe Medical, 1988).

Gynaecology and obstetrics

A journal specializing in the pathology of gynaecology is the *International Journal of Gynecological Pathology* which began publication in 1982.

Books on general pathology of gynaecology and obstetrics include *Gynaecological pathology*, by M. Haines and C. Taylor (3 vols., 3rd edn., Churchill Livingstone, 1987), *Blaustein's Pathology of the female genital tract*, edited by R.J. Kurman (3rd edn., Springer-Verlag, 1987), *Pathology in gynecology and obstetrics*, by C. Gompel and S.G. Silverberg (3rd edn., Lippincott, 1985), *Pathology for gynaecologists*, by H. Fox and C.H. Buckley (2nd edn., Edward Arnold, 1990) and *Novak's Gynecologic and obstetric pathology: with clinical and endocrine relations*, by E.R. Novak and J.D. Woodruff (8th edn., Saunders, 1979).

Atlases include *Atlas of gynaecologic pathology*, by J.D. Woodruff and T.H. Parmley (Lippincott, 1988), *Atlas of gynaecological patho-*

logy, by H. Fox and C. Buckley (MTP, 1982), *Atlas of histopathology of the cervix uteri*, by G. Dallenbach-Hellweg and H. Poulsen (Springer-Verlag, 1990) and *Colour atlas of gynaecological cytology*, by O.A.N. Husain and E.B. Butler (Wolfe Medical, 1989).

There are books on specific aspects of the female system, for example *The endometrium*, by W.B. Robertson (Butterworth, 1981), *Histopathology of the endometrium*, by G. Dallenbach-Hellwig (4th edn., Springer-Verlag, 1988), *Ovarian pathology*, edited by F. Norgales (Springer-Verlag, 1989) and *Pathology of the human placenta*, by K. Benirschke and P. Kaufmann (2nd edn., Springer-Verlag, 1990) while surgical pathology is covered by books such as *Surgical pathology of the endometrium*, by H. Cove (Lippincott,1981), *Surgical pathology of the ovaries*, by P. Russell and P. Bannatyne (Churchill Livingstone, 1989) and *Surgical pathology of the uterine corpus*, by M.R. Hendrickson and R.L. Kempson (Saunders, 1980).

Haematology

Present-day usage restricts the definition of haematology to the study of disorders associated with changes in the cells of the blood or those which affect coagulation, and to diseases of the blood-forming organs.

The word 'haematology' was probably first used in 1743 by Thomas Schwenke in the title of his book *Haematologia, sive sanguinis historia*. Until the 1920s, haematology was a branch of clinical medicine and pathology in which the patients' history and physical examination was supplemented by a study of blood smears and by crude analyses of constituents of the blood. By the 1940s haematology had changed from an essentially morphologic discipline to one that encompasses aspects of cytology, biochemistry, biophysics, molecular and cellular biology, genetics, immunology, pharmacology and oncology. Research in the field has led to some of the most significant advances in the understanding of biology as a whole. The rapid growth of knowledge about disorders affecting the blood and blood-forming organs has moved haematology into a major position in clinical and experimental pathology. It is now difficult to define the boundaries of haematology since the subject encompasses disciplines from molecular biology to the clinical management of malignant disease.

Not surprisingly there are numerous journals covering haematology. These include *Acta Haematologica, Blood*, the journal of the American Society of Hematology which publishes papers describing basic laboratory and clinical investigations included in the broad discipline of haematology, and *British Journal of Haematology* which also publishes original research in clinical laboratory and experimental haematology.

As a result of the magnitude of the subject modern textbooks on haematology tend to be very large and even then, their editors admit, they are not complete. So specialized has the subject become that there are numerous monographs dealing in depth with specific disorders. General textbooks on haematology include *Blood and its diseases*, by I. Chanarin *et al.* (3rd edn., Churchill Livingstone, 1984), *Blood and its disorders*, edited by R.M. Hardisty and D.J. Weatherall (2nd edn., Blackwell Scientific Publications, 1982), *Clinical haematology*, by D.L. Barnard, B.A. McVerry and D.R. Norfolk (Heinemann Medical, 1989) and *Wintrobe's Clinical hematology*, edited by G.R. Lee (9th edn., Lea and Febiger, 1992).

For a better understanding of laboratory haematology as well as the clinical relevance of haematological tests, there is *Blood cells: a practical guide*, by B.J. Bain (Gower Medical, 1988).

There are atlases such as *Atlas of clinical hematology*, by H. Begemann (translated by T.C. Telger) (4th rev. edn., Springer-Verlag 1989), *Atlas of haematology*, by G.A. McDonald, P. James and B. Cruickshank (5th edn., Churchill Livingstone, 1988), *A colour atlas of haematological cytology* by F.G.J. Hayhoe and R.J. Flemans (2nd edn., Wolfe Medical, 1982) and *Colour atlas of paediatric haematology,* by I.M. Hann *et al.* (2nd edn., Oxford Medical, 1990).

Specialist monographs cover topics such as sickle-cell anaemia, thalassaemia and leukaemia. A small selection of these would include *Leukemia: cytology and cytochemistry*, by L. Kass (Lippincott, 1982), *Neoplastic diseases of the blood*, edited by P.H. Wiernik *et al.* (2 vols, Churchill Livingstone, 1985), *Sickle cell disease*, by G.R. Serjeant (Oxford University Press, 1985) and *Thalassemia: pathophysiology and management*, Part A edited by S. Fucharoen *et al.*, Part B edited by P.T. Rowley and N.W. Paul (2 vols, Wiley, 1988).

The history of the rapid development of this discipline is encapsulated in two books by M.M. Wintrobe. The first, *Blood, pure and eloquent* (McGraw-Hill, 1980), tells the story of developments in areas of haematology in the form of essays by people who have been active in the subject. The second, *Hematology, the blossoming of a science* (Lea and Febiger, 1985) is partly autobiographical and also includes some 500 biographies of major contributors to the development of the discipline.

Head and neck

Texts include *Pathology of the head and neck*, by D. R. Gnepp (Churchill Livingstone, 1987).

Heart

Texts include *Colour atlas of adult congenital heart disease*, by L.M.

Shapiro and K.M. Fox (Wolfe Medical, 1990), *Colour atlas of cardiac pathology*, by G. Farrer-Brown (Wolfe Medical, 1977), *Pathology of the heart*, by E.G.J. Olsen (4th edn., Macmillan, 1980) and *Pathology of the heart and great vessels*, edited by B.F. Waller (Churchill Livingstone, 1988).

Liver

There is a considerable amount of literature dealing specifically with the liver. Amongst the general books on the pathology of the liver are *The liver: pathology and pathobiology*, by I.M. Arias (2nd edn., Raven Press, 1988) and *Pathology of the liver*, edited by R.N.M. McSween, P.P. Anthony and P.J. Scheuer (2nd edn., Churchill Livingstone, 1987).There are of course, atlases including *Atlas of liver pathology*, by D.G.D. Wright (MTP, 1982), *Colour atlas of liver disease*, by S. Sherlock and J.A. Summerfield (Wolfe, 2nd edn. 1991) and *Colour atlas of liver pathology*, by R.S. Patrick (*Oxford colour atlases of pathology*, Harvey Miller, 1983). Tumours of the liver are dealt with in *International histological classification of tumours, No. 20; Tumours of the liver, biliary tract and the pancreas* (World Health Organization, 1978).

Liver biopsy also has specialist texts including *Atlas of liver biopsies* by H.E. Poulsen and P. Christoffersen (Munksgaard, 1979), *Biopsy pathology of the liver*, by R.S. Patrick and J.O'D. McGee (2nd edn., Chapman and Hall, 1988) and *Liver biopsy interpretation*, by P.J. Scheuer (4th edn., Baillière Tindall, 1988). Surgical pathology of the liver is covered by *Pathology of the liver and biliary tract*, by B.H. Ruebner and C.K. Montgomery (*Wiley series in surgical pathology*)), Wiley, 1982).

Lung

Texts include: *Atlas of pulmonary pathology*, by A.R. Gibbs and R.M.E. Seal (MTP, 1982)

Biopsy pathology of the bronchi, by E.M. McDowell and T.F. Beals (Chapman and Hall, 1985)

Clinical and experimental pathology of lung cancer, edited by J.G. McVie (Nijhoff, 1986)

International histological classification of tumours, No. 1: Histological typing of lung tumours (2nd edn., World Health Organization, 1981)

The pathology of emphysema, by L. Reid (Lloyd-Luke, 1967)

Pathology of the lung, by H. Spencer (2 vols, 4th edn., Pergamon Press, 1985)

Pulmonary pathology, by D.H. Dail and S.P. Hammar (Springer, 1988)

Pulmonary pathology, by M.S. Dunnill (2nd edn., Churchill Livingstone 1987)

Pulmonary pathophysiology: the essentials, by J.B. West (3rd edn., Williams and Wilkins, 1987)

Surgical pathology of non-neoplastic lung diseases, by A.-L. A. Katzenstein and F. B. Askin (W.B. Saunders, 1990)

Lymph nodes

Texts include *Atlas of lymph node pathology*, by J. Arno (MTP Press, 1980), *Colour atlas of thymus and lymph node histopathology and ultrastructure*, by K. Henry and G. Farrer-Brown (Wolfe Medical, 1981) and *Lymph node biopsy*, by H.L. Ioachim (Lippincott, 1982).

Male reproduction

Texts include *Atlas of male reproductive system pathology* by I.D. Ansell (*Current Histopathology series no. 10*) (MTP Press, 1985) and *Atlas of sperm morphology*, by M.M. Adelman and E.M. Cahill (Raven Press, 1989).

Mouth

Journals relating to the pathology of the mouth include: *Archives of Oral Biology* and *Journal of Oral Pathology*.

A number of very comprehensive general textbooks exist including *Oral pathology*, by J.L. Giunta (3rd edn., Decker, 1989), *Oral pathology: clinical–pathologic correlations*, by J.A. Regezi and J.J. Sciubba (Saunders, 1989) and *Textbook of oral pathology*, by W.G. Shafer *et al.* (4th edn., Saunders, 1983).

A popular undergraduate text which is much shorter and has deliberately omitted discussion of the rarer oral diseases is *Oral pathology*, by J.V. Soames and J.C. Southam (Oxford University Press, 1985).

Atlases are, again, a popular medium. Examples are *Atlas of oral pathology*, by R. B. Lucas and J.W. Eveson (MTP Press, 1985), *Colour atlas of clinical oral pathology* by B.W. Neville *et al.* (Lea and Febiger, 1990), *Colour atlas of oral medicine*, by C. Scully and S. Flint (Lippincott, 1989) *Colour atlas of oral pathology*, by K.W. Lee (Lea and Febiger, 1985), *Atlas of oral pathology*, by R.M. Smith, J.E. Turner and M.L. Robbins (Mosby, 1981).

Oral tumours are covered by *International histological classification of tumours* (World Health Organization); *No. 5; Histological typing of odontogenic tumours, jaw cysts and allied lesions* (1971); *No.7, Histological typing of salivary gland tumours* (1972), *Pathology of tumours of the oral tissues,* by R.B. Lucas (4th edn., Churchill Livingstone, 1982) and *Colour atlas of oral cancers,* by A. Burkhardt and R. Maerker (Wolfe Medical, 1981).

Muscle

Diseases of muscle: a study in pathology, by R.D Adams (3rd edn., Harper and Row, 1975) is a classic monograph on muscle pathology. Other books include *Biopsy pathology of muscle,* by M. Swash and M.S. Schwartz (2nd edn., Chapman and Hall, 1990), *Muscle biopsy: a practical approach* by V. Dubowitz (2nd edn., Baillière-Tindall, 1985), *Muscle pathology,* edited by R.R. Heffner (Churchill Livingstone, 1984), *Pathology of skeletal muscle,* by S. Carpenter and G. Karpati (Churchill Livingstone, 1984) and *Skeletal muscle pathology,* by F.L. Mastalgia and J.N. Walton (Churchill Livingstone, 1982).

Mycoses

Texts include *Atlas of fungal pathology,* by K. Salfelder *et al.* ((*Current histopathology,* Vol. 17) Kluwer Academic, 1990), *Colour atlas and textbook of the histopathology of mycotic diseases,* by F.W. Chandler *et al.* (Wolfe Medical, 1980) and *Medical mycology: a practical approach* by E.G.V. Evans and M.D. Richardson (IRL Press, 1989).

Nervous system

The specialist journals that cover neuropathology, the pathology of the nervous system, include: *Journal of Neuropathology and Experimental Neurology* and *Neuropathology and Applied Neurobiology.*

Some of the books on neuropathology are: *Greenfield's Neuropathology,* edited by J.H. Adams, J.A.N. Corsellis and L.W. Duchen (4th edn., Edward Arnold, 1984), *An introduction to neuropathology,* by J.H. Adams, D.I. Grahm and D.G.F. Harriman (Churchill Livingstone, 1988), *Clinical neuropathology,* by R.O. Weller *et al.* (Springer-Verlag, 1983) and *Histology and histopathology of the nervous system,* edited by W. Haymaker and R.D. Adams (2 vols, C.C. Thomas, 1982).

Atlases include *Atlas of gross neuropathology,* by R.E. Slemmer (Green, 1983), *Atlas of neuropathology,* by H. Okazaki and B. Scheithauer (Gower, 1988), *Atlas of neuropathology,* by M.V. Salmon (MTP, 1981) and *Colour atlas of neuropathology,* by C.S. Treip (Wolfe Medical, 1978).

Nose and sinuses

Texts include *Atlas of ear, nose and throat pathology,* by L. Michaels (Kluwer Academic, 1990) *Colour atlas of E.N.T. diagnosis,* by T.R.

Bull (2nd edn., Wolfe Medical, 1987) and *Diseases of the nose, throat, ear, head and neck*, by J.J. Ballenger (14th edn., Lea and Febiger, 1991) which, as a large textbook contains a considerable amount of pathological material. Others are *Pathology of granulomas and neoplasms of the nose and paranasal sinuses*, by I. Friedmann and D.A. Osborn (Churchill Livingstone, 1982) and *International histological classification of tumours, No. 19: Upper respiratory tract tumours* (World Health Organization, 1978).

Paediatrics

Texts include: *Diseases of the fetus and newborn: pathology, radiology and genetics*, edited by G.B. Reed, A.E. Claireaux and A.D. Bain (Chapman and Hall, 1989), *Fetal and neonatal pathology*, edited by J.W. Keeling (Springer-Verlag, 1987), *Fetal and neonatal pathology: perspectives for the general pathologist*, edited by A.J. Barson on behalf of the Royal College of Pathologists (Praeger Scientific, 1982), *Paediatric pathology*, edited by C.L. Berry (2nd edn., Springer-Verlag, 1989), *Pathology of perinatal brain injury*, by L.B. Rorke (Raven Press, 1982), *Pediatric pathology: a colour atlas and descriptive text*, by N. Boehm (Hanley-Belfus, 1988), *Textbook of fetal and perinatal pathology*, edited by J.S. Wigglesworth and D.B. Singer (Blackwell Scientific Publications, 1989).

Palaeopathology

Texts include: *Ancient diseases: the elements of paleopathology*, by S. Zivanivic, translated by L.F. Edwards (Methuen, 1982) *Archaeology of disease*, by K. Manchester (University of Bradford, 1983), *Diseases of antiquity: a survey of the diseases, injuries and surgery of early populations*, by D.R. Brothwell and A.T. Sandison (C.C. Thomas, 1967), *Palaeopathology: an introduction to the study of ancient evidences of disease*, by R.L. Moodie (AMS Press, 1923, reprinted 1980), *Palaeo-oncology: the antiquity of cancer*, by S. Retsas (Farrand Press, 1986).

Prostate

The journal *Prostate* contains material of pathological interest and there are a number of textbooks on the prostate which also include sections dealing with pathology, for example *The prostate*, by J.P. Blandy and B. Lytton (Butterworth, 1986).

Books more specifically pathological include *Pathology of the prostate*, by D.G. Bostwick (Churchill Livingstone, 1990), *The prostatic cell: structure and function; part A, Morphologic, secretory and biochemical aspects*, edited by G.P. Murphy *et al.* (Alan R. Liss, 1981),

Prostate biopsy interpretation (Biopsy interpretation series), by J.I. Epstein (Raven Press, 1989) and *International histological classification of tumours, No. 22: Prostate tumours* (World Health Organization, 1980).

Radiation

Texts include *Medical effects of ionizing radiation*, by F.A. Mettler and R.D. Mosley (Grune and Stratton, 1985), *Pathology of irradiation*, by C.C. Berdjis (Williams and Wilkins, 1971) and *Radiation histopathology*, by G.W. Casarett (2 vols, CRC Press, 1981).

Skin

Two journals are of particular relevance here, the *American Journal of Dermatpoathology* and the *Journal of Cutaneous Pathology*, while among the books the classic work is *Histopathology of the skin*, by W.F. Lever and G. Schaumburg-Lever (7th edn., Lippincott, 1989). Others include *Colour atlas of histopathology of the skin*, by G. Schaumburg-Lever and W.F. Lever (Lippincott, 1988) (this atlas is designed to be used in conjunction with the textbook), *Biopsy pathology of the skin,* by N. Kirkman (Chapman and Hall, 1990), *Pathology of the skin*, edited by E.R. Farmer and A.F. Hood (Appleton and Lange, 1990), *Pathology of the skin: with clinical correlations*, by F.H McKee (Gower, 1989) and *Primer of dermatopathology*, by A.F. Hood *et al.* (Little, Brown, 1984).

Toxicology

Texts include *Pathology of drug-induced and toxic diseases*, edited by R.M. Riddell (Churchill Livingstone, 1982) and *Principles of toxicological pathology*, by J.R. Glaister (Taylor and Francis, 1985).

Transplantation

In the early years of the 1980s live organ transplantation underwent tremendous development. Clinical transplantation is a major new discipline crossing conventional boundaries within the basic and clinical sciences. Departments of Transplantation have grown up and the discipline of transplantation pathology has developed alongside. Possibly the first book devoted to the subject is *The pathology of organ transplantation*, edited by G.E. Sale (Butterworths, 1990).

Tropical medicine

This is a subject where most of the textbooks on tropical medicine will tend to contain a considerable amount of interest to the pathologist. Included among these are *Manson's Tropical diseases*, by P.E.C.

Manson-Bahr and D.R. Bell (19th edn., Baillière Tindall, 1987) *Clinical tropical diseases* by A.R.D. Adams and B. Maegraith (9th edn., Blackwell, 1989) and *Colour atlas of tropical medicine and parasitology* by W. Peters and H.M. Gilles (3rd edn., Wolfe Medical, 1989).

Books which deal specifically with pathology include *Tropical pathology*, by H. Spencer *et al.* (Springer-Verlag, 1973) and *Pathology in the tropics*, by G.M. Edington and H.M. Gillies (2nd edn., Edward Arnold, 1976).

Urinary tract

Texts include:

Colour atlas of urology, by R.W. Lloyd-Davies, J.G. Gow and R.D. Davies (Wolfe Medical, 1983)

Concise renal pathology (excluding neoplasms), by F.E. Dische (Castle House, 1987)

Immunopathology of renal disease, by C.B. Wilson (Churchill Livingstone, 1988)

Pathological basis of renal disease, by M.S. Dunnill (2nd edn., Baillière Tindall, 1984)

Pathology of the kidney, by R.H. Heptinstall (3 vols, 3rd edn., Little, Brown, 1983)

Pathophysiology of renal disease, by B.D. Rose (2nd edn., McGraw-Hill, 1987)

Renal pathology: with clinical and functional correlations, by C.C. Tisher and B.M. Brenner (2 vols, Lippincott, 1989)

Urologic pathology, by P. Peterson and B. Stein (Lippincott, 1986)

Uropathology, edited by G.S. Hill (Churchill Livingstone, 1989)

Tumours are dealt with in *International histological classification of tumours* (World Health Organization); *No. 25, Kidney tumours* (1981); *No. 10, Histological typing of urinary bladder tumours* (1973).

History of pathology

The first systematic history of the subject in English is *History of pathology*, by E.R. Long (Williams and Wilkins, 1928). The same writer also edited *Selected readings in pathology from Hippocrates to Virchow* (C.C. Thomas, 1929). E. Goldschmid's *Entwicklung und Bibliographie der pathologisch-anatomischen Abbildung* (Hiersemann, Leipzig, 1925) traces the development of pathological anatomical illustration and includes a chronological bibliography of all important publications containing illustrations of pathological conditions and an index of artists, printers and publishers. W. D. Foster published *A short history of clinical pathology* (Livingstone, 1961) and more recently *Pathology as a profession in Great Britain and the early history of the Royal College of Pathologists* (The College, 1982). The early nineteenth century is dealt with in *Morbid appearances: the anatomy of pathology in the early nineteenth century*, by R.C. Maulitz (Cambridge University Press, 1987).

References

Angier J.J., Beck, S.L. and Eyre, H.J. (1990) Use of the PDQ systems in a clinical setting. *Bulletin of the Medical Library Association*, **78**, 15-22.

Hubbard, S.M., Henney, E. and DeVita, V.T. (1987) A computer data base for information on cancer treatment. *New England Journal of Medicine*, **316**, 315-318.

Schipma, P.B. (1988) A CD-ROM database product for oncology. *Journal of the American Society for Information Science*, **39**, 63-66.

CHAPTER THIRTEEN

Medical microbiology

SUSAN A. BLOOMFIELD

Introduction

In the last decade medical microbiology has hit the headlines with incidents of food poisoning caused by Salmonella or Listeria, concern over drinking water quality, outbreaks of meningitis, Legionnaire's disease, Lyme disease and toxic shock syndrome, and, most prominently, the emergence of AIDS. These problems, be they new or established recurrent problems growing in size, have resulted in increasing case reports and research output. The volume and scope of literature has increased in consequence. This chapter reflects these changes and continues the survey of the literature from where it was left off in the third edition of this series by Betty Whyte (1984). For conciseness, some sources which remain useful, particularly historical items and older secondary literature, have not been repeated here.

Scientific organizations play an important role in the advancement of microbiology and several, being important publishers, are referred to in the text. The most prolific publisher in the field is the American Society for Microbiology (ASM). The British equivalents are the Society for General Microbiology (SGM) and the Society for Applied Bacteriology (SAB). All these come together with national societies from other countries in the International Union of Microbiological Societies (IUMS). This works through a network of committees, commissions and federations such as the International Commission on Microbiological Specifications for Foods (ICMSF), the World Federation for Culture Collections (WFCC) and the taxonomy committees. The Federation of European Microbiological Societies (FEMS) exists to encourage communication between European national societies and to facilitate rapid publication of journals.

Many relevant publications are produced by the World Health Organization (WHO) particularly in its series such as *Technical Reports* or *Working Documents*. In Britain, the Department of Health (DoH), formerly the Department of Health and Social Security (DHSS), issues reports and memoranda on all matters of public health. In England and Wales, the Public Health Laboratory Service (PHLS) is the statutory body for the diagnosis, surveillance and control of communicable disease, with a network of laboratories throughout the country and a range of reference and special units, most of which are based at its Central Public Health Laboratory (CPHL) at Colindale in North London. The history of the PHLS is traced in *Microbiology for the public health* by R.E.O. Williams (PHLS, 1985). The Bureau of Hygiene and Tropical Diseases housed at the London School of Hygiene and Tropical Medicine produces some important sources of secondary information and the British Medical Association (BMA) has published some relevant items.

In the USA, the Centers for Disease Control (CDC) in Atlanta have a similar, if broader, role to the PHLS and publish on microbiological, epidemiological and surveillance topics. The American Public Health Association (APHA) compiles a series of excellent diagnostic handbooks.

Microbiology

Primary journals

The number of microbiological journals publishing original contributions continues to increase, with two or three new titles appearing each year. Many of the journals are published by or on behalf of scientific societies. The most notable example in terms of quality and quantity is the ASM. It currently publishes ten serials including *Journal of Clinical Microbiology, Journal of Virology, Applied and Environmental Microbiology, Infection and Immunity* and *Antimicrobial Agents and Chemotherapy*. Other useful titles, which are most likely to be found in general medical libraries, include *Journal of Medical Microbiology, Journal of Clinical Pathology, Journal of Hospital Infection, Journal of Infection* and *Journal of Infectious Diseases*.

Many important microbiological articles are published in leading journals such as *British Medical Journal, The Lancet* and *New England Journal of Medicine*. Others appear in journals concerned with biochemistry, immunology, paediatrics, parasitology, pathology and other specialties. The list which follows includes only journals specific to microbiology and communicable disease, other areas being covered elsewhere in this book.

MICROBIOLOGY

Acta Microbiologica Hungarica
Antonie van Leeuwenhoek Journal of Microbiology
APMIS
Archives of Microbiology
Canadian Journal of Microbiology
Clinical Microbiology Newsletter
Current Microbiology
Diagnostic Microbiology and Infectious Disease
European Journal of Clinical Microbiology and Infectious Diseases
FEMS Microbiology and Immunology
FEMS Microbiology Letters
International Journal of Systematic Bacteriology
Journal of Applied Bacteriology
Journal of Bacteriology
Journal of Clinical Microbiology
Journal of General Microbiology
Journal of Medical Microbiology
Letters in Applied Microbiology
Medical Microbiology and Immunology
Microbial Ecology in Health and Disease
Microbial Pathogenesis
Microbiologica
Microbiology and Immunology
Molecular Microbiology
Research in Microbiology
Systematic and Applied Microbiology
Zentralblatt für Bakteriologie: International Journal of Medical Microbiology
Zentralblatt für Hygiene und Umweltmedizin: International Journal of Hygiene and Environmental Medicine

VIROLOGY

Acta Virologica
Antiviral Chemistry and Chemotherapy
Antiviral Research
Archives of Virology
Intervirology
Journal of General Virology
Journal of Medical Virology
Journal of Virological Methods
Journal of Virology
Research in Virology
Viral Immunology
Virology
Virus Research

MYCOLOGY

Journal of Medical and Veterinary Mycology
Mycopathologia
Mycoses

ENVIRONMENTAL MICROBIOLOGY

Applied and Environmental Microbiology
Canadian Journal of Public Health
Food Microbiology
International Journal of Food Microbiology

Dairy Food and Environmental
  Sanitation

Journal of Food Protection
Journal of Food Science

LABORATORY METHODS

*American Journal of Clinical
  Pathology*
*Archives of Pathology and Laboratory
  Medicine*
Biologicals
Biotechniques
*Canadian Journal of Medical
  Technology*
Clinical Laboratory Science

Journal of Clinical Pathology
Journal of Immunoassay
*Journal of Laboratory and Clinical
  Medicine*
Journal of Microbiological Methods
Laboratory Investigation
Laboratory Medicine
Medical Laboratory Sciences
Molecular and Cellular Probes

COMMUNICABLE DISEASES

American Journal of Epidemiology
American Journal of Public Health
*American Review of Respiratory
  Disease*
Epidemiology and Infection
European Journal of Epidemiology
Genitourinary Medicine
Immunität und Infektion
Infection (Munich)
Infection and Immunity
Infectious Disease Newsletter
International Journal of Epidemiology
*Journal of Epidemiology and
  Community Health*

Journal of Infection
Journal of Infectious Diseases
Journal of Public Health Medicine
Médecine et Maladies Infectieuses
Pediatric Infectious Disease Journal
Public Health
*Scandinavian Journal of Infectious
  Disease*
*Serodiagnosis and Immunotherapy
  in Infectious Disease*
Sexually Transmitted Diseases
Tubercle

AIDS

AIDS
AIDS Forschung
*AIDS Research and Human
  Retroviruses*
*International Journal of STD and
  AIDS*
*Journal of Acquired Immune
  Deficiency Syndromes*

INFECTION CONTROL

American Journal of Infection Control
*Infection Control and Hospital
  Epidemiology*
Journal of Hospital Infection
Journal of Infection Control Nursing

ANTIMICROBIAL THERAPY

*Antimicrobial Agents and
    Chemotherapy
Chemotherapy
International Journal of Antimicrobial
    Agents
Journal of Antimicrobial
    Chemotherapy*

VETERINARY MEDICINE

*British Veterinary Journal
Canadian Journal of Veterinary
    Research
Journal of the American Veterinary
    Medical Association
Research in Veterinary Science
Veterinary Microbiology
Veterinary Record*

Reviews

Review articles by experts appraising the increasing volume of publish-ed original research are a very useful source for keeping abreast with developments. The microbiologist continues to be well served by re-view journals publishing such articles. Recent newcomers to the field are *Reviews in Medical Microbiology* published by Wiley and *Clinical Microbiology Reviews* from the ASM, which complements their more general *Microbiological Reviews*. Other established titles are *Advances in Microbial Physiology, Annual Review of Microbiology, CRC Critical Reviews in Microbiology, Current Topics in Microbiology and Immuno-logy* and *FEMS Microbiology Reviews*. For the virologist *Advances in Virus Research* and *Progress in Medical Virology* were joined in 1991 by the quarterly *Reviews in Medical Virology* from Wiley.

Some journals are more clinically orientated. *Reviews of Infectious Diseases* from the ASM is the largest of all the microbiological review journals in terms of numbers of articles. More specialized examples are *Advances in Pediatric Infectious Diseases* and *Epidemiologic Reviews*. *Current Opinion in Infectious Diseases* aims to review each major area of communicable disease annually. It also publishes annotated lists of key papers and more extensive bibliographies of articles up to 18 months old for each topic.

Some useful series appear sporadically. Examples are *Current Clini-cal Topics in Infectious Diseases,* edited by J.S. Remington and M.N. Swartz (vol.1–, McGraw Hill, 1980–), *Recent Advances in Infection,* edited by D.S. Reeves and A.M. Geddes (No.1–, Churchill Livingstone, 1979–), *Current Topics in AIDS* and *Current Topics in Mycology.*

Retrospective searching: abstracts, indexes and bibliographies

In microbiology, as in the other medical specialties, the principal tools for searching back through the literature are the large databases because of their wide availability and range of coverage of literature. These are discussed in detail in Chapter X and so will only be mentioned briefly here. MEDLINE, with its printed equivalent *Index Medicus*, is the prime source for breadth and depth of scope. EMBASE has a more European bias and its printed version, *Excerpta Medica*, is divided into over 40 subject sections. The most relevant are *4—Microbiology, 17—Public Health, Social Medicine and Hygiene, 26—Immunology, Serology and Transplantation* and *47—Virology.* BIOSIS and its printed *Biological Abstracts* cover many relevent life-science journals excluded from the more clinically biased MEDLINE and EMBASE.

Two more specialized databases contain several files of interest to microbiologists. The LIFE SCIENCES COLLECTION from Cambridge Scientific Abstracts has 18 subject subfiles including microbiology, mycology and virology. These are published as *Microbiology Abstracts*, including mycology, and *Virology Abstracts*. The names of the printed versions of relevant files from the CABI database maintained by CAB International indicates their scope: *Abstracts on Hygiene and Communicable Diseases, Review of Medical and Veterinary Mycology, Dairy Science Abstracts* for the food microbiologist and *Index Veterinarius.* The *Abstracts on Hygiene*, produced by the Bureau of Hygiene and Tropical Diseases, includes books and reports and its signed abstracts are written by experts in the field. Another specialist source for the food microbiologist is *Food Science and Technology Abstracts.*

The DHSS DATABASE contains items relating to health policy and care in the UK and is particularly useful for tracing government reports and grey literature. *Health Service Abstracts*, its published form, is currently rather slow in production. CINAHL, the *Cumulative Index to Nursing and Allied Health Literature*, is useful for articles on infection control.

Many databases including the aforementioned general ones contain items on AIDS. There is a comprehensive list with hints on search terms in the article by Roberts, Shepherd and Wade (1987). Two comprehensive specialist files are the AIDS DATABASE, covering literature from 1984 with some earlier material and produced by the Bureau of Hygiene and Tropical Diseases, and AIDSLINE, containing all AIDS-related citations from MEDLINE.

For tracing historic items the sources are *Index Medicus* published from 1879, the *Referate* section of the *Zentralblatt für Bakteriologie,*

Mikrobiologie und Hygiene with abstracts sections in the earlier volumes of the *Zentralblatt* itself from 1887, the *Bulletin de l'Institut Pasteur* from 1903 and *Index Veterinarius* from 1933.

Fewer bibliographies seem to have been published in recent years than was previously the case. This is due to the growing number and availability of databases. Bibliographies tend to be compiled for areas of emerging interest where the literature is scattered. Some examples are:

AIDS bibliography (National Library of Medicine, 1987) covering 1986 and 1987

Collected papers on AIDS research, 1976–1986 (BIOSIS, 1987)

Cryptosporidium Species and other intestinal coccidia: a bibliography (Bureau of Hygiene and Tropical Diseases, 1987)

Foodborne viruses: a survey of the recent literature, compiled by A.C. Halligan and M.A.E. Auty (British Food Manufacturing Industries Research Association, 1988)

Key references in infectious diseases: an annotated guide, compiled by F.S. Southwick and P.T. Schooley (Churchill Livingstone, 1982) covers 1959–1980

Legionnaires' disease: a bibliography (1981–1985) (Bureau of Hygiene and Tropical Diseases, 1985)

Current awareness

The microbiologist has the choice of a variety of methods for keeping up to date with the literature. *Current Contents, Life Sciences,* containing reprints of a wide selection of contents pages of journals, can be scanned on a weekly basis. This is time-consuming but does retain the element of serendipity in search, an advantage over mechanized searches. Whilst the *Life Sciences* section of *Current Contents* includes the core microbiological journals, the *Clinical Medicine* section exclusively lists some clinical journals in which relevant articles may be found. Both sections are available online or as CURRENT CONTENTS ON DISKETTE (CCOD), weekly floppy discs in 600 or 1200 title versions. The references listed in the journal *Current Opinion in Infectious Diseases,* which was referred to in the section on reviews, are available on discs updated bimonthly from the publisher, Current Science. Subscribing to floppy discs is costly but allows the user to construct and run personalized searches.

The PHLS Central Library at Colindale, North London, produces *PHLS Library Bulletin*, an updating service in the fields of medical microbiology and epidemiology of communicable disease. It lists an average of 350 titles weekly selected from 350 journals. The *Abstracts of the Annual Meeting of the American Society for Microbiology*, abstracts of hundreds of papers and posters presented at this huge meeting, can be referred to as a guide to research in progress.

The explosion of the literature in the field of AIDS has resulted in the appearance of many alerting services from the AIDS worker. *AIDS Information* is published monthly by the Oncology Information Service, University of Leeds Medical and Dental School. References are arranged by subject with abstracts and keywords but indexes are not provided. *AIDS Research Today* is produced monthly from the BIOSIS database. Arrangement is by author with subject and author indexes. *ATIN: AIDS Targeted Information Newsletter* (Williams and Wilkins) has abstracts under eight key subject areas but is considerably more expensive than its European counterparts. Gower's *Current AIDS Literature* lists monthly abstracts from the AIDS DATABASE of the Bureau of Hygiene and Tropical Diseases, London. It is also a good source for books, conference proceedings and grey literature. A specialist publication for the microbiologist, concentrating on diagnosis and transmission of HIV, is the monthly *PHLS HIV Bulletin* listing titles of articles, with keywords, taken from the PHLS Central Library database. Two services are aimed at more general audiences and are more biased to media items than the scientific sources. For health care workers, the Bureau of Hygiene and Tropical Diseases publishes *AIDS Newsletter*, 20 issues a year, and for the general medical and lay audience there is *AIDS Letter*, bimonthly from the Royal Society of Medicine.

As an alternative to scanning published bulletins some researchers prefer to receive lists of references tailor-made to their own requirements on a regular basis. These selective dissemination of information (SDI) services are available from all the databases discussed in the previous section.

Reference works: dictionaries, encyclopaedias and handbooks

The comprehensive, well cross-referenced *Dictionary of microbiology and molecular biology*, by P. Singleton and D. Sainsbury (2nd edn., Wiley, 1987) contains some concise reviews and is an invaluable reference work. *Virology: directory and dictionary of animal, bacterial and plant viruses*, by R. Hull, F. Brown and C. Payne (Macmillan, 1989) is also referenced. Other specialized examples are *Dictionary of medical laboratory sciences*, edited by A.D. Farr (Blackwell Scientific Publications, 1988), *Ainsworth and Bisby's dictionary of fungi*, by D.L. Hawksworth (7th rev. edn., Commonwealth Mycological Institute, 1983) and *A dictionary of epidemiology*, edited by J.M. Last (2nd edn., Oxford University Press, 1988).

CRC Press publishes several comprehensive works. *CRC handbook of microbiology* is edited by A.I. Laskin and H.A. Lechevalier (2nd edn., 9 vols, 1977–1988). Bacteria and associated infections are covered in the first volume, other organisms in the second and biochemistry and physiology in volumes 3 to 8. A condensed version, *CRC practical handbook of microbiology*, edited by W.M. O'Leary, was published in 1989. There are two relevant sections in the *CRC handbook series in clinical laboratory science*, a compilation of diagnostic data, edited by D. Seligson: *Section E—Clinical microbiology* (2 vols, CRC Press, 1977) and *Section H—Virology and rickettsiology* (2 vols, CRC Press, 1978). *CRC handbook of laboratory safety*, edited by A.K. Furr (3rd edn., 1990) covers all general aspects of safety.

Two encyclopaedias useful for historic reference are *Kolle und Wassermann's Handbuch der pathogenen Mikroorganismen*, edited by W. Kolle, R. Kraus and P. Uhlenhuth in 10 multipart volumes (3rd edn., Fischer, 1927–1931) and the MRC's *A system of bacteriology in relation to medicine*, edited by P. Fildes and J.C.G. Ledingham (9 vols, HMSO, 1929–1931).

Textbooks

The definitive text and reference work is the comprehensive and authoritative *Topley and Wilson's Principles of bacteriology and immunity*, edited by M.T. Parker and L.H. Collier (8th edn., 5 vols, Arnold, 1990) with each chapter written by leading experts. The work comprises *Volume 1: General bacteriology and immunity, Volume 2: Systematic bacteriology, Volume 3: Bacterial diseases, Volume 4: Virology* and *Volume 5: Index*. An imaginative approach to the subject from a practical standpoint is *Interpretive medical microbiology*, edited by H.P. Dalton and H.C. Nottebart (Churchill Livingstone, 1986).

Reliable textbooks for students are *Clinical microbiology*, by E.J. Stokes and G.L. Ridgway (6th edn., Arnold, 1987), *Medical microbiology*, by C.G.A. Thomas (Baillière Tindall, 1988) and *A new short textbook of microbial and parasitic infection*, by B.I. Duerden, T.M.S. Reid, J.M. Jewsbury and D.C. Turk (Hodder and Stoughton, 1987). These can be supplemented by referring to *Review of medical microbiology* by E. Jawetz, J.L. Melnick and E.A. Adelberg (18th edn., Appleton and Lange, 1989), a concise compilation of recent advances which is updated every two or three years.

Of the popular textbooks covering the whole of microbiology, two are substantial: *General microbiology*, by R.Y. Stanier, J.L. Ingraham, M.L. Wheelis and P.R. Painter (5th edn., Macmillan, 1987) and *Microbiology*, by B.D. Davis, R. Dulbecco, H.N. Eisen and H.S. Ginsberg (4th edn., Lippincott, 1990). More concise is *Biology of microorganisms*, by T.D. Brock and M.T. Madigan (5th edn., Prentice-Hall, 1988).

Bacteriology

Textbooks and treatises

The comprehensive source is *The bacteria: a treatise on structure and function* published by Academic Press from 1960. The original series editors were I.C. Gunsalus and R.Y. Stanier. Additional volumes were added under the editorship of Gunsalus and then of J.R. Sokatch who has been joined by L.N. Ornston for the most recent volume, vol. XI. Two useful student texts are *Medical bacteriology*, by J.D. Sleigh and M.C. Timbury (Churchill Livingstone, 1990) and *Gillies and Dodds' bacteriology illustrated* by R.R. Gillies (5th edn., Churchill Livingstone, 1984).

Special aspects are covered in the following titles:

Microbial physiology, by A.G. Moat and J.W. Foster (2nd edn., Wiley, 1988)

Survival and dormancy of microorganisms, edited by Y. Henis (Wiley, 1987)

Microbial lipids Vol. 1, edited by C. Ratledge and S.G. Wilkinson (Academic Press, 1988)

Bacterial toxins, by J. Stephen and R.A. Pietrowski (2nd edn., ASM, 1986)

Handbook of endotoxin, edited by R.A. Procter (4 vols., Elsevier, 1984–1986)

Microbial ecology: organisms, habitats, activities, by H. Stolp (Cambridge University Press, 1988)

Microbial genetics is a very important area being the basis of much experimental and diagnostic work. The most recent accounts are *Molecular genetics of bacteria*, by J.W. Dale (Wiley, 1989), *Genetics of microbes*, by B.W. Bainbridge (2nd edn., Blackie, 1987) and *Bacterial plasmids*, by K. Hardy (2nd edn., Van Nostrand Reinhold). Texts on techniques will be covered in the section on laboratory methods. Bacteriophage has received little attention since the classic *Bacteriophages*, by M.H. Adams (Interscience, 1959) other than as a tool in genetics. However R. Calendar has begun editing a series, *The bacteriophages* (vol.1, Plenum Press, 1988).

Pathogenicity is a related important area which has been usefully treated in the following:

Molecular basis of bacterial pathogenesis, edited by B.H. Iglewski and V.L. Clark (Academic Press, 1990)—this is vol. XI of *The bacteria: a treatise on structure and function* (mentioned above)

Mechanisms of microbial disease, edited by M. Schaechter, G. Medoff and D. Schlessinger (Williams and Wilkins, 1989)

Virulence mechanisms of bacterial pathogens, edited by J.A. Roth (ASM, 1988)

Systematics and culture collections

The work elucidating the universally accepted classification scheme is *Bergey's manual of systematic bacteriology*, series editor J.G. Holt (4 vols, Williams and Wilkins, 1984–1989). Thousands of names, many inadequately authenticated, are listed in *Index Bergeyana*, edited by R.E. Buchanan *et al.* (Livingstone, 1966) and its *Supplement*, edited by N.E. Gibbons *et al.* (Williams and Wilkins, 1981). *A dictionary of microbial taxonomy*, by S.T. Cowan and edited by L.R. Hill (Cambridge University Press, 1978) is a readable guide containing a chapter on the history of classification and a bibliography of key works. The International Committee on Systematic Bacteriology (ICSB) of the IUMS is the body responsible for the official naming of bacteria. Its publications include *Approved lists of bacterial names*, edited by V.B. Skerman, V. McGowan and P.H.A. Sneath (ASM, 1980). This is reprinted from the official organ of the ICSB, *International Journal of Systematic Bacteriology*, **30**, 225. Subsequently approved names appear in annual validation lists in the journal.

Culture collections maintain and make available micro-organisms. *CRC practical handbook of microbiology* cited in the section on reference works lists the addresses of the world's major collections on pages 249–250. The UK collection is housed at the Central Public Health Laboratory, Colindale. Its catalogue is entitled *Catalogue of the National Collection of Type Cultures (NCTC): Bacteria, mycoplasmas, typing-bacteriophages. 7th edn.; Catalogue of the plasmid section, NCTC: plasmids, bacteriophages, transposons; Catalogue of the National Collection of Pathogenic Fungi (NCPF): Fungi, yeasts, aerobic actinomycetes* (PHLS, 1989). The equivalent U.S. body is the American Type Culture Collection (ATCC) at Rockville, Maryland. R. Gherna, W. Nierman and P. Pienta edited its *Catalogue of Bacteria, Phages and rDNA Vectors* with an *Index to industrial applications* (16th edn., ATCC, 1985).

Specific organisms

Many works are produced on specific bacteria or genera and their associated infections. The following is a selection of recent works on organisms of particular current medical interest:

Anaerobic infections in humans, edited by S.M. Finegold and W.L. George (Academic Press, 1989)

Bacillus, edited by C.R. Harwood (Plenum Press, 1989)

Bacterial meningitis, edited by J.D. William and J. Burnie (*Beecham Colloquia* No.8, Academic Press, 1987)

Biology of anaerobic microorganisms, edited by A.B. Zehnder (Wiley, 1988)

The biology of the mycobacteria, edited by C. Ratledge, J. Stanford and J.M. Grange (3 vols, Academic Press, 1982–1989)

Brucellosis, edited by M.M. Madkour (Butterworths, 1989)

Campylobacter pylori and gastroduodenal disease, edited by B.J. Rathbone and R.V. Heatley (Blackwell Scientific Publications, 1989)

Clostridia, edited by N.P. Minton and D.J. Clarke (Plenum Press, 1989)

Escherichia coli and Salmonella typhimurium: Cellular and molecular biology, edited by F.C. Neidhardt (2 vols, ASM, 1987)

Foodborne listeriosis, edited by A.L. Miller, J.L. Smith and G.A. Somkuti (Elsevier, 1990)

Legionella infections, by C.L.R. Bartlett, A.D. Macrae and J.T. Macfarlane (Edward Arnold, 1986)

The mycoplasmas, edited by M.F. Barile, S. Razin, J.G. Tully and R.F. Whicomb (5 vols, Academic Press, 1979–1989)

Pasteurella and Pasteurellosis, edited by C. Adlam and J.M. Rutter (Academic Press, 1989)

Pseudomonas: biotransformations, pathogenesis and evolving biotechnology, edited by S. Silver, A.M. Chakrabarty, B. Iglewski and S. Kaplan (ASM, 1990)

Laboratory methods for specific groups of organisms are covered in *Anaerobic infections: clinical and laboratory practice*, edited by A.T. Willis and K.D. Phillips (PHLS, 1988), *A laboratory manual for Legionella*, edited by T.G. Harrison and A.G. Taylor (Wiley, 1988) and *Edwards and Ewing's identification of Enterobacteriaceae*, by W.H. Ewing (4th edn., Elsevier, 1986).

Virology

Textbooks and treatises

Two large works have emerged as the standard reference texts: *Fields' Virology*, edited by B.N. Fields and D.M. Knipe (2nd edn., 2 vols,

Raven Press, 1990) and *Principles and practice of clinical virology*, edited by A.J. Zuckerman, J.E. Banatvala and J.R. Pattison (Wiley, 1987). The encyclopaedic series *Comprehensive virology*, edited by H. Fraenkel-Conrat and R.R. Wagner (19 vols., Plenum Press, 1974–1984) is older but still valuable. The well-referenced *Andrewes' viruses of vertebrates*, edited by J.S. Porterfield (5th edn., Baillière Tindall, 1989) is a compilation of virus characteristics. For students *Notes on medical virology*, by M.C. Timbury (8th edn., Churchill Livingstone, 1986), *Textbook of human virology*, edited by R.B. Belshe (PSG, 1984) and *Textbook of medical virology*, edited by E. Lycke and E. Norrby (Butterworths, 1983) have proved popular. N.J. Dimmock and S.B. Primrose's *Introduction to modern virology* (3rd edn., Blackwell, 1987) emphasizes molecular biology. *Medical virology* by D.O. White and F.J. Fenner (3rd edn., Academic Press, 1986) is strong on viral infections. Veterinary aspects are covered in *Veterinary virology* by F. Fenner, P.A. Bachmann, E.P.J. Gibbs, F.A. Murphy, M.J. Studdert and D.O. White (Academic Press, 1987). Two excellent atlases are *Animal virus structure*, edited by M.V. Nermut and A.C. Steven (Elsevier, 1987) and C.R. Madeley and A.M. Field's *Virus morphology* (2nd edn., Churchill Livingstone, 1988). Pathogenicity has been covered in a series edited by A.L. Notkins and M.B.A. Oldstone, *Concepts in viral pathogenesis* (3 vols., Springer-Verlag, 1984–1989) and *Virus immunity and pathogenesis*, edited by C.A. Mims (Churchill Livingstone, 1985), reprinted from *British Medical Bulletin*, 1985, **41**, 1–102.

Meetings are a source of current research information. An international symposium on medical virology has taken place annually since 1981. Its proceedings are published, latterly by Plenum Press, as *Medical virology*, edited by L.M. de la Maza and E.M. Peterson. To 1990, eight international congresses of virology have been held under the auspices of the Virology Division of the IUMS with published abstracts of the proceedings.

Systematics and culture collections

The International Committee on Taxonomy of Viruses (ICTV) of IUMS is the regulatory body and its reports are published regularly in *Intervirology*. J.L. Melnick reviews the position annually in *Progress in Medical Virology*. Culture collections are listed in *CRC practical handbook of microorganisms* cited in the preceding section on bacteriology. The American Type Culture Collection is one of the largest. Its most recent list is *Catalogue of animal and plant viruses, Chlamydiae, Rickettsiae and virus antisera*, edited by L.E. Benade, D.A. Stevens, N. Elliott and J. Aebig (5th edn., ATCC, 1986).

Specific organisms

There is a wealth of published books on specific viruses and virus groups. The following are comprehensive texts on organisms of especial current interest:

Chlamydia, by P.-A. Mardh, J. Paavonen and M. Puolakkainen (Plenum Press, 1989)

Coxsackieviruses: a general update, edited by M. Bendinelli and H. Friedman (Plenum Press, 1988)

CRC handbook of parvoviruses, edited by P. Tijssen (2 vols., CRC Press, 1990)

Epstein–Barr virus and human disease, edited by P.H. Levine, D.V. Ablashi, M. Nonoyama, G.R. Pearson and R. Glaser (Humana Press, 1987)

Herpes simplex virus, by A. Mindel (Springer-Verlag, 1989)

Infectious mononucleosis, edited by D. Schlossberg (Springer, 1989)

Influenza, by E.D. Kilbourne (Plenum Medical Book Co., 1987)

Retroviruses and disease, edited by H. Hanafusa, A. Pinter and M.E. Pullman (Academic Press, 1989)

Viral hepatitis: biological and clinical features, specific diagnosis, and prophylaxis, by F.B. Hollinger, J.L. Melnick and W.S. Robinson (Raven Press, 1985)

Prions, small infectious particles, have been implicated in bovine spongiform encephalopathy (BSE) which may be transmissible to man. Few books have been published on the subject. In 1987 *Ciba Foundation Symposium no.135* was held and published as *Novel infectious agents and the CNS*, edited by G. Bock and J. Marsh (Wiley, 1988). S.B. Prusiner and M.P. McKinley have edited *Prions: novel infectious pathogens causing scrapie and Creutzfeldt–Jakob disease* (Academic Press, 1987). The DoH and the Ministry of Agriculture, Fisheries and Food have issued the *Report of the Working Party on Bovine Spongiform Encephalopathy*, otherwise known as the Southwood Report (HMSO, 1989).

Laboratory methods in virology

The comprehensive manual for laboratory methods is *Diagnostic procedures for viral, rickettsial and chlamydial infections*, edited by N.J. Schmidt and R.W. Emmons (6th edn., APHA, 1989). E.H. Lennette, a respected author of bench manuals, has edited *Laboratory diagnosis of viral infections* (Dekker, 1985). A useful introduction to methods is *Virology: a practical approach*, edited by B.W.J. Mahy (IRL Press, 1985).

Mycology and parasitology

Fungi, parasites and related organisms have come to prominence in the last decade as agents of opportunistic infections in people with AIDS and other immunocompromised hosts. Parasitology is dealt with in the section on tropical medicine and so only organisms which are encountered in the UK will be considered here. J.W. Deacon's *Introduction to modern mycology* (2nd edn., Blackwell, 1984), *Essentials of medical mycology*, by E.G.V. Evans and J.C. Gentles (Churchill Livingstone, 1985) and *Medical parasitology*, by E.K. Markell, M. Voge and D.T. John (6th edn., W.B. Saunders, 1986) are useful texts.

CAB International issue the *Bibliography of Systematic Mycology* and *Index of Fungi: a List of Names of New Genera*. The National Collection of Pathogenic Fungi in the UK is held at the PHLS Mycological Reference Laboratory, part of the Central Public Health Laboratory. Its catalogue is included with the *Catalogue of the NCTC* referred to in the bacteriology section.

Opportunistic infections are dealt with in J.M.B. Smith's *Opportunistic mycoses of man and other animals* (CAB International, 1989) and *Parasitic infections in the compromised host*, edited by P.D. Walzer and R.M. Genta (Dekker, 1989). Candida, one of the most prevalent pathogens, is comprehensively covered by F.C. Odds in *Candida and candidosis* (2nd edn., Baillière Tindall, 1988). *Oral candidosis*, edited by L.P. Samaranayake and T.W. MacFarlane (Wright, 1990) deals with infection to which the immunocompromised are particularly prone. *Pneumocystis carinii pneumonitis* by W.T. Hughes (2 vols, CRC Press, 1987) is an extensive account of a common and serious infection in AIDS.

Recently there has been an occasional appearance of cryptosporidium or giardia in water supplies in the UK. Literature on these organisms is scant. Examples are *Cryptosporidiosis: Proceedings of the First International Workshop, Edinburgh, 7–8 September 1988*, edited by K.W. Angus and D.A. Blewett (Animal Diseases Research Association, 1989) and *Giardia and giardiasis: biology, pathogenesis and epidemiology*, edited by S.L. Erlandsen and E.A. Meyer (Plenum Press, 1984). J.P. Dubey and C.P. Beattie's *Toxoplasmosis of animals and man* (CRC Press, 1988) examines an infection which can cause problems in pregnancy.

The diagnostic reference work is *Diagnostic procedures for mycotic and parasitic infections*, edited by B.B. Wentworth (7th edn., APHA, 1988). *Diagnosis and therapy of systemic fungal infections*, by K. Holmberg and R.D. Meyer (Raven, 1989) includes the most common pathogens and *Medical mycology: a practical approach*, edited by E.G.V. Evans and M.D. Richardson (IRL Press, 1989) is a handy text.

S.L. Fleck and A.H. Moody's *Diagnostic techniques in medical parasitology* (Wright, 1988) covers organisms likely to be encountered in a UK laboratory.

Environmental microbiology

Recent outbreaks of food poisoning and concerns about water quality together with EC legislation have given increased prominence to this branch of microbiology.

Food

The standard work is *Food microbiology*, by W.C. Frazier and D.C. Westhoff (4th edn., McGraw Hill, 1988). G.J. Banwert's *Basic food microbiology* (2nd edn., Van Nostrand, 1989) is a useful student text. Food poisoning and its prevention are covered in *Food poisoning and food hygiene*, by B.C. Hobbs and D. Roberts (5th edn., Arnold, 1987). In response to recent outbreaks the UK Government has convened the Committee on the Microbiological Safety of Food chaired by Sir Mark Richmond. It has reported in *The microbiological safety of food. Part 1. Report of the Committee to the Secretary of State for Health, the Minister of Agriculture, Fisheries and Food, and the Secretaries of State for Wales, Scotland and Northern Ireland* (HMSO, 1990).

The British Standards Institution (BSI) is in the process of publishing the multipart *BS 5763: British Standard methods for microbiological examination of food and animal feeding stuffs*. The definitive European published text on laboratory methods is still *Isolation and identification methods for food poisoning organisms*, edited by J.E.L. Corry, D. Roberts and F.A. Skinner *(SAB Technical Series No. 17*, Academic Press, 1982). M.L. Speck has edited the American *Compendium of methods for the microbiological examination of foods* (2nd edn., APHA, 1984). The International Commission on Microbiological Specifications for Foods (ICMSF) of the IUMS is working towards a consensus on methods in *Microorganisms in foods* (vol. 1, 2nd edn., University of Toronto Press, 1978; vol. 2, 2nd edn., Blackwell, 1986; vol. 3 Parts I and II, Academic Press, 1980; vol. 4, Blackwell, 1988). *Rapid methods in food microbiology*, edited by M.R. Adams and C.F.A. Hope (Elsevier, 1989) is a useful compilation. On special aspects are the British Standard *BS 4285: Microbiological examination for dairy purposes* (BSI, in progress), *Standard methods for the examination of dairy products*, edited by G.H. Richardson (APHA, 1985) and *Methods for the microbiological examination of fish and shellfish*, edited by B. Austin and D.A. Austin (Ellis Horwood, 1989).

Regulations and notification procedures are given in *Food poisoning: the investigation and control of food infection in England and Wales (DHSS Memo 188/MED*, HMSO, 1982) available from the DoH. Surveillance reports on food poisoning in England and Wales have been published by the PHLS for 40 years, currently appearing in the *Communicable Disease Report* and the *British Medical Journal*. CDC issues annual statistics for the USA.

Water

The official criteria for ensuring drinking water quality in European Community member states are published as *Directive No.80/778/EEC of 15 July 1980 relating to the quality of water intended for human consumption* which appeared in *Official Journal of the European Communities* No.L229, 11. Other EC directives apply to water to be used for abstraction for a drinking water supply *(No.75/440/EEC of 25 July 1975* and *No.79/869/EEC of 9 October 1979)* and officially designated bathing waters *(No.76/160/EEC of 8 December 1975)*. WHO has published *Guidelines for drinking water quality* (3 vols., WHO, 1984–1985). Microbiological tests to be used to ensure that the EC regulations are being met are given in *DHSS Reports on Public Health and Medical Subjects No.71*. Colloquially known as Report 71, this was published by the Department of the Environment, DHSS and PHLS as *The bacteriological examination of drinking water supplies 1982* (5th edn., HMSO, 1983) and is now under revision. BSI is in the process of publishing *BS 6068: Water quality. Part 4. Microbiological methods*. U.S. methods are detailed in *Standard methods for the examination of water and wastewater* (16th edn., APHA, 1985, with a supplement 1988) prepared by the APHA, American Water Works Association and Water Pollution Control Federation. Special aspects are covered in *Laboratory procedures for the examination of seawater and shellfish*, edited by A.E. Greenberg and D.A. Hunt (5th edn., APHA, 1985). Infections are considered in *Waterborne diseases in the United States*, edited by G.F. Craun (CRC Press, 1986).

Disinfection and sterilization

Little has been published in this field since the third edition of the present book. The principal texts are still *Principles and practice of disinfection, preservation and sterilisation*, edited by A.D. Russell, W.B. Hugo and G.A.J. Ayliffe (Blackwell, 1982) and S.S. Block's *Disinfection, sterilization and preservation* (3rd edn., Lea and Febiger, 1983). J.F. Gardner and M.M. Peel's *Introduction to sterilization and disinfection* (Churchill Livingstone, 1986) is a useful starting point and *Hospital hygiene* by I.M. Maurer (3rd edn., Arnold 1985) contains practical advice. The British Medical Association has published a concise guide, *A code of practice for sterilisation of instruments and control of cross infection* (BMA, 1989). The DoH has produced a report on choice of disinfectants, *Report of the Expert Advisory Committee on Biocides* (HMSO, 1989) chaired by Dr. A.E. Wright. A practical booklet *Chemical disinfection in hospitals* by G.A.J. Ayliffe, D. Coates and P.N. Hoffman (PHLS, 1984) is in wide use in many establishments. Standards and practice guidelines for sterilizers and disinfectants are issued by the DoH as *Circulars*, BSI and the U.S. Association for the Advancement of Medical Instrumentation.

Laboratory methods

Laboratory methods have evolved rapidly in recent years with the development of new genetic, molecular and immunological techniques applicable to micro-organisms. This is reflected in the volume of relevant publications being written. Works of general interest only are listed here. Specialist texts for individual organisms or groups are included elsewhere under the appropriate subheadings.

New editions of the standard diagnostic works have appeared in the last few years. The long-awaited update of the well-established UK student text has been published as *Mackie and McCartney Practical medical microbiology*, edited by J.G. Collee, J.P. Duguid, A.G. Fraser and B.P. Marmion (13th edn., Churchill Livingstone, 1989). The complete work is in two volumes and this is the new edition of volume two. Volume one remains as *Mackie and McCartney Medical microbiology, vol. 1—Microbial infections*, edited by J.P. Duguid, B.P. Marmion and R.H.A. Swain (13th edn., Churchill Livingstone, 1978). There are two outstandingly comprehensive U.S. technical reference works. *Diagnostic procedures for bacterial infections*, edited by B.B. Wentworth (7th edn., APHA, 1988) previously included fungal and parasitic infections. These now appear in a separate publication, cited earlier. *Manual of clinical microbiology*, edited by E.H. Lennette, A. Balows, W.J. Hausler and H.J. Shadomy (4th edn., ASM, 1985) is updated by pamphlets on specific methods in the ASM's irregularly published *Cumitechs* series. Other respected texts are *Bailey and Scott's Diagnostic microbiology*, by S.M. Finegold and E.J. Baron (7th edn., Mosby, 1986), E.J. Stokes and G.L. Ridgway's *Clinical microbiology* (6th edn., Arnold, 1987), *Collins and Lyne's Microbiological methods*, by C.H. Collins, P.M. Lyne and J.M. Grange (6th edn., Butterworths, 1989) and D.C. Shanson's *Microbiology in clinical practice* (2nd edn., Wright, 1989).

The definitive atlas for visual identification is *Color atlas and textbook of diagnostic microbiology*, by E.W. Koneman, S.D. Allen, V.R.

Dowell, W.M. Janda, H.M. Sommers and W.C. Winn (3rd edn., Lippincott, 1988) and identification is also covered in *Isolation and identification of micro-organisms of medical and veterinary importance*, edited by C.H. Collins and J.M. Grange *(SAB Technical Series No.21*, Academic Press, 1985). For media there is the manufacturer's directory *The Oxoid manual of culture media, ingredients and other laboratory services* (5th edn., Oxoid, 1982) and the comprehensive *Media for isolation, cultivation, identification, maintenance of medical bacteria. Vol.1*, by J.M. MacFaddin (Williams and Wilkins, 1985). Other important aspects of laboratory practice are covered in *Methods for quality control in diagnostic microbiology*, edited by J.M. Miller and B.B. Wentworth (APHA, 1985) and *Maintenance of microorganisms: a manual of laboratory methods*, edited by B.E. Kirsop and J.J.S. Snell (Academic Press, 1984).

Laboratory techniques are well served in the multivolume compilation *Methods in microbiology* (Academic Press, 1969–) edited originally by J.R. Norris and D.W. Ribbons, and latterly by T. Bergan and Norris, with most volumes on an individual topic. Immunoassays are covered in *Immunological techniques in microbiology*, edited by J.M. Grange, A. Fox and N.L. Morgan *(SAB Technical Series No.24*, Blackwell Scientific Publications, 1987), *Complementary immunoassays*, edited by W.P. Collins (Wiley, 1988), *ELISA and other solid phase immunoassays: theoretical and practical aspects*, edited by D.M. Kemeny and S.J. Challacombe (Wiley, 1988) and *ELISA in the clinical microbiology laboratory*, edited by T.G. Wreghitt and P. Morgan-Capner (PHLS, 1990).

Many guides to genetic manipulation and molecular cloning have been produced. The following have proved popular with microbiologists:

Principles of gene manipulation: an introduction to genetic engineering, by R.W. Old and S.B. Primrose (4th edn., Blackwell, 1989)

Introduction to practical molecular biology, by P.D. Darbre (Wiley, 1988)

Molecular cloning: a laboratory manual, by J. Sambrook, E.F. Fritsch and T. Maniatis (3 vols, 2nd edn., Cold Spring Harbor Laboratory Press, 1989)

A practical guide to molecular cloning, by B. Perbal (2nd edn., Wiley, 1988)

DNA cloning: a practical approach, edited by D.M. Glover (3 vols, IRL Press, 1985–1987)

Monoclonal antibodies against bacteria, edited by A.J.L. Macario and E.C. de Macario (3 vols, Academic Press, 1985–1986)

Making monoclonals: a practical beginner's guide to the production and characterization of monoclonal antibodies against bacteria and viruses, by D.G. Newell, B.W. McBride and S.A. Clark (PHLS, 1988)

Plasmids: a practical approach, edited by K.G. Hardy (IRL Press, 1987)

Other techniques are covered in:

PCR protocols: a guide to methods and applications, edited by M.A. Innis, D.H. Gelfand, J.J. Sninsky and T.J. White (Academic Press, 1990)

Gel electrophoresis of nucleic acids: a practical approach, edited by D. Rickwood and B.D. Hames (2nd edn., IRL Press, 1990)

Gel electrophoresis of proteins, edited by B.D. Hames and D. Rickwood (2nd edn., IRL Press, 1990)

Microbial applications of high-performance liquid chromatography, by D.B. Drucker (Cambridge University Press, 1987)

Computers in microbiology: a practical approach, edited by T.N. Bryant and J.W.T. Wimpenny (IRL Press, 1989)

The *Association of Clinical Pathologists Broadsheets* are a useful series on methods and in the USA, the National Committee for Clinical Laboratory Standards publishes standards and assessments of techniques and specifications for reference materials.

Laboratory safety

The maintenance of safe practice in the handling of pathogens and potentially hazardous substances has always been of prime concern to laboratory workers but emphasis continues to be added to the subject with the wider application of genetic manipulation techniques, the advent of HIV, concern over the prevalence of hepatitis viruses and increasing legal requirements, the Control of Substances Hazardous to Health Regulations (1988) being the most recent in the UK. The key publication for safe handling of pathogens is *Code of practice for the prevention of infection in clinical laboratories and post-mortem rooms*, known as the 'Howie Code', issued by the former DHSS (HMSO, 1978). The Health and Safety Commission (HSC), the body charged with implementing UK regulations, and its Executive, issue helpful guidance publications. Of particular relevance to microbiologists are *A guide to the Health and Safety (Dangerous Pathogens) Regulations 1981* (Booklet HS(R)12, HMSO, 1981) and from the HSC's Health Services Advisory Committee *Safety in Health Service laboratories: hepatitis B. Precautions to minimise the risk of infection from specimens known or suspected to be positive and in the testing of specimens for the presence of hepatitis b antigens or antibodies* (HMSO, 1985) and *Safety in health service laboratories: the labelling, transport and reception of specimens* (HMSO, 1986). The Advisory Committee on Dangerous Pathogens (ACDP) advises the Government on handling micro-organisms as in their report *Categorisation of pathogens according to hazard and categories of containment* (HMSO, 1984) and the Genetic Manipulation Advisory Group (GMAG) advises on genetic engineering through *GMAG Notes*. A well-referenced practical handbook is *Laboratory-acquired infections: history, incidence, causes and prevention*, by C.H. Collins (2nd edn., Butterworths, 1988).

Covering all aspects of safety are *Codes of practice for pathology departments* (Royal College of Pathologists, 1989) and *Safety in clinical and biomedical laboratories*, edited by C.H. Collins (Chapman and Hall, 1988). In the USA, CDC and the National Institutes of Health have produced guidelines on *Biosafety in microbiological and biomedical laboratories* (2nd edn., U.S. Government Printing Office, 1988) and the ASM has published *Laboratory safety: principles and practices*, edited by B.M. Miller, D.Vesley, J.R. Songer *et al.* (1986). The comprehensive *CRC handbook of laboratory safety* cited under reference works is a useful volume.

Communicable diseases

Textbooks

Principles and practice of infectious diseases, edited by G.L. Mandell, R.G. Douglas and J.E. Bennett (3rd edn., 2 vols, Churchill Livingstone, 1990) is the most comprehensive of the standard texts. A.B. Christie's *Infectious diseases: epidemiology and clinical practice* (4th edn., 2 vols., Churchill Livingstone, 1987) covers the common diseases and is a good source of references. Unusually for a major text it is still the work of one author. *Infectious diseases: a modern treatise of infectious processes*, edited by P.D. Hoeprich and M.C. Jordan (4th edn., Lippincott, 1989) is also well thought of. The best account specifically on viruses is *Viral infections of humans: epidemiology and control*, edited by A.S. Evans (3rd edn., Plenum, 1989). Of the student texts *The biologic and clinical basis of infectious diseases* by G.P. Youmans, P.Y. Paterson and H.M. Sommers (3rd edn., W.B. Saunders, 1985) is the most comprehensive and W.E. Farrar and H.P. Lambert's *Infectious diseases* (Gower Medical, 1984) is usefully concise.

Two working handbooks are pocket-sized but full of information. *Control of communicable diseases in man*, edited by A.S. Benenson (14th edn., APHA, 1985), colloquially referred to as the 'Red book', is invaluable and usefully supplemented by *Infection*, by R.T.D. Emond, J.M. Bradley and N.S. Galbraith (2nd edn., Blackwell, 1989) for UK control measures.

The leading atlases are *A colour atlas of infectious diseases*, by R.T.D. Emond and H.A.K. Rowland (2nd edn., Wolfe Medical, 1987) and H.P. Lambert and W.E. Farrar's *Infectious diseases illustrated: an integrated text and colour atlas* (Pergamon, 1982).

Sexually transmitted diseases

Sexually transmitted diseases, edited by K.K. Holmes, P.-A. Mardh, P.F. Sparling and P.J. Wiesner (2nd edn., McGraw-Hill, 1990) has quickly established itself as a reference text. A new comprehensive work is *Sexually transmitted diseases: a textbook of genitourinary medicine*, edited by G.W. Csonka and J.K. Oates (Baillière Tindall, 1990). *Atlas of sexually transmitted diseases*, edited by S.A. Morse, A.A. Moreland and S.E. Thompson (Gower Medical, 1990) takes an interesting epidemiological approach and is well produced with many charts and diagrams. On the clinical side there are D.H.H. Robertson, A. McMillan and H. Young's *Clinical practice in sexually transmitted diseases* (2nd edn., Churchill Livingstone, 1989) and *Genital tract infection in women*, edited by M.J. Hare (Churchill Livingstone, 1988). *Laboratory methods for the diagnosis of sexually transmitted diseases*, edited by B.B. Wentworth and F.N. Judson is a comprehensive manual complemented by the concise *Sexually transmitted diseases: a rational guide to their diagnosis*, edited by A.E. Jephcott (PHLS, 1987) which gives the PHLS approach.

Infection control and hospital-acquired infections

Prevention and containment of nosocomial infections continues to be a problem. An authoritative British text is *Hospital-acquired infection: principles and prevention*, by G.A.J. Ayliffe, B.J. Collins and L.J. Taylor (2nd edn., Wright, 1990). The U.S. viewpoint is given in M. Castle and E. Ajemian's *Hospital infection control: principles and practice* (2nd edn., Wiley, 1987) and *Prevention and control of nosocomial infections*, edited by R.P. Wenzel (Williams and Wilkins, 1987). The official UK guidelines are *Hospital Infection control: guidance on the control of infection in hospitals prepared by the Joint DHSS/PHLS Hospital Infection Working Group* (DHSS, 1988). The DoH issues more specialized advice such as *Guidance for clinical health care workers: protection against infection with HIV and hepatitis viruses. Recommen-*

dations of the Expert Advisory Group on AIDS (HMSO, 1990). The BMA has issued two handy practical books: *Infection control: the BMA guide* (Arnold, 1989) and *A code of practice for the safe use and disposal of sharps* (BMA, 1990). Substantial manuals from professional associations in the USA are the American College of Surgeons: Committee on Control of Surgical Infections' *Manual on control of infection in surgical patients* (2nd edn., Lippincott, 1984) and from the American Practitioners in Infection Control, *The APIC curriculum for infection control practice*, edited by B.M. Soule (2 vols., Kendall/Hunt, 1983). Proceedings of meetings are published by the Infection Control Nurses Association, in their *Yearbook*, and the Hospital Infection Society.

Recent texts on infections include *Hospital infections*, edited by J.V. Bennett and P.S. Brachman (2nd edn., Little, Brown, 1986), A. Pollock's *Surgical infections* with a section on microbiology and immunology by C. Easmon (Arnold, 1987), *Infections in emergency medicine, vol.1*, edited by D. Schillinger and A. Harwood-Nuss (Churchill Livingstone, 1989) and *Infections in the orthopaedic patient*, edited by R. Coombs and R.H. Fitzgerald (Butterworths, 1989).

Other specific infections

Zoonoses, infections transmitted from animals to man, remain of interest. Very comprehensive coverage is given in *CRC handbook series in zoonoses*, edited by J.H. Steele (8 vols, CRC Press, 1979–1984). A useful recent text is *The zoonoses: infections transmitted from animals to man*, by J.C. Bell, S.R. Palmer and J.M. Payne (Arnold, 1988). *Zoonoses and communicable diseases common to man and animals*, by P.N. Acha and B. Szyfres (2nd edn., WHO Pan American Health Organization, 1987) is international in scope.

On infections in children *Textbook of pediatric infectious diseases*, edited by R.D. Feigin and J.D. Cherry (2nd edn., 2 vols, W.B. Saunders, 1987) and *Infectious diseases of children*, by S. Krugman, S.L. Katz, A.A. Gershon and C.M. Wilfert (8th edn., Mosby, 1985) are well established. Particular attention has been paid to infections in the neonate and fetus. J.S. Remington and J.O. Klein have edited *Infectious diseases of the fetus and newborn infant* (2nd edn., W.B. Saunders, 1983) which is complemented by the more specialized *Bacterial infections in the fetus and newborn*, by P.A. Davies and L. Gothefors (W.B. Saunders, 1984) and J.B. Hanshaw, J.A. Dudgeon and W.C. Marshall's *Viral diseases of the fetus and newborn* (2nd edn., W.B. Saunders, 1985). Pregnancy is covered in *Infections in pregnancy*, edited by L.C. Gilstrap and S. Faro (Alan R. Liss, 1990), *Parasitic infections in pregnancy and the newborn*, edited by C.L. MacLeod (Oxford University Press, 1988) and *Virus infection in pregnancy*, edited by M.S. Amstey (Grune and Stratton, 1984). For the other end of the lifespan, B.A. Cunha has edited *Infectious diseases in the elderly* (PSG Publishing, 1988). Treating the immunocompromised is now particularly relevant and *Clinical approach to infection in the compromised host*, edited by R.H. Rubin and L.S. Young has rapidly appeared in a second edition (Plenum Medical, 1988).

Infections of different systems are dealt with in the following:

Enteric infection: mechanisms, manifestations and management, edited by M.J.G. Farthing and G.T. Keusch (Chapman and Hall Medical, 1989)

Respiratory infections: diagnosis and management, edited by J.E. Pennington (Raven Press, 1989)

Neurological infections, by M. Wood and M. Anderson (W.B. Saunders, 1988)

Urinary tract infection in clinical and laboratory practice, edited by R.M. Maskell (Arnold, 1988)

Detection, prevention and management of urinary tract infections, by C.M. Kunin (4th edn., Lea and Febiger, 1987)

Infections in the rheumatic diseases: a comprehensive review of microbial relations to rheumatic disorders, edited by L.R. Espinoza (Grune and Stratton, 1988)

Epidemiology and surveillance

Texts on epidemiology include A.M. Lilienfield and A.B. Lilienfield's *Foundations of epidemiology* (2nd edn., Oxford University Press, 1980) and the clinically orientated *Epidemiology of diseases*, edited by D.L. Miller and R.D.T. Farmer (Blackwell, 1982). A specialist work is *The epidemiology and ecology of infectious disease agents: Proceedings of a Royal Society Discussion Meeting held on 17 and 18 February 1988 (Philosophical Transactions of the Royal Society of London B*, 1988, **321**, 327–607). Abstracts of current research are published in the *CDC Epidemic Intelligence Service Annual Conference.*

Surveillance and regular reporting of the incidence in the community is central to its control. Many countries issue weekly bulletins giving statistics and documenting current outbreaks. The PHLS Communicable Disease Surveillance Centre (CDSC) produces *Communicable Disease Report (CDR)* for England and Wales and the Scottish Home and Health Department issues *Communicable Diseases, Scotland.* Quarterly updatings from both are published in *Journal of Public Health Medicine. On the State of the Public Health: the Annual Report of the Chief Medical Officer of the DoH* contains brief reports on important infections. Statistics are published quarterly by the Office of Population Censuses and Surveys as *OPCS Monitor Series MB2: Infectious Diseases* and cumulated annually by the OPCS and CDSC as *Communicable Disease Statistics (OPCS Series MB2*, HMSO). In the U.S., *Morbidity and Mortality Weekly Report (MMWR)* is issued by CDC. It includes annual surveillance reports on many infections. WHO publishes *Weekly Epidemiological Record (WER)* highlighting incidents from all countries and *World Health Statistics Annual*. N.G. Becker's *Analysis of infectious disease data* (Chapman and Hall, 1989) is a guide to the statistical treatment of data.

Immunity and immunization

The nature of infection and immunity is covered in most works on infectious diseases and in the major microbiological texts. Specialist books are *The pathogenesis of infectious disease*, by C.A. Mims (3rd edn., Academic Press, 1987), J.P. Kreier and R.F. Mortensen's *Infection, resistance and immunity* (Harper and Row, 1990) and *Genetics of resistance to bacterial and parasitic infection*, edited by D. Wakelin and J.M. Blackwell (Taylor and Francis, 1988).

The Joint Committee on Vaccination and Immunisation prepares guidelines for the UK, published annually by the DoH as *Immunisation against infectious disease* (HMSO). WHO issues *International travel and health: vaccination requirements and health advice* annually. A useful general text on immunization is G. Dick's *Practical immunization* (MTP Press, 1986) and for paediatrics there is *British Paediatric Association manual of infections and immunizations in children*, edited by A. Nicoll and P. Rudd (Oxford University Press, 1989). All aspects of vaccination including development and production are covered in S.A. Plotkin and E.A. Mortimer's *Vaccines* (W.B. Saunders, 1988).

Antimicrobial therapy

The final volume of the *CRC handbook of microbiology* covers antibiotics (Vol. 9A, 1988) and antivirals (Vol. 9B, 1988). *The use of antibiotics: a comprehensive review with clinical emphasis*, by A. Kucers and N.McK. Bennett (4th edn., Heinemann Medical, 1987) is the standard clinical manual and D. Greenwood has edited a useful student text, *Antimicrobial chemotherapy* (2nd edn., Oxford University Press, 1989). The mechanism of antibiotic action is considered in T.J. Franklin and G.A. Snow's *Biochemistry of antimicrobial action* (Chapman and Hall, 1989). Specifically on antivirals there are J.S. Oxford and B. Öberg's *Conquest of viral diseases: a topical review of drugs and vaccines* (Elsevier, 1985) and *Antiviral drugs: basic and therapeutic aspects*, edited by R. Calio and G. Nistico (Pythagora Press, 1989).

Methods and documentation of sensitivity testing can be found in *Antibiotics in laboratory medicine*, edited by V. Lorian (2nd edn., Williams and Wilkins, 1986). The drug resistance problem is covered in *Microbial resistance to drugs*, a collection of articles on current research topics, edited by L.E. Bryan (Springer, 1989), A.D. Russell and I. Chopra's *Understanding bacterial action and resistance* (Ellis Horwood, 1990) and *Antibiotic resistance in bacteria*, edited by N. Datta (Churchill Livingstone, 1984, reprinted from *British Medical Bulletin*, 1984, **40**, 1–111). *Program and abstracts of the Interscience Conference on Antimicrobial Agents and Chemotherapy*, published by the ASM, contains hundreds of abstracts summarising up-to-date research from a large annual meeting.

AIDS and HIV

The acquired immunodeficiency syndrome (AIDS) was recognized as a distinct pathological condition in 1981. In 1983 Gallo in the USA proposed that AIDS was caused by a retrovirus, a variant of HTLV-I or II, subsequently called human T-lymphotropic virus type III (HTLV-III). Shortly afterwards Montagnier and his co-workers in Paris reported discovery of a new retrovirus, not closely related to HTLV-I or II, afterwards named lymphadenopathy-associated virus (LAV). Although the controversy over retrovirus characterization and the causative agent continued between these two groups of workers, the generic term human immunodeficiency virus (HIV), recommended by the international nomenclature committee, was widely adopted during 1986–1987. An effective blood test for antibodies to HTLV-III/LAV was announced in 1984. During the mid-1980s as the extent of the AIDS epidemic and its worldwide implications became apparent, increasing research efforts were made with a consequent explosion of published information. In a chapter such as this it is only possible to provide a brief outline of the principal available sources. For more detailed information the reader is referred to the article by Roberts, Shepherd and Wade (1987). This remains useful as the major bibliographic tools had begun publication by the time it was written and are described. It also details search terms to be used to overcome the problems of complex retrovirus nomenclature and of tracing relevant case literature published before the syndrome was characterized. In this chapter, specialist journals have been listed, and secondary sources of information discussed in the retrospective searching and current-awareness sections. This section covers some representative texts, reports and conference proceedings for the scientific and clinical audience. It should be remembered that, as with all specialist topics, much of the important information is published in the major primary general journals and texts.

As introductions to the subject *AIDS: the acquired immune deficiency syndrome*, by V.G. Daniels (2nd edn., MTP, 1987), *ABC of AIDS* reprints of articles from *BMJ* edited by M.W. Adler (*BMJ*, 1987) and the more specialized *The biology of AIDS*, by H. Fan, R.F. Conner and L.P. Villarreal (Jones and Bartlett, 1989) are useful. The October 1988 issue of *Scientific American*, reprinted as *The science of AIDS: readings from Scientific American magazine* (Freeman, 1989), is good background material and has exceptional diagrams and representations of HIV. For historical background there are some useful collections of articles from journals containing the first reports: *AIDS: epidemiological and clinical studies* (Massachusetts Medical Society, 1987) reprinted from issues of *New England Journal of Medicine* 1981–1987, *AIDS: papers from Science, 1982–1985*, edited by R. Kulstad (American Association for the Advancement of Science, 1986) and *Reports on AIDS published in the Morbidity and Mortality Weekly Report, June 1981 through May 1986* (CDC, 1986), which contains 90 reports.

Good general clinical texts are *AIDS: etiology, diagnosis, treatment and prevention*, edited by V.T. DeVita, S. Hellman and S.A. Rosenberg (2nd edn., Lippincott, 1988), *The medical management of AIDS*, edited by M.A. Sande and P.A. Volberding (Saunders, 1988) and *AIDS: pathogenesis and treatment*, edited by J.A. Levy (Dekker, 1989). Atlases are C.F. Farthing, S.E. Brown and R.C.D. Staughton's *A colour atlas of AIDS and HIV disease* (2nd edn., Wolfe Medical, 1988) and *A colour atlas of AIDS in the tropics*, by M.A. Ansary, S.K. Hira, A.C. Bayley, C. Chintu and S.L. Nyaywa (Wolfe Medical, 1989).

Laboratory methods are discussed in *Human immunodeficiency virus infection: laboratory detection and confirmation*, edited by P.D. Swenson (American Health Consultants, 1989). Means of containing the virus are given in *Guidelines on sterilization and disinfection methods effective against HIV* (2nd edn., WHO AIDS Series No. 2, 1989). HIV-related infections are covered in the comprehensive *AIDS and infections of homosexual men*, edited by P. Ma and D. Armstrong (2nd edn., Butterworth, 1989), *Opportunistic infections in patients with the acquired immunodeficiency syndrome*, edited by G. Leoung and J. Mills (Dekker, 1989) and R. Lechtenberg and J.H. Sher's *AIDS in the nervous system* (Churchill Livingstone, 1988). On therapy M. Youle, J. Clarbour, P. Wade and C. Farthing have written *AIDS: therapeutics in HIV disease* (Churchill Livingstone, 1988).

Epidemiology and transmission are discussed in *The epidemiology of AIDS: expression, occurrence, and control of human immunodeficiency virus type 1 infection*, edited by R.A. Kaslow and D.P. Francis (Oxford University Press, 1989). Specific aspects of transmission are considered further in *AIDS, sexual behavior and intravenous drug use*, edited by C.P. Turner, H.G. Miller and L.E. Moses (National Academy Press, 1989) and *AIDS and drug misuse. Part 1. Report by the Advisory Council on the Misuse of Drugs* from the former DHSS (HMSO, 1988). A good introduction to the problem of AIDS in Africa is *AIDS and the Third World* (3rd edn., Panos Publications, 1988) from the Panos Institute, a body which has produced several reports in this field. There has been much discussion on the problem of accurately predicting the incidence of AIDS. It received scholarly consideration at a Royal Society meeting the proceedings of which were edited by D.R. Cox, R.M. Anderson and H.C. Hillier and published as epidemiological and statistical aspects of the AIDS epidemic in *Philosophical Transactions of the Royal Society of London B*, 1989, **325**, 37–187. Actual predictions for the UK are given in the DoH's *Short-term prediction of HIV infection and AIDS in England and Wales: Report of a Working Group* (HMSO, 1988), which is known as the 'Cox Report' after the chairman, and *Acquired immune deficiency syndrome in England and Wales to end 1993: Projections using Data to end September 1989* published by the PHLS CDSC in 1990. Theoretical consideration of statistical methods is given in *Statistical analysis and mathematical modelling of AIDS*, edited by J.C. Jager and E.J. Ruitenberg (Oxford University Press, 1988). Actual statistics are published in the surveillance bulletins listed in the previous section under epidemiology and surveillance.

The issues of confidentiality and testing for HIV and of care of the infected individual have given rise to consideration of ethical and health policy matters. The BMA's Foundation for AIDS has produced guidelines for UK doctors in *HIV infection and AIDS: ethical considerations for the medical profession* (BMA, 1988). A U.S. view is given in *AIDS: the emerging ethical dilemmas*, edited by C. Levine and J. Bermel (Hastings Centre, 1985). Policy issues are covered in *Confronting AIDS: directions for public health, health care and research* from the Institute of Medicine and National Academy of Sciences of the USA (National Academy Press, 1986) and *AIDS: impact on public health and policy. An international forum*, edited by R.F. Hummel *et al.* (Plenum Press, 1987).

Many official guidelines have been produced by government departments, notably the DoH, mostly during the mid-1980s. The principal document for all those working with the virus or with people infected with it is *LAV/HTLV III: the causative agent of AIDS and related conditions. Revised guidelines. June 1986* prepared by the Advisory Committee on Dangerous Pathogens (DHSS, 1986). WHO has two series dedicated to the topic: *WHO AIDS series* and, on the global programme on AIDS, *WHO working documents GPA series*.

Much of the primary research information has been disclosed at conferences. An increasingly large international conference on AIDS has been held annually since 1985. Since the third conference the proceedings have only been available to delegates as Programme and Abstracts volumes. The first was published as an issue of *Annals of Internal Medicine*, 1985, **103**(5) and the second as an issue of *Annales de l'Institut Pasteur, Virologie*, 1987, **138**(1). A.F. Fleming, M. Carballo, D.W. Fitzsimons, M.R. Bailey and J. Mann have edited *The global impact of AIDS: Proceedings of the First International Conference on the Global Impact of AIDS* held in London in 1988 (Alan R. Liss, 1988). A meeting which brought together many UK workers was edited by P. Jones as *Proceedings of the AIDS Conference 1986, Newcastle on Tyne, UK* (Intercept, 1986). A list of research currently in progress is published annually by the Medical Research Council as *AIDS Research*.

As a means of compiling information in a subject specialist field the COMPACT LIBRARY: AIDS DATABASE produced by the Massachusetts Medical Society and available on CD-ROM from Microinfo is a major development in information provision. It contains both primary and secondary sources namely: the 'AIDS Knowledge Base', an electronic textbook prepared by physicians from San Francisco General Hospital and others; the full text of AIDS-related articles from eight leading journals; AIDSLINE, a file of all relevant references from MEDLINE and the Bureau of Hygiene and Tropical Diseases' AIDS DATABASE. It has been received by users with enthusiasm.

History

The first comprehensive account is W. Bulloch's *The history of bacteriology* (Oxford University Press, 1938, reprinted 1960). It has biographical notes and an extensive bibliography and it remains the first point of reference. Bulloch's work covers the subject up to 1900 and the story is then continued in W.D. Foster's *A history of medical bacteriology and immunology* (Heinemann, 1970). *The development of microbiology*, by P. Collard (Cambridge University Press, 1976) is a concise account with histories of topics such as media and sterilization. *Milestones in microbiology*, edited by T.D. Brock (Prentice Hall, 1961, reprinted by ASM, 1975) is an anthology of classic papers, including first descriptions of the Petri dish, the Gram stain and Koch's postulates.

The standard work for virology is *An introduction to the history of virology*, by A.P. Waterson and L. Wilkinson (Cambridge University Press, 1978) which has biographical notes. *The virus: a history of the concept*, by S.S. Hughes (Heinemann, 1977) is a scholarly account of the development of the idea of the virus. An interesting approach is taken in *Portraits of viruses: a history of virology*, edited by F. Fenner and A. Gibbs (Karger, 1988), a series of articles on the history of a virus or group of viruses, each written by an expert and originally published in *Intervirology*. Mycology is covered by a noted authority, C.G. Ainsworth, in his *Introduction to the history of medical and veterinary mycology* (Cambridge University Press, 1986).

Outbreaks of infections were recorded and their causes discussed long before the science of microbiology evolved. C. Creighton's classic *A history of epidemics in Britain* (2 vols, Cambridge University Press, 1891, 1894, reprinted with additional bibliography, Frank Cass, 1965) documents recorded epidemics since A.D. 664. The most recent in a long line of histories is *Plagues and poxes: the rise and fall of epidemic disease* by A.J. Bollet (Demos Publications, 1987). Classics on the practice of epidemiology are M. Greenwood's *Epidemics and crowd diseases* (Williams and Norgate, 1935), which bases the teaching of epidemiology on historical study, and *Epidemiology in country practice* by W.N. Pickles (Wright, 1939), which records individual surveillance in rural Yorkshire in the 1920s and 1930s. Developments in treatment are covered in P.E. Baldry's *The battle against the bacteria—a fresh look* (Cambridge University Press, 1976) and *Infectious diseases: prevention and treatment in the nineteenth and twentieth centuries*, by W.W. Spinks (Dawson, 1978). On vaccination are two books by H.J. Parish published by Livingstone: the scholarly *A history of immunization* (1965) and *Victory with vaccines* (1968), more suitable for the lay reader.

References

Roberts, S., Shepherd, L. and Wade, J. (1987) The scientific and clinical literature of AIDS: development, bibliographic control and retrieval. *Health Libraries Review*,4, 197–218.

Whyte, B.H. (1984) –Medical microbiology. In *Information sources in the medical sciences*, ed. L.T. Morton and S. Godbolt, 3rd edn., pp. 250–280. London: Butterworths.

CHAPTER FOURTEEN

Immunology and transplantation

P. B. MORGAN

Immunology has been described as an eclectic science. More, perhaps, than any other discipline, it typifies modern medicine both by the manner in which it draws on and synthesizes progress in many areas of research, and by its pervasive influence on medical practice through the subsequent application of immunologically-based techniques. During the last 30 years it has moved to centre stage as a science that impinges on almost all areas of medicine, playing a major role in most of the disciplines, bridging the divisions among the traditional specialties, and between the research laboratory and the clinical environment. As a result, while its literature is plentiful and continues to proliferate, it is also very widely scattered. No short review of the subject such as this can do justice to all the material that is available, and the reader should bear in mind that much valuable information can be obtained from sources which at first sight may have little explicit relevance to immunology.

It is tempting to regard immunology as an essentially post-war science, harnessing the insights and techniques provided by the new discipline of molecular biology to give medicine a better understanding of the processes through which the body overcomes, tolerates, or succumbs to disease. This view, while giving well-deserved credit to the enormous advances in immunology witnessed during the last three decades, should not be allowed to obscure the fact that immunology can claim an active history of more than a century. Medical science had stumbled towards a theory of immunity through centuries of popular medical traditions and then, on a more scientific basis, through the series of experiments during the eighteenth century that culminated in Edward Jenner's studies on smallpox vaccination. But the breakthrough came in the 1880s and the following two decades, when immunology grew out of bacteriological research as a distinct science. Louis Pasteur, with his pioneering studies on the prevention of disease, provided a lead for others like Robert Koch to follow. Rival hypotheses on the nature of the immune response were developed, amid high controversy, by Elie Metchnikoff and Paul Ehrlich.

While these early years saw a spectacular surge of interest, debate and controversy regarding theories of immunity, the following period up to the 1940s was one of less dramatic progress. The theories and their practical applications failed to realize early expectations, in spite of some successes in developing vaccines, and the emphasis shifted for a time from immunopathological to immunochemical research. The dominant figure of this era, consolidating the earlier achievements, was Karl Landsteiner. In the immediate post-war decades, further important landmarks were established as the discipline entered another phase, progressing under MacFarlane Burnet's leadership from an immunochemical to an immunobiological science. At this time, too, Peter Medawar's work on transplantation immunology laid the foundations for the eventual development of successful transplantation techniques. The emergence of molecular biology saw immunology undergoing a further transformation, with cellular immunology — the principal theme of the 1960s and 1970s — most recently giving way to molecular immunology. In the mid-1970s, a further milestone was passed, with the development by Georges Köhler and Cesar Milstein of monoclonal antibodies and the introduction of hybridoma technology.

Bibliographical and current-awareness guides

Because the literature is so scattered it follows that, while sources devoted to specific aspects of immunology and transplantation are indeed available, the immunologist must also be prepared to make extensive use of the more general biomedical indexes, abstracts, and current-awareness services: in casting their net more widely, such guides can encompass a range of literature containing relevant material that might otherwise escape notice. A few general sources are briefly mentioned below: for further information on these and other such sources, see Chapters 3 and 5.

The subject of immunological information is treated much more thoroughly than is possible here in *Immunology: an information profile*, by R. and D. Nicholas (Mansell, 1985): this detailed and wide-ranging study is particularly valuable for its account of the information sources

— professional organizations, conferences, and specialist forms of publication like trade catalogues — that exist alongside the more familiar core literature of books and journals.

R. Nicholas is also the author of *Hybridoma technology: an annotated listing of key papers 1975–1985* (Mansell, 1986), while another specialist bibliography of journal articles is *Mind and immunity: behavioural immunology: an annotated bibliography 1976–1982*, edited by S.E. Locke and M. Hornig-Rohan (Praeger, 1983).

A unique sidelight on immunological literature is provided by *The form of information in science: analysis of an immunology sublanguage*, by Z. Harris *et al.* (*Boston Studies in the Philosophy of Science*, Vol. 104, Kluwer Academic, 1989), in which the literature of 1940–65 on the cellular source of antibody is listed and subjected to a linguistic analysis, with the aim of developing a formal tool that can be applied to the conceptual analysis of science.

History

General historical sources are dealt with in detail in Chapter 24, but a few publications merit special mention here. *Morton's Medical bibliography* (Garrison and Morton) 5th edn., edited by Jeremy M. Norman (Gower, 1991) is 'an annotated check-list of texts illustrating the history of medicine', including both books and journal articles: in particular, it has sections devoted to 'Infection, immunology, and serology'; 'Allergy and anaphylaxis'; and — for transplantation — 'Surgery: plastic and reconstructive surgery'. J. Klein's *Immunology: the science of self-nonself discrimination* (Wiley, 1982) includes a bibliography of 'The 100 classic papers', and *A history of immunology*, by A.M. Silverstein (Academic Press, 1989) also has a useful bibliography of seminal publications.

Two periodicals, the *Bibliography of the History of Medicine*, and *Current Work in the History of Medicine: an International Bibliography*, cover both books and journal literature and permit searches of immunological topics by subject heading.

General biomedical coverage

The general bibliographical periodicals all offer some form of subject indexing that enables the literature of immunology and transplantation to be identified. The most relevant titles include *Biological Abstracts* and *Biological Abstracts RRM (Reports, Reviews, Meetings)*; *Current Contents: Life Sciences* for immunology and *Current Contents: Clinical Medicine* for transplantation; *Index Medicus*; and the *Science Citation Index*. The proportion of coverage given to immunology varies slightly, but *Index Medicus* is fairly typical: of the 3500 journals it indexes, about 120 are predominantly immunological.

Specific immunological coverage

The following list outlines publications that are restricted in scope to immunology and related subjects.

> *AIDS* (London). Each monthly issue includes a 'Bibliography of the current world literature' drawn from over 250 journals.
>
> *AIDS Bibliography*. Monthly, from the National Library of Medicine, covering journals, books, and audiovisual materials.
>
> *Allergy*. Eight issues a year each include 'Selected Abstracts' from other journals in related fields.
>
> *Annals of Allergy*. Each monthly issue includes a 'Journal Club' section listing references to recent articles on allergy and immunology selected from about 30 major journals, together with a short test based on these articles.
>
> *ATIN: AIDS Targeted Information Newsletter*. Monthly, supplying a compendium of research articles selected from more than 100 journals.
>
> *BIOSIS/CAS Selects*. A series of bi-weekly publications, including *Allergy and Antiallergy*; *Cancer Immunology*; *Immunochemical Methods*; *Interferon*; *Monoclonal Antibodies*; and *Transplantation*.
>
> *Current Advances in Immunology*. One of the monthly *Current Awareness in Biological Sciences* series, covering journal articles from about 3000 titles.
>
> *Current AIDS Literature*. Monthly, containing citations, most with brief abstracts, of articles published in 1400 journals.
>
> *Current Opinion in Immunology*. Bimonthly, containing review articles on chosen topics with annotated lists of references, as well as a bibliography of world literature covering 80 journals.
>
> *Excerpta Medica: Section 26 — Immunology, Serology and Transplantation*. 30 issues a year, containing abstracts. (Other useful sections, published at varying frequencies, are: *13 — Dermatology and Venereology*; *25 — Hematology*; and *54 — AIDS: Acquired Immune Deficiency Syndrome*.)
>
> *ICRDB Cancergrams*. Among the large number of titles in this series published by the United States International Cancer Research Data Bank are: *Clinical Cancer Immunology and Biological Therapy*; *Immunobiology and Cancer* (issued in various subsections); and *Viral Immunology*.
>
> *Immunology Abstracts*. Monthly, drawn from 5000 source journals scanned for the publisher's database.

Journal of Acquired Immune Deficiency Syndromes. Each bimonthly issue includes a citation index of AIDS literature.
Leeds University Oncology Information Service. Among the monthly titles published in this current awareness series are *AIDS Information*, and *Immunologic Aspects of Cancer.*
Sheffield University Biomedical Information Service (SUBIS). Various titles are published, usually monthly, in this current awareness series for researchers. They include *Antigen–Antibody Reactions; Autoimmune Immunohistochemistry; Complement; Immunologic Receptors; Immunoparasitology; Killer Cells and Cytotoxicity; Leucocytes; Lymphocytes; Lymphokines; Macrophages; Monoclonal Antibodies; Neoplasm Immunology; Phagocytes; Renal Transplantation and Dialysis;* and *Transplantation Immunology.*
Virology and AIDS Abstracts. Monthly, from the same stable as *Immunology Abstracts.*
Zentralblatt für Bakteriologie, Mikrobiologie und Hygiene. 35 issues a year. Abstracts, including a significant number on immunology, in English, German and French.

Forthcoming meetings

Notices of meetings are often published in the main immunological journals, and especially in the official journals of sponsoring organizations. To supplement these sources there is the *CIOMS Calendar of Congresses of Medical Sciences* (Council for International Organizations of Medical Sciences) which is annual and very comprehensive.

Rapid communications

While many journals make some provision for the prompt publication of short reports on research in progress, a few are dedicated to the rapid publication of papers, utilizing camera-ready copy, concentrating on brief communications, and reducing the role of referees. *Immunological Investigations* (bimonthly), and the monthly *Immunology Letters* (official journal of the European Federation of Immunological Societies) are both important examples of this genre. Another group of publications contribute to the task of keeping immunologists up to date with recent developments by adopting a news-orientated approach. They include two monthly titles, *Clinical Immunology Newsletter* and *Immunology Today*, both of which concentrate on topical items. The latter, which also contains some review articles, is available in a special library edition that includes a cumulated end-of-year compendium.

Periodicals

Mainstream immunology titles are already numerous, and continue to multiply: *Ulrich's International periodicals directory* lists over 120 titles under 'Allergology and Immunology', of which about 50 started during the 1980s. To these must be added, not only the specialized abstracts and indexes already discussed, but also some interdisciplinary journals that may be assigned primarily to other fields such as microbiology, communicable diseases, pathology and surgery.

History

While there are no journals devoted solely or in large part to the history of immunology and transplantation, several — notably the *Bulletin of the History of Medicine*, the *Journal of the History of Medicine and Allied Sciences*, and *Medical History* — include relevant material from time to time.

More often, though, articles on historical topics will be found in the broad range of immunological journals, as illustrated by the following selection of general articles:

Billingham, R.E. *et al.* (1984) Reproductive immunology: past, present, and future. *Perspectives in Biology and Medicine*, **27**, 259–275.
Gowans, J.L. *et al.* (1989) Sir Peter Medawar Memorial Symposium, London 1988. *Immunology Letters*, **21**, 1–99 [devoted largely to a retrospect of transplantation immunology].
Kabat, E.A. (1988) Before and after. *Annual Review of Immunology*, **6**, 1–24.
Talmage, D.W. (1988) A century of progress: beyond molecular biology. *Journal of Immunology*, **141** (7, Supplement), S5–S16.

General immunology

The *Journal of Immunology*, official journal of the American Association of Immunologists, is the pre-eminent journal in the subject. It was founded in 1916 as the first English-language journal dedicated to immunology, and dominates the medium as the most cited source of articles on immunological research.

In close attendance are several other major and long-established titles. The *Journal of Experimental Medicine* (1896–) is now, despite its non-specific name devoted almost exclusively to immunological research. *Immunobiology* (first published in 1909 as *Zeitschrift für Immunitätsforschung*, the earliest journal dedicated to immunology) also has a strong research bias, and contains both text and summaries in English. Two even more venerable European journals both originated in microbiology before expanding to embrace immunology: *Medical Microbiology and Immunology* started life in 1886 as *Zeitschrift für Hygiene und Infektionskrankheiten*, and now contains articles in English, German and French; and *Research in Immunology*, now published mainly in English, was established one year later, in 1887, as *Annales de l'Institut Pasteur*.

In recent decades other influential titles devoted to general aspects of immunology have appeared. *Clinical and Experimental Immunology*, one of two journals issued by the British Society for Immunology, has a wide-ranging interest in immunological aspects of the pathogenesis and diagnosis of disease, and also encompasses studies of the normal immune system. The BSI's other and older publication, *Immunology*, is even more general in scope, and includes occasional review articles, both solicited and unsolicited, and book reviews. *Clinical Immunology and Immunopathology* publishes papers, including reviews, on the molecular and cellular basis of immunological disease. These topics are one of the main concerns of *Pathobiology* (a recently-launched merger between *Pathology and Immunopathology* and *Experimental Cell Biology*) which devotes occasional complete issues to a single topic. The *Journal of Experimental Pathology* combines both basic and clinical disciplines in the study of disease and host defence mechanisms. Viewing a similar subject area from a specific angle, *Aging: Immunology and Infectious Disease* presents papers on host defence mechanisms as they relate to the ageing process. *Molecular Immunology* contains papers in a variety of formats, with research reports predominating.

A newcomer to the field, *International Immunology*, is concerned mainly with experimental and theoretical studies. Despite its title, the *Scandinavian Journal of Immunology* is fully international, publishing both research papers and review articles on cellular and molecular immunology; more substantial reviews are issued separately as supplements. The official journal of the Australian Society for Immunology, *Immunology and Cell Biology*, is also international and similarly broad in its coverage. The *Journal of Clinical Immunology*, as its name suggests, covers all aspects of the application of clinical immunology to medical practice.

The *European Journal of Immunology* deals largely with experimental work and, unlike most of the foregoing titles, accepts methodological studies. Papers on laboratory methods form a significant part of the content of both *Journal of Clinical and Laboratory Immunology*, and of *JMCI: Journal of Molecular and Cellular Immunology*.

Cellular mechanisms and related topics receive more attention in a further range of titles. *Cellular Immunology* covers experimental and clinical studies of cell-mediated immunity, both *in vivo* and *in vitro*. *Natural Immunity and Cell Growth Regulation* offers original research on basic cell mechanisms, cloning techniques, and the role of cells in disease. *Inflammation* deals with the cellular response to tissue damage. More general vehicles for cellular studies, such as *Cell Biology International Reports* and *Cell*, also carry papers of immunological interest.

The *Journal of Leukocyte Biology*, the Reticuloendothelial Society's official journal, deals with the lymphoreticular system; while original articles and reviews on specific aspects of thymology and related fields can be found in *Thymus*, which places particular emphasis on the rapid publication of papers. *Lymphokine Research* presents papers on laboratory studies and immunotherapeutic applications of lymphokines and monokines. *Blood*, published for the American Society of Hematology; *Blood Cells*, which devotes each issue to a particular theme; and *Blut*, which publishes articles in German, English and French, are all important sources of papers on immunohaematology. Another group of titles, notably *Immunogenetics*, the *Journal of Immunogenetics*, and *Experimental and Clinical Immunogenetics*, cater for the general field of immunogenetics.

A few journals are devoted to immunological aspects of specific body systems. *Regional Immunology* has a broad scope, publishing original articles, brief reports, and reviews on the immunology of body regions, tissues and organs. *Brain, Behaviour, and Immunity* focuses on interactions between the nervous and immune systems, and a similar field of interest is covered by the *Journal of Neuroimmunology*.

The immunology of reproduction has its own specialist journals, as represented by the *Journal of Reproductive Immunology* (published for the International Society for Immunology of Reproduction), the *American Journal of Reproductive Immunology*, and *Immunology of Reproduction*. Further immunological papers are regularly published in *Fertility and Sterility* and the *International Journal of Fertility*.

Developmental and Comparative Immunology, published for the International Society of Developmental and Comparative Immunology, concentrates on the rapid dissemination of research into the ontogenetic and phylogenetic aspects of immune system maturation. A newcomer to this field, *Developmental Immunology*, promises to fulfil a similar role.

The interrelationships between pharmacology, toxicology and immunology are well covered by three journals, *Immunopharmacology*, the *International Journal of Immunopharmacology*, and *Immunopharmacology and Immunotoxicology*. *Toxicon*, the journal of the International Society on Toxicology, includes studies on the immunological properties of poisons.

Food and Agricultural Immunology publishes original

immunological research with food, agricultural, environmental or veterinary applications. The latter area of interest is also catered for by *Veterinary Immunology and Immunopathology*.

Two general journals which habitually publish immunological papers linking basic research and clinical practice are the American Society for Clinical Investigation's *Journal of Clinical Investigation*, which devotes one of its regular sections to infection, inflammation and immunity, and the European Society for Clinical Investigation's *European Journal of Clinical Investigation*. Even more general in scope, but the source of some of the most important immunological papers, are the major scientific journals such as *The Lancet* and the *New England Journal of Medicine* (especially for clinical topics), and *Nature* and *Science* (both strong in research papers).

Bio/Technology, published monthly, has both news coverage and research papers dealing with the commercial exploitation of living organisms, among which products such as hybridomas and vaccines figure prominently. *Biologicals*, published for the International Association of Biological Standardization, contains original articles, reviews, and patent/licence reports on all biologicals, including monoclonal antibodies and vaccines.

Allergy, hypersensitivity and auto-immunity

Although not devoted exclusively to allergy, the *Journal of Allergy and Clinical Immunology* still ranks as the oldest journal in this field, dating from 1929. Published for the American Academy of Allergy and Immunology, it includes abstracts of papers from the AAAI's annual meeting. The equivalent UK journal, published for the British Society for Allergy and Clinical Immunology, is *Clinical and Experimental Allergy*. Among other titles, *Allergy* contains original papers, reviews and book reviews, and is accompanied by occasional supplements; the *Annals of Allergy* (from the American College of Allergists) has a similar range, as does the *International Archives of Allergy and Applied Immunology*, which emphasizes work that has a direct relevance to clinical practice. *Immunität und Infektion*, which has German articles with English summaries, is concerned largely with allergy and rheumatology.

Additionally, specific aspects of hypersensitivity are featured in a number of titles. *Arthritis and Rheumatism* (issued by the American College of Rheumatology), the *Journal of Rheumatology* and *Clinical and Experimental Rheumatology* all combine experimental and clinical studies. For asthma studies there is the well-established *Journal of Asthma*, and, in paediatrics, two recent specialized titles, the *American Journal of Asthma and Allergy for Pediatricians*, and *Pediatric Asthma,*

Allergy, and Immunology. The *Journal of Autoimmunity* presents research and clinical studies in all aspects of auto-immune diseases. *Complement and Inflammation* covers research into the complement system through original papers and reviews.

Microbiological aspects, including AIDS

The relationship between immunology and microbiology epitomizes the interdisciplinary nature of much immunological activity. Reminding us of immunology's debt to the work of Pasteur and others, it continues to embrace bacteriology, virology (most recently including work on AIDS), the study of infection, epidemiology, and beyond.

APMIS: Acta Pathologica, Microbiologica et Immunologica Scandinavica, published for the Scandinavian Societies for Medical Microbiology and Pathology, is long established: it carries original research papers and has occasional supplements. *FEMS Microbiology Immunology*, a more recent arrival on the scene, includes both original articles and reviews on the host response to infection. It is published by the Federation of European Microbiological Societies as one section, available separately, of the full set of *FEMS Microbiology* titles.

Another corporate publication is *Infection and Immunity*, from the American Society for Microbiology, which includes the immunology of microbial infection as one of its areas of interest. Many of the laboratory and clinical studies on microbiology and infection found in the *Journal of Infectious Diseases* have an immunological theme. *Comparative Immunology, Microbiology and Infectious Diseases* takes a broader view that extends to both medical and veterinary practice, and it also includes a 'New Patents' section listing U.S. patents and patent applications filed under the Patent Co-operation Treaty. *Parasite Immunology* is concerned with research into immunopathological reactions to parasitic infections, while their molecular immunology is one of the fields covered both by *Molecular and Biochemical Parasitology* and by *Experimental Parasitology*.

Antiviral Research contains original and review articles, with the emphasis very much on the former, and includes investigations into the immune response to viral infections and the development of antiviral vaccines, in man and animals. *Viral Immunology* extends its coverage of the same field to include both research and clinical practice, but with a higher proportion of original and review articles. The *Journal of Interferon Research*, published for the International Society for Interferon Research, presents papers on experimental studies and clinical applications. Other more general virological journals, such as *Archives of Virology*, *Virus Research*, the *Journal of Medical Virology* and the *Journal of Virology* (from the American Society for

Microbiology) also regularly contain papers reporting research into immunological aspects. Research, development and use of human and veterinary vaccines are specifically covered by *Vaccine*, which also contains a listing of patent applications.

AIDS research includes a significant body of work on its immunological aspects. Because of the urgency with which AIDS research is being conducted, much of the publishing effort is directed towards rapid dissemination of results, current-awareness surveys, and bibliographical lists. Various features are combined in *AIDS* (London) which carries original papers, a bibliography and statistics. *AIDS Research and Human Retroviruses* confines itself to rapid publication of full and short research communications. The clinical aspects are dealt with more fully in *AIDS Patient Care*. In a more specific field, *Pediatric AIDS and HIV Infection: Fetus to Adolescent* pulls together different specialist interests with the rapid publication of original studies and reviews.

Transplantation

The story behind the advent of successful transplant programmes is not simply one of improved techniques in operative surgery, vital though these have been. It has also depended crucially on progress in controlling graft-versus-host reactions. Transplantation literature reflects these two complementary strands.

The Transplantation Society's journal, *Transplantation*, devotes a substantial part of its contents — original research, reviews, and brief communications — to immunological issues. *Transplantation Proceedings*, sponsored by the same society with a dozen other national and international societies devoted to transplantation, is a vehicle for collections of papers from various meetings. Its scope is very broad, but immunological aspects are well represented. The European Society for Organ Transplantation, in its official publication *Transplant International*, presents both experimental and clinical studies reflecting all the specialties involved in organ transplantation. Experimental studies feature less prominently in *Clinical Transplantation*: here, along with immunological studies, there is also a considerable emphasis on surgical and pathological aspects of clinical practice.

A few journals relating to transplantation of particular organs and cells are also available. An example is *Nephrology, Dialysis, Transplantation*: this title, a continuation of one of the first journals in the field (since the surgical technique of kidney grafts was one of the earliest successes), carries a limited number of immunological studies alongside other papers on renal medicine and surgery. The *Journal of Heart Transplantation*, published for the International Society for Heart

Transplantation, likewise includes papers on both immunological and other aspects of its subject. In *Bone Marrow Transplantation*, considerable weight is attached to experimental studies in both man and animals. *Vox Sanguinis*, published for the International Society of Blood Transfusion, *Transfusion*, the journal of the American Association of Blood Banks and *Transfusion Science* (in which single issues may be monothematic), all include original research and reviews on immunohaematology, transfusion and transplantation.

Other papers on transplantation immunology are to be found in many of the general immunology journals already mentioned in other sections above, and journals devoted to haematology are important additional sources for material on blood transfusion and bone marrow transplantation.

Investigative techniques

Of titles devoted entirely to methodology, the most important is the *Journal of Immunological Methods*, which appears 20 times a year and includes studies of original research, invited reviews, and book reviews. A more recent rival is *Laboratory Immunology*, published twice yearly for the (American) Association of Medical Laboratory Immunologists. Other methodological journals are the *Journal of Immunoassay* and the Ligand Clinical Assay Society's *Journal of Clinical Immunoassay*. *Diagnostic and Clinical Immunology* presents studies on the applications of laboratory techniques and methodologies for diagnostic purposes. A more specific area of diagnostic techniques is covered by *Serodiagnosis and Immunotherapy in Infectious Disease*. The *Journal of Virological Methods* includes techniques for studying the immune response to viruses. *Human Immunology*, from the American Society for Histocompatibility and Immunogenetics, and *Tissue Antigens* are both concerned primarily with histocompatibility testing.

An important source of literature on immunochemical techniques lies in the various journals devoted to clinical biochemistry. Notable among these are two bimonthly titles, the *Annals of Clinical Biochemistry* (published for the Association of Clinical Biochemists), and the Canadian-based *Clinical Biochemistry*, together with the fortnightly *Clinica Chimica Acta*.

Hybridomas and cancer immunology

The development of monoclonal antibodies has opened up new areas of preventive. diagnostic and therapeutic medicine. *Hybridoma* and *Human Antibodies and Hybridomas* both deal with a broad spectrum of experimental research results and clinical diagnostic and therapeutic applications. The diagnostic applications are treated more specifically, through reviews and original reports, as one of the principal techniques covered by *Disease Markers*. *Immunoclones* is a periodic survey of new hybridomas and other immunoclones, produced by CERDIC (the European Centre of Documentation on Immunoclones) for the international Hybridoma Data Bank Network. Current information on sources of new hybrid cell lines is also provided in *Monoclonal Antibody News*.

Cancer Immunology, Immunotherapy covers research and clinical practice in the field of tumour–host interactions, and has extended its scope to embrace other biological response modifications, a topic also covered in more general terms by the *Journal of Biological Response Modifiers*. *Antibody, Immunoconjugates, and Radiopharmaceuticals* takes a holistic approach, through original articles and reviews, to the diagnosis and treatment of cancer. Cancer immunology also features extensively in the large body of general cancer journals, and some — such as *Cancer*, published for the American Cancer Society, and *Cancer Research*, the journal of the American Association for Cancer Research — devote specific sections of their contents to papers with an immunological theme.

Reviews and series

The review format provides a commentary on the recent literature, with summaries and critical evaluations of what has already appeared in original articles. The need for such a service is particularly evident in immunology, not only because there are so many mainstream immunological journals, but also because, as we have seen, much of the relevant literature is scattered among journals devoted to other specialties. While many immunological journals include some reviews either regularly or as occasional features, a number of titles publish little else. They fall broadly into two categories: those published as journals, appearing at regular intervals more than once a year; and those that appear annually or less often, either regularly or irregularly, in edited series.

Review journals

Most review journals devote individual issues to single topics, usually with a guest editor and a number of invited contributors. General immunology is served by *Immunological Reviews* (formerly *Transplantation Reviews*), *Immunology and Allergy Clinics of North America*, and *International Reviews of Immunology*. *Immunologic Research: a Selective Reference to Current Research and Practice* presents a synthesis of scientific results with a strong review element. Reviews of more specific fields are available from *Clinical Reviews in Allergy* and *Springer Seminars in Immunopathology*.

Other titles dispense with the single-topic approach and instead devote each issue to papers on a wide variety of subjects. *Critical Reviews in Immunology* is an important example of this genre, and its stable mates *Critical Reviews in Microbiology* and *Critical Reviews in Oncology/Hematology* also contain papers with an immunological slant. Another journal covering the latter subject is *Hematology Reviews and Communications* (which, though not restricted to reviews, is better suited to them than to rapid communications because of its irregular publication schedule). Regular papers in the field of immunohaematology are also included in *Blood Reviews*. *Immunodeficiency Reviews* focuses on another more specific area of interest.

Reviews and monographic series

The distinction between, on the one hand, edited review series with monothematic volumes and, on the other, numbered series of monographs with a strong review element, is fairly blurred. Sometimes the two distinct forms occur within the same series title. Although the range of titles is considerable, many appear to survive for only a few volumes, or are so unpredictable and infrequent that their status as serials is open to question.

Among the more reliable and influential titles in the review series category, *Advances in Immunology*, edited by F.J. Dixon (Academic Press), is irregular, usually with several volumes a year: volumes 44–47 were published in 1989. Each volume, with its own editor, has about six reviews of specific topics by various authors. The *Annual Review of Immunology*, edited by W.E. Paul *et al.* (Annual Reviews), contains up to 30 reviews of recent literature and current developments, and also provides both a cumulative index to all volumes in the series, and a list of relevant articles that have appeared in volumes of companion titles such as the *Annual Review of Cell Biology* and the *Annual Review of Microbiology* — a reminder, if more were needed, of the eclectic process required when studying the literature of immunology. *The Year in Immunology*, edited by J.M. Cruse and R.E. Lewis Jr (Karger), provides an update on recent literature: latterly, each annual volume has taken a specific theme for its reviews.

As well as the titles that are general in scope, some series relate to narrower subject fields. *Current Topics in AIDS*, edited by M.S. Gottlieb *et al.* (Wiley), includes reviews on immunological aspects: volume 2 appeared in 1989. *Developments in Biological*

Standardization, edited by the International Association of Biological Standardization (Karger), covers aspects of applied immunology such as monoclonal antibodies and vaccines: volume 71 appeared in 1990, frequency varying from one to four volumes in a year. *Lymphokines: a Forum for Immunoregulatory Cell Products*, edited by E. Pick (Academic Press) issues two or three volumes annually, some monothematic while others contain miscellaneous papers. *Reviews on Immunoassay Technology*, edited by S.B. Pal (Macmillan), appears at least once a year (volume 3 in 1989), each issue containing about a dozen papers. *Techniques in Immunocytochemistry*, edited by G.R. Bullock and P. Petrusz (Academic Press), covers recent advances in investigative methodology, with volumes approximately biennial (volume 4 in 1989). *Transplantation Reviews* (formerly *Progress in Transplantation*), is edited by P.J. Morris and N.L. Tilney (Saunders), providing annual topical reviews in clinical transplantation and transplantation biology: volume 2 appeared in 1988.

Among those series that concentrate on monothematic volumes, *Chemical Immunology* (formerly *Progress in Immunology*), edited by K. Ishizaka *et al.* (Karger), publishes several volumes a year, with guest editors supervising important collections of reviews on specific aspects of immunological research: in 1990 it reached volume 49. *Concepts in Immunopathology*, edited by J.M. Cruse and R.E. Lewis Jr (Karger), provides topical overviews of the immunological processes in disease (volume 7 appeared in 1989). *Current Topics in Microbiology and Immunology*, edited by R.W. Compans *et al.* (Springer) has issued more than 160 volumes up to 1990 including both review volumes and conference proceedings. Another series edited for Karger by J.M. Cruse and R.E. Lewis Jr is *Contributions to Microbiology and Immunology*: an irregularly published continuation of *Bibliotheca Microbiologica*, it reflects the growing importance of immunological studies in microbiological research. The *Immunology series* (Dekker), which uses individual volume editors, reviews a wide range of topics that embrace specialties like transplantation and AIDS, and has reached volume 50. *Monographs in Allergy*, edited by L.A. Hanson and F. Shakib (Karger), issues two or three volumes a year (volume 26 in 1989) and consists mainly of conference proceedings.

Conference proceedings have their own important part to play in keeping the reader up to date with recent developments, and a number of series are devoted wholly or substantially to publishing collections of such papers. *Progress in Immunology* (Academic Press) publishes the proceedings of the International Congress of Immunology: volume 6 (1987), edited by B. Cinader and R.G. Miller, contains papers from the sixth Congress. Although not devoted exclusively to immunological topics, the prolific *Advances in Experimental Medicine and Biology*

(Plenum) is a major source of immunological material, several volumes a year carrying the papers of relevant conferences. The same is true of the *UCLA Symposia on Molecular and Cellular Biology* (Alan R. Liss).

Databases

Database versions exist for many of the abstracts, indexes and current-awareness publications listed above. They are usually available online and, in some cases, are also in CD-ROM and diskette format. Full text databases, either on their own or integrated with bibliographical files, are becoming more widely available. In 1991 the IMMUNOCLONE DATABASE (CERDIC) became available on Data-Star and several databases are already available for AIDS literature.

The databases listed below are of particular interest to immunologists. Further guidance on databases in general is provided in Chapter 5, and the quarterly *Directory of online databases* and its companion *Online database selection: a user's guide to the directory of online databases* (Cuadra/Elsevier) can also be used to obtain detailed subject analysis of most of the world's publicly accessible databases.

AIDS (Bureau of Hygiene and Tropical Diseases). A bibliographic database, corresponding in part to *Current AIDS Literature* (see above). (Hosts: BRS, Data-Star, DIMDI)

AIDS ARTICLES FROM COLLEAGUE'S COMPLETE TEXT LIBRARY. Full text articles extracted from books and journals in the Comprehensive Core Medical Library database. (Host: BRS)

AIDS KNOWLEDGE BASE. Full text articles written for the database, together with references to published AIDS literature. (Host: BRS; also available on CD-ROM)

AIDSLINE. A bibliographic database of references, most with abstracts, from MEDLINE and other National Library of Medicine databases. Corresponds to printed *AIDS Bibliography*. (Hosts: BRS; Dialog, NLM)

CURRENT AWARENESS IN BIOLOGICAL SCIENCES. The database from which *Current Advances in Immunology* is produced. (Host: ORBIT)

CURRENT OPINION IN IMMUNOLOGY. The database version of the journal with the same name. (Available on diskette only)

EMBASE. The database version of *Excerpta Medica*. (Hosts: BRS, Data-Star, Dialog, DIMDI; also available on CD-ROM)

LEUCOCYTE TYPING DATABASE IV. An electronic directory of immunoclones, employing data from workshop proceedings which are also published in book form — see the 'Hybridoma' section under 'Books', below (available on diskette only, from IRL)

LIFE SCIENCES COLLECTION. The database from which *Immunology Abstracts* and *Virology and AIDS Abstracts* are produced. (Host: Dialog; also available on CD-ROM)

MEDLINE. The database version of *Index Medicus*. (Hosts: BRS, Data-Star, Dialog, DIMDI, NLM, Télésystèmes-Questel; also available on CD-ROM)

SCISEARCH. The database version of the *Science Citation Index*. (Hosts: Data-Star, Dialog, DIMDI, ORBIT; also available on CD-ROM)

Books

The range of books on immunological and related topics is large and varied. It follows that a survey of this kind must inevitably be highly selective, doing no more than providing pointers to some of the works likely to prove useful. Multi-authored works predominate, and many of the more specialized books are based on conference proceedings.

Dictionaries

Both the *Macmillan Dictionary of immunology*, by F. Rosen *et al.* (Macmillan. 1989), and *A dictionary of immunology*, by W.J. Herbert *et al.* (3rd edn., Blackwell Scientific Publications, 1985), provide a thorough guide to immunological terminology, W.J. Halliday's *Glossary of immunological terms* (Butterworths, 1971), though somewhat dated, is still of interest as its definitions are cross-referenced to a bibliography of nearly 600 source articles. D.K. Male's *Immunology: an illustrated outline* (Churchill Livingstone, 1986) is a dual-purpose pocket-book that serves both as a dictionary of immunology and as a concise revision aid.

Basic and clinical immunology

Among the leading textbooks on the subject, I.M. Roitt's *Essential immunology* (6th edn., Blackwell Scientific Publications, 1988) is an excellent, well-illustrated and regularly revised guide. Another source that is systematically updated is *Basic and clinical immunology*, edited by D.P. Stites *et al.* (7th edn., Prentice-Hall, 1991). W.E. Paul's *Fundamental immunology* (2nd edn., Raven, 1989) is among the most substantial works on the subject. *Fundamentals of immunology and allergy*, edited by R.F. Lockey and S.C. Bukantz, and the same editors' *Principles of immunology and allergy* (both Saunders, 1987) are companion volumes: the former covers the scientific basis, while the latter demonstrates its application to the diagnosis and treatment of immunologic disorders in clinical practice.

An older work that is still noteworthy for its innovative format is *Immunology: the science of self-nonself discrimination*, by J. Klein (Wiley, 1982). Klein's later *Immunology* (Blackwell Scientific Publications, 1989) is a more conventional work that stresses the molecular mechanisms of the immune process, a subject that receives further consideration in *Molecular immunology*, edited by B.D. Hames and D.M. Glover (IRL, 1988). R.E. Langman's *The immune system: evolutionary principles ...* (Academic Press, 1989) adopts an unconventional approach, emphasizing conceptual thinking rather than the experimental basis of immunology. Experimental studies into the immune system of animals are illustrated by *The rabbit in contemporary immunological research*, edited by S. Dubiski (Longman Scientific & Technical, 1987).

Essential immunogenetics, by A.R. Williamson and M.W. Turner (Blackwell Scientific Publications, 1987) brings together a number of interdisciplinary interests. P.N. Plowman's *Haematology and immunology* (Wiley, 1987) provides a concise introduction to this topic. *Immunoglobulin genes*, edited by T. Honjo *et al.* (Academic Press, 1989) and *Immunoglobulins in health and disease*, edited by M.A.H. French *et al.* (MTP, 1986), both look at the role of immunoglobulins, while K.A. Smith has edited *Interleukin 2* (Academic Press, 1988), a review of research into lymphokines in general and IL-2 in particular. Workshop proceedings form the basis of *Natural killer cells: biology and clinical application*, edited by R.E. Schmidt (Karger, 1989). M. Sela has edited a monumental eight-volume treatise, *The antigens* (Academic Press, 1973–87) to provide an exhaustive treatment of this subject.

Among those books that concentrate on clinical applications, *Clinical aspects of immunology*, edited by P.J. Lachmann and D.K. Peters (2 vols, 4th edn., Blackwell Scientific Publications, 1982), is becoming slightly dated but still merits attention as a classic that has not yet been superseded. A more compact work is H. Chapel and M. Haeney's *Essentials of clinical immunology* (2nd edn., Blackwell Scientific Publications, 1988).

The visual element is an important feature of some works. *Understanding medical immunology*, by E.M. Kirkwood and C.J. Lewis (2nd edn., Wiley, 1989), provides a nicely-illustrated introduction to the subject, and includes a new section on AIDS. J.H.L. Playfair's *Immunology at a glance* (4th edn., Blackwell Scientific Publications, 1987) is a short diagrammatic work with accompanying text. Employing a similar approach, but relying even more heavily on a diagrammatic presentation is *The chain of immunology*, by G. Feinberg and M.A. Jackson (Blackwell Scientific Publications, 1983). *Immunology*, by I.M. Roitt *et al.* (2nd edn., Churchill Livingstone, 1989) is a more substantial, finely-illustrated text for which an accompanying slide atlas based on material in the book is also available. The most outstanding pictorial introduction is L. Nilsson's *The body victorious: the illustrated study of our immune system and other defences of the human body* (Faber, 1987), a collection of superb colour photographs and descriptive text.

For students at various levels there is a wide choice. *Introduction to clinical immunology*, by M. Haeney (Butterworths, 1985), is expanded from a series of articles that first appeared in the journal *Hospital Update*, aimed at junior doctors in training. Both postgraduate and medical students will find D.M. Weir's *Aids to immunology* (Churchill Livingstone, 1986) a useful revision text. The same author's *Immunology* (6th edn., Churchill Livingstone, 1988) is designed for the needs of undergraduates, as is the synoptic presentation of W.G. Reeves' *Lecture notes on immunology* (Blackwell Scientific Publications, 1987).

IRL, in association with the British Society for Immunology, have published a number of brief 'In Focus' student guides under the general editorship of D. Rickwood and D. Male. Individual titles include *Complement*, by S.K.A. Law and K.B.M. Reid (1988), *Immune recognition*, by M.J. Owen and J.R. Lamb (1988), *Lymphokines*, by A.S. Hamblin (1988), *Antigen-presenting cells*, by J.M. Austyn (1989), *B lymphocytes*, by G.G.B. Klaus (1990) and *The thymus*, by M. Ritter and N. Crisp (1990).

Some study texts owe their origins to specific university courses in the biological and medical sciences. Examples are B. Davey's *Immunology: a foundation text* (Open University, 1989), based on an Open University course but broadened in scope to appeal to a wider range of students; and the *Textbook of immunopharmacology*, edited by M.M. Dale and J.C. Foreman (2nd edn., Blackwell Scientific Publications, 1989), originating in an undergraduate course at the University of London.

Concise revision guides include Male's dual-purpose dictionary and revision aid, already mentioned in the dictionary section above. *Key facts in immunology*, by D.W. Scott and J.R. Dawson (Churchill Livingstone, 1985) is organized as a structured collection of factual statements rather than a continuous text. R.C. Matthews and J.P. Burnie provide an examination aid for multiple-choice questions in their *MCQ tutor: medical immunology* (Heinemann Medical, 1984). W.W. Yotis, in *Appleton and Lange's Review of microbiology and immunology* (Appleton & Lange, 1989), provides over 700 questions and answers based on U.S. examination practice.

Immunopathology

As its title suggests, S. Sell's *Immunology, immunopathology, and immunity* (4th edn., Elsevier, 1987) is divided into three parts, all broadly emphasizing the contribution of immune mechanisms to human disease. The same author's *Basic immunology: immune mechanisms in health and disease* (Elsevier, 1987) corresponds to the first section of the previous title. An even more substantial work than Sell's is *Immunological diseases*, edited by M. Samter (2 vols, 4th edn., Little, Brown, 1988). *Complement in health and disease*, edited by K. Whaley (MTP, 1987) looks at the role of complement in immune complex disease.

A number of books adopt a regional approach to immunopathology, usually combining a discussion of the underlying pathology with a review of the contribution immunodiagnostic methods can make to clinical investigations and prognosis. Those devoted to respiratory immunology include *Immunology and immunologic diseases of the lung*, edited by R.P. Daniele (Blackwell Scientific Publications, 1988). Works available on gastrointestinal medicine include *Immunopathology of the small intestine*, edited by M.N. Marsh (Wiley, 1987), and *Immunology and immunopathology of the liver and gastrointestinal tract*, edited by S.R. Targan and F. Shanahan (Igaku-Shoin, 1990). This latter work emphasizes the role of the mucosal immune system, a topic reviewed more thoroughly in *Mucosal immunity and infections at mucosal surfaces*, edited by W. Strober *et al.* (Oxford University Press, 1988).

Volume 18 of the series *Contemporary Issues in Nephrology* is devoted to *Immunopathology of renal disease*, edited by C.B. Wilson (Churchill Livingstone, 1988). Dermatological interests are discussed at considerable length in *Immunopathology of the skin*, edited by E. H. Beutner *et al.* (3rd edn., Wiley, 1987). G. Smolin and G.R. O'Connor's *Ocular immunology* (2nd edn., Little, Brown, 1986), and *Immunological aspects of oral diseases*, edited by L. Ivanyi (MTP, 1986) provide further texts on regional specialties. R. Lloyd's *Explorations in psychoneuroimmunology* (Grune and Stratton, 1987) examines the relationship between emotion and the immune system, as does *Depressive disorders and immunity*, edited by A.H. Miller (American Psychiatric Press, 1989). Research into the relationship between diet and resistance to infection is considered in *Nutrition and immunity*, edited by M.E. Gershwin *et al.* (Academic Press, 1985), and in *Nutrition and immunology*, edited by R.K. Chandra (*Contemporary Issues in Clinical Nutrition*, vol. 11, 1988, Alan R. Liss).

Allergy, hypersensitivity and auto-immunity

Allergy: an international textbook, edited by M.H. Lessof *et al.* (Wiley, 1987), and N. Mygind's *Essential allergy: an illustrated text for students and specialists* (Blackwell Scientific Publications, 1986), are both comprehensive treatments of the subject. W.F. Jackson and R. Cerio's *A colour atlas of allergy* (Wolfe Medical, 1988) is a profusely illustrated guide to allergic disorders and their management.

Allergy and asthma: new trends and approaches to therapy, edited by A.B. Kay (Blackwell Scientific Publications, 1989), and Kay's own *Allergy and inflammation* (Academic Press, 1987) concentrate on specific areas of interest. Respiratory allergies are presented visually in G.M. Cochrane and P.J. Rees' *A colour atlas of asthma* (Wolfe Medical, 1989). G.R.V. Hughes' *Connective tissue diseases* (3rd edn., Blackwell Scientific Publications, 1987) gives a thorough account of immunological considerations, while a similar area of interest is covered in depth by *Rheumatology and immunology*, by A.S. Cohen and J.C. Bennett (2nd edn., Grune and Stratton, 1986). C.W. Bierman and D.S. Pearlman review developmental aspects in *Allergic diseases from infancy to adulthood* (2nd edn., Saunders, 1988).

The auto-immune diseases are well catered for through published conference proceedings. Volume 105 in the *UCLA Symposia on Molecular and Cellular Biology* series is *Mechanisms of human hypersensitivity and autoimmunity*, edited by E.J. Goetzl (Alan R. Liss, 1989). Symposium proceedings also form the basis of *Autoimmunity and autoimmune disease* (Ciba Foundation Symposium, 129) (Wiley, 1987), while *T cell activation in health and disease: disorders of immune regulation, infection and autoimmunity*, edited by M. Feldman *et al.* (Academic Press, 1989) originated from a workshop.

Microbiological aspects, including AIDS

An authoritative survey of bacteriological issues can be found within *Topley and Wilson's Principles of bacteriology, virology and immunity*, edited by T. Parker and L.H. Collier (5 vols, 8th edn., Arnold, 1990), in which Vol. 1 edited by A.H. Linton and H.M. Dick, is concerned with *General bacteriology and immunity*. A.J.L. Macario and E. Conway de Macario have edited a multivolume treatise *Monoclonal antibodies against bacteria* (3 vols, Academic Press, 1985–6) which focuses on monoclonal antibodies in the context of a general review of bacterial immunology. *Antimicrobial agents and immunity*, edited by J. Jeljaszewicz and G. Pulverer (Academic Press, 1986) provides a mixture of reviews and research reports. Antiviral mechanisms are discussed in *Clinical aspects of interferons*, edited by M. Revel (Kluwer, 1988).

Research into the development of vaccines is covered in depth by *Vaccines*, edited by S.A. Plotkin and E.A. Mortimer (Saunders, 1988), while a collection of brief reviews first published as articles in *The Lancet* have now been collected and edited by E.R. Moxon as *Modern vaccines: current practice and new approaches* (Arnold, 1990). G. Dick's *Practical immunization* (MTP, 1986) is a concise introduction to the subject, which is dealt with in more detail in *Immunization*, edited by R.K. Root *et al.* (Churchill Livingstone, 1989). *Recent developments in prophylactic immunization*, edited by A.J. Zuckerman (Kluwer, 1989), reviews research into new vaccines.

A.G. Dalgleish and R.A. Weiss have edited *AIDS and the new viruses* (Academic Press, 1990), a collection of topical reviews for virologists and immunologists. Immunological sections are included in *AIDS: etiology, diagnosis, treatment, and prevention*, edited by V.T. DeVita *et al.* (2nd edn., Lippincott, 1988), and in *Clinical aspects of AIDS and AIDS-related complex*, edited by M. Staquet *et al.* (Oxford University Press, 1986). Immunological aspects are also extensively covered throughout the first half of *The AIDS knowledge base: a textbook on HIV disease...*, edited by P.T. Cohen *et al.* (Medical Publishing, 1990), which is the printed version of a computerized database.

Laboratory techniques

Among the general works, the *Handbook of experimental immunology*, edited by D.M. Weir *et al.* (4 vols, 4th edn., Blackwell Scientific Publications, 1986) is an acknowledged standard, while the authoritative *Manual of clinical laboratory immunology*, edited by N.R. Rose *et al.* (3rd edn., American Society for Microbiology, 1986), concentrates on specific laboratory techniques. More recently, H. Zola has edited *Laboratory methods in immunology* (2 vols, CRC, 1990). *Clinical immunology: a practical approach*, edited by H.C. Gooi and H. Chapel (IRL, 1990) excludes research techniques, concentrating on basic methods in immunodiagnosis. Two other books from the same source provide further technical guidance: *Lymphokines and interferons: a practical approach*, edited by M.J. Clemens *et al.* (IRL, 1987), brings together techniques relevant to these closely related areas, and D. Catty has edited *Antibodies: a practical approach* (2 vols, IRL, 1988–9), a laboratory manual for those who produce or work with antibodies. At a more specialist level, H. Zola's *Monoclonal antibodies: a manual of techniques* (CRC, 1987) is a laboratory guide to the different procedures available.

N.J. Bryant, in *Laboratory immunology and serology* (2nd edn., Saunders, 1986), provides a guide for students of medical technology and includes review questions at the end of each chapter. J.C. Jennette has edited *Immunohistology in diagnostic pathology* (CRC, 1989), a thorough review of immunostaining techniques for a variety of diseases. C.R. Taylor's *Immunomicroscopy: a diagnostic tool for the surgical pathologist* (*Major Problems in Pathology*, vol. 19, Saunders, 1986) is a comprehensive treatment of the subject. Pictorial guidance is available from C.D. Ockleford in *An atlas of antigens: fluorescence microscope localisation patterns in cells and tissues* (Macmillan, 1990), and in the *Atlas of diagnostic immunohistopathology*, edited by L.D. True (Gower Medical, 1990).

The range of works on immunochemistry is extensive. Among the general texts, *Immunocytochemistry: modern methods and applications*, edited by J.M. Polak and S. Van Noorden (2nd edn., Wright, 1986) and *Immunochemistry in practice*, by A. Johnstone and R. Thorpe (2nd edn., Blackwell Scientific Publications, 1987) are well-established introductions. More concise guides to the subject are available in L-I. Larsson's *Immunocytochemistry: theory and practice* (CRC, 1988), and in B. Beltz and G.D. Burd's *Immunocytochemical techniques: principles and practice* (Blackwell Scientific Publications, 1989). Specific techniques include J. Clausen's *Immunochemical techniques for the identification and estimation of macromolecules* (*Laboratory techniques in biochemistry and molecular biology*, Vol. 1, Part 3, 3rd edn., Elsevier, 1988) which gives, as appendices, extensive descriptions of the immunochemical methods.

Immunoassay, edited by D.W. Chan (Academic Press, 1987), introduces this standard technique. One specific area of application is dealt with by H. Kangro and J.C. Booth in *Immunoassays in clinical virology* (Butterworths, 1989). For radioimmunoassay procedures, T. Chard's *An introduction to radioimmunoassay and related techniques* (*Laboratory techniques in biochemistry and molecular biology*, Vol. 6, part 2, 3rd edn., Elsevier, 1987) is available, as is *Radioimmunoassay in basic and clinical pharmacology*, edited by C. Patrono and B.A. Peskar (*Handbook of experimental pharmacology*, Vol. 82, Springer, 1987). *Complementary immunoassays*, by W.P. Collins (Wiley, 1988), reviews progress in the development and application of different immunoassay techniques.

Hybridomas and cancer immunology

The main area of immunological activity in oncology arises from the development of hybridoma technology and the use of monoclonal antibodies for therapeutic purposes. J.W. Goding takes a broad view in *Monoclonal antibodies: principles and practice* (2nd edn., Academic Press, 1986), which looks at their production and applications in cell biology, biochemistry and immunology. A wide range of interests is covered by K.C. McCullough and R.E. Spier in *Monoclonal antibodies in biology and biotechnology: theoretical and practical aspects* (Cambridge University Press, 1990).

Recent developments in cancer applications are summarized by *Monoclonal antibodies and immunoconjugates in cancer treatment*, edited by R.W. Baldwin and V.S. Byers (Parthenon, 1989), and by the San Francisco symposium proceedings edited by J.M. Vaeth and J.L. Meyer with the title *The present and future role of monoclonal antibodies in the management of cancer* (*Frontiers of Radiation Therapy and Oncology*, Vol. 24, Karger, 1990). W. Knapp *et al.* have edited *Leucocyte typing IV: white cell differentiation antigens* (Oxford University Press, 1990), the extensive proceedings of a workshop which provided evaluations of about 1100 different monoclonal antibodies. The resultant data are also available on diskette.

Among texts offering a general approach, *Immunology of malignant diseases*, edited by V.S. Byers and R.W. Baldwin (MTP, 1987), is a useful introduction. *Immunity to Cancer II*, edited by M.S. Mitchell (Alan R. Liss, 1989), provides a comprehensive review of tumour immunology from basic concepts to clinical trials. Diagnostic and therapeutic aspects provide the main theme of *Human tumour antigens and specific tumour therapy*, edited by R.S. Metzgar and M.S. Mitchell (Alan R. Liss, 1989).

Other immunotherapeutic agents of interest to oncology are reviewed in *Biological response modifiers: new approaches to disease intervention*, edited by P.F. Torrence (Academic Press, 1985), while research into specific agents and their clinical applications is presented by F.R. Balkwill in *Cytokines in cancer therapy* (Oxford University Press, 1989); in *Immunotoxins*, edited by A.E. Frankel (*Cancer Treatment and Research*, Vol. 37, Kluwer, 1988) and in *Interleukin-2 and killer cells in cancer*, edited by E. Lotzova and R.B. Heberman (CRC, 1989).

Transplantation

While the relevant surgical procedures are sometimes included in books on transplantation, immunological considerations usually predominate. *Graft-vs.-host disease: immunology, pathophysiology, and treatment*, edited by S.J. Bourakoff *et al.* (*Hematology*, Vol. 12, Dekker, 1990), reviews research into graft rejection and immunosuppression. In *Organ transplantation and replacement*, edited by G.J. Cerilli (Lippincott, 1988), a major part of the book is devoted to immunological considerations. Two other works, *Clinical transplantation: current practice and future prospects*, edited by G.R.D. Catto (MTP, 1987), and

Organ transplantation: current clinical and immunological concepts, edited by L. Brent and R.A. Sells (Baillière Tindall, 1989), provide a less detailed approach to the subject, while an even more concise introduction is available in C. Green's *Recent progress in organ transplantation* (Medicine Group, 1988). *Cyclosporin: mode of action and clinical applications*, edited by A.W. Thomson (Kluwer, 1989) reviews all aspects of this important immunosuppressive drug. *Anesthesia and organ transplantation*, edited by S. Gelman (Saunders, 1987), examines immunological problems both in general terms and then by focusing on specific organs in turn.

The individual organs receive fuller consideration in a variety of books. Kidney transplantation, though a well-established procedure, still commands attention through works such as *Kidney transplant rejection: diagnosis and treatment*, edited by G.M. Williams *et al.* (*Kidney disease*, Vol. 7, Dekker, 1986); *Kidney transplantation: principles and practice*, edited by P.J. Morris (3rd edn., Saunders, 1988); and *Renal transplantation*, edited by E.L. Milford (*Contemporary Issues in Nephrology*, Vol. 19, Churchill Livingstone, 1989). Hepatic transplantation has generated a sizeable literature: *Liver transplantation: the Cambridge–King's College Hospital experience*, edited by R.Y. Calne (2nd edn., Grune and Stratton, 1987), reports on a long-term collaborative research and clinical programme. Research is also well to the fore in N. Kamada's *Experimental liver transplantation* (CRC, 1988) and in *Transplantation of the liver*, edited by W.C. Maddrey (*Current Topics in Gastroenterology*, Vol. 1, Elsevier, 1988); while J.W. Williams' *Hepatic transplantation* (Saunders, 1989) looks at problems caused by immunosuppressive drugs.

The *International handbook of pancreas transplantation*, edited by J.M. Dubernard and D.E.R. Sutherland (Kluwer, 1989) gives a comprehensive survey of basic techniques and clinical experience. *Pancreatic transplantation*, edited by C.G. Groth (Saunders, 1988) and *Pancreas transplantation*, edited by L.H. Toledo-Pereyra (Kluwer, 1988), both offer general reviews of recent progress, while J.P. Squifflet's *Pancreas transplantation: experimental and clinical studies* (Karger, 1990) is more selective in its discussion of some of the problems currently under investigation. *Small-bowel transplantation: experimental and clinical fundamentals*, edited by E. Deltz *et al.* (Springer, 1987), provides an introduction to another area of developing expertise.

New trends in heart transplantation, edited by E. Wolner *et al.* (*Bibliotheca Cardiologica*, Vol. 43, Karger, 1988) presents the papers from a Viennese symposium devoted entirely to aspects of rejection and immunosuppression, while M.E. Thompson's *Cardiac transplantation* (Davis, 1990) provides an up-to-date review of current practice. W.A.

Baumgartner and B.A. Reitz, with *Heart and lung transplantation* (Saunders, 1989), and *Heart and heart–lung transplantation*, edited by J. Wallwork (Saunders, 1989), consider one of the multiple-organ techniques now being developed.

Bone marrow transplantation is well represented in the literature. Among recent works, *A guide to bone marrow transplantation*, by H.J. Deeg *et al.* (Springer, 1988), is a useful introduction, while *Bone marrow transplantation*, edited by R. Champlin (Kluwer, 1990) provides more detail. *Recent advances and future directions in bone marrow transplantation*, edited by S.J. Baum *et al.* (Springer, 1988), presents papers from a Tokyo symposium.

Audio-visual aids

Immunology has received little attention from programme producers. The notable exception is *Immunology in focus*, edited by A. Johnstone and J. King (IRL, 1988), a three-volume set of videotapes on basic immunology.

Organizations

Immunology has a number of national and international organizations. The pre-eminent international body is the International Union of Immunological Societies, an umbrella organization for about 30 of the principal national immunological societies. Other major international bodies — some of which have their own official journals — include the International Association of Allergology and Clinical Immunology, the European Federation of Immunological Associations (which publishes *Immunology Letters*), the International Association of Biological Standardization (*Biologicals* and the series *Developments in Biological Standardization*), the International Society of Developmental and Comparative Immunology (*Developmental and Comparative Immunology*), the Transplantation Society (*Transplantation* and *Transplantation Proceedings*), and the International Society of Blood Transfusion (*Vox Sanguinis*).

Many countries in the developed world have, in addition to their premier national societies, a range of other more specialized organizations; and a substantial proportion of all of them also publish at least one official journal. Among the leading English-speaking societies (with their journals listed where appropriate) are:

American Academy of Allergy and Immunology (*Journal of Allergy and Clinical Immunology*)
American Association of Immunologists (*Journal of Immunology*)
American College of Allergists (*Annals of Allergy*)
Australian Society for Immunology (*Immunology and Cell Biology*)
British Society for Allergy and Clinical Immunology (*Clinical and Experimental Allergy*)
British Society for Immunology (*Clinical and Experimental Immunology* and *Immunology*)
British Transplantation Society

One further group of organizations should not be overlooked. The voluntary sector includes non-professional societies that offer advice and support to members of the public with immunologically-related problems such as food and respiratory allergies. In the UK these include Action Against Allergy (which has a *Newsletter*), and the National Society for Research into Allergy (which publishes the journal *Reaction*).

Approaching organizations is not always straightforward, as their main public contact may be an honorary officer who will change from time to time, rendering entries in directories of organizations rapidly obsolete. Where the society in question has an official journal, that will usually be the best source for up-to-date information on the society's current address. In the absence of such assistance, one of the senior national bodies will often have the necessary information.

History

A.M. Silverstein's *A history of immunology* (Academic Press, 1989), is a comprehensive review of the subject, and includes a biographical dictionary. *Milestones in immunology: a historical exploration*, edited by D.J. Bibel (Science Tech, 1988), charts the subject's development by gathering together a collection of key writings by the leading protagonists. The history of immunity also receives attention in an earlier work in a similar format, *Milestones in microbiology*, edited by T.D. Brock (Prentice-Hall, 1961). *Experimental foundations of modern immunology*, by W.R. Clark (3rd edn., Wiley, 1986), outlines the history of the subject by describing landmark experiments in its development. *Nineteen thirty-nine to nineteen eighty-nine: fifty years progress in allergy*, edited by B.H. Waksman (*Chemical Immunology*, vol. 49, Karger, 1990) is a Festschrift for Paul Kallos. Other older historical studies that remain helpful are *A history of medical bacteriology and immunology*, by W.D. Foster (Heinemann, 1970) and *A history of immunization*, by H.J. Parish (Livingstone, 1965).

Briefer introductions to the subject abound. The *Oxford Companion to medicine*, edited by J.N. Walton *et al.* (2 vols, OUP, 1986), contains useful historical summaries on 'Immunology' by J.L. Gowans (Vol. 1, pp. 579–588), and on 'transplantation' by R.Y. Calne (Vol. 2, pp. 1386–1391). Many immunology textbooks contain historical introductions: 'The history of immunology', by A.M. Silverstein, *Fundamental Immunology*, pp. 21–38, edited by W.E. Paul (Raven, 1984), is an authoritative survey.

Biographies of key figures in the history of immunology provide another source. They include: *Dr Jenner of Berkeley*, by D. Fisk (Heinemann, 1959); *Pasteur and modern science*, by R. Dubos (new edition by T.D. Brock, Science Tech, 1988); *Robert Koch: a life in medicine and bacteriology*, by T.D. Brock (Science Tech, 1988); *Paul Ehrlich, scientist for life*, by E. Baumler (Holmes & Meier, 1984); *Karl Landsteiner: the discoverer of the blood groups and a pioneer in the field of immunology*, by P. Speiser and F.G. Smekal (Hollinek, 1975). The modern period is represented by two autobiographies, *Credo and comment: a scientist reflects*, by F.M. Burnet (Melbourne University Press, 1979) and *Memoir of a thinking radish: an autobiography*, by P.B. Medawar (Oxford University Press, 1986).

CHAPTER FIFTEEN

Clinical medicine

D.W.C. STEWART

Medicine, as an applied science, is dependent on many disciplines and the literature of these disciplines plays an important part in the development of the art of medical practice. Clinical medicine is that aspect of the medical sciences concerned directly with the treatment of the patient but in the background is the wide range of specialist subjects which contribute to the understanding of disease processes, their diagnosis, prevention and treatment.

Medicine was described by Stevens (1986) in the *Oxford companion to medicine* as a cultural phenomenon: 'The role of the physician in society is not determined solely, or even primarily, by the array of drugs, scientific methods, and techniques accepted as useful by the international medical community; medical practice has distinctive national characteristics.'

Because clinical medicine and the effectiveness of its practitioners can determine matters, literally, of life and death there has been a long tradition of communication between its exponents and the medically related literature is one of the best developed and diverse of the literatures of applied sciences.

Journals

The periodical literature of medicine is very extensive; most countries of the world publish at least one journal and all of the developed countries produce a wide range. Although the growth in recent years seems to have been great an unpublished study has indicated that the ratio of practising physicians to medical journals in the USA has remained constant over a long period and this may be the case in other countries also.

General clinical medical journals play a variety of roles; they educate, inform, warn, record, advertise, entertain, discuss, debate, politicize, criticize and advise. Some do all of these things, and more, very well. They may aim at the widest definable 'medical' audience or they may concentrate on specific types of doctor such as general practitioners, hospital doctors or clinical researchers while still retaining a broad coverage of medicine. Where the target audience is defined as being international, usually when the journal publishes papers on clinical research, the language of publication will almost certainly be English.

The *Index Medicus: List of Journals Indexed*, is published as a supplement and gives an overview of the 3000 or so medical journals considered important enough for inclusion in the *Index*. These form a selection from the 20 000 or so titles taken by the National Library of Medicine in Bethesda, Maryland, USA. The other major biomedical indexing and abstracting service, *Excerpta Medica*, also publishes a list of the titles it covers. The *Science Citation Index*, dealt with in detail elsewhere, publishes journal lists by subject in its *Journal Citation Reports* together with citation pattern analysis which indicates the relationship of journals to each other and, to a certain extent, their relative importance in their field.

The journal literature of medicine has a two-tiered structure which reflects a dual function. The majority of workers in medicine are practitioners and not researchers; they are concerned with solving existing problems and in the practical application of advances in treatment, and much less in the advancement itself.

One of the most important general medical journals from every point of view, not least for the quality of the writing and editing, is the *New England Journal of Medicine*. It has the highest ratio of citation to article published of any medical journal and ranks also very highly in a table of all scientific journals. Its importance is underlined by the fact that for rapidity of distribution it is printed in both the USA and the UK. Its criteria for publication are extremely rigorous though 85 per cent of the rejected papers are eventually published in other journals. Other important journals of a similar character are the *British Medical Journal, The Lancet*, the *American Journal of Medicine, Journal of the American Medical Association* and *Medical Journal of Australia*; all carry original papers, reviews, commentary on medico-political matters, correspondence and advertising. Very clinically orientated are: *British Journal of Hospital Medicine, Hospital Update, Hospital Practice* and *Update*. *British Medical Bulletin* specializes in publishing monographic issues on major clinical topics, as do the journals in the '*Clinics*' series, published either by Saunders or Baillière.

Important non-English-language European journals are: *Münchener medizinische Wochenschrift, Deutsche medizinische Wochenschrift, Klinische Wochenschrift, Schweizerische medizinische Wochenschrift, Wiener klinische Wochenschrift* and *Presse Médicale.* Several European countries publish general clinical medicine journals in English such as *Danish Medical Bulletin* and *Netherlands Journal of Medicine.*

There has been an increase in the last few years of journals distributed, free of charge on request, to general practitioners and funded largely by advertising. They are increasingly well edited and relevant to problems met in clinical practice and form an important source of current information, though they may not always be taken or retained by libraries. The Medical Tribune publishing group, for example, produce several such as *Respiratory Disease in Practice* and *Dermatology in Practice.*

Clinical practitioners, although not perhaps being involved in research themselves, play an important role through the reporting of pathological conditions, drug side effects and other clinical problems in providing feedback to researchers and the pharmaceutical industry. The case report is an important form of literature in medical reporting and is recognized as making an important contribution to medical progress, in that the alerting to a condition and the description of disease development form important steps towards the understanding of a disease entity. The first report of malformation due to thalidomide appeared as a letter in the *Medical Journal of Australia*, for example, and the importance of case reports – however brief – means that they are often indexed by the major databases and indexing services.

Indexing, abstracting and current awareness

Indexing, abstracting and alerting services in clinical medicine are many and varied and range from a section in a free medical newspaper to weekly contents listings such as *Current Contents: Clinical Medicine.* Both of these will be quite up to date but are less than ideal for making a literature search to solve a clinical problem. The *Index Medicus* appears monthly and indexes the contents of about 3000 journals worldwide. It is the best retrospective search tool and is available not only as a printed publication but as a computer database in several forms including compact disc (CD-ROM). *Excerpta Medica* is published in a number of sections and covers a larger range of journals. It also produces abstracts.

Reviews

Reviews are always valuable in a rapidly developing subject and are especially so in an applied subject such as clinical medicine, which not only takes account of its own advances, but is also affected by advances throughout the basic sciences. The term 'review' here covers a wide range of publications, reflecting once again the differing needs of researcher and practitioner. It embraces the full scholarly review of the literature of a specific topic, the survey of recent progress, and the subject digest by an authoritative writer for the practising clinician.

There is a tendency among clinicians to prefer information which has been screened or digested by other clinicians rather than by information 'specialists' or librarians. The series *Current Medical Literature* published by CML Ltd and the Royal Society of Medicine is aimed specifically at the clinician and covers over 15 subjects each of which has its own publication. Each journal issue lists only papers which have been assessed for their relevance by an editorial team of clinicians. In most cases an abstract or evaluative editorial note, which may be critical of the paper reviewed, is also included.

Current Science Ltd publish a series *Current Opinion in ...* which provide in each issue a number of review articles with an indication of the importance of the articles reviewed; each issue also has an extensive bibliography of the special topic of the issue. Most of the titles published so far are of relevance to the clinician.

General annual review serials are *Advances in Internal Medicine* and *Annual Review of Medicine*. Both of these assume a considerable subject knowledge and are reviews for the postgraduate; both have companion publications in specialist areas. The *Year Book* series also has a volume on most medical specialties with a strong emphasis on clinical medicine (see p. 69).

Conn's Current therapy edited by R.E. Rakel (Saunders, 1992) is not an annual review in the normal sense as references to the literature are not cited, but its objective is to provide the physician with a practical reference source which incorporates the most recent advances in therapy.

Related to orthodox reviews are symposia, which are often produced under pharmaceutical company sponsorship and sometimes not published through conventional channels. Many are published in answer to the need to provide the physician with up-to-date, high-quality information in an easy assimilable form and arise out of meetings focused on practical problems. In this category are the *Clinics* series published by Saunders, each hardbacked issue of which is a separate symposium. They are similar in style and content to *Medical Clinics of North Ameri-*

ca from the same publisher, which was one of the prototypes for this kind of publication. *British Medical Bulletin* is similar in format.

Horizons in Medicine (Baillière Tindall), formerly *Advanced Medicine*, contains the papers presented at the annual conference of the Royal College of Physicians; it provides a high-quality update on a variety of clinically relevant topics. Churchill Livingstone publishes a book series *Recent Advances in* ... with volumes in most specialties as well as general medicine. Frequency has been rather irregular in recent years but plans are in hand for this good quality series to be relaunched with greatly improved frequency.

General textbooks and monographs

With new knowledge being applied and new techniques employed so fast that for something to be in print it must be almost out of date, multi-volume textbooks and monographs belong more to the basic science than to clinical medicine and loose-leaf updatable systems, common in legal literature, have not been a success in medicine. General medical textbooks are usually no more than one or two volumes but some of the single-volume works come with the option of two-volume format, useful both for medical practice collections and medical libraries.

The most important British comprehensive textbook of medicine is the *Oxford textbook of medicine* (formerly Price's) edited by D.J. Weatherall, J.G.C. Ledingham and D.A. Warrell (2nd edn., OUP, 1987) in two volumes. It has also scored a notable first in being the only machine-readable general medical textbook through its CD-ROM edition. Unfortunately this format does not include illustrations or tables but expanded captions are included as partial compensation.

Cecil textbook of medicine edited by James B. Wyngaarden and Lloyd H. Smith, Jr. (18th edn., Saunders, 1988) is the other major heavyweight text and is available in either a one- or-two volume version. *Harrison's Principles of internal medicine*, edited by J.D. Wilson (12th edn., McGraw-Hill, 1991) is an American standard text as is *The principles and practice of medicine*, edited by A. McGhee Harvey *et al.* (22nd edn., Appleton and Lange, 1988) which is the lineal descendant of the text first written by William Osler in 1892 and a standard work of great merit, with most contributors drawn from the staff of the Johns Hopkins University School of Medicine.

Among the more concise and portable general medicine texts are *Davidson's Principles and practice of medicine*, edited by John MacLeod, Christopher Edwards and Ian Bouchier (15th edn., Churchill Livingstone, 1987).

Complementary medicine

Alexis Carrel in *Man the unknown* (London, Hamish Hamilton, 1936) pointed out that 'man is an indivisible whole of extreme complexity' who is not only the complex of parts which might be analysed by scientific techniques, but who is also an unknowable personality with a spiritual consciousness that depends on the integrity of the organism as a whole. Interest in complementary, or alternative, medicine has increased considerably in the UK in recent years; the British Medical Association established a working party which produced a report *Alternative medicine* (BMA, 1986) and the Royal Society of Medicine set up a series of meetings with conventional and alternative practitioners which resulted in a publication *Talking health: conventional and complementary approaches* edited by Sir James Watt (RSM, 1988) which identifies problem areas in the practice both of orthodox scientific medicine and of alternative systems. The acceptance that alternative therapies, though not always scientifically understood, can usefully complement conventional therapy is becoming more widespread and there is now much greater interchange of ideas, particularly with the complementary specialties which have formal recognized training and professional standards of practice.

A good general introduction to most of the alternative therapies in general use in the UK is *Alternative therapies: a guide to complementary medicine for the health professional*, edited by G.T. Lewith (Heinemann, 1985) which covers briefly but authoritatively, acupuncture, manipulation, biofeedback, homoeopathic medicine, and clinical ecology. Many of the references cited are to 'conventional' medical journals and the book is a useful source of information with lists of addresses of alternative medicine organizations. Another useful short text is *Alternative medicines*, edited by J.W. Salmon (Tavistock, 1984) viewing the situation from an American perspective. Acupuncture is dealt with in a most comprehensive way in *Textbook of acupuncture* by Felix Mann (Heinemann, 1987). Dr Mann for many years was the leading British writer on the subject and this book gathers together in one volume and updates four other works. It includes discussion on the theoretical principle of Chinese medicine. Margery G. Blackie's *Classical homoeopathy* (Beaconsfield Publishers, 1986) is one of a series, *Beaconsfield Homoeopathic Library*, which deal in detail with this field.

Journals of significance are *British Homoeopathic Journal, Acupuncture in Medicine* and *Complementary Medical Research*.

Clinical skill

Physical examination has always been the first step towards clinical care. Even though the clinician is now backed up by a vast array of diagnostic techniques such as computed tomography, ultrasound, fetal monitoring, radioimmunoassay, in addition to radiography and laboratory investigation, the skills of clinical examination are essential. Nor are the skills static as advances in knowledge mean that revised or refined interpretations need to be placed on observed signs. There are several very useful books, some of which are purely practical and some discursive and philosophical.

Hutchison's Clinical methods, edited by Michael Swash (19th edn., Baillière Tindall, 1989) is a good introduction to clinical examination, a mine of information and sound advice. Other good introductory texts are *Chamberlain's Symptoms and signs in clinical medicine* by C. Ogilvie and C.C. Evans (11th edn., Wright, 1987) and *Clinical examination*, edited by J. Macleod and J. Munro (7th edn., Churchill Livingstone, 1986); the latter reflects the approach of the Edinburgh Medical School and is designed to complement *Davidson's Principles and practice of medicine*.

Clinical skills: a system of clinical examination by I.A.D. Bouchier and J.S Morris (2nd edn., Saunders, 1982) takes the view that there cannot be an 'introductory' text on the subject with one method of clinical examination for juniors and another for seniors. The principles and techniques are the same regardless of the maturity of the student. The book proceeds from the techniques of the medical interview to a system-by-system treatment, with each section including a brief description of further diagnostic options beyond the clinical examination. This book, and those mentioned above, are all more or less pocket-sized and practical.

More substantial works are *Conn's Current therapy*, edited by R.E. Rakel (Saunders, 1991) which deals in greater depth with uncommon conditions and *French's Index of differential diagnosis*, edited by F. Dudley Hart (12th edn., Wright, 1985) which is arranged by sites or apparent symptoms and runs from 'Abdomen, rigidity of' to 'Yawning'. The index to *French* runs to over 130 pages and provides a wide range of approaches to the interpretation of clinical symptoms.

Current medical diagnosis and treatment 1992, edited by S.A. Schroeder (Appleton and Lange, 1992) is revised annually and is a cross between a handbook of clinical diagnosis and a general textbook of medicine as treatment and, increasingly, disease prevention are covered. It is an excellent quick-reference source particularly geared towards the needs of junior hospital doctors and students.

More discursive books for reading rather than reference are *Medical problem solving* by A.S. Elstein and others (Harvard University Press, 1978), *Clinical judgement* by A.R. Feinstein (Williams & Wilkins, 1967), *Controversy in internal medicine* edited by Franz Ingelfinger, former editor of *New England Journal of Medicine* (Saunders, I:1966;

II:1974) and *Richard Asher talking sense: a collection of papers* edited by Sir Francis Avery Jones (Pitman, 1972).

Metabolic and genetic disorders

Now that the major infectious diseases have been brought under control for the most part increasing emphasis is being placed on the metabolic and genetic factors underlying pathologic conditions and they are of considerable importance in both clinical practice and clinical research.

Sir Cyril Clarke's *Human genetics and medicine* (3rd edn., Edward Arnold, 1987) is a short but useful introduction to the subject of medical genetics as is G.H. Valentine's *The chromosomes and their disorders: an introduction for clinicians* (4th edn., Heinemann). V.A. McKusick's *Mendelian inheritance in man: catalogs of autosomal dominant autosomal recessive, and X-linked phenotypes* (9th edn., 1990, Johns Hopkins University Press) is also an essential reference work for the clinician. *The metabolic basis of inherited disease*, edited by C.R. Scriver and others (6th edn., McGraw-Hill, 1989) remains the most comprehensive work in the field though significantly different from previous editions. Most chapters now have a section on molecular genetics and incorporate much new material and reference lists running to 600 or more per chapter.

Oxford University Press publishes a high-quality series of *Oxford monographs in medical genetics* which have so far covered a wide range of topics from *The genetics of mental disorders* to *The distribution of human immunoglobulin allotypes*.

Specialties

Cardiology

Advances in cardiovascular surgery and therapeutics have led to continuing growth in the literature of cardiology. A substantial amount appears in the quality general medical journals such as the *BMJ*, *NEJM*, *Lancet* and *JAMA*, but the major clinical cardiology journals are: *Journal of the American College of Cardiology, American Journal of Cardiology, British Heart Journal, American Heart Journal, European Journal of Cardiology, Journal of Thoracic and Cardiovascular Surgery, Circulation Hypertension, American Journal of Hypertension, European Heart Journal*.

Cardiovascular research articles of importance appear in: *Basic Research in Cardiology, Cardiovascular Research, Circulation Research, Journal of Molecular and Cellular Cardiology* and *Microvascular Research*.

All the journals published by the American Heart Association are of high quality; their *Modern Concepts of Cardiovascular Disease* is a short topic-a-month style leaflet aimed at the specialist. *Progress in Cardiovascular Diseases* and *Current Problems in Cardiology* provide more extensive topical reviews for the postgraduate and *Yearbook of Cardiology* condenses the year's work in the field into a single volume, though *Current Opinion in Cardiology* is perhaps more useful as it provides a more comprehensive overview at more frequent intervals.

TEXTBOOKS

There are many excellent textbooks, the foremost of which is probably *The heart*, edited by J.W. Hurst (7th edn., 1989) available in either one- or two-volume format (McGraw-Hill). A UK work of almost comparable stature is *Diseases of the heart*, edited by Desmond G. Julian *et al.*, London, Baillière Tindall, 1989. Both works are particularly strong on the diagnosis of cardiac disease. Other major general cardiology texts include: E.N Silber, *Heart disease* (2nd edn., New York, Macmillan, 1987) and Eugene Braunwald (ed.), *Heart disease: a textbook of cardiovascular medicine* (3rd edn., Philadelphia, Saunders, 1988). *Clinical heart disease* by S. Oram (2nd edn., Heinemann, 1981) is a practical text with a strong bedside bias. It is written in a firm, clear, sometimes dogmatic style, and each chapter has a select guide to further reading, often including early classic work — for instance Thomas Lewis's *Mechanism and graphic registration of the heart beat* (3rd edn., Shaw, 1925) and Mackenzie's *The study of the pulse* (Pentland, 1902). Specific areas of cardiology are covered by *Management of heart failure*, edited by D.G. Julian and N.K. Wenger (Butterworths, 1986).

The history of cardiology has been well documented and many of the key publications such as those by Harvey, Withering and Starling have been frequently reprinted. Two of the many books which summarize its progress and the people involved are *A history of the heart and circulation* by F.A. Willius and T.J. Dry (Saunders, 1948) and *Cardiac classics*, edited by F.A. Willius and T.E. Keys (Mosby, 1941), itself reprinted as *Classics of cardiology* (Dover, 1961), which reproduces papers from Harvey to Herrick.

For paediatric cardiology there is *Heart disease in paediatrics* by S.C. Jordan and Olive Scott (3rd edn., Butterworths, 1989) which is a very extensive rewriting of the 1981 edition with much additional coverage of non-invasive diagnostic techniques. It is an excellent introductory text. More comprehensive coverage is provided by *Moss' Heart disease in infants, children, and adolescents*, edited by F.H. Adams *et al.* (4th edn., Williams and Wilkins, 1989).

Many of the North American contributors to *Moss* also contribute to

Paediatric cardiology edited by R.H. Anderson, F.J. Macartney, E.A. Shinebourne and M. Tynan (2 vols, Churchill Livingstone, 1987). Although conceived as a UK text, its scope was enlarged to make its content applicable throughout the world; for example, it includes a chapter on paediatric cardiology in the tropics.

A.E. Becker and R.H. Anderson's *Pathology of congenital heart disease* (Butterworths, 1981) is still useful and is complemented by *Clinical recognition of congenital heart disease* by J.K. Perloff (Saunders, 1987) and by *A colour atlas of adult congenital heart disease* by L.M. Shapiro and K.M. Fox (Wolfe Medical, 1990).

Diagnostic aspects of cardiovascular medicine are covered by *Echocardiography* by Harvey Feigenbaum (4th edn., Lea and Febiger, 1986), a well-illustrated text written in a language 'easily understood by individuals who do not have a background in mathematics, physics or engineering'. It is an important reference source with 200-400 references per chapter. Cardiac catheterization is dealt with in a comprehensive way in Graham Miller's *Invasive investigation of the heart* (Blackwell, 1989) and L. Schamroth's *Introduction to electrocardiography* (7th edn., Blackwell, 1990) covers its field well.

For cardiovascular physiology, *Cardiovascular dynamics* by R.F. Rushmer (4th edn., Saunders, 1976) is still valuable with more comprehensive coverage to be found in the four volumes on the cardiovascular system in the American Physiological Society's *Handbook of physiology*, section 2.

On hypertension Sir George Pickering's *High blood pressure* (2nd edn., Churchill, 1968) and his *Nature of essential hypertension* (Churchill, 1961) are now classics; a comprehensive modern text is *Clinical hypertension* by N.M. Kaplan (4th edn., Williams and Wilkins, 1986). *Classic papers in hypertension*, edited by J.D. Swales (Science Press, 1987) provides a historical review of the development of thought on hypertension and reproduces text of 26 papers from Stephen Hales (1769) to a 1977 paper from *Science*; it is one of a series covering a range of topics.

Clinical haematology

Much of the publication on blood disorders deals with the subject from a laboratory point of view but there is an increasing need for the clinician to be well informed and more clinically orientated material is now appearing. *Clinical hematology* by M.M. Wintrobe *et al.* (8th edn., Lea and Febiger, 1981) and *Hematology* by W.J. Williams *et al.* (4th edn., McGraw-Hill, 1990) are important comprehensive works. De Gruchy's *Clinical haematology in medical practice*, edited by Frank Firkin and others (5th edn., Blackwell, 1989) is, in the span of 500 pages, a superb detailed textbook providing authoritative and complete coverage of clinical haematology. De Gruchy is sparingly illustrated and is complemented by *Clinical haematology illustrated* by A.V. Hoffbrand and J.E. Pettit (Churchill Livingstone, 1987) which brings together in visual form clinical features, pathological processes and differential diagnosis.

The major journals in haematology of importance to the clinician are: *Blood, British Journal of Haematology, Baillière's Clinical Haematology* and *Haematology and Oncology Clinics of North America.* The last two publish extended review articles and are useful updating sources as is *Recent advances in haematology*, edited by A.V. Hoffbrand (Churchill Livingstone) the latest edition of which is No. 5. (1988).

Books dealing with important haematological topics include: *Megaloblastic anaemias* by I. Chanarin (3rd edn., Blackwell, 1990), *Haemolytic anaemias* by J.V. Dacie (4th edn., Churchill Livingstone, 1992), *Sickle Cell Disease* by Graham R. Sergeant (OUP, 1985), *Hypoglycaemia* by Vincent Marks and F. Clifford Rose (2nd edn., Blackwell, 1981) and *Leukemia* by E.S. Henderson (5th edn., Saunders, 1990).

The two most useful histories of the subject are both by M.M. Wintrobe: *Blood, pure and eloquent* (McGraw-Hill, 1980) and *Hematology, the blossoming of a science* (Lea and Febiger, 1985). A collection of *Classic papers in hyperlipidaemia*, edited by J.R. Quiney and G.F. Watts (Science Press, 1989) reprints 35 papers from 1913 to 1988.

Respiratory disease

Emphases in the field of respiratory disease have changed several times this century; early on pulmonary tuberculosis, its prevention and treatment formed a large part of the literature. There has been extensive research, 'ebullient activity' in the words of Professor Cotes, in the basic disciplines of lung mechanics and regulatory gas exchange physiology. Genetic and environmental factors have received increased consideration and the importance of immunological factors in many pulmonary diseases has been extensively investigated. Journals have broadened their scope and many titles have changed. The major clinical journals are *American Review of Respiratory Diseases, Thorax, Chest, Tubercle* and *Respiratory Medicine. Seminars in Respiratory Infections* and *Clinics in Chest Medicine* produce issues devoted to single topics. The clinical immunology and allergy journals are important as well as those dealing with a single disorder such as *Asthma. European Journal of Applied Physiology, Journal of Applied Physiology, European Respiratory Journal* and *Respiration* cover lung function extensively.

The two major comprehensive and current textbooks remain G.L. Baum and E. Wolinsky's *Textbook of pulmonary diseases* in two volumes (4th edn., Little, Brown, 1989), an American multi-author work, and *Crofton and Douglas's Respiratory diseases* by A. Seaton, D. Seaton and A.G. Leitch (4th edn., Blackwell, 1989). The latter retains the character of the earlier editions in that it is written by clinicians for clinicians and is essential reading for thoracic physicians. Earlier editions have been translated into Italian, Spanish and Russian.

Clinical atlas of respiratory diseases by Margaret Turner-Warwick and others (Gower Medical, 1989) is *not* a textbook of respiratory medicine but provides a substantial amount of visual material covering radiographs, pathology, clinical appearances, investigative techniques, therapeutic procedures and more. It is designed specifically to complement the comprehensive textbooks and is a rich source of visual teaching material.

Lung function: assessment and application in medicine by J.E. Cotes (Blackwell, 1979) is the definitive work on the subject which, though mainly physiological, deals also with lung function in disease and lung function variations and reference values. *Disorders of ventilation* by J. Shneerson (Blackwell, 1988) has as its main theme the physiological interpretation of the clinical aspects of disorders of ventilation. It has over 3000 references.

A comprehensive review of the pathologic basis of lung disease with a strong emphasis on clinical features and clinico-pathologic correlations is provided by *Pathology of the lung* by W.M. Thurlbeck (Thieme Medical, 1988) and also by H. Spencer's *Pathology of the lung* (4th edn., Pergamon, 1985).

Respiratory illness in children by P.D. Phelan, L.I Landau, and A. Olinsky (3rd edn., Blackwell Scientific, 1990) is a well-referenced text considerably updated in this edition especially with regard to epidemiology of respiratory infection, asthma and cystic fibrosis. A more comprehensive text is *Kendig's Disorders of the respiratory tract in children*, edited by V. Chernick (5th edn., Saunders, 1990).

Occupational respiratory medicine is in a period of transition with some of the old diseases becoming less common, at least in Western Europe, while others persist and the incidence of some is on the increase. There are two particularly important books in the field *Occupational lung disorders* by W.R. Parkes (2nd edn., Butterworth, 1982) and *Work-related lung disorders* by J.E. Cotes and J. Steel (Blackwell Scientific Publications, 1987).

Recent advances in respiratory medicine, edited by D.C. Flenley and T.L. Petty, No. 4 (Churchill Livingstone, 1986) is a useful update source, though not frequently published.

Gastroenterology

Gastroenterology has a wide literature which involves that of biochemistry, genetics and immunology as well as of digestive disease and nutrition. Much important work will be found in the general clinical medical journals with the general gastroenterology journals being *Gastroenterology, Gut, Digestive Diseases and Sciences, Gastroenterology Clinics of North America, Digestion* and the *American Journal of Gastroenterology*. Important specialist journals, though not always clinically orientated, are *Seminars in Liver Disease, Liver,* and *Diseases of the Colon and Rectum.*

Gastroenterology is particularly well served with updating and review publications with, in addition to *Current Medical Literature, Gastroenterology* section and an *Excerpta Medica* section (No. 48), *Current Opinion in Gastroenterology, Recent Advances in Gastroenterology,* edited by Roy Pounder (Number 8, Churchill Livingstone, 1990) and the annual *Topics in Gastroenterology,* edited by D.P. Jewell and J.A. Snook (Blackwell) which published number 17, 1990.

Gastroenterology by H.L. Bockus in seven volumes (4th edn., Saunders, 1985) is the major, and only, multi-volume textbook but at a cost of over £500 it is to be found in only a few medical libraries. *Textbook of gastroenterology* by I.A.D. Bouchier and others (Baillière Tindall, 1984) has established itself as a good comprehensive textbook, and is now the UK standard work in the field. There are some good shorter texts such as Bouchier's *Gastroenterology* (3rd edn., Baillière Tindall, 1982) and H.J. Dworkin's *Gastroenterology* (Butterworths, 1982).

Diseases of the gut and pancreas, edited by J. J. Misiewicz, R. E. Pounder and C.N. Venables (Blackwell, 1987) has a distinguished list of international contributors, is relevant to both physicians and surgeons and covers both the routine and complex gastrointestinal problems encountered in clinical practice.

A colour atlas of the digestive system by R.E. Pounder, M.C. Allison, and A.P Dhillon (Wolfe Medical, 1989) provides the full range of visual material found in most modern colour atlases: patient photographs, radiographs, endoscopic photographs, histological sections, post-mortem specimens and tomograms. It deals with the digestive system in health and disease but it does not cover the liver and biliary system as this aspect is dealt with in *A colour atlas of the digestive system* by Dame Sheila Sherlock and John Summerfield (Wolfe Medical, 1979).

For normal function *Physiology of the digestive tract* by H.W. Davenport (5th edn., Year Book Medical Publishers, 1982) remains the text of choice; also important is *Physiology of the gastrointestinal tract* edited by L.R. Johnson (2nd edn., Raven, 1987). Both of these are complemented by *Scientific foundations of gastroenterology* edited by W. Sircus and A.N. Smith (Heinemann, 1980) which aims to provide clinicians with a knowledge of advances in the basic medical sciences as they relate to gastroenterology; both normal and pathological conditions are covered.

Morson and Dawson's Gastrointestinal pathology, edited by B.C. Morson et al. (3rd edn., Blackwell, 1990) reflects the development of gastroenterology in recent years and has been considerably enlarged. It underlines the fact that surgical specimens and biopsy material from the gastrointestinal tract account for a considerable proportion of material seen in any department of general histopathology. The book is written for the pathologist but should prove useful to physicians, surgeons and radiologists.

Paediatric gastroenterology, edited by C.M. Anderson, V. Burke and M. Gracey (2nd edn., Blackwell, 1987) is a multi-author work with a wide geographical spread of contributors. It has a substantial section on the development of the small intestine, the problems of infective diarrhoeas and parasitic intestinal infections.

The *Oxford textbook of clinical hepatology* (2 vols., OUP, 1991) edited by Neil McIntyre and four European colleagues, is a work which aims to provide a comprehensive account of both common and rare problems, including the effects of infection on the liver. The definitive postgraduate work on the liver in Britain and (in translation) in many other countries has been for years Sheila Sherlock's *Diseases of the liver and biliary system*. The 8th edition (Blackwell, 1989), completely rewritten, gives extensive coverage to hepatitis, and has a chapter on liver transplantation. It is complemented by Sherlock's *Colour atlas of liver diseases* (2nd edn., Wolfe, 1991). Written for clinicians, *Liver disorders in childhood* by Alex P. Mowat (2nd edn., Butterworths, 1987) covers such topics as developments arising from new knowledge of the mechanisms of physiological jaundice and the role of hepatitis B virus infection in chronic liver disease.

Progress in liver diseases (Volume 9, Saunders, 1990) is one of the most high-powered of the progress reporting publications and has contributions from leading experts in the field of hepatology. It was founded by Hans Popper (1903-1988) and appears at irregular intervals.

Books covering special gastroenterological topics of interest to the clinician include: *Bowel obstruction: differential diagnosis and clinical management* by J.P. Welch (Saunders, 1990), *Hepatology for the clinician: a problem-oriented approach* by S. Beker, (Alan R. Liss, 1989), *Inflammatory bowel disease* by J.B. Kirsner and R.G. Shorter (3rd edn., Lea & Febiger, 1988) and *Disorders of gastrointestinal motility in childhood* by P.J. Milla (Wiley, 1988).

Renal disease

The understanding of the kidney in all its aspects has grown dramatically in recent years resulting in better management of patients through the use, in part, of new diagnostic techniques such as needle biopsy of the kidney and the resulting developments in renal pathogenesis. The complex nature of the kidney, with its relationships to endocrinology, its impact on the functioning of blood vessels, bone marrow and bone and its unique ability to undergo virtually complete recovery of structure and function after severe damage, means that the periodical literature of renal disease has a substantial degree of dispersal throughout general medicine, surgery, laboratory medicine, immunology, and cardiovascular medicine as well as the specialty journals. The most important of these are *Kidney International, Clinical Nephrology, Nephron* (all of which have international editorial boards), *American Journal of Kidney Diseases, American Journal of Nephrology* and *Pediatric Nephrology* (the journal of the International Pediatric Nephrology Association).

Nephrology Dialysis Transplantation incorporates the *Proceedings of the European Dialysis and Transplant Association — European Renal Association* and continues to publish reviews of specific issues. *Advances in Nephrology* has developed from a single hospital-based publication (from the Necker Hospital, Paris) to an annual review volume of international importance.

In addition to specifically renal publications the journals of urology are also of importance though many are written specifically for urological surgeons.

The kidney by B.M. Brenner and F.C. Rector (3rd edn., Saunders, 1986) in two volumes covers most aspects of the field and cites over 23 000 references. It does not, however, deal with some topics such as membrane transport which have not significantly changed since the previous edition in 1981. Nevertheless there is a substantial introductory section on normal renal function. *The kidney: physiology and pathophysiology* by D.W. Seldin and G. Giebisch (Raven, 1985), also in two volumes' covers similar ground but with more extensive coverage of, for example, normal renal regulation of electrolytes.

Hugh de Wardener's *The kidney: an outline of normal and abnormal function* (5th edn., Churchill Livingstone, 1985) was, with its first edition in 1958, the first book on clinical nephrology. Now that there are encyclopaedic works such as the two mentioned above, de Wardener has aimed to produce a deliberately small book intended for 'those who are interested in the subject'. It is authoritative and well written and has become something of a classic; it covers all the major disorders of the kidney.

Scientific foundations of urology, edited by G.D. Chisholm and W.R. Fair (3rd edn., Heinemann and Year Book, 1990) is one of the few titles in the series to publish further editions, reflecting the rapidity of change in the field. While it deals with the whole field of urology and is aimed at urological surgeons, it complements the major texts in both nephrology and urology.

Renal pathology, with emphasis on aetiology and pathogenesis, is covered in three volumes by R.H. Heptinstall in *Pathology of the kidney* (3rd edn., Little, Brown, 1983); the book is particularly well referenced.

Books on special topics are: *Kidney electrolyte disorders* by J.C. Chan and J.R. Gill (Churchill Livingstone, 1990), *The nephrotic syndrome* edited by J.S. Cameron and R.J Glasscock (Dekker, 1988), *Acute renal failure*, edited by B.M. Brenner and J.M. Lazarus (2nd edn., Churchill Livingstone, 1988), *A primer of water electrolyte and acid–base syndromes* by E. Goldberger (7th edn., Lea & Febiger, 1986), *The genetics of renal tract disorders* by M. d'A. Crawfurd (OUP, 1988), and *The kidney and hypertension in diabetes mellitus*, edited by C.K. Mogensen (Nijhoff, 1988) forms part of a series *Topics in Renal Medicine*.

Endocrinology and metabolism

Clinical endocrinology is a subspecialty of clinical medicine concerned with understanding, diagnosing, and treating disorders of the endocrine glands. It also encompasses the study and treatment of disorders involving other organs which secrete hormones such as the hypothalamus (vasopressin, oxytocin), the kidney (renin, erythropoietin), the heart (atriopeptins) and the liver (somatomedins). Metabolism is closely related in that it is concerned with disorders relating to intermediary metabolism of carbohydrates (e.g. diabetes mellitus) and lipids as well as nutritional problems of all kinds including obesity and malnutrition. There tends to be no clear dividing line between the literatures of basic and clinical endocrinology and many of the journals cover both aspects.

Endocrine Reviews is the most important journal in the field, publishing substantial reviews in all areas of experimental and clinical endocrinology. The Society for Endocrinology publishes *Journal of Endocrinology* and *Journal of Molecular Endocrinology*.

Other important titles are *Endocrinology, Journal of Clinical Endocrinology and Metabolism, Clinical Endocrinology* and *Metabolism*. Specific special topics are covered by *Diabetes, Diabetes Care, Diabetologia, Journal of Pediatric Endocrinology* and *Journal of Inherited Metabolic Disease. Recent Progress in Hormone Research* constitutes the proceedings of the annual Laurentian Hormone Conference; it is an important annual review as each year all aspects of the field are covered in depth and consistent quality has been maintained since the series started in 1947.

The two major texts are *Williams' Textbook of endocrinology*, edited by J.D. Wilson and D.W. Foster (Saunders,1985) and *Endocrinology*, edited by L.J. DeGroot (2nd edn., Saunders, 1989) in three volumes.

Both aim to form a bridge between the clinical medicine and basic sciences aspects of endocrinology. The nature of the subject requires a multi-author approach and the books have, respectively, 52 and 230 contributors, with an overlap of fourteen. A good shorter text is R. Hall's *Fundamentals of clinical endocrinology* (4th edn., Churchill Livingstone, 1989).

Clinical endocrinology: an illustrated text, edited by G.M. Besser and A.G. Cudworth (Gower, 1987) assembles a distinguished group of writers to produce what is both an atlas and a visual image teaching resource as it was produced in conjunction with a *Slide atlas of endocrinology*. It includes illustrations of clinical manifestations of endocrine disorders as colour photographs, radiographs, computed tomography scans, karyotypes etc. in addition to particularly clear colour diagrams of, for example, androgen action on a target cell. *A colour atlas of endocrinology* by R. Hall, D. Evered and R. Greene (Wolfe, 1979) deals mainly with clinical features but has very little text.

Metabolic control and disease, edited by P.K. Bondy (8th edn., Saunders, 1980), formerly *Duncan's Diseases of metabolism*, is a comprehensive text which covers metabolic disorders better than any other text but a useful, shorter work is *The inherited metabolic diseases* by J.B. Holton (Churchill Livingstone, 1987).

The thyroid gland from anatomy through physiology and function to disease is covered in great detail in *Werner's The thyroid*, edited by S.H. Ingbar and L.E. Braverman (5th edn., Lippincott, 1986); a third of the 1500 pages is devoted to normal function and the book is an essential clinical text. *Thyroid function and disease* by G.N. Burrow, J.K. Oppenheim and R. Volpe (Saunders, 1989) provides a shorter text on the subject.

The standard work on diabetes is *Ellenberg and Rifkin's Diabetes mellitus*, edited by Harold Rifkin and D. Porte (4th edn., Elsevier, 1990). There are 20 chapters on the basic physiology of metabolism and pathophysiology of diabetes and its complications and a further 40 chapters on diagnosis, epidemiology and treatment. The complications of diabetes are important to all clinicians; H. Keen and J. Jarrett's *Complications of diabetes* (2nd edn., Arnold, 1982) covers topics such as diabetic pregnancies and skin disorders associated with diabetes. *Diabetic neuropathy*, edited by P.J. Dyck and others (Saunders, 1987) is a short but thorough textbook on the subject which is, in effect, updated by *Diabetic Neuropathy*, edited by J. Ward and Y. Goto (Wiley, 1990) which covers all aspects of current research in a symposium format.

Special aspects of endocrinology and metabolism are dealt with in:

The spleen: structure, function and clinical significance, edited by A.J. Bowdler (Chapman and Hall, 1990)

Genetic and metabolic disease in pediatrics edited by J.K. Lloyd and C.R. Scriver (Butterworths, 1985)

The pituitary, edited by C. Beardwell and G.L. Robertson (Butterworths, 1981)

Autoimmune endocrine disease, edited by T.F. Davies (Wiley, 1983)

Disorders of porphyrin metabolism by M.R. Moore *et al.* (Plenum, 1987)

Recent advances in endocrinology and metabolism No.3, edited by C.R.W. Edwards and D.W. Lincoln (Churchill Livingstone, 1989) provides a good overview of developments.

HISTORY

Endocrinology has recently attracted historians. For many years the only history was Sir Humphry Rolleston's *The endocrine organs in health and disease* (OUP, 1936). V.C. Medvei's *History of endocrinology* (MTP, 1982) acknowledges the importance of Rolleston's work and aims to complement it; it is illustrated and contains a separate section of biographies of endocrinologists. The American Physiological Society has published *Endocrinology: people and ideas*, edited by S.M. McCann (1988) which deals with twentieth-century developments. F. Mercke's *History and iconography of endemic goitre and cretinism* (MTP Press, 1984; originally published in German in 1971) reviews both descriptions in the medical literature and in creative writing, has substantial sections on historical demography and has a large number of high-quality illustrations.

Dermatology

Although mortality is very low, the incidence of skin diseases is relatively high and some conditions can create a great deal of morbidity. There may be personal or occupational implications for the patient with a skin disorder and these may lead to depression and anxiety. In addition to disorders which are limited to the skin, hair and nails, many systemic diseases present with a cutaneous manifestation. These include connective-tissue diseases such as scleroderma, dermatomyositis, and lupus erythematosus, as well as various internal malignancies.

The existence of these diseases causes some degree of scatter of dermatological publication into immunology journals but it does not present a significant problem in terms of access to the literature. There is a relatively small number of journals, most of good quality, and mainly orientated towards the clinical practitioner. In order of citation frequency the main titles are *Journal of Investigative Dermatology*, *Archives of Dermotology*, *Journal of the American Academy of Dermatology*, *British Journal of Dermatology* and *Contact Dermatitis*. *Cutis* is a useful journal for the practitioner, and research and special topics are covered by *Acta Dermato-Venereologica*, *American Journal of Dermatopathology*, *Journal of Cutaneous Pathology*, *Clinical and Experimental Dermatology* and *Pediatric Dermatology*.

The scientific basis of dermatology has expanded considerably since Rothman's *Physiology and biochemistry of the skin* (1954), the first work to attempt to review all of skin biochemistry and physiology. *Biochemistry and physiology of the skin*, edited by L.A. Goldsmith (2 vols, OUP, 1983) deals also with the anatomy of the skin, especially as revealed by the electron microscope and there are sections on the changes in structure during normal human neonatal development. *Physiology and pathophysiology of the skin*, edited by A. Jarrett was published in nine volumes from 1973 to 1986 (Saunders); it contains more detail than is needed in the normal clinical situation but is nevertheless an important work.

Skin signs of systemic disease by I.M. Braverman (Saunders, 1981) deals with the important area of diseases whose symptoms appear as cutaneous conditions such as the connective-tissue disorders like lupus erythematosus and the endocrine and metabolic diseases.

The definitive text on skin diseases is *Textbook of dermatology*, 'the Rook book', edited by A. Rook and others in four volumes (5th edn., Blackwell, 1991). It integrates for the physician the increasing knowledge of the biology of the skin and pathological processes. As comprehensive, and marginally better in terms of illustrations, is the American equivalent *Dermatology in general medicine*, edited by T.B. Fitzpatrick and others (3rd edn., McGraw-Hill, 1987); it has specific colour atlas sections. *Andrew's Diseases of the skin* by H.L. Arnold, R.B Odom and W.D. James (8th edn., Saunders, 1990) is an excellent single-volume text particularly clinically orientated 'for desk top rather than library use'. Emphasis is placed on accessible recent references in the leading clinical dermatology journals.

Good colour atlas coverage of skin conditions is provided by *A colour atlas of dermatology* by G.M. Levene and C.D. Calnan (Wolfe, 1984) and by *Atlas of clinical dermatology* by A. du Vivier (Churchill Livingstone, 1986). A pocket atlas *Dermatology of black skin* by A. Basset, B. Liataud and B. Ndiaye, translated from the French by Andrew Pembroke (OUP, 1986) deals particularly with the clinical signs which are significantly different in black patients from the classic textbook descriptions based on white patients. As with other atlases, they are designed to supplement the comprehensive textbooks.

Pathology of the skin by P. H. Kee (Gower, 1989) is intended to give histopathologists a source of clinical information but it is also directed at dermatologists with an interest in dermopathology. Very much a bench book with full colour clinical and histologic photographs, photomicrographs and diagrams, it has considerable more text than atlases.

The workplace is now recognized as a major source in the development of skin disorders not only from the point of view of chemicals which may be involved but also from the nature of the working environment. The greater range of complex chemical formulations used in everyday products from cosmetics to preservatives has seen, in spite of improved labelling, increases in the contact dermatoses. *Contact dermatitis* by Etain Cronin (Churchill Livingstone, 1980) and *Contact dermatitis* by A.A. Fisher (3rd edn., Lea & Febiger, 1986) are written with the clinician in mind and both are arranged by causative agent. Fisher is more extensively referenced but neither is illustrated. Both of these books cover industrial dermatology but more detailed treatment is provided in H.I. Maibach's *Occupational and industrial dermatology* (2nd edn., Year Book Medical, 1987) and in R.M. Adams' *Occupational skin disease* (2nd edn,, Saunders, 1990). Both are arranged by agent but Adams also provides a chapter by job description.

Other books on special topics are:

Essential paediatric dermatology by J.L. Verbov (Clinical Press, 1989)

Practical paediatric dermatology by W.L. Weston (2nd edn., Little, Brown, 1985)

Skin disorders in the elderly, edited by B.E. Monk *et al.* (Blackwell, 1988)

Histopathology of the skin by W.F. Lever and G. Schaumberg-Lever (7th edn., Lippincott, 1990)

Management of blistering diseases, edited by F. Wojnarowska and R.A. Briggman (Chapman and Hall, 1990)

Diseases of the nails and their management, edited by R. Baran and R.P.R. Dawber (Blackwell, 1984)

The nails in disease by P.D. Samman and D.A. Fenton (4th edn., Heinemann, 1986)

Diseases of the hair and scalp by A. Rook and R. Dawber (Blackwell, 1982)

Acne by W.J. Cunliffe (Dunitz, 1989)

Textbook of psoriasis, edited by P.D. Mier and P.C.M. van de Kerkhof (Churchill Livingstone, 1986)

The urticarias, edited by R.H. Champion *et al.* (Churchill Livingstone, 1985)

Life threatening dermatoses by P.A. Krusinski and F.P. Flowers (Year Book, 1987)

Rheumatology

Over a hundred different disorders are currently classified as rheumatic diseases and though some are rare others affect millions of people and have been known for thousands of years, possibly being the oldest of identifiable chronic pathologic conditions. The range of conditions is so great that the term 'rheumatism' effectively lacks meaning. The International League against Rheumatism offers the definition

> Rheumatology is a branch of medicine concerned with a heterogeneous group of diseases and disorders commonly affecting the locomotor system. They may arise from primary pathologic processes in connective tissue structures, from disorders of their function, or as a manifestation of systemic disease. Their common denominator appears to be involvement of connective tissue. Although joints appear to be the main site of symptoms, the arthritis is only one component of a constitutional illness of considerable complexity.

The complexity of the condition reflects itself in the interdisciplinary nature of the literature with very strong linkage between the mainstream rheumatology publications and immunology, biochemistry, cell biology, and tissue research as well as clinical and experimental medicine.

The leading research journals are *Arthritis and Rheumatism*, the official publication of the American College of Rheumatology, and the *British Journal of Rheumatology*, the organ of the British Society for Rheumatology. Both cover the field fully and include clinical practice and case reports. *Seminars in Arthritis and Rheumatism* is of similar status but also specializes in publishing special symposia supplements. *Rheumatic Disease Clinics of North America* and *Annals of the Rheumatic Diseases* are important titles with a more clinical emphasis; there are only about ten other titles in the field. The *Current Opinion* series is represented by *Current Opinion in Rheumatology* which provides extensive reviews and literature bibliographies organized on a special subject basis with qualitative evaluations of the papers listed though the speed of indexing can be a little slow. *Rheumatology* is an annual review publication and *Recent advances in rheumatology* edited by J.M.H. Moll and R.D. Sturrock (No.4, Churchill Livingstone, 1986) is part of the occasional review series whose frequency is expected to increase in the future.

The diversity of disciplines bearing on the rheumatic diseases means that the task of producing a 'comprehensive' textbook is one not lightly to be undertaken and there are but three in the field: *Textbook of rheumatology* by W.N. Kelley (3rd edn., Saunders, 1989), *Arthritis and allied conditions* by D.J. McCarty (11th edn., Lea & Febiger, 1989) and *Copeman's Textbook of the rheumatic diseases*, edited by J.T. Scott (6th edn., Churchill Livingstone, 1986). The first two are American, the last British. McCarty contains a particularly extensive section on the scientific basis of rheumatic disease. A specific book on this aspect is *Scientific basis of rheumatology*, edited by G. S. Panayi (Churchill Livingstone, 1982) though it is in need of updating.

Rheumatology in clinical practice by J.M.H. Moll (Blackwell, 1987) is intended as a textbook for postgraduate physicians and bridges the gap between the comprehensive works noted above and the basic introductory texts; it has an extensive section of historical background.

Textbook of paediatric rheumatology by J.T. Cassidy and R.E. Petty (2nd edn., Churchill Livingstone, 1990) provides a comprehensive but focused source of information, extensively supported by references, for physicians. *Paediatric rheumatology update*, edited by P. Woo, P.H. White and B.M. Ansell (OUP, 1990) is the proceedings of a meeting held in 1989 which highlights major issues including differential diagnosis.

Special subjects or approaches are covered by:

Atlas of clinical rheumatology by P.A. Dieppe *et al.* (Oxford, 1986)

Kidney in rheumatic disease, edited by P. Bacon and N.M. Hadler (Butterworths, 1982)

Heart in rheumatic disease, edited by B.A. Ansell and P.A. Simkin (Butterworths, 1984)

Lung in rheumatic diseases, edited by G.W. Cannon and G.A. Zimmermann (Dekker, 1990)

Arthritis and society: the impact of musculoskeletal diseases, edited N.K Hadler and D.B. Gillings (Butterworths, 1985)

Dubois' Lupus erythematosus by D.J. Wallace (3rd edn., Lea & Febiger 1987)

Rheumatic diseases and the heart by J.A Cosh and J.V Lever (Springer, 1988)

Connective tissue diseases by G.R. Hughes (3rd edn., Blackwell, 1987)

Autoimmune rheumatic diseases by J. Morrow and D. Eisenberg (Blackwell, 1987)

Neurology

Neurology is a great stronghold of clinical medicine but, like rheumatology, complexity makes it difficult to define; it overlaps very much with psychiatry and cannot be separated from neurophysiology and the brain sciences generally and embraces neuropathology. The clinical neurologist is, therefore, more affected now than in the past by the work of the neuroscientist and the literature is becoming increasingly interconnected. While the clinical neurologist is a physician whose special concern is with the diagnosis and treatment of disorders of the nervous system, patients often present with psychiatric conditions or neurological sequelae of physical injury.

The literature of neurology is extensive and reflects the diversity of the subject and the developing specialties within the field. There are now only a few journals which attempt to provide total coverage of three or more related areas such as the *Journal of Neurology, Neurosurgery and Psychiatry*, an important title. The other main clinical neurology journals are:

Acta Neurologica Scandinavica

Annals of Neurology

Archives of Neurology

Brain

Journal of Nervous and Mental Disease

Journal of Neurological Sciences

Journal of Neurology

Neurology

Neuropathology and Applied Neurobiology

Several topics have good quality specialist journals such as:

Developmental Medicine and Child Neurology, Epilepsia, Headache, Pain and *Stroke*.

INDEXING AND ABSTRACTING SERVICES

As with many other subjects there are fewer special indexing publications than in the past as the ready availability of computer-based services provides rapid access to current literature citations. *Excerpta Medica; Section 8: Neurology and Neurosurgery* is still the main indexing and abstracting source in the field generally with *Current Opinion in Neurology and Neurosurgery* providing an index, selective abstracts and topic reviews covering the whole of the literature in a twelve month cycle. Specialist abstracting journals are *Muscular Dystrophy Abstracts* and *Epilepsy Abstracts*. Several of the primary journals have short current-literature sections. *Developmental Medicine and Child Neurology* publishes an annual bibliography arranged by topics and covering books as well as journal articles.

REVIEWS

The *Yearbook of Neurology and Neurosurgery* provides a good overview of clinical neurology while *Annual Review of Neuroscience* covers in depth the literature of selected major research topics. *Recent Advances in Clinical Neurology*, edited by Christopher Kennard (No. 6, Churchill Livingstone, 1990) relates basic research to the needs of the clinician in selected subjects such as the neural basis of pain and therapeutic developments in epilepsy. Conference proceedings, reviews and monographs appear in several named series. One such is *Research Publications of the Association for Research in Nervous and Mental Diseases* (ARNMD). These are the proceedings of its annual conference and cover a wide range of topics, including the scientific and the psychiatric. A most important series of this kind is *Advances in Neurology* (Raven Press), publishing high-quality, authoritative, review monographs such as *Neurobehavioral Problems in Epilepsy* (vol. 55, 1991).

A publication which is both a primary and a secondary source is the *Handbook of Clinical Neurology*, edited by P.J. Vinken, G.W. Bruyn and H.L. Klawans (Elsevier, 1968–). Forty-four volumes were published in the original series with a revised series starting with volume 45 in 1984 and planned to produce 27 volumes — volume 14(58) appeared in 1990. The work is very much in the tradition of the great handbooks of the earlier years of this century and is an invaluable reference source both for quality of writing and editing and the range of sources cited. The revised series is not a second edition but rather complements the original work many of whose volumes will be valid for some considerable time.

The progress of neurology, more than of some other disciplines, is signposted by great names and their stories can provide the key to its bibliography. An entry point is *Founders of neurology: one hundred and forty-six biographical sketches ...* edited by W. Haymaker and F. Schiller (2nd edn., C.C. Thomas, 1970), supported by *Neurological classics*, compiled by R.H. Wilkins and I.A. Brody (Johnson Reprint Corp. 1973), which gathers together some good classic descriptions in translation, previously published in *Archives of Neurology*.

TEXTBOOKS

There are several good textbooks. The acknowledged classic Britain text remains *Brain's Diseases of the nervous system*, edited by Sir John Walton (9th edn., Oxford University Press, 1985); it is comprehensive in its coverage and is intended both for the postgraduate and the medical student. The fundamentals of clinical neurology are covered in more detail by the complementary work *Brain's Clinical neurology*, edited by Sir Roger Bannister (6th edn., Oxford University Press, 1985). *Essen-*

tials of neurology by Lord Walton (6th edn., Churchill Livingstone, 1989) is a readable basic textbook with an emphasis on clinical examination and treatment. *Contemporary neurology*, edited by M.J.C. Harrison (Butterworths, 1984) gathers a series of papers first published in the *British Journal of Hospital Medicine* with a strong clinical emphasis at MRCP examination level.

Scientific basis of clinical neurology, edited by Michael Swash and Christopher Kennard (Churchill Livingstone, 1985) discusses current concepts in the neurosciences in relation to the practice of clinical neurology while *Neurology in general medicine*, edited by Michael Aminoff (Churchill Livingstone, 1989) deals particularly with the problems of a neurological nature which may be encountered by non-neurologists and provides a guide to the neurological aspects of general medical disorders and forms a bridge between neurology and other medical specialties.

Special topics are covered by some of the neurological volumes in the Butterworths International Medical Review Series such as *Movement disorders–2*, edited by C.D. Marsden and S. Fahn (Butterworths, 1987) and by:

Neurological Examination in clinical practice by E.R. Bickerstaff and J.A. Spillane (5th edn., Blackwell Scientific Publications, 1989)

The genetics of neurological disorders by M. Baraitser (2nd edn., 1990)

Parkinson's Disease, edited by G.M. Stern (Chapman and Hall, 1990)

Neurological emergencies by E.M.R. Critchley (Saunders, 1988)

A textbook of epilepsy, edited by A.D. Laidlaw (3rd edn., Churchill Livingstone, 1988)

McAlpine's Multiple sclerosis, edited by W.B. Matthews (2nd/4th edn., Churchill Livingstone, 1990)

Wolff's Headache and other head pain, edited by Donald J. Dalessio (5th edn., Oxford University Press, 1987)

The management of motor neurone disease, edited by G.M. Cochrane (Churchill Livingstone, 1987)

Migraine: clinical, therapeutic, conceptual and research aspects, edited by J.N. Blau (Chapman and Hall, 1987)

Clinical Electroencephalography, edited by L.G. Kiloh *et al.* (4th edn., Butterworths, 1981)

Textbook of pain, edited by P.D. Wall and Ronald Melzac (2nd edn., Churchill Livingstone, 1989)

Disorders of voluntary muscle, edited by Sir John Walton (5th edn., Churchill Livingstone, 1988)

HISTORY

The doctrine of the nerves by J.D. Spillane (Oxford University Press, 1981) is a history of neurology whose intention is to show the newcomer to neurology the lie of the land. It can be recommended as a good modern history of the subject.

Medical otorhinolaryngology

Otorhinolaryngology (or otolaryngology) developed over the last hundred or so years as ear, nose and throat surgery (see p. 421). As the need for specialization within the surgical aspects of the field grew and as more conditions became amenable, through the development of new drugs, to non-surgical treatment, the concept of medical otorhinolaryngology emerged with a large amount of medical treatment being delivered by general practitioners.

The main journals in the field are: *American Journal of Otolaryngology, Annals of Otology, Rhinology and Laryngology, Archives of Oto-rhino-laryngology, Clinical Otolaryngology, Journal of Laryngology and Otology* and *Otolaryngologic Clinics of North America*.

The standard textbook in this multi-faceted area remains *Scott-Brown's Otolaryngology*, edited by Alan G. Kerr (5th edn., 6 vols, Butterworth, 1987). Formerly known as *Scott-Brown's Diseases of the ear, nose and throat*, its title change reflects the increased emphasis on topics such as audiology to which a volume is devoted. Volume one is entitled 'Basic sciences' and covers, in addition to anatomy and physiology, speech generation and reception, deglutition, respiration physiology, immunology and chemotherapy. Paediatric otolaryngology has an individual volume reflecting the fact that disorders of the food- and air-passages and of the head and neck generally are among the most common encountered by health professionals caring for children.

Diseases of the nose, throat and ear by I.S. Hall and B.H. Colman (13th edn., Churchill Livingstone, 1987) is a very much more concise book for the student and practitioner. *Dilemmas in otolaryngology* edited by D.F.N. Harrison (Churchill Livingstone, 1988) deals with a number of problems over which there is considerable confusion including the pros and cons of some tests and of the surgical approach to certain conditions. Paediatric otorhinolaryngology is dealt with in depth in *Pediatric otolaryngology*, edited by C.D. Bluestone (2nd edn., 2 vols, Saunders, 1990) where particular emphasis is placed on differential diagnosis.

Occasional updating is provided by *Recent advances in otolaryngology*, edited by R.F. Gray and J. A. Rutka (No. 6, Churchill Livingstone, 1988); other useful titles are: *Mawson's Diseases of the ear*, edited by Harold Ludman (5th edn., Arnold, 1988), *Otitis media in infants and children* by C.D. Bluestone and J.O. Klein (Saunders, 1988), *Logan Turner's Diseases of the nose, throat and ear* edited by A.G.D. Maran (10th edn., Wright, 1988), *Tinnitus* by J.W.P. Hazell (Churchill Livingstone, 1987) and *Dizziness* by Tony Wright (Croom Helm, 1988).

Medical ophthalmology

The importance of sight for survival in primitive societies, coupled with the visibility and accessibility of the organ of sight, the eye, has meant that its diseases have been studied and treated, both medically and surgically, from the very beginnings of medicine. The eye can be affected by a wide range of conditions from simple disorders of the lids through errors of refraction and accommodation such as myopia, to complex conditions whose origins do not lie in the eye itself such as diabetic retinopathy. The eye is also subject to injury, tumours, inflammation, genetic defects and degeneration leading to loss of vision in later life. The condition of the eye may also be an indicator of a systemic disorder which, like sarcoidosis for example, may involve the eye in about 25 per cent of cases. Approaches to ophthalmic disorders therefore, can vary from the preventive to the surgical (see p. 420) and include the wide range of corrective procedures provided by opticians. However, all aspects of the care of sight require practitioners to have a good understanding of the nature of the eye, its disorders and the way in which non-ophthalmological diseases can present with ophthalmic symptoms.

The leading journals in clinical ophthalmology are *British Journal of Ophthalmology*, *American Journal of Ophthalmology*, *Archives of Ophthalmology* and *Eye*. *Recent Advances in Ophthalmology*, edited by S.I. Davidson (No. 8, Churchill Livingstone, 1991) updates on new developments; it will, like all other titles in the series, be published annually from 1991.

All the main textbooks on ophthalmology have substantial sections on the anatomy and physiology of the eye, on the physiology of vision and sometimes on ophthalmic optics. *Physiology of the eye* by Hugh Davson (5th edn., Macmillan, 1990) is a single-volume treatment of the subject which provides a detailed source of reference for both the clinician and the researcher.

Parsons' Diseases of the eye by S.J.H. Miller (18th edn., Churchill Livingstone, 1990) has short, clear chapters ranging from embryology through immunopathology of the eye to the prevention of blindness and the hygiene of vision. In spite of the view of the author that the book is unlikely to be of interest to a UK family doctor because of inadequate ophthalmic out-patient training, it is a very reliable classic. Particularly relevant to the clinician are *The eye in general medicine*, edited by F.C.

Rose (Chapman and Hall, 1983) and *Clinical ophthalmology*, edited by
S.J.H. Miller (Wright, 1987).

The complex relationship between the eye and medicine generally is
dealt with concisely in *The eye in systemic disease* by J.J. Kanski and
D.J. Thomas (2nd edn., Butterworth, 1990), one of an increasing number of titles on the topic.

The glaucomas are an important group of disorders arising from various causes and there is a substantial literature on them. *Becker-Shaffer's
Diagnosis and therapy of the glaucomas*, edited by H.D. Hoskins and
M.A. Kass (6th edn., Mosby, 1989) has been the standard work for a
number of years; *The glaucomas*, edited by Robert Rich and others in
two volumes (Mosby, 1989) is also a comprehensive work. Glaucoma
and many other eye diseases can be inherited to some extent; *Goldberg's Genetic and metabolic eye disease* edited by W.A. Renie (2nd
edn., Little, Brown, 1986) provides good coverage.

Most ophthalmology books are well illustrated; useful diagnostic atlases are *Atlas of ophthalmology* by M.G. Glasspool (MTP, 1982) and
Colour atlas of opthalmological diagnositics by M.A. Bedford (2nd
edn., Wolfe, 1987). Special aspects are covered by *Thyroid eye disease*
by D.H. Char (2nd edn., Churchill Livingstone, 1990) and *Pediatric
ophthalmology* by David Taylor (Blackwell, 1990).

Geriatrics

Demographic changes, particularly in Western Europe and North
America, in the proportion of elderly in the population are placing
greater demands for expertise in geriatric medicine on family doctors
and on practitioners in many of the specialties, including psychiatry.
The specialty of geriatric medicine is of increasing importance and with
its growth, or perhaps ahead of it, have been significant advances in the
study of the biology of ageing. Geriatric medicine, or clinical gerontology, has been defined as the branch of general medicine concerned
with the health and the clinical, social, preventive, and remedial aspects
of illness in the elderly. The elderly are defined by WHO as aged between 60 and 74, while the 'aged' are 75 and over; geriatric medicine is
concerned with these two groups.

As the care of the elderly medically and socially is influenced very
much by the values of society, the literature of geriatrics, in contrast to
that of gerontology, is culturally dependent. This is not to say that a
U.S. textbook is not relevant in the UK though its approach to some aspects of geriatric medicine may differ significantly from that of an
equivalent UK book to a greater extent than, say, a paediatric text
might.

Textbook of geriatric medicine and gerontology, edited by J.C.

Brocklehurst (3rd edn., Churchill Livingstone, 1985, 4th edn. in preparation) and *Principles and practice of geriatric medicine*, edited by M.S.J. Pathy (Wiley, 1985) are two substantial textbooks which address all aspects of the subject, with Brocklehurst being the established text. Both works are well referenced and also deal with theories of ageing and with medical and community care. Both books are British and they have several contributors in common including Professor A.N. Exton-Smith, whose *Practical geriatric medicine*, edited with M.E. Weksler (Churchill Livingstone, 1985) is a good clinical text of just under 500 pages, or half the length of the other two. There are many short general texts in geriatric medicine such as *The care of the elderly in general practice* by M.K. Thompson (Churchill Livingstone, 1984).

Medicine in old age is a series published by Churchill Livingstone each volume of which deals with a specific aspect of geriatric medicine which includes some of the following titles: *Prevention of disease in the elderly*, edited by J.A. Muir Gray (Churchill Livingstone, 1985); *The psychiatry of late life*, edited by R. Levy and Felix Post (Blackwell, 1982); *Psychological assessment of the elderly*, edited by J.P. Wattis and I. Hindmarch (Churchill Livingstone, 1988); *Geriatric psychiatry*, edited by E.W. Busse and D.G. Blazer (American Psychiatric Press, 1989); *The neurology of the elderly* by R.B. Godwin-Austen and J. Bendall (Springer, 1990); *Delirium in the elderly* by James Lindesay and others (OUP, 1990).

There are relatively few journals in the field; the leading titles with a clinical emphasis are *Age and Ageing, Geriatrics, Journal of the American Geriatrics Society* and *Journal of Gerontology. Advanced Geriatric Medicine*, edited by J.G. Evans and F.I. Caird (Number 7, Wright, 1988) is the proceedings of a regular course and is a useful updating source as are *Recent Advances in Psychogeriatrics* edited by Tom Arie (Number 2, Churchill Livingstone, 1991). *Recent Advances in Geriatric Medicine* edited by Bernard Isaacs (Number 3, Churchill Livingstone, 1985) may produce a new volume in 1991.

Nutrition

An understanding of the nutritional requirements of healthy individuals and how these requirements can change in disease is an important element of a physician's skill. Food in even its simplest form is complex and contains, in addition to the nutrients, many chemically identifiable substances which may cause reactions in the consumer of the food. Even in prosperous countries malnutrition still exists but today it more often arises through the inappropriateness of diet rather than from lack of food. There is a considerable number of diseases which are directly caused by dietary deficiency and there are problems of slow growth in poorly nourished children. The family doctor needs to be able to identify deficiencies in diet through the assessment of nutritional status and to put in place appropriate action to restore a healthy status. Nutritional requirements can change with the onset of disease so that adjustments to diet have to be made; for example, vitamin D needs to be increased in patients with renal disease and the use of certain drugs may also call for nutritional adjustments. The increasing use of processed foods makes this task even more difficult, particularly in situations where manufacturers are not obliged to include detailed statements of composition as is still the case in the UK with manufactured infant-feed preparations some of which have been shown to be deficient in protein.

Davidson's Human nutrition and dietetics by R. Passmore and M.A. Eastwood (8th edn., Churchill Livingstone, 1986) is a substantial introductory account of the role of nutrition and dietetics in promoting health and in preventing and treating disease. It is a well-referenced work which includes a detailed listing of food tables for a number of countries, diet sheets and analysis of commercially available oral and tube feed preparations. *Nutrition in the clinical management of disease*, edited by J.W.T. Dickerson and Harry A. Lee (2nd edn., Arnold, 1988) places particular emphasis on the diseases, or conditions, which require nutritional management.

McCance and Widdowson's The composition of foods by A.A. Paul and D.A.T. Southgate (4th edn., HMSO, 1978) was originally published in 1940 as *Medical Research Council Special Report No. 297* and is the authoritative work on the subject, providing in tabular form the composition of all foods available in the UK including proprietary brands from 'Mars Bars' to 'Oxo' cubes. It is updated and expanded by a series of supplements on specific topics such as 'Immigrant foods' (1985) and 'Milk products and eggs' (1989) with others in preparation. The supplements are now published jointly by the Royal Society of Chemistry and the Ministry of Agriculture, Fisheries and Food; there are also computer software packages containing the data available. The book and the supplements also contain recipes. Paediatric aspects of nutrition are covered by *Clinical nutrition in paediatric disorders* by Donald Bentley and Margaret Lawson (Baillière Tindall, 1988) and *Diets for sick children* by D.E.M. Francis (4th edn., Blackwell, 1987).

Food allergy and intolerance, edited by J. Brostoff and S.J. Challacombe (Baillière Tindall, 1987) is a substantial work of 61 chapters and over 80 contributors, providing a scientific basis for the clinical observation and treatment of the problems caused by food allergies. There is particular emphasis on the factors underlying food allergy with 16 detailed chapters on basic mechanisms and an extensive section on the diagnosis of food-allergy problems.

Nutritional standards and the history of food and nutrition in the UK are provided by:

Human energy requirements: a manual for planners and nutritionists by W.P.T. James and E.C. Schofield (OUP, 1990)

The dietary and nutritional survey of British adults, commissioned jointly by the Ministry of Agriculture, Fisheries and Food and the Department of Health (HMSO, 1990)

Height, health and history: nutritional status in the United Kingdom, 1750–1980 by R. Floud and others (CUP, 1990)

Diet and health in Modern Britain, edited by D.J. Oddy and D.S. Miller (Croom Helm, 1985)

Clinical nutrition journals include *American Journal of Clinical Nutrition, British Journal of Nutrition, European Journal of Clinical Nutrition, Journal of Nutrition* and *Nutrition Reviews* and are supplemented by special aspect titles such as *International Journal of Eating Disorders, Journal of Pediatric Gastroenterology and Nutrition, Journal of the American Dietetic Association* and *Nutrition and Cancer. Annual Review of Nutrition* provides a regular overview of recent developments.

CHAPTER SIXTEEN

Diagnostic radiology

MAUREEN FORREST

Radiology differs from the other medical sciences since it has no apparent antecedents in the ancient world. It is a direct consequence of the scientific and technological discoveries of the nineteenth and twentieth centuries and its development reflects the advances in these fields. It is, consequently, a highly dynamic discipline to which new techniques are constantly being added. In order to study the literature, it is necessary to have a basic understanding of the terminology which is itself constantly evolving and has complex relationships which are full of pitfalls for the unwary. For example, 'imaging' which used to refer to techniques which displayed images on screens, has now become largely synonymous with the broader term 'radiology'; emission tomography is part of nuclear medicine but nuclear magnetic resonance is not. The term 'radiology' itself only emerged after various alternatives, such as skiagraphy and actinography, had been discarded and it has an equally popular synonym, the eponymous roentgenology, which is widely used in the USA and Europe. Radiology has two main applications: diagnostic and therapeutic. This chapter covers the diagnostic function and includes interventional radiology.

History

Radiology was conceived from principles laid down in the seventeenth and eighteenth centuries and its birth can be dated precisely as 8 November 1895 when Wilhelm Röntgen, Professor of Physics at the University of Würzburg, first observed the phenomenon of the x-ray, a discovery for which he was awarded the Nobel Prize in 1901. The technique aroused great public interest in the UK where it was exhibited in the music halls, became the subject of satirical verses in *Punch* and was demonstrated to the Prince of Wales. The medical profession adopted it immediately and the Roentgen Society, a forerunner of the British Institute of Radiology, was established in 1897. Today, as then, it is a multidisciplinary society and membership is open to all persons interested in radiology and allied subjects. Roentgenology was the preferred name for the new science, in deference to the discoverer, but it fell from favour in the UK during World War I when it was replaced by the less emotive 'radiology'. The Royal Society of Medicine Section of Radiology, which developed from the British Electrotherapeutic Society, was established in 1931 and the Royal College of Radiologists, previously the Faculty of Radiologists, came into being in 1975. A detailed account of these events is given in *Pioneers and early years: A history of British radiology* by E.H. Burrows (Colophon, 1986).

Radiology quickly became an established branch of medicine and improved x-ray techniques and equipment were introduced. Postwar research, founded on military technology, led to the introduction of major new systems based largely on the research of the eminent Curie family. Marie and Pierre Curie discovered naturally-occurring radioactivity which formed the basis of nuclear medicine and radiotherapy. Pierre Curie also discovered the piezo-electric effect on which ultrasound is based and distinguished various kinds of magnetism which led to the development of magnetic resonance imaging. They were awarded the Nobel Prize for Physics in 1903 and Marie Curie received the Nobel Prize for Chemistry in 1911. Their daughter, Irène, and her husband, Frédéric Joliot were awarded the Nobel Prize in 1935 for their discovery of artificial radioactivity which is used today. Another Nobel laureate, Georg von Hevesy, invented the tracer method which used isotopes to show plant and animal function and is now used in nuclear medicine. By the 1960s, ultrasound and radionuclide imaging were widely used and 1973 saw the announcement of computed tomography, a discovery which earned Godfrey Hounsfield and Allan Cormack the Nobel Prize in 1979. The most recently developed system is magnetic resonance imaging which was developed from atomic research carried out at the end of World War II. Pioneering work was done at Nottingham University but the first magnetic resonance imaging technique is attributed to Paul Lauterbur who generated the first two-dimensional image of a proton in 1973. The high cost of the equipment required for this process has slowed down its introduction as a standard procedure in hospitals but its use has grown during the last decade. It is now widespread in the USA and is becoming more common in the UK.

Further reading on the history of radiology is provided by *History of x-rays and radium* by R.F. Mould (IPC Building & Contract Journals, 1980). The definitive work is *Trail of the invisible light: from x-strahlen to radiobiology* by E.R.N. Grigg (C.C. Thomas, Springfield, 1965). Detailed coverage of the history of tomography appears in *From the watching of shadows* by S. Webb (Adam Hilger, 1990). *Medicine's new vision* by H. Sochurek (Mack Publishing, Easton, PA, 1988) is a layman's guide to the subject which also includes some historical information.

Textbooks and monographs

Radiologists tend to rely on a small core collection rather than a wide-ranging selection of titles. Several general standard works exist of which four or five are outstanding. Recently publishers have concentrated on the specialized fields of the specific techniques; a significant number of titles have appeared but the standard works have yet to be established and the selection of titles is more subjective. An important factor in building a collection is the high production cost of the good quality half-tone illustrations which are so essential in this subject.

A number of comprehensive standard works are published which include all the radiological techniques and their applications. They are major publications, usually in several volumes and are very expensive. In the forefront of these is *Diagnostic radiology: an Anglo-American textbook of imaging*, edited by R.G. Grainger and D.J. Allison (2nd edn., Churchill Livingstone, 1991). Published in three volumes, it is designed as a working bench book in which 119 contributors from both sides of the Atlantic describe the different techniques of radiology, followed by sections on the applications of the techniques arranged by systems of the body.

Almost as popular is *A textbook for radiology and imaging*, edited by D. Sutton (2 vols, Churchill Livingstone, 1987) which has a similar arrangement. *Paul and Juhl's Essentials of radiologic imaging* (5th edn., J.B. Lippincott, 1987) is used widely in the USA. *Correlative imaging* by M.P. Sandler *et al.* (Williams and Wilkins, 1989) compares and discusses the applications of the different techniques. In *Roentgen signs in diagnostic imaging* by I. Meschan (4 vols, 2nd edn., W.B. Saunders, 1987) the emphasis is on conventional radiology and computed tomography. A major revision of a standard work published under the auspices of the President and Council of the Royal College of Radiologists is currently in progress. This textbook, formerly entitled *A textbook of x-ray diagnosis*, is now published under a revised title: *A textbook of radiological diagnosis* (5th edn., H.K. Lewis, 1984–). Each volume has separate editors; Volumes 1, 2 and 4 have been published so far. *Text-

book of radiology by C.E. Putman and C.E. Ravin (3 vols, W.B. Saunders, 1988) is another multi-volume work. *Diagnostic challenges in radiology* by S.R. Baker (J.B. Lippincott, 1988) aims to re-acquaint radiologists with an approach to the assessment of plain films. *Complications in diagnostic imaging*, edited by G. Ansell and R.A. Wilkins (2nd rev. edn., Blackwell Scientific Publications, 1987) is a standard work covering the not uncommon problem of adverse reactions in patients caused by contrast media and drugs used in imaging techniques.

Building and extending a radiology department — a practical guide to planning and project management by D.J. Manton *et al.* (Royal Society of Medicine Services, 1988) is an up-to-date source for those setting up or developing a department.

Atlases

Atlases are of major importance to the radiologist. *Atlas of normal roentgen variants that may simulate disease*, by T.E. Keats (4th edn., Year Book Medical Publishers, 1988) covers a particularly important aspect since the radiologist must be able to recognize all possible normal presentations if he is to produce a correct assessment of abnormalities. Equally important is *Atlas of normal developmental roentgen anatomy* by T.E. Keats and T.H. Smith (2nd edn., Year Book Medical Publishers, 1977). *Clinical imaging: an atlas of differential diagnosis* by R. L. Eisenberg (3rd edn., Heinemann Medical, 1988) is an outstanding work with high-quality photographs. *A colour atlas of human anatomy* by R. M. H. McMinn and R.T. Hutchings (2nd edn., Wolfe Medical, 1988) is an example of a good general anatomical atlas which is a basic requirement for the radiologist. *Sectional anatomy by MRI/CT* by G.Y. El-Khoury *et al.* (Churchill Livingstone, 1990), *Atlas of radiological anatomy* by J. Weir and P. Abraham (2nd edn., Churchill Livingstone, 1986) and *Basic atlas of sectional anatomy with correlated imaging* by W.J. Bo *et al.* (2nd edn., W.B. Saunders, 1990) are other recommended titles. *Normal anatomy for multiplanar imaging*, by B. Raval *et al.* (2 vols, Williams and Wilkins, 1987), *Atlas of anatomic correlation in CT and MRI* by P. Gerhardt and W. Frommhold (Georg Thieme, 1988) and *Atlas of axial, sagittal and coronal anatomy (with CT and MRI)*, edited by A.J. Christoforidis (W.B. Saunders, 1988) are further valuable sources.

Student textbooks

Radiology is an integral part of the medical school curriculum and there are a number of textbooks which are designed to provide the medical student with a good, basic grounding in the subject. An excellent overview, with clear explanations of the various techniques is given in

Diagnostic imaging by P. Armstrong and M.L. Wastie (2nd edn., Blackwell Scientific Publications, 1987). *An introduction to clinical imaging* by D. L. Dixon and L.M. Dugdale (Churchill Livingstone, 1988), *Clinical radiology for medical students* by K.T. Evans *et al.* (Butterworths, 1987) and *Radiology and imaging for medical students* by D. Sutton (Churchill Livingstone, 1988) are further examples of clearly-presented introductions to the subject.

Qualified doctors studying for the fellowship examination of the Royal College of Radiologists are fortunate in having an excellent guide available. This low-cost spiral bound publication is *Radiology study guide for passing the fellowship* by K. Simpkins, R. Bartlett and D. Parker (3rd edn., 1987) available from David Parker, c/o X-Ray Secretaries, Dawson Floor, Leeds General Infirmary, Leeds LS1 3EX, price £5.00 including postage. It is divided into two parts: part 1 gives advice on how to prepare for and tackle the examination; part 2 consists of a list of selected references. Its highly practical, common-sense approach provides all the information the candidate requires to support his clinical knowledge and the excellent reading list provides librarian and student alike with a clear insight into the literature. Its fragile format makes it unsuitable for a lending collection but its cost makes it an essential purchase for the individual candidate and a good value reference tool for the library. One of the outstanding textbooks recommended in this guide is *Aids to radiological differential diagnosis* by S. Chapman and R. Nakielny (2nd edn., Baillière Tindall, 1990) which, although not illustrated, is an excellent, clearly-presented guide to the subject with references for further reading given at the end of each chapter. Other useful titles which post-date the guide are *MCQs on diagnostic imaging* by J.E. Dacie (Churchill Livingstone, 1988) and *Imaging in clinical practice* by A.G. Chalmers *et al.* (Edward Arnold, 1988).

Techniques

NUCLEAR MEDICINE

This technique differs from other types of diagnostic imaging since it is used to show physiological function rather than morphology. It employs radioactive isotopes which emit gamma-rays as they decay and which are tagged to specific substances which concentrate selectively in different parts of the body. This method includes emission tomography in which a gamma-camera moves round the patient to produce sectional images on a computer, similar to x-ray computed tomography. *Freeman and Johnson's Clinical radionuclide imaging* by L.M. Freeman and P.M. Johnson (3 vols, Grune and Stratton, 1984–85) is a major work on the subject and *Practical nuclear medicine*, edited by P.F. Sharp and

H.G. Gemmell (IRL Press, 1989), is also a favoured text. A *Clinical manual of nuclear medicine* by J.M. Walker and D. Margouleff (Appleton-Century-Crofts, 1984), *Practical nuclear medicine*, edited by P.F. Sharp *et al.* (IRL Press, 1990), *Textbook of nuclear medicine* edited by J. Harbert *et al.* (2 vols, 2nd edn., Lea and Febiger, 1984) and *Sensitivity and specificity of gamma scintigraphic procedures* by M.L. Goris (Year Book Medical Publishers, 1985) are other useful titles. *An atlas of clinical nuclear medicine* by I. Fogelman and M. Maisey (Martin Dunitz, 1988) and *Atlas of nuclear medicine*, edited by D. Van Nostrand and S. Baum (J.B. Lippincott, 1988) are well-produced atlases.

ULTRASOUND

In diagnostic ultrasound, very high frequency sound is directed into the body from a transducer placed in contact with the skin on which a jelly-like substance has been smeared to aid acoustic contact. The high-frequency signal produces an image of interfaces which reflect the sound on to a screen. The technique is non-invasive and so is particularly valuable for fetal monitoring. *Clinical diagnostic ultrasound* by E. Barnett and P. Morley (Blackwell, 1985) is an excellent textbook. A basic introduction is provided by *Diagnostic ultrasound principles, instruments and exercises* by F.W. Kremkau (3rd edn., W.B. Saunders, 1989), *Practical ultrasound*, edited by R.A. Lerski (IRL Press, 1988) and *Basic clinical ultrasound* by H.B. Meire and P. Farrant (British Institute of Radiology, 1982).

Doppler ultrasound is used to show speed of movement, for example the flow rate of blood through the heart or blood vessels. *Doppler ultrasound: physics instrumentation and clinical applications* by D.H. Evans *et al.* (Wiley, 1989) and *Clinical applications of Doppler ultrasound* by K.J.W. Taylor *et al.* (Raven Press, 1988) give a good insight into the subject.

COMPUTED TOMOGRAPHY

CT scanners are complex machines which use an enhanced version of conventional x-rays. The x-ray tube moves round the patient and the image, which is derived from hundreds of measurements of x-ray absorption, is displayed on a grid on a computer monitor. A view of the tissues in cross-section is produced on which the organs are not superimposed. *Computed body tomography: with MRI correlations* by J.K. Lee *et al.* (2nd edn., Raven Press, 1989) is a standard work. *Computed, tomography of the whole body*, edited by J.R. Haaga and R.J. Alfidi (2nd edn., Mosby, 1988) is a comprehensive work in two volumes. Other notable titles are *Computed tomography of the body: a radiological and clinical approach* by J.E. Husband and I.K. Fry (Macmillan,

1985), *Whole body computed tomography: practical image analysis* by O.H. Wegener (Karger, 1983) and *Computed tomography review*, edited by J. Husband (Churchill Livingstone, 1989). *Computed tomography in the evaluation of trauma* by M.P. Federle and M. Brant-Zawadzki (2nd edn., Williams and Wilkins, 1986) and *Computed tomography in trauma* by B.D. Toombs and C.M. Sandler (W.B. Saunders, 1987) cover the application of the technique in trauma.

MAGNETIC RESONANCE IMAGING (MRI)

Originally known as nuclear magnetic resonance (NMR), this technique was subsequently renamed to the present, less emotive one. It is the latest technique to be introduced and is based on the use of a magnetic field which causes the protons in the hydrogen atoms of the body to align with the magnetic force and then relax to their original position in the field, after being excited by an applied radio frequency. The speed and volume of their return is assessed and measured by a computer which displays a diagnostic image on a monitor. Views can be taken in cross-section (axial), front to back (coronal), from side to side (sagittal) or even obliquely. The patient lies in a gantry in which a large circular magnet is housed. No ionizing radiation is involved and the technique is non-invasive. Its main applications to date are in the brain and musculoskeletal systems. *Clinical magnetic resonance imaging*, by R.R. Edelman and J.R. Hesselink (W.B. Saunders, 1990) and *Magnetic resonance imaging of the body*, edited by C.B. Higgins and H.H. Ricak (Raven Press, 1987) are generally considered to be the leading works. *Clinical magnetic resonance imaging*, edited by V.M. Runge (J.B. Lippincott, 1990), *Manual of clinical magnetic resonance imaging* by J.P. Heiken *et al.* (Raven Press, 1986), *Magnetic resonance imaging: principles and applications* by D.M. Kean and M.A. Smith (Heinemann, 1986) and *Magnetic resonance imaging* by D.R.C. Stark (Mosby, 1988) are other recommended titles. In *Biomedical magnetic resonance imaging: principles, methodology and applications*, edited by F.W. Wehrli *et al.* (VCH Publishers, 1988) the emphasis is on the technology.

INTERVENTIONAL RADIOLOGY

Radiologists are now able to follow up their diagnoses by carrying out various procedures, under imaging control, which modify or replace surgery. These include occluding vessels, draining abscesses and obtaining biopsy samples. *Interventional radiology*, edited by R.F. Dondelinger *et al.* (Georg Thieme, 1990) is a major work with multicontributors. Other general titles are *Techniques in diagnostic imaging* by G.H. Whitehouse and B.S. Worthington (2nd edn., Blackwell, 1990), *Interventional radiology* by C.A. Athanasoulis *et al.* (W.B. Saunders,

1982), *Interventional ultrasound*, edited by J.P. McGahan (Williams and Williams, 1990) and *Atlas of interventional radiology* by C. Cope *et al*. (J.B. Lippincott, 1990). Emergency techniques are covered in *Emergency interventional radiology* by M.P. Neal *et al*. (Little, Brown, 1989). *Intravascular ultrasound* by N. Bom and J. Roelandt (Kluwer Academic Publishers, 1989) discusses techniques to support interventional procedures. *Angiography: vascular and interventional radiology* by H.L. Abrams (2 vols, 3rd edn., Little, Brown, 1983) is a major work on an important aspect of the subject.

Like physicians, radiologists tend to specialize in specific systems of the body and approach the literature from their specific viewpoint. The following section gives a selection of important textbooks under system divisions.

RADIOGRAPHY

Radiography is a separate, para-medical discipline which is concerned with the positioning of the patient and the production of the image. The literature of the subject is not covered in this chapter but mention must be made of the definitive work *Clark's Positioning in radiography*, edited by R.A. Swallow *et al*. (11th edn., Heinemann, 1986) which covers radiographic technique and two other useful titles: *Radiographic imaging* by D.N. Chesney and M.O. Chesney (4th edn., Blackwell Scientific Publications, 1989) a basic textbook on photographic and imaging processes and *Equipment for diagnostic radiography* by E. Forster (MTP, 1985).

PHYSICS

Hospital physicists are mainly concerned with the monitoring of radio-isotopes and the calibration of the equipment, quality assurance and safety. *Christensen's Physics of diagnostic radiology* by T.S. Curry, III *et al*. (4th edn., Lea and Febiger, 1990) is a major work. Basic coverage is given in *Physics for radiologists* by P.P. Dendy and B. Heaton (Blackwell Scientific Publications, 1987), *Basic physics for medical imaging* by E.G.A. Aird (Heinemann, 1988), *The physics of medical imaging*, edited by S. Webb (Adam Hilger, 1988) and *Principles of radiological physics* by R.J. Wilks (2nd edn., Churchill Livingstone, 1987). The Institute of Physical Sciences in Medicine (formerly the Hospital Physicists Association), produces a valuable series of handbooks on specific topics.

Specific areas; obstetrics and gynaecology; paediatrics

CARDIOTHORACIC SYSTEM

Comparative cardiac imaging, edited by B.H. Brundage (Aspen, 1990) is a major work which includes coloured illustrations. Another useful title is *Clinical cardiac radiology* by K. Jefferson and S. Rees (2nd edn., Butterworth Scientific Publications, 1980). *Magnetic resonance imaging of congenital heart disease* by B.D. Fletcher and M.D. Jacobstein (Mosby, 1988) covers anatomic, angiographic and echocardiographic correlations. Specialized techniques are covered in *Pocket atlas of cardiac and thoracic MRI* by J.J. Brown and C.B. Higgins (Raven Press, 1989), which is useful for training purposes, *Nuclear cardiovascular imaging. Current clinical practice*, edited by M.J. Guiberteau (Churchill Livingstone, 1990), *Guide to cardiac ultrasound* by R.M. Donaldson and C. Westgate (King and Worth, 1985), *Clinical application of cardiac digital angiography*, edited by G.B.J. Mancini (Raven Press, 1988) which has an extensive bibliography and *CT and MRI of the thorax*, edited by E.A. Zerhouni (Churchill Livingstone, 1990). *Non-invasive diagnosis of peripheral vascular disease*, edited by W.R. Felix Jr. (Raven Press, 1988) covers the peripheral vascular system.

Imaging of diseases of the chest by P. Armstrong *et al.* (Year Book Medical Publishers, 1990) is a major work. *Diagnosis of diseases of the chest* by R.G. Fraser and J.A.P. Pare (vols 1 and 2, 3rd edn., W.B. Saunders, 1987–89) is another standard work which is currently being revised. Nuclear medicine applications are discussed in *Pulmonary nuclear medicine* by M.K. Loken (Appleton and Lange, 1987). *Magnetic resonance imaging of the thorax* by M. Sperber and M.C. Kaiser (Warren H. Green, 1987) is an authoritative guide to this application of magnetic resonance imaging which is still at an early stage of development.

GASTROENTEROLOGY

Gastrointestinal radiology: a pattern approach by R.L. Eisenberg (2nd edn., J.B. Lippincott., 1990) provides a good general source on the subject. *Radiology of the esophagus* by D.N. Hupscher (Georg Thieme, 1988) concentrates on contrast radiology and has exhaustive, up-to-date reference lists. *Diagnostic imaging of the liver, biliary tract and pancreas: data analysis and diagnostic procedures* by S. Sakuma *et al.* (Springer-Verlag, 1987) also has high-quality illustrations. *Imaging of the liver, pancreas and spleen*, edited by R.A. Wilkins, published for the Royal College of Radiologists (Blackwell Scientific Publications, 1990), *Ultrasonography of the spleen*, edited by J-N. Bruneton (Springer-Verlag, 1988), *Dynamic radiology of the abdomen: normal and pathologic anatomy* by M.A. Meyers (3rd edn., Springer-Verlag, 1988) and *Intraoperative ultrasonography in hepato-biliary and pancreatic surgery: a practical guide*, edited by G. Gozzetti *et al.* (Kluwer Academic Publishers, 1989) are more specialized sources. *Small bowel radiology: introduction and atlas* by G. Antes and F. Eggemann (Springer-Verlag, 1988) and *X-ray differential diagnosis in small bowel disease: a practical approach* by J.L. Sellink (Kluwer, 1988) are also recommended.

GENITO-URINARY TRACT

The kidney is covered by *Radiology of the kidney* by A.J. Davidson (W.B. Saunders, 1985), *Clinical renal imaging* by W.R. Cattell *et al.* (Wiley, 1989) which is based on clinical experience and *Evaluation of renal function and disease with radionuclides: the upper urinary tract*, edited by M.D. Blaufox (2nd edn., Karger, 1989) which gives very detailed coverage and has high-quality illustrations, and *Techniques and indications in radiology: kidney and urinary tract* by S. Lange (Georg Thieme, 1987) is a well-produced inexpensive pocket guide. *Alimentary tract radiology* by A. R. Margulis and H. J. Burhenne (2 vols, 4th edn., Mosby, 1988) is the standard work on the subject. *Clinical pelvic imaging*, edited by A.C. Friedman *et al.* (Mosby, 1990) is a comprehensive work covering all aspects of the subject. *Clinical urography: an atlas and textbook of urological imaging*, edited by H.M. Pollack (3 vols, W.B. Saunders, 1990) is a new major work. *Uroradiology* by T. Sherwood (Blackwell Scientific Publications, 1980) is a highly-recommended, well-written introduction. Specific sources on ultrasound include *Genitourinary ultrasound: a text/atlas* by B.G. Coleman (Igaku-Shoin, 1988) and *Ultrasound of the prostate* by M. Rifkin (Raven Press, 1988). AIDS is covered by *Radiology of AIDS, edited by M.P. Federle et al.*, which includes extensive up-to-date references.

HEAD AND NECK

Recommended general titles include *Head and neck imaging. Handbooks of diagnostic imaging* by J.M. Unger (Churchill Livingstone, 1987) and *Computed cranial and spinal imaging: a practical introduction* by J.M. Stevens, *et al.* (Heinemann Medical, 1987). *Magnetic resonance imaging and computed tomography of the head and spine* by C.B. Grossman (Williams and Wilkins, 1990) and *Computed tomography of the head and neck* by T.H. Newton *et al.* (Raven Press, 1988) cover more specialized techniques. There are several atlases available notably *MRI of the brain, head, neck and spine. A teaching atlas of clinical applications* by J. Valk (Martinus Nijhoff, 1987), *Magnetic resonance imaging: atlas of the head, neck and spine* by C.M. Mills *et al.*

(Lea and Febiger, 1988), *Cranial and spinal magnetic resonance imaging. An atlas and guide* by D.L. Daniels *et al.* (Raven Press, 1987) and the smaller *Pocket atlas of head and neck MRI anatomy* by R.R. Lufkin and W.N. Hanafee (Raven Press, 1989). *Essential radiology in head injury: A diagnostic atlas of skull trauma* by D. Mok and L. Kreel (Heinemann, 1988) is relatively inexpensive and deals with a difficult subject in a straightforward manner. Tumours are covered by *MRI/CT and pathology in head and neck tumours: A correlative study*, edited by R. Chisin (Kluwer Academic Publishers, 1989) and *Computed tomography and magnetic resonance tomography of intracranial tumours: a clinical perspective*, edited by E. Kazner *et al.* (2nd edn., Springer Verlag, 1989). *Diagnostic imaging of the nose and paranasal sinuses* by G.A.S. Lloyd (Springer-Verlag, 1988) is a new major specialized work. *Maxillofacial imaging* by A.M. Delbalso (Saunders, 1990) and *Panoramic radiology*, edited by O.E. Langland *et al.* (Lea and Febiger, 1989) give good coverage of specific aspects.

MAMMOGRAPHY

Following the Forrest report: *Breast Cancer Screening: Report to the Health Ministers of England, Wales, Scotland and Northern Ireland* (HMSO, 1986) a mass screening programme for early detection of carcinoma of the breast has been introduced in the UK. *Breast cancer detection; mammography and other methods in breast imaging*, edited by W. Bassett and R.H. Gold (2nd edn., Grune and Stratton, 1987) and *Handbook of breast imaging*, edited by M.E. Peters *et al.* (Churchill Livingstone, 1989) provide good coverage of present techniques; *Teaching atlas of mammography* by L. Tabar and P.B. Dean (2nd edn., Thieme, 1985) is an invaluable atlas for the screening mammographer. The use of ultrasound is covered in *Ultrasound mammography* by B-J. Hackeloer *et al.* (Springer-Verlag, 1989) and *Sonomammography: an atlas of comparative breast ultrasound* by P.B. Guyer and K.C. Dewbury (Wiley, 1987).

MUSCULO-SKELETAL SYSTEM

Imaging techniques play a major role in the diagnosis of problems affecting the musculo-skeletal system. A number of standard works are available of which the most outstanding is the definitive, multi-volume *Diagnosis of bone and joint disease* by D. Resnik and G. Niwayama (6 vols, 2nd edn., W.B. Saunders, 1988). Another important title is *Craniospinal magnetic resonance imaging*, edited by S.J. Pomeranz (W.B. Saunders, 1989) which has an extensive bibliography. *Imaging techniques in orthopaedics*, edited by C.S.B. Galasko and I. Isherwood (Springer-Verlag, 1989) is a good general guide to the subject. Other authoritative titles are *Radiology of skeletal trauma* by L.F. Rogers (2 vols, Churchill Livingstone, 1983), *Radiology of skeletal disorders: exercises in diagnosis* by R.O. Murray *et al.* (4 vols, 3rd edn., Churchill Livingstone, 1989), *Roentgen diagnosis of diseases of the bone* by J. Edeiken and P.J. Hodes (2 vols, 4th edn., Williams and Wilkins, 1989) and *Radiology of bone diseases* by G.B. Greenfield (5th edn., J.B. Lippincott, 1990). Specialized works include *Radiology of the foot and ankle*, edited by T.H. Berquist (Raven Press, 1988), *Magnetic resonance imaging of the knee* by J.H. Mink *et al.* (Raven Press, 1987), *Magnetic resonance of the spine* by D.R. Enzmann *et al.* (C.V. Mosby Co., 1990) and *Imaging anatomy of the knee region* by H. Sick and J-L. Burquet (J.F. Bergmann Verlag, 1988) which is a useful source for computed tomography and magnetic resonance imaging applications. *MRI (musculoskeletal system)* by J. Beltran (J.B. Lippincott, 1990) and *Anatomy and MRI of the joints: a multiplanar atlas*, edited by W.D. Middleton and T.L. Lawson (Raven Press, 1988) also concentrate on magnetic resonance imaging. *An atlas of planar and SPECT bone scans* by I. Fogelman and B.D. Collier (Martin Dunitz, 1989) is a superb atlas; *Atlas of skeletal dysplasias* by R. Wynne-Davies *et al.* (Churchill Livingstone, 1985) is a major work; *An atlas of radiological interpretation: the bones* by J.F. Calder and G. Chessell (Wolfe Medical, 1988) is a more modest but valuable source.

NEUROLOGY

Good general coverage is provided by *Brain imaging: techniques and applications*, edited by N.A. Sharif and M.E. Lewis (Ellis Horwood, 1989) and *Imaging of the nervous system*, edited by P. Butler (Springer-Verlag, 1990). This subject is now a major area of application for magnetic resonance imaging and notable titles include *Magnetic resonance imaging of the central nervous system*, edited by M. Brant-Zawadzki and D. Norman (Raven Press, 1987) and *Magnetic resonance imaging in diseases of the nervous system: an introduction* by I. Moseley (Blackwell Scientific Publications, 1988).

OBSTETRICS AND GYNAECOLOGY

Ultrasound is the major radiological technique used in this field since it is non-invasive and so can be used without fear of harming the fetus. *Obstetric ultrasound: how, why and when* by P. Chudleigh and J.M. Pearce (Churchill Livingstone, 1986) is a concise introduction to the subject; *Ultrasound diagnosis in obstetrics and gynaecology* by M. Hansmann *et al.* (Springer-Verlag, 1985) is another general source. *Sectional fetal anatomy in ultrasound* by A. Standach (Springer-Verlag, 1987) has high-quality illustrations. *Obstetrical measurements in ultra-*

sound: a reference manual by A.B. Kurtz and B.B. Goldberg (Year Book Medical Publishers, 1988) contains comprehensive up-to-date references and may well become the standard work. *Ultrasound of the infant brain (Clinics in Developmental Medicine, 92)* by M.I. Levene *et al.* (Blackwell Scientific Publications, 1985) gives excellent coverage of this specialized aspect.

PAEDIATRICS

The definitive work on the subject is *Pediatric x-ray diagnosis: an integrated imaging approach*, edited by J. Caffey (2 vols, 8th rev. edn., Year Book Medical Publishers, 1985) which also has a condensed version *Essentials of Caffey's Pediatric x-ray diagnosis*, edited by F.N. Silverman and J.P. Kuhn (Year Book Medical Publishers, 1990) aimed at general radiologists. Other recommended titles include *Imaging of the newborn infant and young child* by L. Swischuk (3rd edn., Williams and Wilkins, 1988), *Paediatric diagnostic imaging* by C. Gyll and N. Blake (Heinemann, 1985), *Diagnostic imaging in paediatrics* by I. Gordon (Chapman and Hall, 1987) and *Pediatric ultrasonography* by C.K. Hayden and L.W. Swischuk (Williams and Wilkins, 1987). *Clinical paediatric uroradiology* by J.A. Aaronson and B.J. Cremin (Churchill Livingstone, 1984) is a major work and *Radiological atlas of pulmonary abnormalities in children* by E. B. Swingleton *et al.* (2nd edn., W.B. Saunders, 1988) provides excellent illustrations. Computed tomography applications are covered in *Pediatric body CT* by A. Daneman (Springer-Verlag, 1987) and *Paediatric body computed tomography* by M.J. Siegel (Churchill Livingstone, 1988). *Diagnostic imaging of child abuse* by P.K. Kleinman (Williams and Wilkins, 1987) covers an important subject area.

Abstracts and indexes

Radiology is well-represented in the major secondary sources for the medical sciences: *Index Medicus, Excerpta Medica, Current Contents* and the *Science Citation Index*, all of which are now available in hard copy, online and compact disc forms. Detailed descriptions of these sources appear in Chapters 3 and 5. Radiology receives detailed coverage in the *MeSH* headings of *Index Medicus* where a range of terms for the different techniques are given. The subheading 'radiography', combined with the term for the required organ, region or disease, is preferred for references on diagnosis.

Excerpta Medica provides two relevant sections: *Section 14: Radiology* and *Section 23: Nuclear Medicine*. The coverage of this publication, although more selective than *Index Medicus*, is far wider in its range of material since it includes books, reports and conference proceedings in addition to periodical articles. *Current Contents* remains the most up-to-date general source for periodical literature and the *Science Citation Index* provides a unique means of tracing related literature through the citations of a known reference. Specialized sources include *Applied Health Physics Abstracts and Notes*, a UK publication which issues four parts a year containing abstracts covering the world literature, conferences and unpublished reports in all aspects of the subject; the abstracts are coded to a keyword index and subject and author indexes are produced. The U.S. publication *Current Opinion in Radiology* contains review articles which provide an overview of specific subjects together with annotated references and bibliographies. Recommended reading lists, in which the references are ranked in order of importance, are given. *Radiology*, the official journal of the Radiological Society of North America, publishes an annual supplement, the *RSNA Index to Imaging Literature*, which provides author and subject indexes to 35 major radiology journals; the index covers the volumes for the previous three years.

Annuals, reviews and series

These publications provide valuable reviews of the subject which incorporate the rapid new developments so characteristic of the field. As serial publications they are hybrids between books and periodicals and may often be classified in either category depending on the approach of a particular library. Single titles in a series usually stand alone as complete publications which may be purchased separately rather than by subscription to the general title of which they are a part. However, despite the complications of their form, they are useful sources of current data. Churchill Livingstone publishes a number of excellent series all of which can be recommended: *Recent Advances in Radiology and Medical Imaging* appears irregularly and provides a good overview of developments. In *Clinics in Diagnostic Ultrasound*, also published irregularly, each title is a monograph on a particular topic and is published as a separate work. *Contemporary Issues in Computed Tomography and Contemporary Issues in Nuclear Medicine* are fine series providing current data on specific topics. *Handbooks of Diagnostic Imaging* is a series which started in 1987 and now has three titles. Raven Press publishes *Magnetic Resonance Annual* and *Nuclear Medicine Annual* which provide yearly reviews on subjects of current interest. A third title *Ultrasound Annual* mutated in 1988 to become the journal *Ultrasound Quarterly*. The Year Book Series offer *Year Book of Nuclear Medicine* and *Year Book of Diagnostic Radiology* which contain abstracts of major articles with editorial comments. *Progress in Medical Ultrasound* published by Excerpta Medica gives comprehensive reviews and comments and includes extensive bibliographies. *Frontiers in European Radiology*, published by Springer-Verlag, provides a communication link with continental developments.

Journals

Journals are a particularly important information source since the potential of the new technologies is still being explored. Practitioners have always recognized the need for rapid dissemination of information and the first radiology journal appeared four months after Roentgen's discovery was announced. This journal, entitled *Archives of Clinical Skiagraphy*, is now published under the title *The British Journal of Radiology* and is the official journal of the British Institute of Radiology. It is published monthly and includes abstracts of the proceedings of the Institute. The American equivalent is *Radiology*, the journal of the Radiological Society of North America. Review journals and those which devote each issue to a specific topic are of major importance since they provide, in effect, a series of up-to-date monographs on the latest developments in each section of the subject. Prominent amongst this group are the 'Seminars' publications: *Seminars in Ultrasound, CT and MR, Seminars in Nuclear Medicine* and *Seminars in Roentgenology* (W.B. Saunders) and *Seminars in Interventional Radiology* (Thieme Medical Publishers) are published quarterly and cover the state of the art and new advances in specific subject areas. Similarly, each issue of *Annals of the ICRP* consists of a report on a particular radiation protection topic; this journal is not confined to medicine but covers all aspects of the subject. *CRC Critical Reviews in Diagnostic Imaging* provides in-depth reviews on specific subjects. *Clinics in Diagnostic Ultrasound* and *Radiologic Clinics of North America* are similar important titles. *Current Problems in Diagnostic Radiology* aims to bring the general radiologist up to date with developments in the specialties. *Nuclear Medicine Communications* is a rapid-communications journal which reports good research and clinical work.

A selection of the major journals, covering all aspects of diagnostic radiology and including some leading foreign-language titles, is given in Table 16.1.

Table 16.1. *Diagnostic radiology journals*

Acta Radiologica
American Journal of
  Neuroradiology
American Journal of
  Roentgenology
Annales de Radiologie
Annals of Nuclear Medicine
  (Japan)
Annals of the ICRP
Applied Radiation and Isotopes
Australasian Radiology
British Journal of Radiology
Cardiovascular and
  Interventional Radiology
Clinical Imaging
Clinical Nuclear Medicine
Clinical Physics and
  Physiological Measurement
Clinical Radiology
Computerized Medical Imaging
  and Graphics
CRC Critical Reviews in
  Diagnostic Imaging
Current Opinion in Radiology
Current Problems in Diagnostic
  Radiology
Diagnostic Imaging
European Journal of Nuclear
  Medicine
European Journal of Radiology
Gastrointestinal Radiology
Health Physics
Investigative Radiology
Journal Belge de Radiologie
Journal de Radiologie
Journal of Clinical Ultrasound
Journal of Computer Assisted
  Tomography
Journal of Interventional
  Radiology

Journal of Medical Imaging
Journal of Nuclear Medicine
Journal of Radiological
  Protection
Journal of the Canadian
  Association of Radiologists
Journal of Thoracic Imaging
Journal of Ultrasound in
  Medicine
Magnetic Resonance in Medicine
Medical Physics
Neuroradiology
Nuclear Medicine and Biology
Nuclear Medicine
  Communications
Pediatric Radiology
Physics in Medicine and Biology
Radiation Research
Radiographics
Radiography Today
Radiologia Medica
Radiologic Clinics of North
  America
Radiological Protection Bulletin
Radiology
RöFo (Fortschritte auf dem
  Gebiete der Röntgenstrahlen
  und der neuen bildgebenden
  Verfahren
Seminars in Interventional
  Radiology
Seminars in Nuclear Medicine
Seminars in Roentgenology
Seminars in Ultrasound, CT and
  MR
Skeletal Radiology
Ultrasonics
Ultrasound in Medicine and
  Biology
Urologic Radiology

Quality assurance

The Government White Paper *Working for patients* (HMSO, 1989) has highlighted the value of quality assurance but radiologists have always recognized the need to maintain standards in their highly technical, potentially dangerous discipline. The World Health Organization provides guidance in *Quality assurance in diagnostic radiology* (WHO, 1982) and *Quality assurance in nuclear medicine: a guide prepared following a workshop held in Heidelberg 17-21 November 1980* (WHO, 1982). The British Institute of Radiology has produced guidelines covering all imaging techniques: *Assurance of quality in the diagnostic x-ray department* issued by the Quality Assurance Working Group of the Diagnostic Methods Committee of the British Institute of Radiology (B.I.R., 1988) and *Technical and physical parameters for quality assurance in medical diagnostic radiology* (B.I.R., 1989). Other useful sources include *Practical guide to quality assurance in medical imaging* by B.M. Moores *et al.* (Wiley, 1987) and *The clinician's guide to diagnostic imaging: cost effective pathways* by Z.D. Wossman (Raven Press, 1987). *Quality assurance and image artifacts in magnetic resonance imaging* by R. James *et al.* (Little, Brown, 1988) provides guidance in these specialized techniques.

Safety regulations

Since radioactive materials are fundamental to radiology, the protection of both patient and practitioner is of prime importance and safe practice is governed by legislation supported by expert guidelines. In the UK, the relevant Acts of Parliament are the Radioactive Substances Acts 1948 and 1960 and the Health and Safety at Work Act 1974 together with Statutory Instrument No. 1333 The Ionising Radiations Regulations 1985 in which the permitted dose limits are laid down. These limits are now qualified by additional guidance produced by the Health and Safety Commission *Draft Approved Code of Practice, Part 4: Dose Limitation — Restriction of Exposure. Additional Guidance on Regulation 6 of the Ionising Radiations Regulations 1985 (IRR85)* (Health and Safety Executive, 1990). This draft, which is expected to be adopted in 1991, was produced as a result of *Interim Guidance in the Implications of Recent Revisions of Risk Estimates and the ICRP 1987 Como Statement — NRPB — GS9* (National Radiological Protection Board, 1987). More general guidance on the application of IRR85 is contained in *Health and Safety Commission. Approved Code of Practice Parts 1 & 2. The Protection of Persons Against Ionising Radiation Arising From Any*

Work Activity. Pt. 3. Exposure to Radon. Another Statutory Instrument — Ionising Radiation (Protection of Persons Undergoing Medical Examination or Treatment) Regulations 1988 (S.I. 1988 No. 778) is a national implementation of EEC Directive 84/466/Euratom. Further guidance is provided by the Department of Health which issues circulars and guidelines on specific aspects of safe practice in hospitals. There are also a number of British Standards Institution specifications covering equipment and procedures.

Safety and protection are constantly monitored and researched by a network of national organizations brought together in the International Commission on Radiological Protection. This body was founded in 1928 to be a forum in which representatives of the national bodies could meet to disseminate information and to produce general guidance. Its communication channel is *Annals of ICRP* which consists of a number of single documents, published irregularly. Notable amongst these are *Protection against ionizing radiation from external sources used in medicine (ICRP Publication 33). Annals of the ICRP 1982 9, 1* and *Protection of the patient in diagnostic radiology (ICRP Publication 34). Annals of the ICRP 1982 9, 2/3*. The UK is represented on the Commission by members of the National Radiological Protection Board (NRPB) which was created in 1970 following the Radiological Protection Act. Its function is to give advice, to conduct research and to provide technical services in the field of radiation protection. Since 1977 it has been required to give advice on the application in the UK of standards recommended by international bodies including the EEC and to specify Energy Reference Levels of dose. Its documents contain both formal advice on standards of protection and guidance on their application in practice. *Guidance notes for the protection of persons against ionising radiations arising from medical and dental use* (HMSO, 1988) which was produced by NRPB in conjunction with the Health and Safety Executive and the Departments of Health for the UK, contains a comprehensive list of Acts, regulations and reports issued by NRPB and other relevant bodies. Recently, it has produced a joint report with the Royal College of Radiologists *Patient dose reduction in diagnostic radiology (Documents of the NRPB Vol. 1, No. 3, 1990)* which contains important revised guidance on dose levels and procedures. The equivalent American body is the U.S. National Council on Radiation Protection and Measurements. Two of its major reports are *Medical x-ray, electron beam and gamma-ray protection for energies up to 50 MeV (equipment design, performance and use). NRCP Report No. 102* and *Radiation protection for medical and allied health personnel NRCP Report No. 105*. The United Nations has also issued an important report which brings together international practice: *Sources, effects and risks of ionizing radiation:* issued by the United Nations Scientific Committee on the

Effects of Atomic Radiation 1988, Report to the General Assembly, with annexes (United Nations, 1988).

The British Radiological Protection Association was formed in 1965 to represent the interests of members of existing UK radiological societies at an international level through the International Radiation Protection Association. In collaboration with the British Institute of Radiology it has produced two useful manuals which give guidance on the responsibilities of the practitioner: *Radiation protection of the patient: A manual of good practice. Pt. 1: Diagnostic radiology*, edited by W. A. Langmead (British Institute of Radiology, n.d.) and *Radiation protection of the patient in nuclear medicine: A manual of good practice*, edited by W.A. Langmead (OUP, 1983).

Acknowledgements

Among the many friends and colleagues who have given me help and support, I should like to thank four people without whose expert advice this chapter could not have been written. They are: Mrs. Gunnel Ingham, Librarian, British Institute of Radiology, Mr. David Perry, Librarian, National Radiological Protection Board, Dr. Basil Shepstone, University Department of Radiology and Dr. David Lindsell, Department of Radiology, John Radcliffe Hospital, Oxford. I am indebted to Victoria Churchward for her skill and tolerance in typing this manuscript. I should also like to remember Jenny Wade, late Librarian of the MRC Clinical Research Centre, Harrow, whose illness and subsequent death prevented her from writing this chapter. The example of her high professional standards and the quality of her work have always been before me as a model and an encouragement in completing this work which I dedicate to her.

CHAPTER SEVENTEEN

Psychiatry

M. GUHA

Psychiatry is defined in *Butterworths' Medical dictionary* as 'The branch of medicine dealing with disorders involving mental life and behaviour'. It is, therefore, by Butterworths' definition, a medical discipline. It differs, however, from many of the other medical disciplines discussed in this book in that it overlaps substantially with non-medical disciplines and professions. It is the only area of 'medical' practice in which the English law (and that of many other countries) lays down statutory powers for social workers and nurses. A substantial proportion of relevant therapeutic work within the health service is carried out by occupational therapists and by clinical psychologists. To an even greater extent, outside the health service, the treatment of disorders involving mental life and behaviour is carried out by qualified, but not necessarily medically-qualified, psychoanalysts, and by counsellors from a very wide range of backgrounds. It would therefore be more true to say that psychiatry is a multidisciplinary subject dealing with disorders involving mental life and behaviour. The multidisciplinary nature of psychiatry has considerable effects on the psychiatric librarian, who will have to deal with readers from a wide range of backgrounds, whose literary interests cover the subject range of half a university library. An inquiry regarding 'schizophrenia', for example, might be for a look at Nijinsky's drawings (in the collection of psychotic art at Bethlem Royal Hospital), or for the neuroanatomy of the right cerebral hemisphere, or for the latest developments in molecular pharmacology, or for a sociological analysis of the distribution of schizophrenia by region, income group or social class, or even, be from a philosopher firmly convinced that there is no such thing — that what we are looking at is merely an artefact of society.

Figure 17.1 shows the main areas and topics covered by psychiatry and its related disciplines. The material quoted in the present chapter is for the most part confined to the 'inner circle', with fewer side glances towards medicine and biology, which are covered by other sections of the book, than towards the behavioural and social sciences, with which the user of medical literature may be less familiar. This chapter, therefore, can only touch on some portions of the wide range of literature used by psychiatric readers.

The difference between psychiatry and the rest of medicine should not be over-emphasized to the extent of ignoring the basic medical literature. The medical information sources discussed elsewhere in this book all, potentially, have something to contribute to psychiatry — the existence of *Psychological Abstracts*, for example, does not mean that psychiatrists should not use *Index Medicus* as a first port of call when looking for journal papers.

Classification and definition

The care of the sick can be redefined as the correction of abnormalities. In most medical specialties 'abnormalities' are so obvious as not to require a definition — a child with measles or with a broken leg differs from a 'normal' child in such a clear-cut way that no medical practitioner is going to spend much time on the problem of differentiating 'normal' from 'abnormal'. One only has to consider the implications of declaring someone to be unfit to plead to a criminal charge because of being 'of unsound mind' or of deciding whether particular sexual practices are criminal deviations, or of differentiating between an 'alcoholic' and a 'social drinker', to appreciate that things are very different in psychiatry. Definition is of particular importance, because psychiatrists do have certain legal powers entitling them to treat patients against their will (something that is highly unusual in most branches of medicine), so the definition of a disorder must be precise enough to stand up to legal inspection.

A further problem in definition is that, although the word 'cancer' probably causes more shock and horror in lay hearers than any other single medical term, most illnesses do not carry any great social stigma, while psychiatric illnesses still do. A public figure who has a heart attack or an ulcer can happily admit to the illness, and gain public sympathy for being clearly overworked. A 'nervous breakdown' (let alone, say, an 'alcohol problem') from the same cause is much more likely to be hushed up. This has helped lead to a rapid turnover of termi-

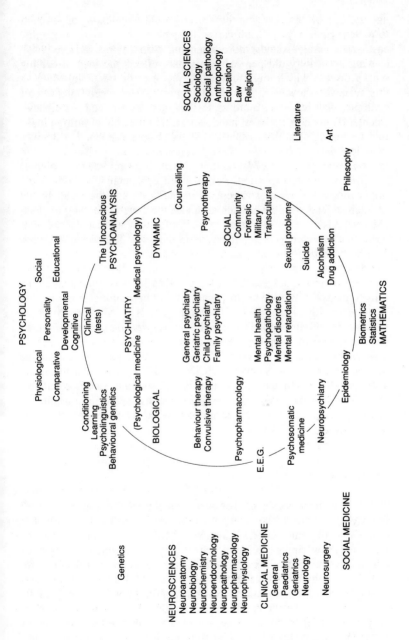

Figure 17.1 Psychiatry and its related disciplines (adapted from Elliott, 1971)

nology. In part, the changing terminology reflects changing approaches to patient care. Saying 'I am caring for patients with Alzheimer's disease' not merely sounds more imposing than saying 'I have a job looking after dotty old people' but it also reflects the idea of dealing with a disease which might ultimately prove to be treatable. Much of this turnover, however, is just euphemistic. The term 'idiocy', for example, was replaced, more or less in turn, by 'mental deficiency', 'mental retardation', 'mental handicap', and at the time of writing looks like becoming 'learning disability'. This change happened so rapidly that the *American Journal of Mental Deficiency* actually changed title to the *American Journal on Mental Retardation* in the middle of a volume.

Given the strong social stigma attached to mental illness, the legal implications of defining someone as mentally ill, and the broad spread of interests and opinions subsumed under the general heading of 'Psychiatry', it is scarcely surprising that classification, and the definition of terms, are regarded as being of crucial importance. The core publication here is the *Diagnostic and statistical manual of the American Psychiatric Association* currently in a revised version (1987) of its third edition, and known universally as DSM-III-R. DSM-III was published at the same time as the World Health Organization *International classification of diseases*, 9th edn. (ICD-9). The publication of DSM-IV is scheduled to coincide with that of ICD-10, so the 'R' was inserted as an intermediate publication, to keep them in sequence. It should be noted that these classification schemes are very different. The DSM categories cannot be seen as an extension of those of ICD. DSM-III-R has been translated into a number of languages, and, in spite of its strong American cultural bias, seems to be generally regarded as authoritative, at least in the sense of being regarded as the common base on which to ground any arguments about classification.

Dictionaries

There are a considerable number of dictionaries which cover portions of the psychiatric field. The most authoritative is probably the *Psychiatric dictionary* (6th edn., by R.J. Campbell, OUP, 1989), which is my first resort for answering general psychiatric enquiries, in spite of some of its curious idiosyncrasies regarding the length and amount of detail in entries, and regarding cross-referencing (the McNaughton Case, for example, is indexed under 'Rule, McNaughton' but not under 'McNaughton'). The sixth edition was produced following the publication of DSM-III-R, so it can be assumed that the seventh will follow DSM-IV. This is the only general dictionary of psychiatry to have produced more than a couple of editions. The Association's *American psychiatric glossary* (6th edn., American Psychiatric Press, 1988) can be used as a very simple dictionary however, also incorporating the DSM-III-R nomenclature, and is possibly more suitable for use by non-psychiatrists. H. Walton's *Dictionary of psychiatry* (Blackwell, 1985) is another small basic dictionary, with an English and ICD-9 bias rather than U.S. and DSM-III-R bias.

There is no classification scheme in psychology to compare directly with DSM-III-R. The nearest equivalent is the American Psychological Association *Thesaurus of psychological index terms* (5th edn., 1988) which lists psychological terms both by relationship and in alphabetical order. This acts as the authority file for *Psychological Abstract* and its related on-line and compact disk versions, in the same way that the *MeSH* headings do for *Index Medicus*.

There seem to be more dictionaries of psychology than dictionaries of any other subject. The most informative, though already in need of some updating, is probably the *Encyclopedic dictionary* (edited by R. Harre and R. Lamb, Blackwell, 1983) and the handiest for personal use is the *Penguin dictionary of psychology* (rev. edn. 1985). Others which can be recommended are the *Macmillan dictionary of psychology* (edited by Stuart Sutherland, 1989) which falls somewhere between the first two in size and depth, and is particularly useful for its coverage of terms on the hard science, rather than the social science fringes of psychology; the *Dictionary of concepts in general psychology* (edited by J.A. Popplestone and M.W. McPerson, Greenwood Press, 1988), which acts as a useful counterbalance to Sutherland in being more social-science based; and the *Longman dictionary of psychology and psychiatry* (1984). Portions of the *Social science encyclopedia* (Routledge, 1988) have been published separately in the Social Science Lexicons series. These include *A lexicon of psychology, psychiatry and psychoanalysis* (1988) and *Social problems and mental health* (1988). Though the publisher can be criticized for publishing bits of the same text in two different forms, this does bring portions of a major reference work down to student price levels.

The psychotherapies, and, in particular, psychoanalysis, present considerable problems to the lexicographer, in that terms are used differently, and often polemically by different writers. Stuart Sutherland's bias against psychoanalysis, for example, renders his dictionary entertaining, but virtually useless for a study of this field. Sue Walrond-Skinner's *Dictionary of psychotherapy* (1986) is a good basic dictionary for the whole field of psychotherapy, mediating calmly between different schools of thought whose use of terminology has often been the basis for bitter wrangling. J. La Planche and J.B. Pontalis' *The language of psychoanalysis* (new edition, 1988) provides the best guide to the language of psychoanalysis in particular. The neurosciences present a different lexicographical problem, in that they are developing so rapidly as to make dictionaries out of date practically as soon as they are printed. As well as the general scientific reference works discussed in Chapter 4, the most current dictionary in the field at the time of writing is D.M. Goodwin's *Dictionary of neuropsychology* (Springer, 1989).

Directories

Psychiatrists are doctors, and can therefore be traced through the appropriate medical directories. The British Association of Psychotherapists publishes a *Roster*, which is 'for members only'. The British Psychological Association has recently received a Royal Charter and now publishes a directory which includes its members' professional interests, making it possible to trace clinical psychologists. The American Psychiatric Association and the American Psychological Association both publish massive biographical directories of all their members, and the *International directory of psychologists exclusive of the USA* (edited by K. Pawlik, 4th edn., Elsevier, 1985) gives at least some information about 32 000 non U.S. psychologists.

Encyclopaedias and general reference works

It should be emphasized again that all general medical reference works are likely to be of value to readers in search of psychiatric information. Among specialized reference works the *International encyclopaedia of psychiatry, psychology, psychoanalysis and neurology*, in 12 volumes plus a 1983 update, edited by Wolman (Van Nostrand Reinhold, 1977) is, of course, already dated as regards terminology, but is nevertheless a very useful reference tool covering the whole field. There are a number of encyclopaedias of psychology available, and at least one major work is in preparation. The *Encyclopedia of psychology* edited by R.J. Corsini (4 vols, Wiley, 1984) is currently useful. This is also available in one-volume form (Wiley, 1987), produced by cutting the length of many of the entries and removing the bulk of the historical, biographical and bibliographical material. The *Oxford companion to the mind* (edited by R.L. Gregory, OUP, 1987) and the *Encyclopedic dictionary of psychology* (mentioned above) are also good reference tools.

Information relevant to psychiatry can also be found in specialized encyclopaedias in other academic fields. The *Social science encyclopedia* (mentioned above) is only the latest in a series of scholarly works in the field, most notable among which are the *International encyclopedia of the social sciences* (17 vols, Macmillan, 1968) and its predecessor, the *Encyclopedia of the social sciences* (15 vols, Macmillan, 1930). These last two are complementary, rather than being a new edition replacing an old one. It is necessary to use both to cover the historical development of a subject. A surprising range of useful information can also be found in the *Encyclopedia of philosophy* (8 vols, Macmillan, 1967).

Biochemical and pharmacological reference tools of immense importance to psychiatry will have been covered in chapters 8 and 10 of this book, and so will not need to be mentioned here. Attention should be drawn however to the *Encyclopedia of neuroscience* (2 vols, Birkhauser, 1987) as a major reference work in a rapidly-changing field, and to the *Encyclopedia of statistical sciences* (9 vols, Wiley, 1982–88) as a useful source of information on epidemiological research methods.

Handbooks

The preface to the *Handbook of psychiatry* (5 vols, CUP, 1982–5) under the general editorship of Michael Shepherd, enthusiastically quotes the late Lord Taylor as saying that modern British psychiatry is 'largely the product of the Maudsley Hospital'. As this handbook is also largely a product of the Maudsley Hospital it should have pride of place in this section. The *American handbook of psychiatry* (2nd edn., 8 vols, Basic Books, 1974) is now very dated, but *Psychiatry* (Lippincott, 1985–) under the editorship of J.O. Cavenar is in three loose-leaf volumes, which facilitates updating, and can be used as the DSM-III based equivalent to it.

The neurosciences are particularly well catered for in handbooks, the most notable (if only for sheer size) being the *Handbook of clinical neurology* (Elsevier, 1969–, currently in 56 volumes). The others particularly worth mentioning here are Lajtha's *Handbook of neurochemistry* (2nd edn., Plenum, 1982–5, 10 vols), the *Handbook of chemical neuroanatomy* (Elsevier, 1983–) and the *Handbook of psychopharmacology*, edited by Iverson *et al.* (Plenum, 1975–) currently in 21 volumes.

The social sciences and psychology are less well represented in this category of publication, but mention must be made of the *Handbook of social psychology*, 3rd (in fact 4th) edition (Random House, 1985), if only for its extraordinary reduction to two volumes, from five in the previous edition.

Major textbooks

As might be expected, the use of textbooks at a postgraduate level varies with the orientation of the reader. The neuroscientists make very little use of books, while the more social-science-based psychologists use them extensively. In particular there are some areas of psychotherapy and of psychology in which the main medium for publishing is the book rather than the journal, and there are psychoanalysts with half-a-dozen books to their credit (or discredit) who have never published any journal papers. In general it does seem likely that psychiatrists are much more book-orientated than members of other medical disciplines. Medical libraries in some other specialties can survive with virtually no books as long as they keep up their journal subscriptions, and even then will find a sizeable proportion of their potential readership making little or no use of their facilities. Psychiatrists tend to use libraries, and are more likely to use books when they are in them.

Among the most heavily used basic psychiatric texts are the 'Essentials', the 'Companion', and the 'Oxford', from the UK, and the 'Comprehensive', the 'Harvard' and the 'APA' from the USA: The *Essentials of postgraduate psychiatry* (edited by P. Hill *et al.* 2nd edn., Grune and Stratton, 1986) represents the Maudsley Hospital viewpoint, in the same way that the *Handbook of psychiatry* (mentioned above) does. The *Companion to psychiatric studies* (edited by R.E. Kendell and A.K. Zealley, 4th edn., Churchill Livingstone, 1988) by contrast hails from Scotland and has few English contributors. The *Oxford Textbook of psychiatry* (edited by M. Gelder *et al.*, 2nd edn., OUP, 1989) is, of course, self-explanatory in its point of origin.

The fifth edition of the *Comprehensive textbook of psychiatry* 2 vols, edited by H.I. Kaplan and B.J. Sadock (Williams and Wilkins, 1989) was, of course, brought out to follow up DSM-III-R. It stands at the head of a sort of family of books, including the *Synopsis of psychiatry*, a one-volume abridgement for serious students, *Clinical psychiatry*, which extracts portions for use by busy practitioners, and the *Study guide and self examination review for the synopsis of psychiatry*, which is a crammer for examination-passers. The *New Harvard guide to psychiatry* (edited by A.M. Nicholi, Belknap Press, 1988) is the successor to the *Harvard guide to modern psychiatry*. All the contributors come from Harvard Medical School (which is comparatively easy to arrange when one considers that Harvard has over 1800 psychiatrists on its staff!). The *American Psychiatric Press textbook of psychiatry* (edited by J.A.Talbott *et al.*, APP, 1988) is similar in general outlines and approach to the *Comprehensive textbook*, but less than half the size. If only one U.S. textbook can be purchased, the *Comprehensive textbook* is recommended.

In the neurosciences, mention must be made of *Basic neurochemistry* (edited by G. Siegel *et al.*, 4th edn., Raven Press, 1989), *Greenfield's neuropathology* (4th edn., by J.H. Adams *et al.*, Edward Arnold, 1984) *Merritt's Textbook of neurology* (8th edn., by L.P. Rowland, Lea and Febiger, 1990) and *Diseases of the nervous system* (by A.K. Asbury *et al.*, 2 vols, W.B. Saunders/Heinemann, 1986). All these are multi-authored works. Among single-authored books pride of place should go to *Organic psychiatry* by W.A. Lishman (2nd edn., Blackwell, 1987) which, though now much plagiarized, was originally a unique text bridging the gap between neurology and psychiatry.

Massive multi-authored textbooks have materialized in some of the specialized fields within psychiatry. In child psychiatry *Child and adolescent psychiatry* (edited by M. Rutter and L. Hersov, 2nd edn., Blackwell, 1985) is the major established text, and forensic psychiatry has recently produced the *Principles and practice of forensic psychiatry* (edited by R. Bluglass and P. Bowden, Churchill Livingstone, 1990). Other areas, such as addiction research, and the psychiatry of old age are, however, still waiting for the massive multi-authored textbook treatment.

In general the more psychoanalytic and more social-science-based areas of psychiatric work are so fragmented that it is difficult to pinpoint the 'major texts' among the vast range of literature on offer. For Freudian psychoanalysts, of course, the basis of their work is the *edition of the complete psychological works of Sigmund Freud*, translated from the German under the general editorship of James Strachey, in 24 volumes (Hogarth Press, 1953–1974) which contains a sizeable proportion of the three million or so words which Freud is said to have published. The final volume, the *Index and Bibliography* is a major reference tool in its own right. The *Collected works* of Jung have similarly been published in 20 volumes edited by Sir Herbert Read *et al.* (Routledge, 1957–1979). Among major book series in the field the International Psycho-Analytic Library (Hogarth Press) stands out as a highly-regarded source of academic texts. Psychoanalysts are so deeply divided into different schools of thought, each named after its original perpetrator, that any list of 'major texts' would simply be a list of the major practitioners in the field.

The Royal College of Psychiatrists has issued a series of *Reading lists in psychiatry* in pamphlet form, and also a *List of books suitable for a psychiatric library* (3rd edn., 1987) which are of some, limited, assistance in selecting from the wide range of books available. For the guidance of trainee psychiatrists the College has published a *Reading list for trainees: general psychiatry* (1990).

Irregular serials and annuals

'Advances in ... ', 'Annual Progress in' and 'Current Researches in' abound in psychiatry, as in other medical disciplines. It is not possible to list all those relevant to psychiatry, but mention should be made of the *Year Book of Psychiatry and Applied Mental Health* (Year Book), and also of the American Psychiatric Association's *Review of Psychiatry* (American Psychiatric). The latter has only been going for eight years, but has already proved to be a very useful review series. In the psychological field the *Annual Review of Psychology* (Annual Reviews) is the main general review, and, for certain clinical applications, *Progress in behaviour modification* (Sage) should be noticed. There are relatively few publications in the social sciences which are of importance here, apart from *Sociological methodology* (Jossey-Bass), which is a useful review of statistical and epidemiological research methods.

The neurosciences are particularly well served in this area, starting obviously, with the *Year Book of Neurology and Neurosurgery* and the *Annual Review of Neuroscience*. There are also a number of publications which are really mainly conference proceedings, but which should, perhaps, rate a mention in this section, such as *Advances in Neurology* (Raven Press), *Clinical Neurosurgery* (Williams and Wilkins) and *Advances in Epileptology* (Raven).

There are a very large number of review series relevant to child psychiatry. Attention is drawn to *Annual Progress in Child Psychiatry and Child Development* (Brunner/Mazel), *Clinics in Developmental Medicine* (MacKeith Press), *The Psychoanalytic Study of the Child* (Yale University Press) and the *Minnesota Symposia on Child Psychology* among many which could be mentioned here.

Sources of bibliographic information

The bulk of the world's psychiatric journal literature is covered by *Index Medicus* and its online and the compact disk derivatives, discussed elsewhere in this book. These should, therefore be the first sources of bibliographic information to be searched when looking for relevant journal papers. Similarly, the various sections of *Excerpta Medica*, and its EMBASE offshoots cover most of the field, most notably, of course, *Section 32 — Psychiatry, Section 8 — Neurology and Neurosurgery, Section 40 — Drug Dependence, Alcohol Abuse and Alcoholism, Section 37 — The Drug Literature Index* and *Section 50 — Epilepsy Abstracts*.

The most useful source of information about journal papers in psychology is *Psychological Abstracts*, and its electronic equivalent. *Psychological Abstracts* is more complicated to use than *Index Medicus*. Abstracts are published in broad subject order, with detailed cumulative author and subject indexes. The time lag for papers appearing in *Psychological Abstracts* is very much greater than that for *Index Medicus*, so it is less useful for keeping completely up to date. A problem in getting access to *Psychological Abstracts* is expense. In both its printed and electronic forms it is far more expensive than *Index Medicus*, which is likely to deter medical libraries with restricted budgets. Nevertheless, it is the second most useful source of bibliographic information in fields related to psychiatry.

There are numerous other bibliographic sources, both printed and electronic, which can be used to trace materials relevant to psychiatrists, varying from the 'hard science' biological and pharmacological databases, to tools such as *Applied Social Sciences Index and Abstracts (ASSIA), the Philosophers Index* (Educational Resources Information Centre), and *Sociological Abstracts*. It should be noted, for example, that relevant material appears both in the *Science Citation Index* and in the *Social Sciences Citation Index*, and that it is not always easy to decide in which of them marginal material will be found. In general it will be found that the nearer the topic is to 'hard science' the easier it is to search for in such bibliographic tools, owing to the difficulties involved in accurately defining terms in the social sciences.

Journal papers in psychoanalysis are listed both by author and by subject in the *Chicago Psychoanalytic Literature Index* (published quarterly and cumulated annually). Older, historical publications in psychoanalysis are best traced in Grinstein's *Index of psychoanalytic writings* (14 vols, International Universities Press, 1956–1975). Mention should also be made of the *Concordance to the standard edition of the complete works of Sigmund Freud* (edited by S. Guttman *et al.*, 6 vols, G.K. Hall, 1980) which is a (KWIC) index to virtually every word Freud ever used. This publication interestingly demonstrates the way in which the psychoanalytic terminology changed and developed over the years, even in the writings of its founder.

A problem in dealing with the social sciences is that 'social scientists are willing to publish in the form of journal papers, but prefer to read in the form of books' (Guha, 1971). This has led to a form of publication largely confined to psychology and the social sciences — the 'collected readings'. Journal papers which are often not easily accessible in their original form are collected by subject and republished in book form, often in cheap paperbacks aimed at the student market. A handy guide to older publications in this form is the North East London Polytechnic's *Psychology reading catalogue* (2 vols, G.K. Hall, 1976). More recently the American Psychological Association has started

PsycBOOKS (annual, 1987–) to index both complete books on psychological subjects and chapters or papers in edited collections. A useful list of whole books only can be found in the *Bibliographic guide to psychology* (G.K. Hall, annual) which lists the psychology books catalogued during the past year by the Library of Congress and the New York Public Libraries.

Journals

As with all medical specialties, journals play the most important role in the dissemination of psychiatric information. There is an enormous number of psychiatric journals, and the number is growing practically daily. Of the general psychiatric journals, six are consistently in the top 1000 scientific publications world-wide picked up by the *Science Citation Index*. These are currently, in order of rank: *Archives of General Psychiatry; American Journal of Psychiatry; British Journal of Psychiatry; Psychological Medicine; Journal of Nervous and Mental Disease; Acta Psychiatrica Scandinavica.*

The most dramatic changes over the past decade have been the rise of *Psychological Medicine* from outside the top 1000 in 1977 to being in the top 500 by 1987 (Lloyd and Fletcher, 1989), and the relative decline of *Acta Psychiatrica Scandinavica*. The latter journal has recently reshaped itself, with substantial non-Scandinavian representation on the editorial board, presumably in order to reverse this slight relative decline. (The word *relative* should be emphasized). As far as can be judged from the Institute for Scientific Information's *Journal Citation Reports*, the extent to which all the above mentioned journals are being cited in the world's non-psychiatric scientific and medical literature is increasing steadily, indicating a steadily increasing acceptance of psychiatric research by non-psychiatrists.

Other general psychiatric journals include the *American Journal of Orthopsychiatry, Biological Psychiatry, Canadian Journal of Psychiatry, Comprehensive Psychiatry, Hospital and Community Psychiatry, Journal of Behavior Therapy and Experimental Psychiatry, Journal of Psychiatric Research, Journal of Psychosomatic Research, Psychiatric Clinics of North America, Psychiatric Quarterly, Psychiatry Research, Psychosomatic Medicine and Psychiatry*. There are also a number of journals devoted to the study of specific groups of disorders which are largely the province of psychiatrists, ranging from *Suicide and Life-Threatening Behaviour* to the *International Journal of Eating Disorders*. The long-established *Schizophrenia Bulletin* has recently been joined by *Schizophrenia Research*, indicating a growth of interest in this core problem. The *Psychiatric Bulletin* of the Royal College of Psychiatrists is the main UK news journal, and *Psychiatric News* is the newspaper of the American Psychiatric Association. The psychiatric journal literature, like that of most medical and scientific subjects, has now reached the size where it is unmanageable, and some form of review journal is essential. Several have been started, of which *Current Opinion in Psychiatry*, Vol. 1, 1988, from the Royal College of Psychiatrists, seems to be the most promising.

Much of the classic literature in psychiatry is in German, and, to a lesser extent, in French. Some understanding of these languages is necessary to study the early history of the subject, and was, until recently, necessary to study the subject at all (see, for example, Critchley, 1975). This pre-eminence has died out with the general development of English into the universal language of science. Thus even the *Archiv für Psychiatrie und Nervenkrankheiten*, founded in 1868, and still now having a predominantly German editorial board, had to change in 1984 to *European Archives of Psychiatry and Neurological Sciences*, and, by volume 238, 1988–9, published its first volume in which all the papers were in English.

In addition to the wide range of general psychiatric journals, of which the above mentioned are only the most heavily-used, many general medical journals publish papers of importance to psychiatrists. In addition, most of the sub-specialties mentioned above have their own specialized journals, and also use materials published in non-medical scientific and social journals

Special divisions of psychiatry

Alcoholism and addiction

There is a vast literature on this subject. Some of it follows the standard bio-medical pattern, but a greater proportion is social science based. A high proportion of publications in this field consist of ephemera and 'grey' literature, for which bibliographic control is very difficult.

In the study of alcoholism and addiction, the most heavily cited journals, among the large number published, are *Alcohol and Alcoholism – Clinical and Experimental Research*, the *American Journal of Drug and Alcohol Abuse*, the *British Journal of Addiction*, the *International Journal of the Addictions*, and the *Journal of Studies on Alcohol*.

Child psychiatry

Again, child psychiatry is a subject which is inevitably interwoven with the social sciences, with education, with development psychology, and with the study of mental retardation, and whose literature overlaps into all these fields. The core journals are the *Journal of Child Psychology* and *Psychiatry* and the *Journal of the American Academy of Child and Adolescent Psychiatry*, with the *Journal of Abnormal Child Psychology*, the *Journal of Adolescence, Child Development and Development Medicine and Child Neurology* (which also publishes bibliographic information).

Family and marital therapy

Among a large number of non-medical social work, counselling and guidance journals, often of an ephemeral appearance there are: the *Journal of Family Therapy*, the *Journal of Marital Therapy, the Journal of Marriage and the Family, Child Abuse and Neglect* and *Family Therapy Networker*.

Forensic psychiatry

This subject presents a major problem to the medical librarian in that, although it is clearly a 'medical' subject, its reading matter is as closely involved with law, and with criminology, as with medicine: the *British Journal of Criminology, Medicine, Science and the Law*, the *Bulletin of the American Academy of Psychiatry and The Law* and the *Howard Journal of Criminal Justice*. The *Journal of Forensic Psychiatry* started in 1990, so it is, perhaps, too early to see if it will be a success. Forensic medicine journals seem to publish very little of relevance to forensic psychiatrists — the general social science, criminology and penology, and law journals are much more relevant.

Geriatric psychiatry

A development in recent years has been the drawing up of distinctions between 'normal' and 'abnormal' ageing, with the concomitant development of a distinctive psychiatry of old age. Demographic trends in Western societies seem likely to make this an area of increasing interest in the near future. The literature has been largely incorporated in existing publications on the problems of normal ageing up till now, but a distinctive literature is beginning to develop in its own right.

Important journals are The *Neurobiology of Aging*, and the more recent *International Journal of Geriatric Psychiatry*, but much relevant material is still published in general journals such as *Age and Ageing*, and the *Journals of Gerontology* (the *s* was recently introduced presumably to upset our alphabetical filing order).

Mental retardation

Within the general area of psychiatry, dealing with the mentally handicapped has been, and still is, the area which gets the least resources and support. Much of the older literature especially, is social-science based, concerned with 'keeping' rather than with 'curing'. The principal periodical are the *American Journal of Mental Retardation,* the *Journal of Autism and Developmental Disorders* and *Journal of Learning Disabilities,* the *Journal of Mental Deficiency Research,* and various educational publications, such as the *Journal of Special Education.*

NEUROLOGY

Neurology separated itself from psychiatry to become part of clinical medicine. There is considerable evidence to suggest that the two are moving back together again. Diseases such as epilepsy and the various movement disorders, disorders of the brain, and the effects of head injury are of at least as much concern to the neuropsychiatrist as to the neurologist.

There are a vast number of neurological journals, many of them being both bulky and expensive. The *Annals of Neurology,* the *Archives of Neurology, Brain, Brain Research* (in all its numerous parts), the *Journal of Neurology, Neurosurgery and Psychiatry* and *Neurology,* are all important general journals of neurology, along with specialized journals such as *Epilepsia,* and surgical journals such as the *British Journal of Neurosurgery* and the *Journal of Neurosurgery.* Neurological subjects are reviewed in *Current Opinion in Neurology and Neurosurgery.* Development in scanning techniques which are of major importance in this field are discussed in *Electroencephalography and Clinical Neurophysiology* (both parts), and in *Neuroradiology.*

The neurosciences

The understanding of the biochemical, pharmacological, physiological and genetic bases of psychiatric disorders has been one of the areas in which the scientific literature has grown most rapidly in recent years. The search for organic bases of mental disorders has drawn psychiatry, neurology and clinical medicine closer, creating a distinctive neuropsychiatric literature. The development of pharmacological methods of treating and controlling mental illness has been a major factor in the change of emphasis from incarceration to treatment in the community. This is also reflected in the growth of the pharmacological literature, which now forms a large proportion of all psychiatric reading-matter. The *Nature* new journals issue of 28 September 1989 mentioned, for example, 22 new journals in the neurosciences that were not being taken by the Institute of Psychiatry library. This explosion of information is one of the factors which seems to be taking psychiatry into the biomedical mainstream. The information sources discussed in Chapters 8 and 10 of this book are, therefore, of major importance for psychiatrists.

The neurosciences present particular problems in that the range of journals is so vast, and seems to be increasing. There are *Endocrinology*, *Neuroendocrinology* and *Psychoneuroendocrinology*, for example, or, *Pharmacopsychiatry* and *Psychopharmacology*. In spite of this plethora of specialized journals much of the literature is still published in general scientific journals, such as the *Biochemical Journal*, *Cell*, or the *Proceedings of the National Academy of Sciences*. The most heavily cited neuroscience journals at the moment seem to be the *Journal of Neurochemistry*, the *Journal of Neuroscience* and *Neuroscience*, with *Neuron* as the most promising of the newcomers and *Trends in Neurosciences* as the best research review. Similarly, in psychopharmacology, the most frequently-used journals entirely devoted to the subject are probably *Neuropharmacology* and *Psychopharmacology*, but a high proportion of the relevant literature is still published in general journals such as *Journal of Pharmacology and Experimental Therapeutics*, or the *British Journal of Clinical Pharmacology*.

Psychoanalysis

Psychoanalysis has its own history and its own distinctive professional literature, entirely separate from medicine, even though many of its practitioners have been medically trained. The literature is enormous— it forms a huge proportion of all the non-fiction books published annually, and fades off into various forms of popular psychology, philosophy, fantasy and mysticism. As psychiatry seems to be moving more into the medical mainstream, psychoanalysis seems to be moving in the opposite direction, away from the medical model of 'treating patients' towards a social work model of 'helping clients'.

Psychoanalysis and psychotherapy, though more book-based than most 'medical' subjects, have produced a large number of journals. The most heavily cited Freudian journals are the *International Journal of Psycho-analysis* and the *International Review of Psycho-analysis* (as cited, incidentally, in the *Social Sciences Citation Index* rather than in the *Science Citation Index*). The chief Jungian journal is the *Journal of Analytic Psychology*, the Adlerian is the *Journal of Individual Psychology*, the followers of Michael Balint have the *Journal of the Balint Society*, etc. Among the psychotherapeutic journals worth mentioning are the *American Journal of Psychotherapy*, *Psychotherapy* and the *International Journal of Group Psychotherapy*.

Psychology

Clinical psychologists are not medically trained, but their work is very closely involved with psychiatry as a medical subject, both in diagnosis, by the administration of tests and measures, and in therapy. Psychology has a very large specialized literature of its own. Though some of it is outside the scope of this book, a high proportion is of some potential interest to anyone working in the psychiatric field.

In spite of the wide interest in the subject, comparatively few psychological journals reach the top 1000 most cited journals in the *Science Citation Index*. It is suspected that this is partly because their citations spread over into the social sciences, and so are not picked up, but mainly due to the fact that papers are spread over a vast range of psychological journals, a high proportion of which are likely to carry some papers of relevance to psychiatry. The American Psychological Association surveyed its members when starting the abstracting journal *PsycSCAN: Clinical Psychology*. They picked out 22 journals of particular relevance. These include, apart from journals already mentioned, *Behaviour Research and Therapy, British Journal of Clinical Psychology, Clinical Psychology Review, Cognitive Therapy and Research, Journal of Abnormal Psychology, Journal of Behavioral Medicine, Journal of Clinical and Experimental Neuropsychology, Journal of Clinical Psychology, Journal of Consulting and Clinical Psychology* and the *Journal of Personality Assessment*, but there are a large number of others of relevance to psychiatry. Rather than attempt to summarize these here, interested readers are referred to a reader's guide, such as D.H. Borchardt and R.D. Francis' *How to find out in psychology* (rev. edn., 1986, Pergamon).

It is, incidentally, interesting to note that in both psychiatry and psychology quite a number of highly-ranked journals are of British origin. This seems to support the suggestion of Martin *et al.* (1987) that psychology and the behavioural sciences are areas of work in which Britain is still relatively strong.

Social and community psychology

Although psychiatry as a discipline appears to be moving towards general medicine, the mode of treatment appears to be moving in the opposite direction, with the change from treating psychiatric patients in the 'hospital' (a medical title, even if 'asylum' was originally a more appropriate name) to treating them 'in the community'. The change to treatment in the community, which is common to most Western societies at the moment, is leading to an increased interest in the social sciences literature, to literature relating to the treatment of psychiatric disorders by general practitioners, and to the literature relating to treatment by non-clinicians.

Social and community psychiatry is a vast field, and, virtually by definition, much of the literature is published in general medical journals, and in social science journals such as *Social Science and Medicine*. The core psychiatric journals in the field are *Hospital and Community Psychiatry, International Journal of Social Psychiatry* and *Social Psychiatry and Psychiatric Epidemiology.*

Social workers, occupational therapists, nurse therapists, etc.

All these groups of trained staff have distinctive, and increasingly important roles to play in the treatment of psychiatric disorders. Psychiatric nursing as a specialty grew out of the old asylum attendants, and has in the past been sharply separated from traditional nursing. Recent developments in nursing education are integrating the specialized training courses much more closely with general nurse training, just as, in the early 1970s the development of the general Certificate of Qualification in Social Work (CQSW) brought the mental health social workers into the mainstream of the social work profession. All these groups have a small highly specialized literature of their own, which is gradually developing into part of the literature of their own general professions. Much of this literature is outside the strict scope of this book, but there is a considerable overlap of interests which should be noted.

Transcultural psychiatry

Many of the nineteenth- and early twentieth-century psychiatrists were keenly interested in anthropology. This early interest faded away, and much of the literature of psychiatry from the last half-century is written on the assumption that Western culture is the only culture worth considering. The existence of large immigrant groups in most Western societies, and the rise of nationalism in the Third World have combined to increase an interest in the effects of culture on psychiatric illness, which is reflected in a small, dispersed, but rapidly growing literature.

The most established journals in transcultural psychiatry are *Culture, Medicine and Psychiatry*, and the review journal *Transcultural Psychiatric Research Review*. Again, many papers relevant to this subject are published in journals outside the normal range of 'medicine'—in anthropological, social work and sociological publications. Many of the journals dealing with race relations are ephemeral and difficult to track down.

Law

Any clinician may, on occasion be required to act as an expert witness, or play some other professional role in a law court. Psychiatrists, however, are required to do so far more frequently than practitioners in any other area of medicine. Most psychiatric libraries obviously cannot afford to provide a full legal information service, but, nevertheless, some idea of the sources of legal information is desirable.

English law is based on acts of Parliament, implemented in detail by Statutory Instruments (which are a form of delegated legislation), and, above all, interpreted by precedents laid down in legal cases.

All acts are published individually by HMSO, and annually in the Public General Acts. The best source of information on acts in force is *Halsbury's Statutes of England* (4th edn., published 1989; individual volumes are replaced as appropriate), updated by a cumulative supplement to the end of the previous year, and a 'Noter-up Service' for recent changes. It is essential to use all three—the volume, the supplement and the noter-up, to find out which parts of a statute are still in force.

Statutory instruments are all published individually by HMSO, listed by subject in the *List of Statutory Instruments*, and cumulated in *Halsbury's Statutory Instruments*.

Along with statutory instruments should be considered the problem of departmental circulars and other non-parliamentary papers. These are not necessarily published by HMSO, and can be difficult to track down. *British Official Publications Not Published by HMSO* (Chadwyck-Healey, bimonthly, cumulated annually) is a handy guide to finding out the existence of these documents. They, of course, date very rapidly. In fact the major problem facing any library attempting to maintain a current legal information service is that of ensuring that obsolete material is removed promptly.

Case law is very difficult to trace. Law reports are published in a wide variety of newspapers and professional journals. The index to the *All England Law Reports* and the *Current Law Case Citators 1947–1976*, updated by the case citator published in the journal *Current Law*, are the major sources for general law. The *Criminal Appeal Reports* are obviously the most useful for criminal case law reports, including a lot of appeals involving psychiatrists.

A particular problem to be considered is that of tracing tribunal cases. The establishment of the welfare state led to the creation of a large number of tribunals set up to resolve disputes in specific areas. The most important of these, from a psychiatric point of view are the Mental Health Review Tribunals, established under the Mental Health Act 1959, and reconstituted under the 1983 Act, to safeguard detained patients. Most decisions of tribunals are not publicly reported, though many of the important decisions of the Social Security Commissioners are published individually by HMSO and are cumulated in the *Reported Decisions of the Social Security Commissioners*.

Lexis

LEXIS is much more than an equivalent to MEDLINE. It is an online service which contains the full text of all acts and statutory instruments in
force, a huge number of case reports, tax material, European law (including case reports, such as those raised under the European
Convention on Human Rights, which can be of considerable importance
to psychiatrists), U.S., Commonwealth and French law reports, and the
full text of a number of major law journals. It is, of course, phenomen-
ally expensive. It is highly unlikely that any medical library will have
direct access to it, but its existence should be noted here.

The most useful tool in the field of law and psychiatry is *Mental
Health Services—Law and Practice*. This has been published by Shaw
and Sons since 1949, but for the 1986 edition, edited by Larry Gostin, is
in loose-leafed form, to allow for up-dating, as the law changes. Its appendices include the Mental Health Act 1983, as amended, all the
relevant Statutory Instruments, the Mental Health Tribunal Rules, and
the relevant departmental circulars. This, plus a good textbook on criminal law, such as J.C. Smith and B. Hogan, *Criminal Law* (6th edn.,
Butterworth, 1988) and one on the law of evidence, such as the redoubt-
able Archbold *Pleading, evidence and practice in criminal cases* (36th
edn., Sweet and Maxwell, 1984) or J.A. Andrews and M. Hirst, *Criminal evidence* (Waterlow, 1987), together with subscriptions to one or
two journals such as *Medicine, Science and the Law* and the *British
Journal of Criminology* should form an adequate base.

Epidemiological and statistical data

The following official publications, available from HMSO, are the basic
sources of epidemiological information for England and Wales. Details
of statistical information sources for Scotland and Northern Ireland can
be found in the Central Statistical Office *Guide to official statistics* (5th
edn., HMSO, 1990):

> The *Annual Abstract of Statistics* contains nearly 400 tables,
> giving annual data for approximately the previous 11 years, and
> covers all aspects of economic, social and industrial life. *Social
> Trends* is the most useful general description of UK society,
> focusing on current policy concerns. The *General Household
> Survey* is a continuous sample survey of 13 000 private
> households. These three form the basis for answering general
> enquiries about life in the UK today.
> The *In-Patient Statistics from the Mental Health Enquiry for
> England* gives, separately, for psychiatric hospitals and units,

mental handicap hospitals and units, and, the special hospitals, details of admissions, discharges, and resident patients. Analyses are provided by sex, age, order of admission, diagnostic group, source of referral, recommended outcome, legal status, duration of stay, etc.

The *Faculties and Services of Mental Illness and Mental Handicap Hospitals in England* details, both for individual mental illness and mental handicap hospitals and units, and for Regional Health Authorities, numbers of beds, resident patients, out-patients and day patients (showing number of new patients and total attendances), admissions, discharges, deaths, and numbers of staff (medical, nursing, other professional, and domestic).

The *Health and Personal Social Services Statistics for England* includes data from the Mental Health Enquiry analysing, both for mental illness and for mental handicap, admissions by age and sex, order of admission, diagnosis, discharges, deaths, and resident patients by length of stay. Numbers of registered private and voluntary homes, local authority day centres, homes and hostels for mentally ill and mentally handicapped, and their staffing are also shown.

The *Personal Social Services Statistics* includes data for each local authority in England and Wales on the mentally ill, the mentally handicapped, residential care, adult training centres, day centres and workshops.

Adult Training Centres for the Mentally Handicapped and Day Centres for the Mentally Ill, the Elderly and the Younger Physically Handicapped and the *Residential Accommodation for Mentally Ill and Mentally Handicapped People* are both published by the Department of Social Security, and provide data by local authority on day centres and hostels, respectively.

Criminal Statistics, England & Wales analyses notifiable offences recorded by the police, and sentences. *Judicial Statistics, England & Wales* contains data on the civil and criminal business of the courts, and of some tribunals. The number of cases dealt with by other tribunals can be found in the *Annual Report of the Council on Tribunals*.

Offences of Drunkenness, England & Wales, and the *Statistics of the Misuse of Drugs in the United Kingdom*, both of which are published as summary reports with supplementary tables, give the official figures for the study of addiction.

International and transcultural comparisons of epidemiological information in psychiatry are difficult and contentious. The increased acceptance of the ICD and DSM definitions should make comparisons easier, but, in many countries, the available statistical information is so sketchy as to be virtually unusable. Cultural differences as to the social acceptability of various mental disorders, different forms of additive and sexual behaviour, practices such as suicide, etc. create grave difficulties for epidemiologists. The World Health Organization made an attempt to overcome this, in the case of a particular group of disorders with the *International pilot study of schizophrenia* (1974), and its Expert Committee on Mental Health has produced a considerable number of technical reports which throw some light on particular problems.

Such relevant comparative statistical information as exists can be found in the United Nations *Statistical Yearbook* and the *Demographic Yearbook*. The United Nations also publishes a number of specialized report series, such as the publications of the International Narcotics Control Board, and the United Nations Social Defence Research Institute.

The World Psychiatric Association includes in its statutes a statement of purpose which includes the co-ordination, on a world-wide scale, of the activities of its member societies. This has not, however extended into the gathering of information on a comparative basis. Most of its activities seem to involve the organization of international congresses, and the occasional pressure on countries that are too blatantly misusing psychiatry for the purposes of political repression.

The country which publishes the most detailed statistical information on psychiatric disorders is almost certainly the USA. A convenient summary of the information sources currently available, and their development, can be found in R.W. Redick *et al., History of the U.S. National Reporting Program for Mental Health Statistics* (National Institute of Mental Health, 1986).

Psychological tests

Testing—the defining of 'normality' and the measuring of individual deviations from it—forms an important part of clinical psychological work. Tests do present some particular bibliographic problems. In order to preserve their effectiveness, test manuals are not normally available on the open market, they are not normally stocked in libraries, and they are not normally available through the inter-library loans system (a fact which many psychiatrists and clinical psychologists find curiously difficult to accept). The tools for tracing and selecting tests are, however, important. The most useful of these is the *Mental Measurements Yearbook*. This was started in 1938, by Oscar Buros, and, in spite of its title, only reached its 10th edition in 1989. A more rapid publication rate is promised for the future. The yearbook lists tests in alphabetical order, with indexes by name, publisher, scoring method and subject, with detailed critical reviews and bibliographic references. The yearbooks themselves are not cumulative, but Buros published cumulative indexes to the earlier volumes under the title *Tests in print*. Another similar venture is *Test critiques*, edited by D.J. Keyser and R.C. Sweetland, currently in five volumes (Test Corporation of America, 1984–6). The largest UK supplier of tests is NFER-Nelson, whose published catalogues form a useful guide.

A problem with tests is that many are not published as such, but are duplicated by their designers for use in their own particular clinical services. The *Directory of unpublished experimental measures* edited by B.A. Goldman and W.L. Osborne in four volumes so far (Human Sciences Press, 1974–) attempts to index these, though it is, obviously, very incomplete.

One of the earliest applications of computers, in any field whatsoever, was for scoring psychological tests—Hollerith punched cards were being used for this purpose in the early 1920s, because testing is the numerical representation of individual characteristics, and because test scoring is a mind-numbingly tedious operation. As computers have become more flexible they are being used for test operations which would not be feasible in any other form, such as tests in which the pattern of questions is altered in response to the answers to earlier questions. Computer-based tests are indexed in the *Psychware sourcebook*, edited by S.E. Krug (3rd edn., Test Corporation of America, 1988).

History

The disciplines considered in this chapter stem from three different groups of professions — the lunatic asylum keepers, the barber surgeons, and the philosophers. Some idea of the history of these groups is necessary in order to appreciate the distribution of the literature. Clearly no hard line can be drawn between those individuals who act as custodians, those who attempt a physical cure, and those who think about the processes of the human mind. There is no intrinsic reason why someone providing secure accommodation for a few lunatics should have to be medically qualified, but even at their worst, asylum keepers seem to have tried to do something to cure, as well as keep, their patients (although the treatments — flogging, blood-letting, cold-water immersions, brandy, opium, locking people up in the dark, and various bizarre diets, seem inhuman today). Similarly, Sigmund Freud, the founder of the psychoanalytic method of thinking about the human mind was originally medically trained, as a neurologist. Nevertheless, the distinction between the psychiatrist, the neurologist, and the psychoanalyst remains, and this distinction is reflected in the literature, and in the popular mind. The contrasting public images of the psychiatrist loading patients with drugs to render them docile and then locking them up under some compulsory order in a remote asylum, the brain surgeon with his unimaginable dexterity, and the infinitely wise psychoanalyst stroking his beard and somewhat understanding the underlying implications of every word uttered by the patient on the couch, are still potent.

Doctors always seem to have had more confidence in dealing with a visible disorder than in 'ministering to a mind diseased' conditions which other doctors cannot cure and which cannot be attributed to 'a virus' tends to be regarded as 'psychosomatic' until some organic basis is found. Thus, for example, anorexia in adolescent girls is currently a matter for psychiatrists to deal with. If or when some hormonal or dietary cause is isolated, it will become the preserve of paediatricians or dieticians.

A great deal has been published on the history of psychiatry. Texts relating to mental illness, from Hippocrates onwards, have been collected by C.E. Goshen in *The documentary history of psychiatry* (Vision Press, 1967) and, especially, by R. Hunter and I. MacAlpine in *Three hundred years of psychiatry 1535–1860* (OUP, 1963). British psychiatry is well covered by D. Leigh, *The historical development of British psychiatry*, Volume 1 (Pergamon, 1961) (Volume 2 has not yet appeared). Eighteenth- and nineteenth-century asylums have had a peculiar fascination for historians, so there is a wide range of books on the subject, among which can be noted W.L. Parry-Jones, *The trade in lunacy* (Routledge, 1972) and A.T. Scull, *Museums of madness* (Allen Lane, 1979). There are many histories of individual hospitals, ranging from the imposing and ornamental (such as A. Foss and K. Trick *St Andrew's Hospital Northampton: the first one hundred and fifty years* (Granta, 1959) to the unobtrusive but informative (such as R. Cooper and J. Bird, *The burden: fifty years of clinical and experimental neuroscience at the Burden Neurological Institute* (White Tree Books, 1989). It is curious to note however, that the only history of the Bethlem Royal Hospital was published in 1914, and that no history of the Maudsley Hospital has yet been published (though an outstanding bio-bibliography of its founders has recently appeared — M. Collie, *Henry Maudsley: Victorian psychiatrist* (St Paul's Bibliographies, 1988). Roy Porter has been publishing at least one book a year on the history of psychiatry, and W.F. Bynum *et al.* have edited *The anatomy of madness* (in three volumes so far) (Tavistock Press, 1985–), a collection of essays. They are publishing a journal, *History of Psychiatry*. At the moment, the main journal in the field is the *Journal of the History of the Behavioral Sciences*.

As might be expected of such highly personal subjects, both psychology and psychoanalysis are very well documented, mainly in a biographical form. The book series *A history of psychology in autobiography*, now published by W.H. Freeman, collects autobiographies, which supplement L. Zusne's *Names in the history of psychology* (Wiley, 1975), and individual biographies exist for most of the well-known practitioners, usually written either by disciples or detractors. The outstanding work of discipleship, of course, is Ernest Jones' *Sigmund Freud* (3 vols, Hogarth Press, 1953–57). Innumerable books have subsequently been written by detractors probing for the feet of clay beneath the flowing robes which Jones draped around the subject.

As might be expected from such impersonal subjects, very little has been published about the history of the neurosciences, and what little there is tends to be hidden in general textbooks and journals.

Aside from general medical collections, such as those of the Wellcome Institute, the largest collections of material relating to the history of psychiatry can be found in the Bethlem Royal Hospital Museum and Archives, in the library of the Royal College of Psychiatrists, and in the library of the Institute of Psychiatry (which includes the Mayer-Gross Collection). Mayer-Gross was a German psychiatrist who escaped from Nazi Germany with thousands of rare books. Copies of many of these were burnt as being 'Jewish Science' in Germany, so they are not easily obtained elsewhere, and the Hunter-MacAlpine Collection which has been acquired by Cambridge University Library. The largest collections of materials relating to the history of psychoanalysis are in the Freud Museum and Archives, and in the Institute of Psychoanalysis library.

Future trends

It seems likely that psychiatry is growing closer to neurology and the rest of clinical medicine, which is leading to a closer involvement with the general biomedical literature. The neurosciences seem to be the most promising of all current areas of scientific research, both in the understanding of the biochemical and genetic bases of behaviour, and in the pharmacological treatment of disorders of behaviour. Psychotherapy, on the other hand, seems to be moving away from the medical model towards a social work/social science type of literature. The treatment of the mentally ill in the community is becoming more widespread, which seems likely to lead to the expansion of a separate forensic and social psychiatry literature.

References

Borchardt, D.H. and Francis, R.D. (1986) *How to find out in psychology.* Oxford: Pergamon Press.

Critchley, M. (1975) The training of a neurologist (reprinted in *The divine banquet of the brain*, Raven Press, 1979, pp. 178–182).

Elliot, C.K. (1971) *A guide to the documentation of psychology.* London: Clive Bingley.

Guha, M. (1971) Literature use by European sociologists. *International Library Review*, **4**, 445.

Lloyd, G.G. and Fletcher, A.E. (1989) Citation trends of general psychiatric journals. *Psychological Medicine*, **19**, 15–18.

Martin, B.F. et al. (1987) The continuing decline of British science. *Nature*, **330**, 123–126.

CHAPTER EIGHTEEN

Surgery and anaesthesia

A.M. RODGER

Surgery

While the basic principles of the craft of surgery remain the same, scientific and technical progress has created new areas of surgical specialties which have undergone rapid development in recent years. Over the past few decades the emphasis has moved from infectious complications to the new techniques in cardiac and transplant surgery. The relevance of computerized information to surgical practice has increased not only in the field of information retrieval but also in the areas of diagnosis and teaching as well as in the wider issues of audit. Some of the most dramatic changes in recent years have been the range of anti-rejection drugs and the reduction in the operative treatment of some carcinomata in favour of chemotherapy. Complications have been reduced by the introduction of better techniques and materials. This, however, is a change in emphasis only because advances in treatment nearly always provide new problems, as in antibiotic therapy where the causative organisms of infection develop strains resistant to existing medication. Both the rapid progress in surgical research and the wide range of specialties limit the utility of textbooks of general surgery. Most of the primary information is found in the journal literature and the stocks of many medical libraries now consist predominantly of journals, which are the main source of new surgical information, and of review articles which survey recent developments in specialized subjects. The journal reader is aided by abstracting services which provide a summary of the most outstanding contributions to the journal literature. Information on progress in surgical specialties may also be obtained from monographs, i.e. books dealing with one selected topic, and from publications in book form which aim to present advances in particular aspects of surgery. The journal remains the principal source for the dissemination of new information.

Journals

In addition to the many journals catering for the specialist, there are a number which carry articles on all aspects of surgery. These are usually nationally or geographically orientated, e.g. *Acta Chirurgica Scandinavica, American Journal of Surgery, American Surgeon, Australian and New Zealand Journal of Surgery, British Journal of Surgery, European Surgical Research, World Journal of Surgery* and *Surgical Clinics of North America*, the last concentrating on a single topic per issue.

Other journals of a similar type are produced which are without a national emphasis in the title but whose content may reflect the country of origin. Sometimes such commercially-produced journals are the official organ of a society or group. Examples here are *Annals of Surgery* (official publication of the American Surgical Association), *Archives of Surgery* (official publication of the International Cardiovascular Society and Western Surgical Association), *Journal of Surgical Research* (official organ of the Association for Academic Surgery), *Surgery* (Journal of the Society of University Surgeons) and *Surgical Forum*. This last is hardly a journal in the accepted sense. It is an annual publication and takes the form of the Proceedings of the American College of Surgeons Forum on fundamental surgical problems.

There are weekly medical publications which not only disseminate news and current research, but also carry articles of surgical import. Such journals include the *British Medical Journal, The Lancet, Journal of the American Medical Association* and the *New England Journal of Medicine*. Yet another group of journals is published under the aegis of a single institution, often with an international reputation. Among such journals are *Annals of the Royal College of Surgeons of England, Journal of the Mount Sinai Hospital, Journal of the Royal College of Surgeons of Edinburgh* and *Mayo Clinic Proceedings*.

As with most other areas of medicine, the journals together constitute the most important source of surgical information, covering as they do communications regarding new discoveries, reviews of the literature or state-of-the-art appraisals, case reports, and advances in techniques.

Indexes and Abstracts

To peruse regularly even a selection of journals is too time-consuming for the individual. For bibliographic search purposes *Index Medicus* is the most widely used aid in terms of the printed word. Access to the MEDLINE computer database allows searching of files back to 1966 when a manual search is considered insufficient or inappropriate. Many such indexing and abstracting services are also available on CD-ROM which gives the flexibility of a computer search without the need to have traditional online facilities.

In surgery the most comprehensive abstracting service is provided by *Excerpta Medica* (see page 56). There are over 50 sections and those most relevant to surgery are: *Surgery* (Section 9); *Neurology and Neurosurgery* (Section 8); *Plastic Surgery* (Section 34); *Orthopedic Surgery* (Section 33); *Cardiovascular Diseases and Cardiovascular Surgery* (Section 18); *Cancer* (Section 16); *Gastroenterology* (Section 48); *Chest Diseases, Thoracic Surgery and Tuberculosis* (Section 15); *Urology and Nephrology* (Section 28); *Oto-rhino-laryngology* (Section 11); *Ophthalmology* (Section 12). *International Abstracts of Surgery* is published as part of the monthly journal *Surgery, Gynecology and Obstetrics*. About 4000 abstracts appear each year, arranged anatomically and indexed biannually.

Abstracts and reviews of relevant literature are published in certain specialty journals, e.g. *Diseases of the Colon and Rectum, British Journal of Urology* and *Journal of Pediatric Surgery*.

The *Audio Digest of Surgery* appears twice monthly in audio cassette form and it is produced by the Audio Digest Foundation which in turn is a subsidiary of the California Medical Association.

The plethora of journals and the increasing number of new ones launched each year make a speedy alerting service difficult to maintain. A reasonable international cover is provided by *Current Contents: Life Sciences* and *Current Contents: Clinical Medicine* which between them provide the reader with the tables of contents of virtually all the major journals.

Reviews

The review publication is a useful way of keeping track of recent advances or trends in certain areas of medicine and surgery. Review publications are invaluable guides, not only to workers whose specialty may be the subject reviewed but also to specialists in ancillary fields, keeping them up to date with major developments. Many such publications concentrate on specific topics and examples of these are mentioned in the relevant sections. One such publication of general surgical interest is *Recent advances in surgery* — 13, edited by R.C.G. Russell (Churchill Livingstone, 1988) which contains comprehensive reviews of a variety of topics including major trauma, breast cancer and paediatric surgical gastroenterology. The book also includes a comprehensive review of new plastic-surgery techniques by Ian Jackson. Year Book Medical Publishers of Chicago, Illinois, specialize in the production of just such a publication not only for the general surgeon but also catering for a range of specialties. Of interest to the general surgeon is the series *Advances in surgery* of which the latest is *Advances in surgery — 23*, edited by R. Tomkins *et al.*, which has contributions on a variety of topics of current interest such as advances in microsurgery, septic shock and the early detection of breast cancer. Also from the same stable is the series of *Year Books of Surgery* under the general editorship of S.I. Schwartz. The 1990 *Yearbook* is published in September of that year. The 1989 edition covers shock, wound healing, transplantation, aspects of oncology as well as a variety of other topics. It should be noted however that the series has a distinctly American bias. *Progress in surgery* volume 3, edited by I. Taylor (Churchill Livingstone, 1989) is one of an occasional series aimed at the surgical trainee as well as keeping the established surgeon informed on recent developments. A notable example of this type of publication is the series *Current surgical practice* of which the latest is Volume 5, edited by J. Hadfield, M. Hobsley and T. Treasure (Edward Arnold, 1990). This series comprises a selection of lectures given at the Royal College of Surgeons of England and emphasizes areas of surgery in which there have been important advances in recent years.

Textbooks

GENERAL SURGERY

The single-volume textbook covering all aspects of surgery suffers from the faults expected of a textbook that deals with evolving and diversifying subject matter; principally obsolescence, often before publication, and uneven weighting when attempting to discuss all specialties. Nevertheless such works are essential as basic training manuals. There are a number of textbooks of high reputation, gained through the popularity of successive editions with generations of students. One of the best known is *Bailey and Love's Short practice of surgery*, revised by A.J.H. Rains and C.V. Mann (20th edn., Lewis, 1988). *Current surgical diagnosis and treatment*, edited by L.W. Way (8th edn., Prentice Hall, 1988) is a popular U.S. textbook with an international reputation. It is comprehensive and deals with specialized subjects as well as filling the requirements of a basic text. One of the notable features of this book through successive editions is the currency of its references. It might be of more use to the undergraduate than the fellowship candidate although the latter will find the up-to-date references a good guide to further reading. Useful for general revision are *Lecture notes on general surgery* by H. Ellis (7th edn., Blackwell, 1987) and *Lee McGregor's Synopsis of surgical anatomy* by G.A.G. Decker and D.J. Du Plessis (12th edn., Wright, 1986). A useful book for background reading for FRCS candidates is *Scientific foundations of surgery*, edited by J. Kyle and L.C. Carey (4th edn., Heinemann, 1989).

OPERATIVE SURGERY

A standard work for many years has been *Hamilton Bailey's Emergency surgery*, edited by H.A.F. Dudley (11th edn., Wright, 1986). This title is now well established as a practical guide. The book advises when to operate and when not, and how to proceed in emergencies. It is especially valuable to the surgeon working in isolation. *Farquharson's Textbook of operative surgery*, edited by R.F. Rintoul (6th edn., Churchill Livingstone, 1986) is a standard work for those working for higher surgical qualifications.

General surgical operations, edited by R.M. Kirk and R.C. Williamson (2nd edn., Churchill Livingstone, 1987) is a practical manual for the general surgeon. The essential reference work for the library shelves is the series *Operative surgery* under the general editorship of C. Rob and R. Smith (4th edn., Butterworths, 1984–). This comprises a multi-volume series with each volume being compiled by a specialist editor. The latest section 'Paediatric Surgery' is in fact only in its second edition (Butterworths, 1988). Of use to postgraduates is the series *Tutorials in surgery* (Pitman).

Intensive care

The development of the intensive care unit (ICU) is a relatively modern phenomenon which allows for the concentration of specialized skills and resources in one team. Practice varies and in some hospitals the recovery room which may be viewed as a subdivision of intensive care is used for all postoperative procedures while in others only patients who have undergone strenuous or prolonged surgery are listed for time in recovery. As surgical and medical treatment advances, patients who some years ago might have had a very poor prognosis, now find that there are procedures available to them. To this extent intensive or critical care, as it is also known, are due to be expanding areas of concern.

Among the journals which cover this field are: *Anaesthesia and Intensive Care; Critical Care Clinics; Critical Care Medicine; Intensive Care Medicine; Anästhesie, Intensivtherapie, Notfallmedizin; Current Anaesthesia and Critical Care.*

There are a number of review publications. Two of the British reviews are *Recent advances in critical care medicine — 3*, edited by I.M. Ledingham (Churchill Livingstone, 1988) and the series *Clinics in critical care medicine* of which the latest is No. 15, *Fluids, electrolytes and acid–bases*, edited by G.T. Shires (Churchill Livingstone, 1988).

There are a number of textbooks dealing with different aspects of intensive care. One of the best and most popular in the area of trauma is *Principles of trauma care* by G. Shires (3rd edn., McGraw Hill, 1985). This is a comprehensive text and should be consulted by anyone with an interest in this field. *Anaesthesia and intensive care: practical procedures* by Neil Soni (Heinemann, 1989) is, as the title suggests, primarily a practical manual. It contains excellent summaries of procedures and clear illustrations. There are appendices of useful information at the end of the book and it is thoroughly recommended especially to the new practitioner in this field. Paediatric intensive care is not yet a generally recognized subject specialty in the UK as it is in the USA, nevertheless it forms a large part of critical care work and *Pediatric intensive care*, edited by E. Nussbaum (2nd edn., Futura Publishing, 1989) can be recommended as a current authoritative work albeit with an American bias, especially in those sections dealing with ethical and legal considerations.

Orthopaedics

The correction of diseases and injuries to the locomotor system forms a major branch of surgery and here dramatic changes have taken place in the organization and techniques employed in accident surgery, and, in particular, the management of trauma. There have been rapid developments in the use of artificial prostheses for hip, hand and knee joints.

JOURNALS

In addition to the general surgical journals listed at the beginning of this chapter, a number of journals cater specifically for the orthopaedic surgeon. The most important of these are *Acta Orthopaedica Scandinavica, Orthopedic Clinics of North America, Journal of Bone and Joint Surgery* (UK and U.S. editions), *Journal of Trauma, Injury: The British Journal of Accident Surgery, Spine, Journal of Orthopaedic Research* and the *Journal of Orthopaedic Trauma. Injury* and the *Journal of Trauma* carry a short selection of abstracts relating to orthopaedics.

The video *Journal of Orthopedics* is published by W.B. Saunders in conjunction with the American Academy of Orthopedic Surgeons. Each volume contains six issues and each issue has four video cassette presentations.

REVIEWS

There are several survey publications in orthopaedics including *Recent advances in orthopaedics — 5* edited by A. Catterall (Churchill Livingstone, 1987). In particular articles dealing with the fixation of prostheses without cement, and clean air and the use of antibiotics in surgery have been well received. There is also the *Year Book of Ortho-*

pedics, edited by C.B. Sledge (Year Book Medical Publishers, 1989). An occasional series is *Current problems in orthopaedics* of which the latest is *Arthroscopic management of the knee* by D.J. Dandy (Churchill Livingstone, 1987).

TEXTBOOKS AND MONOGRAPHS

The most comprehensive work is *Campbell's Operative orthopaedics*, edited by A.H. Crenshaw (7th edn., C.V. Mosby, 1987). This four-volume work is priced beyond the individual's pocket but it is a must for the medical library shelves as it is generally regarded as the definitive reference work. Other general works which may be considered as essential reading are *A system of orthopaedic fractures* by A.G. Apley (6th edn., Butterworths, 1984). This work is notable for both the clarity of the text and the illustrations. It is recommended reading for FRCS examinations. *Mercer's orthopaedic surgery* edited by R.B. Duthie and G. Bentley (8th edn., Arnold, 1983) is essential library material and a standard reference work, as is *Watson-Jones Fractures and joint injuries*, edited by J.N. Wilson (6th edn., Churchill Livingstone, 1982). For the personal collection *Standard orthopaedic operations* by J.C. Adams (3rd edn., Churchill Livingstone, 1985) and *Lecture notes on orthopaedics and fractures* by T. Duckworth (2nd edn., Blackwell Scientific Publications, 1984) are recommended. Last but by no means least is one of the most popular books on the subject of orthopaedics, *Clinical orthopaedic examination* by R. McRae (3rd edn., Churchill Livingstone, 1990).

Some recommended texts on regional orthopaedic surgery are *Surgery of the foot* by R.A. Mann (5th edn., Mosby, 1985) and *The principles of hand surgery* by F.D. Burke, D.A. McGrowther and P.J. Smith (Churchill Livingstone, 1989). Although it is over 10 years since the last edition, *Injuries of the knee joint* by I.S. Smillie (5th edn., Churchill Livingstone, 1978 is a classic work.

Paediatric surgery

The information sources contained in the chapter on paediatrics (page 471) are appropriate also to paediatric surgery. Abstracts are published in *Excerpta Medica*, Section 7: *Pediatrics and pediatric surgery*. Review publications dealing with medical paediatrics also contain certain information for the surgeon, e.g. the series *Pediatric and adolescent medicine*, formerly *Modern problems in pediatrics* edited by D. Branski (Karger). Other publications of this type are *Advances in pediatrics* of which the latest is volume 36 (Year Book Publishers, 1989). Butterworths International Reviews series has a paediatric section, Volume 3 in this series being *Pediatric nutrition: theory and practice*, edited by G.C. Arneil and J. Metcoff (Butterworths, 1985).

Monographs and textbooks on paediatric surgery include *Paediatric surgery* by L. Spitz and H. Homewood Nixon (4th edn., Butterworths, 1988). This is one of the comprehensive Rob and Smith's *Operative surgery* series. Useful companion sets are *Paediatric emergencies*, edited by J.A. Black (2nd edn., Butterworths, 1987) and *Neonatal emergencies*, edited by J. Black and M. Whitfield (2nd edn., Butterworths, 1988). *Neonatal surgery* by J. Lister and I.M. Young (3rd edn., Butterworths, 1989) is the latest edition of a book which has become well established since it first appeared over 20 years ago. Of more specialized interest is *Pediatric neurosurgery; surgery of the developing nervous system*, edited by R. McLurin *et al.* (2nd edn., Saunders, 1989) which has been produced under the auspices of the paediatric section of the American Association of Neurological Surgeons and as such provides a detailed account of the current position in paediatric neurosurgery although with a distinct U.S. bias. One area which has seen rapid progress over the last few years is that of paediatric cardiology and *Fetal and neonatal cardiology*, edited by W.A. Long (Saunders, 1990) covers this topic.

Thoracic and cardiovascular surgery

The primary specialist journals in this section are the *American Journal of Cardiology, Journal of the American College of Cardiology, Journal of Cardiovascular Surgery, Journal of Thoracic and Cardiovascular Surgery, Scandinavian Journal of Thoracic and Cardiovascular Surgery, Thorax* and *Annals of Thoracic Surgery*.

The American Journal of Cardiology publishes abstracts of the conference proceedings of the American College of Cardiology, usually in advance of presentation. Also the American Heart Association publishes occasional monographs under the series title, *Cardiovascular surgery*. Another new series has been launched under the heading of *Current topics in cardiovascular medicine* of which the most recent is *Coronary and peripheral angiography and angioplasty* by D.R. Leachman and R.D. Leachman (Edward Arnold, 1989). A U.S. text with a comprehensive survey of the current treatment of coronary artery disease is the *1989 Year Book of vascular surgery*, edited by J.J. Bergan and J.S.T. Yao. The same publishers also produce the *Year book of Vascular Surgery*.

Two books of note in Rob and Smith's *Operative surgery* series are *Thoracic and cardiac surgery*, edited by J.W. Jackson and D.K.C. Cooper (4th edn., Butterworths, 1986) and *Vascular surgery*, edited by J.A. DeWeese (4th edn., Butterworths, 1985). The former was originally two separate volumes but is now issued as a set. A recent textbook is *General thoracic surgery* by T.W. Shields (3rd edn., Lea and Febiger, 1989). At £100 it is priced more for the library than the individual market but it is recommended for the library shelves as one of the up-to-date texts on the subject. Other recent works in this area are *Vascular surgery*, edited by H. Hainovici (3rd edn., Appleton and Lange, 1989). This is a rapidly-expanding field of research and this edition comes five years after the previous one. Recent developments in vascular imaging and laser therapy are well covered. In general the book is pitched at the level of the experienced vascular surgeon. The value of *Vascular surgery* by G. Herbert and R.J.A.M. Van Dongen (Springer, 1989) is that it provides a European perspective on its subject. There are contributions from the Netherlands, Austria, Germany and Switzerland and each chapter is written by an acknowledged expert in his or her field. On the whole the translations are excellent and the references are as would be expected, mainly from European journals. Two atlases have been recently produced and are worthy of consideration. *Atlas of general thoracic surgery* by M.M. Ravitch (Academic Press, 1988) is by an internationally known thoracic surgeon. Over 100 operations and procedures are described and copiously illustrated. *A colour atlas of surgical management of venous disease* by C.V. Ruckley (Wolfe, 1988) is a practical guide with high-quality illustrations and has been well received.

Aortic surgery, edited by J.J. Bergan and J.S.T. Yao (Saunders, 1989) is not only a multi-authored review but also a good and well-referenced practical guide. The editors have an international reputation as vascular surgeons.

Neurosurgery

The neurosurgeon tends to work in a distinct field with emphasis on head injuries and lesions of the intervertebral disk which require close co-operation with the orthopaedic surgeon. There are a number of journals concerned with this specialty, particularly: the *Journal of Neurology; Neurosurgery and Psychiatry; Journal of Neurosurgery; British Journal of Neurosurgery; Clinical Neurology and Neurosurgery*; and *Clinical Neurosurgery*.

Relevant information is also to be found in: *Acta Neurologica Scandinavica; Archives of Neurology; Brain; Diseases of the Nervous System; Electroencephalography and Clinical Neurophysiology; European Neurology; Journal of Neurological Sciences; Neurology*.

In non-book format the publishers W.B. Saunders produce the *Video Journal of Neurosurgery*. Each volume consists of six issues, each issue containing four video presentations. Review publications include the

Neurosurgical Review which is published approximately every four years by Walter de Gruyter on behalf of the German Society of Neurosurgeons. Two other series published by Springer are *Advances and Technical Standards in Neurosurgery*, of which the latest is Volume 16 for 1988. The series *Advances in neurosurgery* has now reached Volume 17 (1989) and deals with the prognosis for head injuries, microsurgery and a discussion on brain death. A further new series from the same publisher is *Advances in Neurotraumatology* which is published on behalf of the Neurotraumatology Committee of the World Federation of Neurological Societies. The series is now up to Volume 3, *Cerebral contusions, lacerations and haematomas* edited by R.A. Frowein (Springer, 1990). The American Congress of Neurosurgeons publishes its annual proceedings under the title *Clinical Neurosurgery*. The series has now reached volume 37 and is published on behalf of the society by Williams and Wilkins. Standard textbooks and monographs in neurosurgery include *Neurosurgery* edited by L. Symon, D.G. Thomas and K. Clark (4th edn., Butterworths, 1989). *Neurological emergencies* by S.D. Shorvon (Butterworths, 1988) is a practical guide for junior doctors in accident and emergency departments. It deals with the standard topics that might be expected of a book of this type including coma, meningitis, stroke, haemorrhage, head injury and spinal cord dysfunction. Although last published some seven years ago, *An introduction to neurosurgery* by B.W. Jennett remains an excellent basic textbook and is highly recommended. Another text catering for a similar market is *Essentials of neurosurgery* by R. Hayward (Blackwell, 1980). A standard work in this area is *Northfield's Surgery of the central nervous system*, edited by J.D. Miller (2nd edn., Blackwell Scientific Publications, 1987).

Ophthalmic surgery

This specialty is well served in the number of serial publications which cater for practitioners. *Acta Ophthalmologica, American Journal of Ophthalmology, Annals of Ophthalmology, Archives of Ophthalmology, British Journal of Ophthalmology, Cornea, Current Eye Research, Developments in Ophthalmology, Eye, International Ophthalmology Clinics, Journal of Clinical Neuro-ophthalmology, Journal of Ocular Therapy and Surgery, Ophthalmic Surgery* and *Transactions of the American Ophthalmological Society*. There are also a number of foreign-language journals including *Journal Français d'Ophtalmologie, Ophtalmologie* and *Vestnik Oftalmologii (Moscow)*.

Abstracts are covered by *Excerpta Medica*, Section 12 (Ophthalmology). Review publications include *Advances in ophthalmic, plastic and reconstructive surgery*. Volumes 6 and 7 of this series comprise *Orbital trauma*, part 1, and *Orbital trauma*, part 2, edited by S.L. Bosniak (Pergamon Press, 1987). As well as providing an overview of current techniques there are reprints of classic papers. The *Acta Concilium Ophthalmologicum* are the published proceedings of meetings held by the International Federation of Ophthalmological Societies. Articles in this publication are in English, French and German. The *Année Therapeutique et Clinique en Ophtalmologie* is published annually by Fueri-Lami, Marseille. Butterworths International Review series have a section on Ophthalmology of which *Glaucoma* by J. McAlister and R. Wilson is number 3 in the series (Butterworths, 1986). *Developments in Ophthalmology* is published twice yearly by Karger with text in both German and English. Every five years the *Transactions of the European Ophthalmological Society Congress* are published by Academic Press.

Stallard's Eye surgery, edited by M.J. Roper-Hall (7th edn., Butterworths, 1989) is an up-to-date standard UK reference work as is *Ophthalmic surgery*, edited by T.A. Rice, R.G. Michels and W.J. Stark (4th edn., Butterworths, 1984). This book is part of Rob and Smith's *Operative surgery* series. Ophthalmic surgery lends itself to practical guide by illustration and an example of this is the series *Atlas of ophthalmic surgery* of which Volume 2 is *Cornea, glaucoma, lens*, edited by K. Heilmann and D. Paton (Georg Thieme, 1987). Like the previous volume in this series which dealt with *Lids, orbits and extraocular muscles* (Georg Thieme, 1985) this series is characterized by superb illustrations coupled with a clear and concise text. A recent U.S. orientated textbook is *Surgery of the eye*, edited by S.R. Woltman *et al.* (Churchill Livingstone, 1987). This is a two-volume work and the contributors are mainly from the USA.

Manual of cataract surgery by R.M. Sinskey and J.V. Patel (Churchill Livingstone, 1987) is a book aimed at the surgeon beginning his surgical training and gives a clear account of extracapsular cataract technique.

Ear, nose and throat surgery

Journals include *Acta Oto-laryngologica, Acta Oto-Rhino- Laryngologica, American Journal of Otolaryngology, Annales d'Oto-laryngologie et de Chirurgie Cervico-Faciale, Annals of Otology, Rhinology and Laryngology, Archives of Otolaryngology, Archives of Oto-rhino-laryngology (Berlin), Ear, Nose and Throat Journal, HNO* (Berlin); this last has text in German with index and summaries in English and German *Journal of Laryngology and Otology, Laryngoscope, Otolaryngologic Clinics of North America, Otolaryngology – Head and Neck Surgery* and *Vestnik Otorinolaringologii (Moscow)*.

Abstracts are to be found in *Excerpta Medica*, Section 11, and since

January 1989 a selection of relevant abstracts from a variety of journals has appeared in each issue of the *Journal of Laryngology and Otology*. *Advances in Oto-Rhino-Laryngology* (Karger) is an intermittent review publication under the series editorship of C.R.P Faltz. Butterworths International Medical Review Series has *Otolaryngology* Volume 2, *Plastic reconstruction in the head and neck*, edited by T.R. Bull and E.N. Myers (Butterworths, 1986). Another review publication is *Recent advances in otolaryngology — 6*, edited by R.F. Gray and J.A. Rutka (Churchill Livingstone, 1988). This edition includes information on the contribution made to ENT by developments in physics and technology. It should be noted however that there is very little information on the subspecialty of rhinology in this particular volume. The current volume in the yearbook series is *Year Book of Otolaryngology – head and neck surgery 1989*, edited by M. Paparella and B. Bailey (Year Book Publishers, 1989).

The *Ear*, edited by J.C. Ballantyne and A. Morrison (4th edn., Butterworths, 1986) is part of the Rob and Smith's *Operative surgery* series. Probably one of the best known books is *Logan Turner's Diseases of the nose, throat and ear*, edited by A.G.D. Maran (10th edn., John Wright, 1988). Because of its popularity in the Middle East and Asia the book also includes pathologies rarely seen in Europe. Also there is *Diseases of the nose, ear and throat* (13th edn., Churchill Livingstone, 1987). This is, as it describes itself on the title page, a handbook for students and practitioners. The definitive encyclopaedic reference work on this subject is *Scott-Brown's Otolaryngology*, edited by A.G. Kerr and J. Groves (5th edn., Butterworths, 1987). This set comprises six volumes, each one by a separate editor. The topics covered in each volume are by turn basic sciences, adult audiology, otology, rhinology, laryngology and paediatric otolaryngology. Another standard work is *Mawson's Diseases of the ear*, edited by H. Ludlum (5th edn., Edward Arnold, 1988). This edition has been radically updated and enlarged since the last edition nearly 10 years previously. Laser surgery is a technique used more and more and developments are summarized in *Lasers in otolaryngology*, edited by J.A.S. Chapman and G.T. Simpson (Chapman and Hall, 1988). This book is modestly priced and will be especially popular with the new generation of surgeons.

Plastic surgery

This is a very distinct and arguably one of the oldest branches of surgery. Burn injuries remain one of the main reasons for surgical repair as do hand injuries and the repair of cleft lip and palate. Immunological research is of paramount importance to the plastic surgeon, especially in the areas of skin homografts and cartilage grafts.

JOURNALS

The specialist journals include *Acta Chirurgiae Plasticae, British Journal of Plastic Surgery, Burns, Journal of Maxillo-Facial Surgery, Hand Clinics, Plastic and Reconstructive Surgery*, which carries a selection of international abstracts, and the *Scandinavian Journal of Plastic and Reconstructive Surgery*.

REVIEWS

One of the current review publications is *Recent advances in plastic surgery — 3*, edited by I.T. Jackson and B.C. Sommerlad (Churchill Livingstone, 1985). Another occasional series began with *Advances in plastic and reconstructive surgery*, Volume 1 edited by M.B. Habal (Blackwell, 1984). There have been no further issues of this series so far and the best section in this volume is Ian Jackson's chapter on the treatment of cleft palates. Year Book Medical Publishers produce the *Year Book of Plastic and Reconstructive Surgery*, the last issue being Volume 5 (1989), edited by M.B. Habal.

TEXTBOOKS

The latest and most comprehensive text is a multi-volume work *Plastic surgery*, edited by J.G. McCarthy (8 vols, Saunders, 1990). The current cost is up to £600 which destines the set for only the larger libraries with budgets to match but the volumes are available for sale on an individual basis at around £90 each. An excellent basic textbook is *Fundamental techniques of plastic surgery and their surgical application* by I.A. McGregor (8th edn., Churchill Livingstone, 1989). This book has proved itself essential reading for surgical training through successive editions and it has maintained a high standard of clear text and illustration since it first appeared over twenty years ago. *Operative plastic and reconstructive surgery*, edited by J.N. Barron and M.N. Saad (Churchill Livingstone, 1980-1981) is a three-volume work, the first two dealing with general plastic and reconstructive techniques while the third is devoted to surgery of the hand. In the *Operative surgery* series there is *Plastic surgery*, edited by J. Watson and R.M. McCormack (4th edn., Butterworths, 1986). Another comprehensive but concise work is *Plastic surgery: a concise guide to clinical practice*, edited by W.C. Grabb and J.W. Smith (3rd edn., Little, Brown, 1980) which is designed for senior students and surgeons in training. More specialized current monographs include *Plastic surgery in infancy and childhood*, edited by J. C. Mustarde and I.T. Jackson (3rd edn., Churchill Livingstone, 1988) and *Textbook of ophthalmic plastic and reconstructive surgery* by R. Kohn (Lea and Febiger, 1988). One of the most rapidly developing fields is that of hand surgery and there is a journal devoted to developments in this area. Nevertheless there are a number of books which deal comprehensively with the subject. One of the most recent is *Principles of hand surgery* by F.D. Burke, D.A. McGrowther and P.J. Smith (Churchill Livingstone, 1990). This is recommended for trainees in hand surgery and deals with principles rather than practical applications which are dealt with in *The practice of hand surgery*, edited by D.W. Lamb, G. Hooper and K. Kuczynski (2nd edn., Blackwell, 1988). A definitive and exhaustive work on the subject is *Operative hand surgery* edited by D.P. Green (3 vols, 2nd edn., Churchill Livingstone, 1988).

Urological surgery

Some of the principal journals of interest to the urological surgeon are the *British Journal of Urology, Journal of Urology, Urologic Clinics of North America, Nephron, Scandinavian Journal of Urology and Nephrology*. An up-to-date review series is *Recent Advances in Urology —4*, edited by W.F. Hendry (Churchill Livingstone, 1987). Less up to date but also recommended is *Current trends in Urology — 5*, edited by M.I. Resnick (Williams and Wilkins, 1985).

There are several comprehensive textbooks of surgical urology. Some of the best known are *Campbell's Urology*, edited by P.C. Walsh *et al.* (5th edn., W.B. Saunders, 1985) and *Operative urology* by J. Blandy (2nd edn., Blackwell, 1986). This latter is a step-by-step manual of instruction in the basic operations of urologic surgery. As part of the *Current operative surgery* series, there is *Urology* by A.R. Mundy (W.B. Saunders, 1987). This is a short textbook comprising about 200 pages but the information is concise and direct. Background reading for surgical Fellowship candidates is provided by *Scientific basis of urology* by A.R. Mundy (Churchill Livingstone, 1987). Other texts are *Current therapy in genitourinary surgery*, edited by M.I. Resnick and E. Kursh (B.C. Decker, 1987). This comprises a series of short (average 4 – 6 pages) contributions by acknowledged experts on a wide range of sub-topics. It is a reasonably comprehensive survey but there are no references provided. *New techniques in urology*, edited by R.W. DeVere White and J.M. Palmer (Futura Publishing, 1987) although now not so current is a good survey of modern techniques. The book is in four parts — renal calculi, new urological instrumentation, diagnosis and new technologies in patient management.

Abdominal surgery

The preserve of the general surgeon includes abdominal surgery, and relevant articles are to be found in the standard surgical journals, as well as in the specialist serials such as *Digestive Diseases and Sciences,*

American Journal of Gastroenterology, Diseases of the Colon and Rectum, Gastroenterology, Gut and the *Journal of Abdominal Surgery.*

Each month the *American Journal of Gastroenterology* publishes a *World Literature Review* which provides an abstract and comment on selected articles in other serial publications. Selective abstracts are provided by *Excerpta Medica, 48: Gastroenterology. Modern techniques in surgery (abdominal surgery)* is published on average annually by Futura Publications.

Some of the books currently available in this area of surgery are the following: *Maingot's Abdominal operations*, edited by Seymour I. Schwartz and Harold Ellis (2 vols, 9th edn., Appleton and Lange, 1989). This is the standard authoritative work on the subject. *Manual of lower gastrointestinal surgery* by C.E. Welch, L.W. Ottinger and J.P. Welch (Springer, 1980) is one of a series from this publisher under the general title of *Comprehensive manuals of surgical specialities*. A work which can be recommended for postgraduate study is *Surgery of the alimentary tract* by R.T. Shackleford and G.D. Zuidema (5 vols, 2nd edn., W.B. Saunders, 1988). A short concise 'pocket' book is *Cope's Early diagnosis of the acute abdomen*, edited by W. Silen (17th edn., OUP, 1987). Another text which can be unreservedly recommended is *Surgery of the anus, rectum and colon* by J.C. Goligher (5th edn., Baillière Tindall, 1984). Among the more specialized texts is *Surgery of the liver and biliary tract*, edited by L.H. Blumgart (Churchill Livingstone, 1988) and *Surgery of the gall bladder and bile ducts* by Lord Smith of Marlow and S. Sherlock (2nd edn., Butterworths, 1981).

Anaesthesia

The scope of anaesthetics has travelled far from the concept of the ether bottle, and now includes a more sophisticated range of anaesthetic agents, and changes in the method of induction, including intravenous anaesthetic drugs and relaxants. Improved methods as well as advances in physiology and pharmacology have enabled the surgeon to gain access to deeper structures and to explore more extensively and with greater safety than before. The modern anaesthetist must have a considerable knowledge, anatomical and functional, of the respiratory, cardiovascular and nervous system. Metabolism, excretion and endocrine function also have aspects related to the efficient practice of anaesthetics. Techniques have become specialized for anaesthetists in oto-rhino-laryngology, dental surgery, pulmonary operations, neurosurgery, ophthalmology and electroconvulsive therapy. Special care units — respiratory and coronary — and intensive care therapy units now involve a major contribution from the anaesthetist. The principal

English-language journals of anaesthesia are: *Acta Anaesthesiologica Scandinavica; Anaesthesia; Anesthesia and Analgesia; Anesthesiology; Anaesthesia and Intensive Care; British Journal of Anaesthesia; European Journal of Anaesthesiology; Anaesthesia* contains *Anaesthetic Literature*, which is a classified list of recent articles pertaining to anaesthetics. This journal also carries reviews of appropriate audio-visual material available.

Abstracting and indexing services

These include *Excerpta Medica*, Section 24: *Anesthesiology*, and *Anesthesia Abstracts*. *Anesthesiology Bibliography* is a quarterly service provided by the National Library of Medicine in the USA through the Wood Library Museum of Anesthesiology, and is useful as a quick-reference tool.

Textbooks and monographs

Comprehensive textbooks have the disadvantage of being out of date often by the time of publication, but they do have the merit of gathering together current, concepts and practice in one or two volumes. One of the most popular and widely consulted texts in the UK is *General anaesthesia*, edited by J.F. Nunn, J.E. Utting and B.R. Brown (5th edn., Butterworths, 1989). Another comprehensive textbook is *Anaesthesia*, edited by R.D. Miller (3rd edn., Churchill Livingstone, 1990). Two shorter texts are *Textbook of anaesthesia*, edited by G. Smith and A.R. Aitkenhead (2nd edn., Churchill Livingstone, 1990) and *Manual of anesthesia* by J.C. Snow (Little, Brown, 1983). Both of these last two can be recommended for students and trainee anaesthetists. *The Scientific foundations of anaesthesia*, edited by C. Scurr and S. Feldman (3rd edn., Heinemann, 1982) may be recommended to those taking higher examinations in anaesthesia. There are a number of good monographs dealing with anaesthesia under a variety of conditions and varying occasions and, while there are many such monographs, among the more recent and well received are *Principles and practice of regional anaesthesia*, edited by J.A.W. Wildsmith and E.M. Armitage (Churchill Livingstone, 1987), *Handbook of epidural anesthesia and analgesia*, edited by B.G. Corvino and D.B. Scott (Grune and Stratton, 1985), and *Pediatric anesthesia*, edited by G.A. Gregory (2nd edn., Churchill Livingstone, 1989).

History

Surgery

Probably the best known source of historical information is *Morton's Medical Bibliography* by L.T. Morton (5th edn., edited by J.M. Norman, Gower, 1991). The National Library of Medicine in the USA produces a *Bibliography of the History of Medicine* which is retrospectively available in five-year cumulations. There are several good texts in the history of surgery. Two relatively recent publications are the *Rise of surgery* by O.W. Wangensteen and S.D. Wangensteen (Dawson, 1978) and *The healers, a history of medicine in Scotland* by D. Hamilton (Canongate, 1981). Older standard texts include *The history and literature of surgery* by J.S. Billings (Argosy Antiquarian, 1970), a reprint of a classic text initially published in 1895 as part of *A system of surgery* by F. S. Dennis. *An introduction to the history of surgery* by R.H. Meade (Saunders, 1970) is useful as a basis for further study and contains an excellent bibliography. *Great ideas in the history of surgery* by L.M. Zimmerman and J. Veith (Baillière, Tindall and Cox, 1962) contains extracts from antiquarian texts and verbatim reports as they originally appeared. *Milestones in modern surgery* by A. Hurwitz and G.A. Degenshein (Cassell, 1958) is dependent upon U.S. authors' concept of a 'milestone', but the criteria used for selection ensure a reasonable survey. *The development of modern surgery* by F.E. Cartwright (Arthur Baker, 1967) covers the last 150 years and is designed for the lay reader as well as the student of medical history. A classic which has been reprinted and is again available since its appearance 50 years ago is *A short history of surgery* by D'Arcy Power (New York, AMS Press, 1981). Information on the history of surgery is also to be found in the histories of some of the great institutions, e.g. *The Royal College of Surgeons of England – A history* by Z. Cope (Blond, 1959) and in the biographies of famous surgeons. A useful source of biographical information is contained in *Bailey and Bishop's Notable names in medicine and surgery* revised by H. Ellis (4th edn., H.K. Lewis, 1983).

In addition to the volumes already cited, there are a number of books dealing with the historical aspect of surgical specialties. Examples of this type are *History of urology* by L.S. Murphy (C.C. Thomas, 1972) an exhaustive treatise on the subject. *A history of the acute abdomen* by Z. Cope (OUP, 1965) is a compact work crammed with well-organized information and *A history of thoracic surgery* by R. Meade (Blackwell, 1961) runs to 1000 pages and carries an extensive bibliography. Plastic surgery is served by *The source book of plastic surgery*, by F. McDowell (Williams and Wilkins, 1977). However no résumé of the history of this specialty would be complete without mention of

McDowell Indexes of plastic surgery, edited by F. McDowell (Williams and Wilkins, 1977–1981). This monumental five-volume work covers citations in journal or book from 900 BC to 1976 and must rank as an astonishing piece of historical research.

Anaesthesia

The last few decades have seen some considerable developments in anaesthesia and this comparatively recent history is covered by *Anaesthesiology progress since 1940* by E.M. Papper, S.H. Ngai and L.C. Mark (University of Miami Press, 1973). An earlier period is dealt with in *Essays on the first hundred years of anaesthesia* by W.S. Sykes (Churchill Livingstone, 1982). *Foundations of anesthesiology* by A. Faulconer and T.E. Keyes (C.C. Thomas, 1965) is a compilation of some 150 reprints of famous papers on anaesthesia and related topics. Another compilation of first-hand accounts is *Milestones in anesthesia* by F. Cole (University of Nebraska Press, 1965) which covers the period 1665 – 1940. *The evolution of anaesthesia*, by M.H. Armstrong Davidson (John Sherratt, 1965) is a history in which the author sets out to dispel some of the 'romantic myths' of the 'conquest of pain'. B.M. Duncum's *The development of inhalation anaesthesia* (OUP, 1947) deals with the period 1846 – 1900. An earlier work which has been updated by additional material is *History of surgical anesthesia* by T.E. Keys (Krieger, 1978). One recent volume is *The history of anaesthesia*, edited by R.S. Atkinson and T.B. Boulton (Parthenon, 1987), this being the proceedings of the Second International Conference on the History of Anaesthesia. In conclusion the history of the extensive range of anaesthetic equipment is explored in *The development of anaesthetic apparatus* by K.B. Thomas (Blackwell, 1975). This is a history based on the Charles King Collection of the Association of Anaesthetists of Great Britain and Ireland.

CHAPTER NINETEEN

Obstetrics and gynaecology

PATRICIA C. WANT

The specialty of obstetrics and gynaecology concerns the human reproductive process in all its aspects. More specifically it includes pregnancy and its complications, fetal medicine, artificial reproduction and the control of fertility as well as diseases of women. The Royal College of Obstetricians and Gynaecologists officially recognizes four sub-specialties: reproductive medicine, fetal medicine, gynaecological urology and gynaecological oncology. All are covered in this chapter together with related subjects, such as human genetics, that are not addressed elsewhere. Emphasis has been placed on the more important sources, and complementary titles appear only as a guide to further reading. Where very little material has been published, titles are listed with no attempt at discrimination. Undergraduate texts are included where appropriate.

Indexes and abstracts

The primary printed bibliographical source, *Index Medicus* with annual cumulations, is described elsewhere (p. 52). Indexes and abstracts of a more specialized nature are also available as follows:

A current-awareness publication, *Ad Referendum: Obstetrics and Gynaecology* (Solihull: Infomed, 1982–), comprises contents lists of some 12 or so core journals in the specialty. It is published bimonthly and distributed free of charge by the sponsor to interested members of the medical profession. *Core Journals in Obstetrics/Gynecology* (Amsterdam: Excerpta Medica, 1977–) contains abstracts of original articles from approximately 12 key specialist periodicals plus five leading general medical journals; these appear some 4–6 weeks after journal receipt. Issues are published monthly with a combined June/July issue and each has an author and subject index. A companion series, *Core Journals in Clinical Endocrinology* first appeared in 1982.

Bibliography of Reproduction: a Monthly Listing of the Literature in Vertebrate Reproductive Biology and Clinical Science (Cambridge: Reproduction Research Information Service, 1963–) is an official publication of the Society for the Study of Fertility (UK), the Society for the Study of Reproduction (USA), the Australian Society for Reproductive Biology and the Blair Bell Research Society (UK). Coverage includes books and theses, as well as periodicals, some scanned directly, others covered indirectly by means of *Index Medicus* and *Current Contents*. Published monthly, in two volumes per annum, each issue carries author and animal indexes and each volume a subject index referring the researcher to individual citation numbers. It is more up to date than *Index Medicus* and designed for current, rather than retrospective, searching. Several thousand journals are covered and 50 per cent of the papers indexed are in foreign languages, translations of the titles being provided. Entries are grouped under broad subject headings and each paper is cited in only one place and allotted a serial number which may be given as a cross-reference elsewhere. Papers quoting more than 40 references are marked with an asterisk. Within each subject section books and monographs are listed first followed by papers in hierarchical order from humans through to fishes. Addresses of authors are included wherever possible. The absence of cumulated author indexes hampers any attempt at retrospective searching by name but patient scanning through a few monthly issues can sometimes yield results with citations not indexed elsewhere. Special subject bibliographies are included in certain issues and are also available separately. A useful list of future meetings pertaining to reproductive biology is issued regularly. The publishers also operate a literature searching service, 'Repro-Search', from a database which in 1990 contained over 120 000 references indexed since 1983 and which grows at a rate of approximately 1400–1800 additional citations per month. References from 1963 onwards, some 300 000 from an earlier information store, can be searched on application via the original system.

The most comprehensive abstracting publication in this subject field is *Excerpta Medica; Section 10: Obstetrics and Gynecology* (Amsterdam, 1948–). This appears in two volumes per annum, each comprising ten issues, with accompanying author and keyword subject indexes which are cumulated in the last issue of each volume. Abstracts are usually short and may comprise the summary already published at source. This useful publication occasionally eliminates the need to pursue the original paper. Section 3: *Endocrinology*; Section 22: *Human Genetics* and Section 28: *Urology and Nephrology* are of related interest. The *Year Book of Obstetrics and Gynecology* (Chicago: Year Book Medical Publishers, 1902–) has appeared under various titles, the subjects initially being separated. It may contain a review paper in addition to the normally substantial summaries and occasional accompanying editorial comment. An attempt is made at approximate subject grouping which is helpful in reviewing recent work on a particular topic. The companion volume, *Year Book of Perinatal Neonatal Medicine* first published in 1987 has a similar format. *Obstetrical and Gynecological Survey* (Baltimore: Williams and Wilkins, 1946–) provides, as the title suggests, a survey of the specialist literature. Each monthly issue contains from one to three review articles in addition to substantial summaries of important papers. Editorial comment accompanies each summary, often at length. Each December issue comprises a five-year cumulative author and subject index to both reviews and abstracts and provides a useful quick reference guide to recent literature.

The International Abstracts of Surgery section of *Surgery, Gynecology and Obstetrics* (Chicago: American College of Surgeons) appears in the latter publication from 1913, Volume 16 onwards. It contains signed abstracts on the 'Surgery of the female reproductive system' which is subdivided into: uterus and adnexa; ovaries; external genitalia; pregnancy and complications; and placenta, fetus and newborn. Emphasis is on general surgery, however, and the periodical itself cannot be regarded as a primary source in the subject field of obstetrics and gynaecology. The abstracts are therefore of limited value since non-subscribers are unlikely to take the trouble to check through them. A new, more specialized publication, is *Obstetric Anesthesia Digest* (Wichita, KA: Obstetric Anesthesia Digest Inc., 1981–). It appears quarterly and contains summaries of key papers together with critical commentaries. Obstetric anaesthetists may find it a useful addition to their personal library, and the thin volumes occupy little shelf space.

Similar publications originate overseas. These include: *Berichte über die gesamte Gynäkologie und Geburtshilfe sowie deren Grenzgebiete* (Berlin: Deutsche Gesellschaft für Gynäkologie, 1923–); *Meditsinskii Referativnyi Zhurnal* (Moscow, 1957–); *Gynäkologische Rundschau* (Basle: Karger, 1964–); *Rassegna Bibliografia della Stampa Ostetrico-Ginecologia* (Rome, 1949–) and *Sekai Sanfujinka Soran* [*Survey of World Obstetrics and Gynaecology*] (Tokyo, 1958–).

Dictionaries

Although it may not be considered a dictionary in the usual sense of the term, *Obstetric-gynecologic terminology*, edited by E.C. Hughes (Davis, 1972) falls within this category and is a most useful reference tool. Arranged by subject rather than alphabetically the index provides the key to the whole. A brief definition is provided, together with known synonyms for each term, and entries are on the whole more detailed than those found in conventional medical dictionaries. A polyglot dictionary, prepared by N.C. Louros, is *Obstétrique et gynécologie; glossaire des termes obstétricaux et gynécologiques en français, latin, anglais, russe, allemand, espagnol, italien, grec* (Elsevier, 1964). A selection of dictionaries intended for midwives have been published, the most recent being *Baillière's midwives dictionary* (7th edn., by Vera Da Cruz and Margaret Adams, Baillière Tindall, 1983).

Directories

Directories have a limited life and even those updated at regular intervals may not be totally reliable. A selection of the more useful directories is as follows: *Royal College of Obstetricians and Gynaecologists, Register of Fellows and Members* (RCOG, 1966–) which was included in the *Annual Report* through 1964 and is currently published biannually. Arrangement is alphabetical, with separate sections for Fellows and Members containing names of practitioners within the main towns of the countries represented.

For the USA, the equivalent source is the American College of Obstetricians and Gynecologists' *Directory of Fellows, with Office Committees* (Washington, D.C., ACOG) which is regularly updated. Continental publications include *Gynäkologen deutscher Sprache. Biographie und Bibliographie* (Stuttgart, 1928–) published under a succession of titles.

Journals

Many important papers will, of course, be found in leading general medical journals and few specialist libraries would lack copies of the *British Medical Journal*, *The Lancet*, or *New England Journal of Medicine* for example. Periodicals devoted specifically to obstetrics and gynaecology and closely associated subjects now exist in abundance, however, and the tide shows no sign of receding with the addition of anything from two to six or so new titles each year with some claim to consideration for inclusion in stock. Listed below, and grouped very approximately by subject, are a selection of those titles most likely to be encountered by the librarian, the emphasis with certain exceptions being on Britain and American publications. A number of newer titles which at present may not easily be traced in check-lists elsewhere have also been included for information. The cited year refers to the first issue of the most recent form of the title.

Obstetrics, gynaecology and fetal medicine

Acta Obstetricia et Gynecologica Scandinavia, Stockholm (1926–)

American Journal of Obstetrics and Gynecology, St. Louis, MO (1920–)

Archives of Gynaecology and Obstetrics, Heidelberg (1987–)

Asia-Oceania Journal of Obstetrics and Gynaecology, Tokyo (1980–)

Australia and New Zealand Journal of Obstetrics and Gynaecology, Melbourne (1961–)

Baillière's Clinical Obstetrics and Gynaecology, Oxford (1975–)

Biology of Reproduction, Champaign, IL (1969–)

British Journal of Obstetrics and Gynaecology, Oxford (1975–)

Clinical Obstetrics and Gynaecology, Hagerstown, MD (1958–)

Contemporary Ob/Gyn, Oradell, NJ (1975–)

Contemporary Reviews in Obstetrics and Gynaecology, London (1988–)

Early Human Development, Limerick (1977–)

European Journal of Obstetrics, Gynaecology and Reproductive Biology, Amsterdam (1973–)

Fetal Medicine Review, Sevenoaks, Kent (1989–)

Geburtshilfe und Frauenheilkunde, Stuttgart (1939–)

Gynecology and Obstetrici Investigation, Basle (1978–)

Gynecologic Oncology, Duluth, MI (1972–)

Human Reproduction, Oxford (1986–)

International Journal of Gynecological Pathology, New York (1982–)

International Journal of Gynaecology and Obstetrics, Limerick (1969–)

International Journal of Prenatal and Perinatal Studies, Carnforth, Lancs (1989–)

International Urogynaecology Journal, London (1990–)

Journal of Gynecologic Surgery, New York (1989–)

Journal of Obstetrics and Gynaecology, Basingstoke, Hants (1980–)

Journal of Perinatal Medicine, Chicago, IL (1968–)
Journal of Perinatology, E. Norwalk, CT (1989–)
Journal of Reproductive Immunology, Limerick (1980–)
Journal of Reproductive Medicine, St. Louis, MO (1968–)
Maturitas, Limerick (1979–)
Minerva Ginecologica, Turin (1950–)
Obstetrics and Gynecology, New York (1953–)
Obstetrics and Gynecology Clinics of North America, Philadelphia, PA (1987–)
Placenta, London (1980–)
Prenatal Diagnosis, Chichester, W. Sussex (1977–)
Seminars in Perinatology, Duluth, MI (1977–)
Surgery, Gynecology and Obstetrics, Chicago, IL (1905–)
Ultrasound in Obstetrics and Gynecology, Carnforth, Lancs (1991–)
Zeitschrift für Geburtshilfe und Perinatologie, Stuttgart (1972–)
Zentralblatt für Gynäkologie, Leipzig (1877–1944; 1947–)

Infertility and contraception

Acta Europaea Fertilitatis, Rome (1969–)
British Journal of Family Planning, London (1977–)
Contraception, Stoneham, MA (1970–)
Fertility and Sterility, Birmingham, AL (1950–)
Infertility, New York (1978–)
International Journal of Fertility, Port Washington, NY (1955–)
Journal of In-Vitro Fertilization and Embryo Transfer, New York (1984–)
Journal of Reproduction and Fertility, Cambridge (1960–)
Reproduction, Fertility and Development, Melbourne (1989–)

Endocrinology

Acta Endocrinologica, Copenhagen (1948–)
Clinical Endocrinology, Oxford (1972–)
Endocrinology, Baltimore, MD (1917–)
Gynecological Endocrinology, Carnforth, Lancs (1987–)
Journal of Clinical Endocrinology and Metabolism, Baltimore, MD (1941–)

Journal of Endocrinology, Bristol (1939–)

Seminars in Reproductive Endocrinology, New York (1983–)

Human genetics

American Journal of Human Genetics, Baltimore, MD (1949–)

Annals of Human Genetics, Cambridge (1954)

Journal of Medical Genetics, London (1964–)

Serials and series

Certain regularly published series and serials provide reviews on selected topics within the subject field. Extensive bibliographies may be included. A title popular with postgraduate specialists is *Progress in Obstetrics and Gynaecology* edited by J.W.W. Studd (Churchill Livingstone, Volume 8, 1990). Content is divided equally between the two subject fields and chapters are contributed by specialists on topics of current interest. *Recent Advances in Obstetrics and Gynaecology* (edited by John Bonnar, Churchill Livingstone, Volume 16, 1990) has appeared irregularly since 1947 under various editors and is useful whilst current. A similar publication, originating from the USA, devoted solely to gynaecology, is M.L. Taymor and J.H. Nelson's *Progress in Gynecology* (Grune and Stratton, Volume 7, 1983), but no more recent edition has been announced. *Clinical Obstetrics and Gynecology*, containing a selection of papers on two or three key topics, was first published in 1958 and appeared quarterly. Two separate *Clinics* titles are now available, one UK, one U.S., succeeding the popular *Clinics in Obstetrics and Gynaecology*. These are, respectively, *Baillière's Clinical Obstetrics and Gynaecology* (Baillière Tindall 1987–) and *Obstetrics and Gynecology Clinics of North America* (Saunders, 1987–). The former is a core journal for postgraduate students preparing for primary examinations in the specialty in the UK since most of the contributors are known specialists in their subject field. Both titles appear quarterly and are available individually or on a combined subscription at a reduced rate. A small number of more specialized publications may be mentioned in this category such as: *Reviews in Perinatal Medicine*, edited by E.M. Scarpelli and E.V. Cosmi (Volume 1, Liss, 1977, in progress); *Clinics in Perinatology* (Volume 1, Saunders, 1974, in progress) which is similar in format to the aforementioned *Clinics in Obstetrics and Gynaecology* and *Oxford Reviews of Reproductive Biology* (OUP, Volume 1, 1979 in progress). Perinatology Press (Ithaca, New York) publish a number of titles in the following series: *Reproductive and Perinatal Medicine; Research in Perinatal Medicine* and *Animal Models in Fetal Medicine*. Certain publications appear in series but may also be separately advertised as monographs cited under author and volume title. One of the examples most likely to be encountered is *Contributions to Gynecology and Obstetrics* (Karger, 1961–).

Textbooks and monographs

The subject headings adopted in the following pages form only approximate divisions with logical progression from general to specific. Books on more than one subject are normally allotted the earliest appropriate placing without subsequent repetition.

Subjects often overlap since obstetrics, which concerns the pregnant state, often goes hand in hand with gynaecology, which addresses the diseases of women. It is not within the scope of this chapter to cover these subjects comprehensively at all levels, so texts intended for nurses and laywomen will only be mentioned from time to time where such information may be helpful. Midwifery is a subject field in its own right and will not be covered here except for certain representative texts. Unless otherwise specified, material is generally intended for postgraduate use.

Combined texts

Standard reference works include: *Dewhurst's Integrated obstetrics and gynaecology for postgraduates* (4th edn., Blackwell, 1986), edited by C.R. Whitfield; *Obstetrics and gynecology* by J.R. Willson and others (7th edn., Mosby, 1983) and *Danforth's Obstetrics and gynecology*, edited by J.R. Scott with 65 contributors (6th edn., Lippincott, 1990). Among the smaller paperbacks available are: *Contemporary obstetrics and gynaecology*, edited by G. Chamberlain (Butterworths, 1988); J. Willocks and J.P. Nielsen's *Obstetrics and gynaecology* (4th edn., Churchill Livingstone, 1990) in the 'Student Notes' Series: R.S. Ledward's *Handbook of obstetrics and gynaecology: a guide for housemen* (Wright, 1986); *Undergraduate obstetrics and gynaecology*, edited by M.G.R. Hull, G. Turner and D.N. Joyce (2nd edn., Wright, 1986); Sir Stanley Clayton and J.R. Newton's *Pocket obstetrics and gynaecology* (11th edn., Churchill Livingstone, 1988). D. Llewellyn-Jones' *Fundamentals of obstetrics and gynaecology*: vol. 1, *Obstetrics*; vol. 2 *Gynaecology* (5th edn., Faber, 1990) and B.G. Wren and R.A. Lobo's *Handbook of obstetrics and gynaecology* (3rd edn., Baillière, 1989). Useful texts for foundation studies for primary examinations are: *Scientific foundations of obstetrics and gynaecology*, edited by E.E. Philipp and M. Setchell (4th edn., Butterworth–Heinemann, 1991); *Scientific basis of obstetrics and gynaecology*, edited by R.R. MacDonald (3rd edn., Churchill Livingstone, 1985) and T. Chard and R. Lilford's *Basic sciences for obstetrics and gynaecology* (3rd edn., Springer, 1990) which is available in paperback. For many years *Obstetrics and gynaecology in the tropics and developing countries* by J.B. Lawson and D.B. Stewart (Arnold, 1967) has provided required reading in this more specialized field. The long awaited new edition is currently in preparation. *The Proceedings of the XIIth World Congress of Gynaecology and Obstetrics* (Rio de Janeiro, October, 1988) are available in a series of six volumes which may be purchased individually or as a boxed set under the title *Advances in Gynecology and Obstetrics*, edited by P. Belfort, J.A. Pinotti and T.K.A.B. Eskes (Parthenon, 1989). The volumes contain selected contributions and titles are as follows: vol. 1: Fertility, Sterility and Contraception; vol. 2: Fetal Physiology and Pathology; vol. 3: Gynaecological Cancer; vol. 4: Maternal Physiology and Pathology; vol. 5: Pregnancy Termination and Labour; vol. 6: General Gynecology.

The following is a selection of titles produced as aids to candidates for the various RCOG examinations. For the MRCOG Part 1, V.R. Tindall's *Multiple choice tutor: basic sciences in obstetrics and gynaecology* (Heinemann, 1987) which incorporates both first and second series in a single volume, is helpful; also T. Chard and R. Lilford's *MRCOG Part 1* (Springer, 1987). G.M. Stirrat's *Aids to obstetrics and gynaecology: for MRCOG Part 2* (2nd edn., Churchill Livingstone, 1987) and V.R. Tindall, R.H. Martin and R.W. Burslem's *Preparation and advice for the MRCOG* (Churchill Livingstone, 1989) relate to Part 2. *Notes for the DRCOG* by P. Kay (2nd edn., 1988) is suitable as an aid to revision at Diploma level as is *Preparation and revision for the DRCOG* by J. Rymer and others (Churchill Livingstone, 1990).

OBSTETRICS

Two substantial textbooks have recently filled a gap in the UK market; these are *Obstetrics*, edited by Sir Alec Turnbull and G. Chamberlain (Churchill Livingstone, 1989) and *Principles of obstetrics* by B.M. Hibbard (Butterworths, 1988) which last may be purchased individually or in a boxed set with a companion volume on gynaecology by V.R. Tindall (q.v). *Williams' Obstetrics* by F.G. Cunningham and others has now reached an 18th edition (Prentice Hall, 1989) and is the equivalent U.S. text. Also available are *Clinical obstetrics* edited by C.J. Pauerstein (Wiley, 1987) and S.G. Gabbe, J.R. Niebyl and J.L. Simpson's *Obstetrics: normal and problem pregnancies* (Churchill Livingstone, 1986). A less substantial but well-known publication is *Obstetrics by ten teachers* edited by T.L.T. Lewis and G. Chamberlain (15th edn., Arnold, 1990). Student texts include: G.V.P. Chamberlain, C.R. Gibbings and Sir John Dewhurst's *Illustrated textbook of obstetrics* (Lippincott,

1988); *Obstetrics illustrated* by A.W.F. Miller and R. Callander (4th edn., Churchill Livingstone, 1989); G.V.P. Chamberlain's *Lecture notes on obstetrics* (5th edn., Blackwell, 1984) and *Obstetrics pocket consultant* by G.M. Stirrat (2nd edn., Blackwell, 1986). The main textbooks for midwives are: *Myles' Textbook for midwives*, edited by V. Ruth Bennett and Linda K. Brown (11th edn., Churchill Livingstone, 1989), and *Mayes' Midwifery: a textbook for midwives* (11th edn., Baillière Tindall, 1987) by Betty Sweet. T.F. Redman has produced a fourth edition of *Lecture notes on midwifery* (Wright, 1985) for student midwives.

An impressive two-volume work edited by I. Chalmers, M. Enkin and M.J.N.C. Keirse, *Effective care in pregnancy and childbirth* (OUP, 1989), over 1500 pages in length, contains the contributions of 98 authors from 13 countries who between them have amassed the available evidence concerning perinatal care, particularly respecting the results of randomized controlled trials. The results and conclusions presented in this highly important contribution to the literature have been condensed into a small volume available in paperback, entitled *A guide to effective care in pregnancy and childbirth* by M. Enkin, M.J.N.C. Keirse and I. Chalmers (OUP, 1989). Full bibliographies appear only in the main volume. The basic analyses are incorporated into the *Oxford database of perinatal trials* (Oxford Electronic Publishing) which contains over 5000 published reports, plus details of unpublished, ongoing and planned trials in this field. Data are updated at six-monthly intervals. Of particular value are the 300 or so overviews (meta-analyses) of trials containing editorial commentaries, graphs and tables which are updated or rewritten as necessary. Obstetric complications are dealt with in Ian Donald's *Practical obstetric problems* (5th edn., Lloyd-Luke, 1979) now somewhat out of date but still of interest. R.F. Zacharin's *Obstetric fistula* (Springer, 1988) is the only in-depth study of this subject.

Books concerning emergencies in obstetrics are as follows: *Essential management of obstetric emergencies* by T.F. Baskett (Wiley, 1985), a new edition being in preparation; *Obstetric emergencies*, edited by G.I. Benrubi (Churchill Livingstone, 1990); R.W.M. Baldwin and G.C. Hanson's *The critically ill obstetric patient* (2nd edn., Farrand Press, 1989) and D.M.F. Gibb's *Common obstetric emergencies* (Butterworth-Heinemann, 1991), a quick reference work for junior registrars and midwives. Texts on multiple pregnancy and birth are to be found in the 'Pregnancy' section of this chapter.

Very little has been produced to date on audit of obstetrical and gynaecological services but the Royal College of Obstetricians and Gynaecologists has recently established an Audit Unit in Manchester which will report in due course. Meanwhile two publications from the American College of Obstetricians and Gynecologists are attracting interest, namely *Quality assurance in obstetrics and gynecology* (7th edn.,

ACOG, 1989) and *Standards for obstetric-gynecologic services* (7th edn., ACOG, 1989). The National Audit Office's Report (HC 297) by the Comptroller and Auditor General on *Maternity services* (HMSO, 1990) should be noted in connection with examination of provision of existing facilities in the UK and implementation of good practice.

GYNAECOLOGY

Jeffcoate's Principles of gynaecology (5th edn., Butterworths, 1987), edited by V.R. Tindall, is a leading reference text. It may be purchased separately or in a boxed set with its companion volume on *Obstetrics* by B.M. Hibbard (q.v.).U.S. sources include: *Novak's Textbook of gynaecology* by H.W. Jones III, A. Colston Wentz and L.S. Burnett (11th edn., Williams and Wilkins, 1988); *Kistner's Gynecology: principles and practice*, edited by K.J. Ryan, R. Barbieri and R. Berkowitz (5th edn., Year Book Medical Publishers, 1990); *Principles and practice of clinical gynaecology*, edited by N.G. Kase, A.B. Weingold and D.M. Gershenson (2nd edn., Churchill Livingstone, 1990) and the large paperback *Green's Gynecology: essentials of clinical practice* by D.L. Clarke-Pearson and M.Y. Dawood (Little, Brown, 1990). Also useful is *Gynaecology by ten teachers*, edited by T.L.T. Lewis and G. Chamberlain (15th edn., Arnold, 1990) which has appeared regularly since 1919 when it bore the title *Diseases of women*. V.R. Tindall has compiled a short *Colour atlas of clinical gynaecology* (Wolfe, 1981) which appeared in a soft-cover edition in 1988. Other recent titles include: T.R. Varma's *Clinical gynaecology* (Arnold, 1990); *Practical gynaecology* edited by D.T.Y. Liu and G.C.L. Lachelin (Butterworths, 1989) and *Lecture notes on gynaecology* by Dame Josephine Barnes and G. Chamberlain (6th edn., Blackwell, 1988). One or two texts have been written specifically for general practitioners, a recent example being A. McPherson's *Women's problems in general practice* (2nd edn., OUP, 1988). J.M. Monaghan and D. Ireland's *Common gynaecological emergencies* (Wright, 1988) addresses this more specific aspect of gynaecological practice. *Everywoman: a gynaecological guide for life* by D. Llewellyn-Jones (5th edn., Faber, 1989) is intended for the laywoman.

Obstetrics and gynaecology in adolescence and paediatric gynaecology

Unless the reader is particularly interested in the sociological aspects of adolescent pregnancy the majority of available titles contain little of interest to the clinician. An exception is *Adolescent obstetrics and gynecology*, edited by A.K.K. Kreutner and D.R. Hollingsworth (Year Book Medical Publishers, 1978) which contains a large section on the subject; also J.K. Russell's *Early teenage pregnancy* (Churchill Livingstone, 1982). *Teenage mothers and their partners* by Madeleine Simms and Christopher Smith (Research Report No. 15, HMSO, 1986) presents the results of a survey in England and Wales and may be of interest for statistical purposes. Certain gynaecological disorders encountered in childhood are unusual and it may be helpful to refer additionally to older sources. Recent titles are: *Dewhurst's Practical paediatric and adolescent gynaecology* by D.K. Edmonds (2nd edn., Butterworth, 1989); *Paediatric and adolescent gynaecology* by S.J.H. Emens and D.P. Goldstein (3rd edn., Churchill Livingstone, 1990) and Sir John Dewhurst's *Female puberty and its abnormalities* (Churchill Livingstone, 1984). *The gynaecology of childhood and adolescence* by J.W. Huffman, Sir C. John Dewhurst and V.J. Capraro (2nd edn., Saunders, 1981) is now over ten years old but still of value for reference purposes.

Female reproductive anatomy and physiology

A standard specialist text, sadly out of print but still available for reference in some libraries, is *Gynaecological and obstetrical anatomy* by C.F.V. Smout, F. Jacoby and E.W. Lillie (4th edn., Lewis, 1969). C.W.F. Burnett's *Anatomy and physiology of obstetrics; a short textbook for students and midwives* revised by M.M. Anderson (6th edn., Faber, 1979) is apparently still available.

Clinical physiology in obstetrics, edited by F.E. Hytten and G.V.P. Chamberlain (Blackwell, 1980), formerly entitled *The physiology of human pregnancy*, is an important source of information although some sections require updating. Another useful reference work of approximately the same vintage is R.P. Shearman's *Human reproductive physiology* (2nd edn., Blackwell, 1979). A more recent publication by a U.S. author, D.H. Riddick, is *Reproductive physiology in clinical practice* (Thieme, 1987). Less substantial, but useful for undergraduates is *Essential reproduction* by M.H. Johnson and B.J. Everitt (3rd edn., Blackwell, 1988). The comprehensive multi-volume *Marshall's Physiology of reproduction*, edited by G.E. Lamming, concerns comparative physiology. A fourth edition is in the process of publication, volumes being revised one by one. Two of the six anticipated volumes have already appeared and Volume 3 should be available from Churchill Livingstone in 1991. The International Federation of Gynaecology and Obstetrics (FIGO) have recently produced a three-volume illustrated handbook for teaching purposes entitled *The FIGO manual of human reproduction* (Parthenon, 1989) under the general editorship of A. Rosenfield and M.F. Fathalla. Volumes are individually edited and available separately under the following titles: Volume 1: *Reproductive physiology*; Volume 2: *Family planning*; Volume 3: *Reproductive health: global issues.* Supportive sets of colour slides are also available; approximately 200 slides per set. If slides are purchased the accompanying volume is supplied without extra charge.

DIAGNOSIS

(See also 'Prenatal diagnosis', p. 457.) Since the early 1980s literature on the use of ultrasound for obstetrical and gynaecological diagnosis has abounded, most titles originating from the USA. The following list comprises some of the better-known titles:

Ultrasound in obstetrics and gynecology, by P.A. Athey and F.P. Hadlock (2nd edn., Mosby, 1985)

Ultrasound in perinatal care edited by M.J. Bennett (Perinatal Practice, 1) (Wiley, 1984)

Atlas of obstetrical ultrasound (Lippincott, 1988) by C. Benson, T. Jones and M. Lavery

Ultrasonography in obstetrics and gynecology (2nd edn., Saunders, 1988) by P.W. Callen

Obstetric ultrasound: how, why and when by P. Chudleigh and J.M. Pearce (Churchill Livingstone, 1986)

The principles and practice of ultrasonography in obstetrics and gynecology, 4th edn. (Appleton and Lange, 1990) by A.C. Fleisher and others

Ultrasound diagnosis in obstetrics and gynecology by M. Hansmann, B.J. Hackeloer and A. Staudach (Springer, 1985)

Diagnostic ultrasound applied to obstetrics and gynecology (2nd edn., Harper and Row, 1987) by R.E. Sabbagha

Practical guide to gynecological and obstetrical ultrasound (2nd edn., Butterworth, 1988) by E. Vuillard, M. Vital and P. Dubbins

There is growing interest in vaginal ultrasound. Recent publications include:

Endosonography in obstetrics and gynaecology by G. Bernaschek and others (Springer, 1990)

Transvaginal color Doppler: a comprehensive guide to transvaginal colour Doppler sonography in obstetrics and gynecology by A. Kurjak (Parthenon 1990)

Transvaginal sonography (Heinemann, 1988) by I.E. Timor-Tritsch and S. Rottem

Among the titles concerning endoscopy and peritoneoscopy are some well-produced atlases including: E. Burghardt's *Colposcopy cervical pathology: textbook and atlas* (Thieme, 1984); R. Cartier's *Practical colposcopy* (3rd edn., Churchill Livingstone, 1982) and A.G. Gordon and B.V. Lewis's *Gynaecological endoscopy* (Chapman and Hall, 1988). Other titles include: M. Borten's *Laparoscopic complications* (Dekker, 1986); J.F. Hulka's *Textbook of laparoscopy* (Grune and Stratton, 1985); M.S. Baggish, J. Barbot and R.F. Valle's *Diagnostic and operative hysteroscopy* (Year Book Medical Publishers, 1989); A.M. Siegler and H.J. Lindemann's *Hysteroscopy: principles and practice* (Lippincott, 1984); and *Operative gynaecologic endoscopy*, edited by J.S. Sanfilippo and others (Springer, 1989).

Concerning cytology, a well-presented volume is *Clinical cytotechnology* by D.V. Coleman and P.A. Chapman (Butterworths, 1989) which concerns the principles and practice of clinical cytology for all with a major interest in the field.

O.A.N. Husain and E.B. Butler's *A Colour Atlas of gynaecological cytology* (Wolfe Medical, 1989) may also be useful for reference.

Very little has been published recently on diagnostic radiology but the following title may be of interest to some: *Exposure of the pregnant patient to diagnostic radiations: a guide to medical management* (Lippincott, 1985) by L.K. Wagner, R.G. Lester and L.R. Saldana.

PATHOLOGY

A familiar reference book, Haines and Taylor's *Gynaecological pathology* has recently been greatly expanded and updated and now includes obstetrics. Edited by H. Fox, the 3rd edition (2 vols, Churchill Livingstone, 1987) is entitled *Obstetrical and gynaecological pathology*. Another sizeable well-illustrated and very useful reference work is *Blaustein's Pathology of the female genital tract*, edited by R.J. Kurman (3rd edn., Springer, 1987). A standard U.S. reference work is *Novak's Gynecologic and obstetric pathology* by E.R. Novak and J.D. Woodruff (8th edn., Saunders, 1979). J.D. Woodruff and T.H. Parmley's *Atlas of gynecologic pathology* (Gower, 1988) is well illustrated, largely in colour, and emphasis is on histopathology although some clinical photographs and diagrams have been included.

Recent titles dealing with infections and benign disorders are as follows:

Genital tract infection in women edited by M.J. Hare (Churchill Livingstone, 1988)

Infection in the female by W.J. Ledger (2nd edn., Lea and Febiger, 1986)

Clinical infection in obstetrics and gynaecology by A.B. Maclean (Blackwell, 1990)

Pelvic pain in women: diagnosis and management by I. Rocker (Springer, 1990)

Infectious diseases of the female genital tract by R.L. Sweet and R.S. Gibbs (Williams and Wilkins, 1990)

AIDS in obstetrics and gynaecology: the Proceedings of the 19th Study Group of the RCOG edited by C.N. Hudson (RCOG/Springer, 1988)

Gynaecological oncology is now a recognized sub-specialty. General texts are listed below; those relating to specific organs can be found in the appropriate sections:

H.R.K. Barber *Manual of gynecologic oncology* (2nd edn., Lippincott, 1989)

R. Barua *Tumours of the female lower genital tract: classification and pathology* (Springer, 1990)

P. Belfort, J.A. Pinotti, T.K.A.B. Eskes (eds) *Gynecological cancer* (Parthenon, 1989). *Advances in Gynecology and Obstetrics, 3*

M. Coppleson *Gynecologic oncology: fundamental principles and clinical practice* (2 vols, Churchill Livingstone, 1981)

P.J. Disaia and W.T. Creasman (eds) *Clinical gynecologic oncology* (3rd edn., Mosby, 1988)

S.B. Gusberg, H.M. Shingleton, G. Deppe (eds) *Female genital cancer* (Churchill Livingstone, 1988)

E. Hernandez and N.B. Rosenshein *Manual of gynecologic oncology* (Churchill Livingstone, 1989)

R.C. Knapp and R.S. Berkowitz (eds) *Gynecologic oncology* (Macmillan, 1986)

P. Kolstad *Clinical gynaecologic oncology: the Norwegian experience* (Universitetsforlaget, 1986)

C.P. Morrow *Synopsis of gynecologic oncology* (3rd edn., Wiley, 1987)

J.H. Shepherd and J.M. Monaghan (eds) *Clinical gynaecological oncology* (Blackwell, 1985)

SURGERY

Established UK texts are *Bonney's Gynaecological surgery* by J.M. Monaghan (9th edn., Baillière Tindall, 1986), *Gynaecology and Obstetrics* (4th edn., Butterworth, 1987) in the *Operative surgery* series produced by C. Rob and Sir Rodney Smith, also edited by Monaghan, and *Shaw's Textbook of operative gynaecology* (5th edn., revised by J. Hawkins and C.N. Hudson, Churchill Livingstone, 1983). S.L. Stanton has edited *Principles of gynaecological surgery* (Springer, 1987) and

J.M. Monaghan has recently produced *Complications in the surgical management of gynaecological and obstetrical malignancy* (Baillière, 1989). An impressive series of colour atlases, six volumes in all, have been prepared by D.H. Lees and A. Singer. Under the title *Colour atlas of gynaecological surgery* (Wolfe, 1978–1982) the following three volumes have now appeared in a new edition (1986–89): Vol. 1, *Vaginal operations*; Vol. 2 *Abdominal operations for benign conditions;: and Vol. 3 Operations for malignant disease*. New editions of *Surgery of vulva and lower genital tract* (Vol. 4), *Infertility surgery*, (Vol. 5) and *Surgery of conditions complicating pregnancy* (Vol. 6) are not yet available. Reference works originating from the USA are *Te Linde's Operative gynecology* of which the new (7th) edition is imminent, to be edited by J.D. Thompson and J.A. Rock and *Atlas of pelvic surgery* by C.R. Wheeless Jr (2nd edn., Lea and Febiger, 1988). Also available are: B.J. Masterson's *Manual of gynecologic surgery* (Springer, 1989); *Strategies in gynecologic surgery* edited by H.J. Buchsbaum and L.A. Walton (Springer, 1986) in the series *Clinical perspectives in obstetrics and gynecology*; W.R. Keye's *Laser surgery in gynecology and obstetrics* (2nd edn., Year Book Medical Publishers, 1989), M.S. Baggish's *Basic and advanced laser surgery in gynecology* (Appleton-Century-Crofts, 1985), D.H. Nichols' *Reoperative gynecologic surgery*, (Mosby–Year Book Medical Publishers, 1991) and A.J. Penfield's *Gynecologic surgery under local anesthesia* (Urban and Schwarzenberg, 1986). The standard UK text concerning obstetrics is *Munro Kerr's Operative obstetrics*, edited by P.R. Myerscough (10th edn., Baillière, 1982). An alternative text from the USA is *Douglas-Stromme's Operative obstetrics* by F.P. Zuspan and E.J. Quilligan (5th edn., Appleton & Lange, 1988).

THERAPEUTICS

Some of the better known recent titles are as follows:

G. Deppe (ed.) *Chemotherapy of gynecologic cancer* (2nd edn., Wiley-Liss, 1990)

T.K.A.B. Eskes and M. Finster *Drug therapy during pregnancy* (Butterworths, 1985)

D.F. Hawkins *Drugs and pregnancy: human teratogenesis and related problems* (2nd edn., Churchill Livingstone, 1987)

R.S. Ledward *Drug treatment in gynaecology* (Butterworths, 1984)

R.S. Ledward, D.F. Hawkins and L. Stern *Drug treatment in obstetrics* (2nd edn., Chapman and Hall, 1990)

R.S. Leward *Prescribing in pregnancy: a guide to the use of medicine in pregnancy* (Media Medica, 1989)

E.J. Quilligan and F.P. Zuspan, (Wiley, 1989) *Current therapy in obstetrics and gynecology* (3rd edn., Saunders, 1990)

Female reproductive organs: normal and abnormal

UTERUS AND CERVIX

Only the more recent publications are cited here. These are few in number compared with those mentioned in this book's previous edition of this chapter to which the reader is referred if older material is likely to be of interest for reference purposes.

Biology of the uterus, edited by R.M. Wynn and W.P. Jollie (2nd edn., Plenum, 1989) provides comprehensive coverage of its subject. The new edition contains additional chapters and numerous references. A more recent offering is *Uterine function: molecular and cellular aspects* (Plenum, 1990), edited by M.E. Carsten and J.D. Miller.

Pathological aspects are covered in: D.V. Coleman and D.M.D. Evans' *Biopsy pathology and cytology of the cervix* (Chapman & Hall, 1988); *Atlas of histopathology of the cervix uteri* (Springer, 1990) edited by G. Dallenbach-Hellweg; and H. Paulsen and G. Dallenbach-Hellweg's *Histopathology of the endometrium* (4th edn., Springer, 1987).

Malignant conditions and their management are dealt with in: E.A. Surwit and D.S. Albert's *Endometrial cancer* (Kluwer, 1989), which is Volume 49 in the series *Cancer Treatment and Research;* S. Li and E. Wang's *Endometrial carcinoma* (Springer; People's Medical Publishing House, Beijing, 1990), translated from the Chinese; M.R. Hendrickson and R.L. Kempson's *Surgical pathology of the uterine corpus* (3rd edn., Saunders, 1990); and *High dose rate afterloading in the treatment of cancer of the uterus, breast and rectum* (Urban & Schwarzenberg, 1988), edited by H. Vahrson. Techniques of abdominal and vaginal hysterectomy are covered in considerable detail in the standard textbooks and atlases of gynaecological surgery described earlier. It may also be useful to note one or two publications intended for patients, such as S. Haslett and M. Jennings' *Hysterectomy and vaginal repair* (Beaconsfield Publishers, 1988) and E. Phillipp's *Hysterectomy*, updated periodically and available from the BMA in its *Family doctor publication* series.

Endometriosis by J.A. Chalmers (Butterworths, 1975) has been succeeded by a number of more up-to-date monographs but is worth noting as a source of information on endometriosis occurring in unusual sites as the author has carefully reviewed earlier literature. Recent titles include: *Endometriosis*, edited by E.A. Wilson (Liss, 1987); R.S. Schenken's *Endometriosis: contemporary concepts in clinical management* (Lippincott, 1989) and D.T. O'Connor's *Endometriosis* (Churchill

Livingstone, 1987), a compact review of the subject. The most up-to-date account, edited by R.W. Shaw, is *Endometriosis*, Volume 1, in the series *Advances in reproductive endocrinology* (Parthenon, 1990).

OVARY

The three-volume study, *The ovary*, by Lord Zuckerman and B.J. Weir (2nd edn., Academic Press, 1977) is now somewhat outdated but worth noting. Information on the many and varied ovarian tumours can be found in H. Fox and F.A. Langleys *Tumours of the ovary* (Heinemann, 1976), and G. Teilum's *Special tumours of ovary and testis* (2nd edn., Munksgaard, Lippincott, 1976) and *Tumors and tumorlike conditions of the ovary* edited by L.M. Roth and B. Czernobilsky (Churchill Livingstone, 1985). W. Futterweit's *Polycystic ovarian disease* (Springer, 1984) contains over 1000 references and provides a very useful contribution to the subject which can be updated from journal literature as required. Ovarian cancer is, of course, a major topic of concern and an area of on-going research. G. Blackledge and K.K. Chan's *Management of ovarian cancer* (Butterworths, 1986) is one of the more useful monographs. A year later the Royal College of Obstetricians and Gynaecologists published the proceedings of its 17th Study Group as *Ovarian cancer — the way ahead*, edited by F. Sharp and W.P. Soutter (RCOG, 1987). Probably the most important new publication is *Ovarian cancer: biological and therapeutic challenges*, edited by F. Sharp, W.P. Mason and R.E. Leake (Chapman and Hall Medical, 1990). The volume comprises papers, presentations and discussions by a panel of international experts at the 2nd Helene Harris Memorial Trust Biennial International Forum on Ovarian Cancer and provides a useful overview of current work. Other titles pertinent to the subject are: M.S. Piver's contribution to the *Current reviews in obstetrics and gynaecology* series entitled *Ovarian malignancies: the clinical care of adults and adolescents* (Churchill Livingstone, 1983); *Clinical pathology of the endocrine ovary* by J. de Brux (MTP, 1984) and *Surgical pathology of the ovaries* (Churchill Livingstone, 1989), by P. Russell and P. Bannatyne.

FALLOPIAN TUBES

Literature on microsurgical technique in connection with tubal sterilization or restoration of fertility appears elsewhere in this chapter. Those interested in fallopian tube structure and function, or pathology, may be referred to *The fallopian tube: basic studies and clinical contributions* (Futura, 1986), edited by A.M. Siegler and R.H.F. Hunter's *The fallopian tubes* (Springer, 1988) or to two much earlier monographs: C.J. Pauerstein's *The fallopian tube: a reappraisal* (Lea and Febiger, 1974) and J.D. Woodruff and C.J. Pauersteins' *The fallopian tube: structure, function, pathology and management* (Williams and Wilkins, 1969). Information on fallopian tube neoplasms is best obtained from journal literature.

VULVA AND VAGINA

An excellent monograph entitled *The vulva* (Churchill Livingstone, 1988), edited by Constance M. Ridley is a recommended source of information providing a comprehensive study of pathological conditions in addition to chapters on, for example, anatomy and embryology. J. Hewitt, M. Pelisse and B. Paniel have produced a colour atlas, *Pathology of the vulva* (McGraw-Hill, 1990) with editions in English, French, Italian and Spanish, whilst a good reference text is provided in J.W. Reagan and Y.S. Fu's *Pathology of the uterine cervix, vagina and vulva* (Saunders, 1989), Volume 21 in the series *Major problems in pathology*. *Benign diseases of the vulva and vagina* (3rd edn., Year Book Medical Publishers, 1989) by R.H. Kaufman, E.C. Friedrich and H.L. Gardner is useful for reference as is *Vaginal surgery* (3rd edn., Williams & Wilkins, 1989) edited by D.H. Nichols and C.L. Randall *Malignant disease of the vulva* (Churchill Livingstone, 1982) by the late Stanley Way remains an important contribution to the literature. Two further titles are relevant to this general section, W. Mendling's *Vulvovaginal candidiasis: theory and practice* (Springer, 1987) and *Bacterial vaginosis*, edited by P.A. Mårdh and D. Taylor-Robinson (Almquist and Wiksell, 1984).

OVULATION, MENSTRUATION AND THE MENOPAUSE

Ovulation

A reasonably comprehensive text, now somewhat outdated is *Human ovulation: mechanisms, prediction, detection and induction* (North-Holland, 1970) by E.S.E. Hafez. Similarly, *Follicular maturation and ovulation* (Excerpta Medica, 1982), edited by R. Rolland and others is no longer readily available. Nonetheless, they may be worth noting considering the limited number of books available on the subject. A little more current is *Ovulation and its disorders* (MTP, 1984) edited by W. Thompson, R.F. Harrison and J. Bonnar containing papers from the XIth World Congress on Fertility and Sterility, Dublin, June 1983; also P.G. Crosignani's *Induction of ovulation* (Baillière, 1990) and R.L. Collins' *Ovulation induction* (Springer, 1991), a basic text but one which includes accounts of the newer agents now in use. *Chronic hyperandrogenic anovulation* (Parthenon, 1990), edited by H.J.T.C. Benninck, may be of use to specialists.

Menstruation

S.L. Israel's *Diagnosis and treatment of menstrual disorders and sterility* (5th edn., Harper and Row, 1967), the last of a series of editions of this standard textbook, is now superseded by any number of more specialized monographs in both of these subject areas. D.T. Baird and E.A. Michie have edited Volume 25 in the *Serono Symposia Publication* series entitled *Mechanism of menstrual bleeding* (Raven Press, 1985) and M.G. Brush and E.M. Goudsmit are the editors of *Functional disorders of the menstrual cycle* (Wiley, 1988). The premenstrual syndrome has become a topic of greater interest in recent years. K. Dalton's work is well known, and her book *The premenstrual syndrome and progesterone therapy* (2nd edn., Heinemann, 1984) was one of the earliest to appear. Useful recent titles are: P.M.S. O'Brien's *The premenstrual syndrome* (Blackwell, 1987); *The premenstrual syndrome* (Churchill, 1988), edited by L.H. Gise, Volume 2 in the series *Contemporary issues in obstetrics and gynaecology*; W.R. Keye's *The premenstrual syndrome* (Saunders, 1988), and the older but more comprehensive *Premenstrual syndrome and dysmenorrhea* (Urban and Schwarzenberg, 1984), edited by M.Y. Dawood, J.L. McGuire and L.M. Demers.

Menopause

The menopause, edited by H.J. Buchsbaum (Springer, 1983) is a useful monograph but one of the best recent sources is *The menopause*, edited by J.W.W. Studd and M.I. Whitehead (Blackwell, 1988). Also useful is the volume of published proceedings of a Scientific Meeting of the Royal College of Obstetricians and Gynaecologists entitled *HRT and osteoporosis*, edited by J.O. Drife and J.W.W. Studd (Springer, 1990), with contributions from leading specialists. Other publications include: *The menopause: comprehensive management* (2nd edn., Collier Macmillan, 1988) by B. Eskin; *Menopause: physiology and pharmacology* (Year Book Medical Publications, 1986), edited by D.R. Mishell, Jr.; *The medical management of menopause and premenopause: their endocrinogic basis* (Lippincott, 1984) by W.B. Cutler and C.R. Garcia and *Update on hormonal treatment in the menopause* (Karger, 1989), edited by M. L'Hermite which contains contributions from international experts. The proceedings of the Fifth International Congress on the Menopause, 1987, edited by L. Zichella, M. Whitehead and P.A. Van Keep have appeared in a volume entitled *The climacteric and beyond* (Parthenon, 1988). Specialists in this subject field contribute regularly to the journal literature to which readers should be directed for 'state of the art' information on, for example, developments in hormone therapy and its applications. A popular book with the public, which perhaps deserves mention, is Wendy Cooper's *No change: a biological revol-*

ution for women (3rd edn., Arrow Books, 1988), advocating hormone replacement therapy.

FERTILIZATION AND EMBRYOLOGY

Fertilization

Anyone interested in a comprehensive study of fertilization can be directed to *Fertilization: comparative morphology, biochemistry and immunology*, edited by C.B. Metz and A. Monroy (2 vols, Academic Press, 1967–1969). However, most readers will be interested only in very recent material, particularly in view of the rapid advances made in recent years in the field of assisted reproduction, the subject of a subsequent section in this chapter (p. 456).

Among the best-known embryology textbooks are J. Langman's *Medical embryology* (Williams and Wilkins, 1990) which has now reached its sixth edition, by T.W. Sadler, and K.L. Moores *The developing human: clinically orientated embryology* (4th edn., Saunders, 1988). Two recent texts also worth noting are *Pathology of the human embryo and previable fetus* (Springer, 1990), edited by D. Kalousek and others and *The embryo: normal and abnormal development and growth* (Springer, 1991), edited by M.G. Chapman, J.G. Grudzinskas and T. Chard, in which leading researchers describe recent contributions to the subject.

PREGNANCY, MULTIPLE PREGNANCY AND MISCARRIAGE

Pregnancy

The most comprehensive reference work available is R.G. Edwards' *Conception in the human female* (Academic Press, 1980) produced by one of the pioneers of *in vitro* fertilization. Topics covered include sexual differentutation, regulation of reproduction, human sexuality, fertilization, implantation and related themes. It also contains a section on legal and ethical matters. A wide choice of books on pregnancy is now available to the laywoman and the latest offerings are to be found in most bookstores. However, it may be worth noting the popular *Pregnancy book* produced by the Health Education Authority (1988) in A4 format, with paper covers, helpfully illustrated and revised from time to time as appropriate. It also contains a two-page appendix of addresses of societies and associations which librarians may find useful for reference. Preconceptional care, a subject once addressed only in isolated articles in the periodical literature, is now the subject of two sizeable texts, *Prepregnancy care: a manual for practice* edited by G. Chamberlain and J. Lumley (Wiley, 1986) and *Medical counselling before pregnancy* (Churchill Livingstone, 1988), edited by D.R. Hollingsworth and R. Resnik. *Pregnant women at work* (Royal Society of Medicine; Macmillan, 1984), edited by G. Chamberlain and *Exercise in pregnancy* edited by R. Artal-Mittelmark, R.A. Wiswell and B. Drinkwater (2nd edn., Williams and Wilkins, 1990) are similarly devoted to topics of emerging interest. Where antenatal care is concerned the once authoritative *Browne's Antenatal care* which reached its 11th edition in 1978, has not reappeared in a new edition and a comparable source is not readily available although Marion Hall's *Antenatal care* (Baillière, 1990) is worth noting. Nutrition in pregnancy is a topic of on-going interest, one of the most recent sources being *Nutrition in pregnancy and lactation* by B. Worthington-Roberts and S.R. Williams (4th edn., Mosby, 1989). On a similar theme, Barbara Thompson and her colleagues have produced a most interesting comparative study comprising two social, obstetric and dietary studies of married primigravidae in Aberdeen entitled *Having a first baby: experiences in 1951 and 1985 compared* (Aberdeen University Press, 1989).

Multiple pregnancy

Multiple pregnancy is a perpetual topic of interest and two recent publications should be noted, *Twinning and twins*, edited by I. MacGillivray, D. Campbell and B. Thompson (Wiley, 1988) which originates from a centre specializing in the field, and the monograph *Quadruplets and higher multiple births* by M.M. Clay (MacKeith Press/Blackwell, 1989). No. 107 in the series *Clinics in developmental medicine*, is a rich source of available documentation to date; relevant associations support groups and study centres are listed for information. Another useful study is the report on *Triplets and higher order births* (HMSO, 1990), edited by B.J. Botting, A. MacFarlane and F.V. Price.

Miscarriage

Miscarriage and associated conditions are addressed in the following publications: *Early pregnancy loss–mechanisms and treatment*, the Proceedings of the 18th RCOG Study Group, 1987 (Springer, 1988) edited by R.W. Beard and F. Sharp; *Spontaneous and recurrent abortion* (Blackwell, 1986), edited by M.J. Bennett and D.K. Edmonds; *Early pregnancy failure* (Churchill Livingstone, 1990) by H.J. Hughes and T. Lind and *Pregnancy loss: medical therapeutics and practical considerations* (Williams and Wilkins, 1987) edited by J.R. Woods Jr. and J.L. Esposito.   Finally, a recent publication on post-partum depression should be mentioned: *Depression after childbirth: how to recognize and treat postnatal illness* (2nd edn., OUP, 1989) by Katharina Dalton, an author with a special interest in this field.

Various general texts on the medical and surgical complications of pregnancy are available and it is helpful to have two or even three of these for reference purposes in a large library in order to cover most of the disorders which may be encountered in clinical practice. A text popular with postgraduates is *Medical disorders in obstetric practice*, edited by M. de Swiet (2nd edn., Blackwell, 1989). *Medical and surgical problems in obstetrics*, edited by M. Brudenell and P.L. Wilds (Wright, 1984) contains contributions from known specialists on subjects such as diabetes, drugs in pregnancy, immunological disorders and many others; Rovinsky and Guttmacher's substantial *Medical, surgical and gynecologic complications of pregnancy*, edited by S.H. Cherry, R.L. Berkowitz and N.G. Kase, first appeared in 1960 (Williams and Wilkins, 3rd edn., 1985). It is divided into 23 general sections, each with sub-sections of from one to seven chapters, a total of 61 chapters in all; the main sections include, for example: cardiovascular disorders; renal system, neurology, neoplastic disorders and gynecologic problems. Unusually, a chapter is even devoted to dental problems! Another large volume is *Principles of medical therapy in pregnancy*, edited by N. Gleicher (Plenum, 1985).

Arrangement is again by main subject groups such as metabolic diseases, hormonal diseases, and infectious diseases, the chapters being further grouped by sub-sections in some cases. *Medical complications during pregnancy*, by G.N. Burrow and T.F. Ferris (Saunders, 1988) contains a total of 24 chapters on selected disorders. L.A. Cibils' *Surgical diseases in pregnancy* (Springer, 1990) addresses the problems confronted by the gynaecological surgeon in treating the pregnant patient. Finally, some readers may be interested in the more specific *Pregnancy, autoimmunity and connective tissue disorders* (OUP, 1990), edited by J.S. Scott and H.A. Bird.

A growing selection of monographs is available on specific pregnancy complications including the following examples:

Parasitic infections in pregnancy and the newborn edited by C.L. McLeod (OUP, 1988)

Fetal alcohol syndrome: an annotated bibliography by E.L. Abel (Praeger, 1986)

Diabetes complicating pregnancy: the Joslin Clinic method, edited by J.W. Hare (Liss, 1989)

Carbohydrate metabolism in pregnancy and the newborn, IV, edited by H.W. Sutherland, J.M. Stowers and D.W.M. Pearson (Springer, 1989)

Psychological disorders in obstetrics and gynaecology, edited by R.G. Priest (Butterworths, 1985)

Suicide in pregnancy, by G.J. Kleisner and W.M. Greston (Wright, 1984)

Immunobiology of normal and diabetic pregnancy, edited by D. Andreani and others (Wiley, 1990)

Hypertension and pregnancy, by J.M. Sullivan (Year Book Medical Publishers, 1986)

Trauma and pregnancy, edited by C.E. Haycock (PSG, 1985)

Pregnancy, diabetes and birth: a management guide, by D.R. Hollingsworth (Williams and Wilkins, 1984)

Infections in pregnancy, by L.C. Gilstrap (Wiley-Liss, 1990)

Extrauterine pregnancy, edited by A. Langer and L . Iffy (PSG, 1986)

Controversies in diabetes and pregnancy, edited by L. Jovanovic (Springer, 1988)

Cardiac problems in pregnancy: diagnosis and management of maternal and fetal disease, edited by U. Elkayam and N. Gleicher (2nd edn., Wiley, 1990)

Drugs, alcohol, pregnancy and parenting, edited by I.J. Chasnoff (Kluwer, 1988)

Smoking and reproductive health, by M.J. Rosenberg (Wright, 1987)

Cardiovascular diseases and pregnancy, by O.M. Eliseev (Springer, 1988)

Pregnancy and renal disorders, edited by G.R.D. Catto (Kluwer, 1985)

The kidney in pregnancy, by V.E. Andreucci (Nijhoff, 1986)

Diabetic pregnancy, by M. Brudenell and M. Doddridge (Churchill Livingstone, 1989)

Pain and reproduction, edited by F. Facchnetti and others (Parthenon, 1988)

Neurological disorders of pregnancy, by P.J. Goldstein (Futura, 1986)

Blood disorders in pregnancy, edited by R.K. Laros Jr. (Lea and Febiger, 1986)

Management of the diabetic pregnancy, edited by B.S. Nuwayhid and others (Elsevier, 1987)

Motherhood and mental illness 2: causes and consequences, edited by R. Kumar and I.F. Brockington (Wright, 1988)

Epilepsy, pregnancy and the child, edited by D. Janz and others (Raven Press, 1982)

Coagulation problems during pregnancy, by E.A. Letsky (Churchill Livingstone, 1985)

Psychological disorders in obstetrics and gynaecology, by M. Oates (Baillière, 1990)

Hypertension in pregnancy (Handbook of hypertension, 10), edited by P.C. Rubin (Elsevier, 1988)

Gestational diabetes, by P.A.M. Weiss and D.R. Coustan (Springer, 1988)

Diabetes and pregnancy, by P. Chahal and D.F. Hawking (Butterworths, 1989)

Neurology and pregnancy (Major problems in pathology, 7), by J. Donaldson (Saunders, 1989)

INFERTILITY AND ASSISTED REPRODUCTION

Infertility

Perhaps the most comprehensive work on infertility with over 50 contributors is the third edition of Behrman and Kistner's *Progress in infertility* (Little, Brown, 1988), edited by G.W. Patton. Other general works on the subject include *Infertility, male and female*, edited by V. Insler and B. Lunenfeld (Churchill Livingstone 1986), *Infertility: a comprehensive text*, by M. Seibel (Appleton and Lange, 1989), *Infertility: a clinicians' guide to diagnosis and treatment*, by M.L. Taymor (2nd rev. edn. of *Infertility*, Plenum, 1990) and *Reproductive failure*, edited by A.H. DeCherney (Churchill Livingstone, 1986). Also worth noting is the second edition of *The infertile couple*, edited by R.J. Pepperell, B. Hudson and C. Wood (Churchill Livingstone, 1987) which is said to be a successor to the U.S. Behrman and Kistner. Recent topics of current interest are dealt with in Volume 4 of *Modern trends in infertility and conception control*, edited by E.E. Wallach and R.D. Kempers (Year Book Medical Publishers, 1988), *Recent advances in the management of infertility* by C. Chen, S.L. Tan and W.C. Cheng (McGraw-Hill, 1989), *The management of infertility* by J.L. Yovich and G. Grudzinskas (Heinemann Medical, 1990), and *Advances in assisted reproductive technologies*, edited by S. Mashiach, Z. Ben-Rafael, N. Laufer and J.G. Schenker (Plenum, 1990). An all-round account of infertility and its diversifications is provided by *Current therapy of infertility 3*, edited by C.R. Garcia, L. Mastroianni, J.R.D. Amelar and L. Dubin (Decker, 1988). *Advances in fertility and sterility: Proceedings of the XIIth World Congress on Fertility and Sterility, 1986*, is available in six volumes, each on a specific topic and each with different editors. The series is edited by S.S. Ratnam and E.S. Teoh (Parthenon, 1987). *Recent developments in fertility and sterility Proceedings of the XIIIth World Congress on Fertility and Sterility, 1989 are also available in six volumes and edited by Y. Boutaleb and A. Gzouli (Parthenon, 1991). A specific aspect is covered by Ultrasound and infertility*, edited by A. Kurjak (CRC Press, 1989). Surgery, including microsurgery, is the subject of a number of publications such as J.J. Stangel's *Infertility surgery* (Appleton and Lange, 1990), *Reproductive surgery* edited by A.H. DeCherney and M.L. Polan (Year Book Medical Publishers, 1987) and G.W. Patton and R.W. Kistner's *Atlas of infertility surgery* (2nd edn., Little, Brown, 1984). Tubal disease and surgery are covered by G. Sotrel's *Tubal reconstructive surgery* (Lea and Febiger, 1990) and *Tubal infertility* by I.A. Brosens and A.G. Gordon (Gower, 1989).

Assisted reproduction

In-vitro fertilization and embryo transfer and research are now established techniques. They were the subject of government debate in the Warnock Report in *Report of the Committee of Inquiry into Human Fertilisation and Embryology* (HMSO, 1984) and the *Human Fertilisation and Embryology Act 1990* (HMSO, 1990). D. Morgan and R.G. Lee have produced *Blackstone's Guide to the Human Fertilisation and Embryology Act 1990* (Blackstone Press, 1991). A recent *British Medical Bulletin* (1990, **46** (3)) was devoted to the techniques, outcome, ethics and other areas of the subject — 'Assisted Human Conception'. Two of the first publications devoted to this subject are *In vitro fertilization and embryo transfer*, edited by E.S.E. Hafez and K. Semm (MTP, 1982), and *Implantation of the human embryo: Proceedings of the Second Bourn Hall Meeting*, edited by R.G. Edwards, J.M. Purdy and P.C. Steptoe (Academic Press, 1985). Bourn Hall's contribution to the field is continued in *The Bourn Hall Textbook of in vitro fertilization and assisted reproduction*, edited by P.R. Brinsden and P.A. Rainsbury (Parthenon, 1991). The story of the events leading to the birth of Louise Brown, the first 'test-tube baby' is told in R.G. Edwards and P.C. Steptoe's book *A matter of life: the story of a medical breakthrough* (Hutchinson, 1980) written to appeal to the general public. Other publications on the subject are A. Trounson's *In vitro fertilisation and embryo transfer* (Churchill Livingstone, 1985) and the second edition of *Clinical in vitro fertilization* (Springer, 1988), edited by C. Wood and A. Trounson. GIFT is the subject of a publication edited by G.L. Capitanio, R.H. Asch, I. DeCecco and S. Croce entitled *GIFT: from basic to clinics* (Raven, 1990). Male infertility is the subject of such works as *Contemporary management of impotence and infertility*, edited by E.A. Tanagho, T.F. Lue and R.D. McClure (Williams and Wilkins, 1988), *Human spermatozoa in assisted reproduction*, edited by A.A. Acosta (Williams and Wilkins, 1989), T.B. Glovers *Human male fertility and semen analysis* (Academic Press, 1990) and *Common problems in infertility and impotence* by J. Rajfer (Year Book Medical Publishers, 1990). Two publications by A. Jequier are also worth mentioning: *Infertility in the male* (Churchill Livingstone, 1986) which is number 11 in the series

Current reviews in obstetrics and gynaecology and *Semen analysis: a practical guide* (Blackwell, 1986) written with J. Crich.

Prenatal diagnosis and genetics

A Working Party of the Royal College of Physicians has produced a report on *Prenatal diagnosis and genetic screening: Community and service implications* (RCP, 1989) which examines key issues such as genetic counselling, future developments, ethical aspects and ethnic minorities. It includes appendices giving lists of centres, organizations and support groups. A selection of books and monographs on prenatal diagnosis are:

Prenatal diagnosis and prognosis by R. Lilford (Butterworths, 1990)

Prenatal diagnosis of congenital anomalies by R. Romero (Appleton and Lange, 1987)

Prenatal diagnosis in obstetric practice, edited by M.J. Whittle and J.M. Connor (Blackwell, 1989)

Congenital malformations: antenatal diagnosis, perinatal management and counseling, by J.W. Seeds and R.G. Azizkhan (Aspen, 1990)

First trimester fetal diagnosis, edited by M. Fraccaro, G. Simoni and B. Brambati (Springer, 1985)

Chorion villus sampling, by D.T. Liu, E.M. Symonds and M.S. Golbus (Chapman and Hall, 1987)

A practical guide to chorion villus sampling, edited by D.T.Y. Liu (OUP, 1991)

The following titles may be noted in connection with genetic counselling and the study of medical genetics generally:

Principles of medical genetics, edited by T.D. Gelehrter and F.S. Collins (Williams and Wilkins, 1990)

Practical genetic counselling by P. Harper (3rd edn., Wright, 1988)

The new genetics and clinical practice by D.J. Weatherall (3rd edn., OUP (1990)

Principles and practice of medical genetics, edited by A.E.H. Emery and D.L. Rimoin (2 vols, Churchill Livingstone, 1983)

Elements of medical genetics by A.E.H. Emery (6th edn., Churchill Livingstone, 1983)

Genetics in obstetrics and gynecology by J.L. Simpson and others (Grune and Stratton, 1982)

Perinatal medicine, fetus and neonate

In recent years, numerous texts have appeared dealing with the general topic of perinatal medicine. A substantial volume consisting of about 1200 pages is *Maternal–fetal medicine: principles and practice* (2nd edn., Saunders, 1989) by R.K. Creasy and R. Resnik. It is divided into substantial sections, such as 'Fetal diagnostic and treatment modalities' and 'Maternal and fetal pathophysiology' which are in turn divided into sub-sections each containing a chapter, or chapters, by specialists. *Perinatal medicine* by G. McClure, H. Halliday and W. Thompson (Baillière Tindall, 1988), representing the two specialties of paediatrics and obstetrics, is intended for the use of all from medical students upwards interested in the management of mother and infant and the rationale of related decision making. *Fetal medicine–1*, edited by C. Rodeck (Blackwell, 1989) is the first of an intended regular series of reviews in this field.

M.A. England has produced *A colour atlas of life before birth: normal fetal development* (Wolfe, 1983) and F. Cockburn has edited *Fetal and Neonatal Growth* (Wiley, 1988), Volume 5 in the *Perinatal practice* series. In the following year the proceedings of the 20th Study Group of the Royal College of Obstetricians and Gynaecologists appeared entitled *Fetal growth* (RCOG/Springer, 1989) edited by F. Sharp and R.B. Fraser and R.D.G. Milner. *Fetal and neonatal development* edited by C.T. Jones (Perinatology Press, Ithaca, N Y, 1988), Volume VII of the series *Research in perinatal medicine*, contains the proceedings of an International Meeting devoted to perinatal science. A further text worth noting is *Fetal physiology and medicine: the basis of perinatology* (2nd edn., Dekker, 1984) edited by R.W. Beard.

The following titles concern fetal welfare and fetal monitoring: *Fetal well being: physiological basis and methods of clinical assessment* (CRC Press, 1990) by M. Katz, I. Meizner and V. Insler; *A practical guide to fetal heart rate monitoring* by P.L. Wood and H.G. Dobbie (Macmillan 1988); *Fetal monitoring: physiology and techniques of antenatal and intrapartum assessment* (OUP, 1989), edited by J.A.D. Spencer, which includes a chapter on medico-legal aspects and C. Kleinman's *Fetal echocardiography: principles and applications* (Futura, 1990). G. Chamberlain's *Modern antenatal care of the fetus* (Blackwell, 1990) provides broader coverage of this important subject. Fetal growth retardation is a topic of on-going concern and the following are relevant: *Intrauterine growth retardation: pathophysiology and clinical management* (McGraw-Hill, 1984) by Chin Chu Lin and M.I. Evans; *Intrauterine growth retardation: a practical approach* (Year Book Medical Publishers, 1989) edited by T.L. Cross and R.J. Sokol and A. Kurjak's *Fetal growth retardation: diagnosis and treatment*

(CRC Press, 1989). More generally, a useful text is M.R. Harrison, M.S. Golbus and R.A. Fills *The unborn patient: prenatal diagnosis and treatment* (2nd edn., Saunders, 1990).

Fetal and neonatal pathology (Springer, 1987) edited by J.W. Keeling is well referenced and illustrated with 587 figures. Another substantial text, extensively illustrated with good bibliographies is *Diseases of the fetus and newborn: pathology, radiology and genetics* (Chapman and Hall, 1989), edited by G.B. Reed, A.E. Claireaux and A.D. Bain; also *Infectious diseases of the fetus and newborn* (3rd edn., Saunders, 1990) by J.S. Remington and J.O. Klein. A smaller, but very useful monograph, covering topics such as perinatal listeriosis and HIV in the newborn, appearing in the *Perinatal practice* series, is entitled *Infection in the newborn* (Wiley, 1990), edited by J. De Louvois and D. Harvey. New on the market is a well-presented reference work of over 1300 pages, available in a boxed set of two volumes, edited by J.S. Wigglesworth and D.B. Singer, entitled *Textbook of fetal and perinatal pathology* (Blackwell, 1991).

Prematurity and low birth weight are addressed in the following publications: *Prematurity* edited by V.Y.H. Yu and E.C. Wood (Churchill Livingstone, 1987); *The baby under 1000 g*, edited by D. Harvey, W.I. Cooke and G.A. Levitt (Butterworths, 1989) and *Sequelae of low birthweight: the Vancouver study* (MacKeith Press/Blackwell/Lippincott, 1986), edited by H.G. Dunn, No. 95/96 of *Clinics in Developmental Medicine*. R. Carr-Hill and C. Pritchard's *The development and exploitation of empirical birthweight standards* (Macmillan, 1985) contains sections on, for example, birthweight trends since 1950, birthweight surveys and material and statistical methods. *Craig's Care of the newly born infant* by T.L. Turner and others (8th edn., 1988) is an established text on the subject.

PLACENTA AND FETAL MEMBRANES; TROPHOBLASTIC TUMOURS

Placenta

Although out of print it is worth noting the existence of the beautifully produced large-quarto volume by J.D. Boyd and W.J. Hamilton, *Human placenta* (Macmillan, 1970), an authoritative study containing a historical introduction and extensive bibliography. Later publications include *Placental physiology: structure and function of fetomaternal exchange* by J.J. Faber and K.L. Thornburg (Raven Press, 1983) and *Fetal nutrition, metabolism, and immunology: the role of the placenta* (Plenum, 1984), edited by R.K. Miller and H.A. Thiede. A new edition has recently appeared of a useful reference text, 870 pages, by K. Benirschke and P. Kaufmann entitled *Pathology of the human placenta* (2nd edn., Springer, 1990). E.V.D.K. Perrin has edited *Pathology of the placenta*

(Churchill Livingstone 1984) and D.R. Shanklin has produced a comprehensive monograph entitled *Tumors of the placenta and umbilical cord* (Dekker, 1990). *Amniotic fluid: research and clinical application*, edited by D.V.I. Fairweather and T.K.A.B. Eskes (2nd edn., Excerpta Medica, 1978) is now dated but remains an important reference source.

Tumours

Many of the major published sources of information on choriocarcinoma and other trophoblastic tumours are similarly some years old, but are worth noting if updated with published papers. These include K.D. Bagshawe's *Choriocarcinoma: the clinical biology of the trophoblast and its tumours* (Arnold, 1969), W.W. Park's *Choriocarcinoma: a study of its pathology* (Heinemann, 1977) which also contains a brief historical introduction and R. Hertz's *Choriocarcinoma and related trophoblastic tumors in women* (Raven Press, 1977) which contains material on hydatidiform mole as well as choriocarcinoma. A useful new work is *Gestational trophoblastic disease*, edited by A.E. Szulman and H.J. Buchsbaum (Springer, 1987) in the series *Clinical perspectives in obstetrics and gynecology*.

LABOUR, DELIVERY AND PAIN RELIEF

Labour and delivery

The management of labour, edited by J. Studd (Blackwell, 1985) is a leading text in respect of current practice. A similar publication, originating from the USA is *Management of labor*, edited by W.R. Cohen and E.A. Friedman (2nd edn., Aspen, 1988). E.A. Friedman is also the co-author, with R.K. Neff of *Labour and delivery: impact on offspring* (Wright, 1987). Oxorn-Foote: *Human labor and birth* (5th edn., Appleton-Century-Crofts, 1986) by Harry Oxorn is a substantial handbook, but the following titles are more representative of UK practice: *A manual of labour ward practice* by J.M. Pearce and S.A. Steel (Wiley, 1987); *Labour ward manual* by D.T.Y. Liu and D.V.I. Fairweather (Butterworths, 1985) and *A practical guide to labour management* by D. Gibb (Blackwell, 1988). F.A. Al Azzawi has produced *A colour atlas of baby delivery* (Wolfe Medical, 1990), an illustrated practical reference manual and Janet Balaskas, pioneer of the Active Birth movement, outlines its history and promotes alternative delivery methods in *New active birth: a concise guide to natural childbirth* (Unwin, 1989). More specific aspects are addressed in K. O'Driscoll and D. Meagher's *The active management of labour: the Dublin experience* (2nd edn., Baillière Tindall, 1986); D. Langnickel's *Problems of the pelvic passageway* (Springer, 1987), *Risks of labour* edited by J.W. Crawford (Wiley, 1985), Volume 2 in the series *Perinatal practice*; also *Preterm labor*, edited by M.G. Elder and C.H. Hendricks (Butterworths, 1981) and *Preterm birth: causes, prevention and management*, edited by F. Fuchs and P.G. Stubblefield (Macmillan, 1984).

Until recently no comprehensive text on caesarean section has been available. This situation has now been remedied with the publication of the very useful *Cesarean delivery*, edited by J.P. Phelan and S.L. Clark (Elsevier, 1988), its 39 chapters devoted to every conceivable aspect of the subject, including an introductory section on its history.

Other methods of operative delivery are covered in J.P. O'Grady's *Modern instrumental delivery* (Williams and Wilkins, 1988) which contains a comprehensive historical introduction and Dennen's *Forceps deliveries* (3rd edn., Davis, 1989) by P.C. Dennen. Both represent U.S. practice. J. Chalmers has written an informative little monograph entitled *The ventouse: the obstetric vacuum extractor* (Lloyd-Luke, 1971), worth noting as background reading on this subject.

Pain relief

Pain relief in labour is a topic well represented in the literature. Two useful UK texts are J.S. Crawford's *Principles and practice of obstetric anaesthesia* (5th edn., Blackwell, 1984) and D.D. Moir's *Obstetric anaesthesia and analgesia* (3rd edn., Baillière, 1986) containing a historical introduction. A third title worth noting is the more recent *Problems in obstetric anaesthesia* (Wiley, 1987), edited by Barbara Morgan, Volume 3 in the series *Perinatal practice*. Barbara Morgan is herself the editor of a new series entitled *Controversies in obstetric anaesthesia* first published in 1990 (Arnold) and based on a series of debates at Queen Charlotte's Hospital; a second volume is scheduled to appear shortly. Amongst other recent titles are S. Ramanathan's *Obstetric anesthesia* (Lea and Febiger, 1988) and S. Datta's *Anesthetic and obstetric management for high risk pregnancy* (Year Book Medical Publishers, 1990).

Sterilization, contraception and abortion

STERILIZATION

There are few recent publications on the subject of sterilization and sterilization reversal but older texts can be supplemented by reference to recent chapters in publications and journal literature. Female sterilization is dealt with in A.J. Penfield's *Female sterilization by minilaparotomy or open laparoscopy* (Urban and Schwarzenberg, 1980) and *Female sterilization. An overview with emphasis on the vaginal route and the organization of a sterilization program* (Wright, PSG; 1982) by H.P. Brown and S.N. Schanzer. Reversal is dealt with in *Reversibility of Fe-*

male Sterilization edited by I.A. Brosens and R.M.L. Winston (Academic Press/Grune and Stratton, 1978).

CONTRACEPTION

The theory and practice of contraception is a topic of interest to general practitioners as well as practising clinicians in obstetrics and gynaecology and is covered by a variety of texts such as J.F. Porter's *The control of human fertility: a text for health professionals* (2nd edn., Blackwell, 1987), *Textbook of contraceptive practice* by M. Potts and P. Diggory (2nd edn., CUP, 1983), *Contraception: the facts* by P. Bromwich and T. Parsons (2nd rev. edn., OUP, 1990) and M. Filshie and J. Guillebaud's *Contraception: science and practice* (Butterworth, 1989). Guillebaud is also the author of a general work for the laywoman *Contraception: your questions answered* (Pitman, 1985). Current techniques, ethical and practical aspects are dealt with in *Family planning*, edited by A. Rosenfield, M.F. Fathalla and C. Indriso which is volume 2 of *The Figo manual of human reproduction* (Parthenon, 1989). Other works of interest include *Family planning handbook for doctors*, edited by R.L. Kleinman (6th edn., IPPF, 1988), *Handbook of family planning*, edited by N. Loudon (2nd rev. edn., Churchill Livingstone, 1991) and *Handbook of contraception and abortion* (Little, Brown, 1989) by R.T. Burkman. Immunological aspects are covered by *Immunological factors in human contraception*, edited by S. Shulman and F. Dondero (Field Educational Italia, Acta Medica, 1983), G.P. Talwar's *Immunology of contraception* (Arnold, 1980) and *Immunological aspects of reproduction and fertility control*, edited by J.P. Hearn (MTP, 1980). Among publications devoted to individual methods of contraception are *Intrauterine contraception* (4th edn., IPPF, 1977), edited by R.L. Kleinman, *Biomedical aspects of IUD's*, edited by H. Hasson, E.S.E. Hafez and W.A. Van Os (MTP, 1985), J. Marshall's *Planning for a family: an atlas of mucothermic charts* (2nd edn., Faber, 1979) and J. Guillebaud's *The pill* (3rd edn., OUP, 1984), the latter aimed at the laywoman. The story of the development of the pill over the past 30 years is described in A.D.G. Gunn's *Oral contraception in perspective: thirty years of clinical experience with the pill* (Parthenon, 1987) while the current interest in the pill and cancer is the subject of *Oral contraceptives and breast cancer: the implications of present findings for informed consent and informed choice* (Parthenon, 1989), edited by R.D. Mann. A WHO organized symposium is also of note. *Contraception and mechanisms of endometrial bleeding*, edited by C. D'Arcangues, I.S. Fraser, J.R. Newton and V. Odlind (CUP, 1990). More detailed information on all aspects of family planning can be obtained from the International Planned Parenthood Federation, the Family Planning Association, or the Margaret Pyke Centre.

ABORTION

There are few recent texts on abortion techniques as opposed to legal and sociological aspects. *Abortion* by D.M. Potts, P.L. Diggory and J. Peel (CUP, 1977) provides an all-round view of the subject. Among more recent publications are A. Bygdeman's *Medical induction of abortion* (Baillière, 1990), *Second trimester pregnancy termination* (Leiden University Press, 1982) edited by M.J.N.C. Keirse, J. Bennebroek Gravenhorst, D.A.F. van Lith and M.P. Embrey, *Voluntary termination* (Leiden University Press, 1982), edited by M.J.N.C. Keirse, J. Bennebroek Gravenhorst, D.A.F. van Lith and M.P. Embrey, *Voluntary sterilization: an international fact book* by J.A. Ross, S. Hong and D.H. Huber (Association for Voluntary Sterilization, 1985) and E.S.E. Hafez's *Voluntary termination of pregnancy* (MTP, 1984). A review of the history of abortion legislation is provided by J. Keown's *Abortion, doctors and the law: some aspects of the legal regulation of abortion in England from 1803–1982* (CUP, 1988). There are a variety of publications concerned with ethical problems but a specifically Christian viewpoint is provided by *Abortion: the personal dilemma* by R.F.R. Gardner, a Christian gynaecologist (Paternoster Press, 1972).

Female endocrinology

A comprehensive general text is *Williams' Textbook of endocrinology* (7th edn., Saunders, 1985) edited by J.D. Wilson and D.W. Foster whilst the slim publication *Essentials of endocrinology* (2nd edn., Blackwell, 1988) edited by J.L.H. O'Riordan and others is helpful for revision purposes. For the specialist a major reference work of some 750 pages is *Clinical reproductive endocrinology*, edited by R.P. Shearman (Churchill Livingstone, 1985) but MRCOG candidates and others are likely to find G.C.L. Lachelin's more recent *Introduction to clinical reproductive endocrinology* (Butterworth–Heinemann, 1991) a more useful source of information. Two established titles are *Reproductive endocrinology: physiology, pathology and clinical management* by S.S.C. Yen and R.B. Jaffe (2nd edn., Saunders, 1986) and *Gynecologic endocrinology*, (4th edn., Plenum, 1987) edited by J.J. Gold and J.B. Josimovich, whilst contributions from international specialists appear in *Advances in gynecological endocrinology* (2 vols, Parthenon, 1989) edited by A.R. Genazzani and others. A.R. Genazzani has also edited, with A. Volpe and F. Facchnetti, a volume of Congress Proceedings entitled *Gynecological endocrinology* (Parthenon, 1987). M. Dalton's *Gynaecological endocrinology: a guide to understanding and management* (Macmillan,

1989) is a concise contribution to the literature for the use of junior doctors. More specialized monographs are available as follows:

LHRH and its analogues: their use in clinical practice by R.W. Shaw and J.C. Marshall (Wright, 1989)

LHRH analogues in gynaecology, edited by I. Brosens, H.S. Jacobs and B. Runnebaum (Parthenon, 1990)

The cause and management of hirsutism, edited by R.B. Greenblatt, V.B. Mahesh and R.D. Gambrell (Parthenon, 1987)

Endocrinology of pregnancy, edited by F. Fuchs and A. Klopper (3rd edn., Harper and Row, 1983)

Endocrinology of pregnancy by S. Franks, in Baillière's *Clinical endocrinology and metabolism* series (Baillière Tindall, 1990).

Endocrine disorders in pregnancy by S. Brody and K. Ueland (Appleton and Lange, 1988)

Clinical gynecologic endocrinology and infertility by L. Speroff, R.H. Glass and N.G. Kase (4th edn., Williams and Wilkins, 1988)

Female urology

Clinical gynecologic urology, edited by S.L. Stanton (Mosby, 1984) contains contributions from well-known specialists and includes numerous illustrations. A very useful introductory text which contains references and guides to further reading is *Introduction to clinical gynaecological urology* (Butterworth-Heinemann, 1990) by J.R. Sutherst, M.I. Frazer, D.H. Richmond and B. Haylen. *Micronutrition: The Proceedings of the 21st Study Group of the Royal College of Obstetricians and Gynaecologists, October 1989* (RCOG/Springer, 1990) appear in a volume edited by J.O. Drife, P. Hilton and S.L. Stanton. A useful source of information on the general subject of urodynamics entitled *Urodynamics: principles, practice and application* (Churchill Livingstone, 1984) is edited by A.R. Mundy, T.P. Stephenson and A.J. Wein. Other volumes dealing specifically with female urological disorders and their management include: *The unstable bladder* (Wright, 1989), edited by R.M. Freeman and J. Malvern; *Surgery of female incontinence* (2nd edn., Springer, 1986) edited by S.L. Stanton and E.A. Tanagho; *Clinical gynaecological urology* (Blackwell, 1983) by M. Asmussen and A. Miller and *Female urinary incontinence: Proceedings of an Educational Course Held at the Royal College of Obstetricians and Gynaecologists, June 1989* (RCOG, 1990) edited by G.J. Jarvis. *Incontinence and its management* (2nd edn., Croom Helm, 1980), edited by D. Mandelstam is a handy reference source for nurses.

Statistics

Statistical inquiries can present a decided challenge even to a specialist librarian. Most of the standard sources of national and international statistics are well known, but it may be helpful to draw attention to those considered useful in the particular context of this chapter. The *World Health Statistics Annual*, produced by WHO, is of limited value but the international comparisons may be useful on occasion. For example, in 1989, under the heading *Global Overview*, figures 5 and 6 relate respectively to 'Women attended during pregnancy, according to level of development, 1986–88' and 'Women attended during delivery, according to level of development, 1986-88'. Certain columns in the sections concerning natality and causes of death can provide helpful general data though perhaps not always the degree of detailed analysis that the specialist requires. Publications of the Office of Population Censuses and Surveys are described elsewhere (see pp.83 and 202). The statistical tables of particular interest are Series FM1 (Births); DH1, DH2, DH3 (Mortality); MB1 (Cancer); MB3 (Congenital Malformations) and AB (Abortion). Formerly, Series AB was published as *Supplement on Abortion to the Registrar General's Statistical Review of England and Wales*, and is a source of detailed figures back to April, 1968, when the Abortion Act 1967 came into effect. *Population trends*, published quarterly by HMSO since 1975, contains appended tables of annual and, in some cases, more recent quarterly statistics which include figures relating to abortion, births and perinatal mortality. The publication also includes articles on aspects of population studies which occasionally have a bearing on obstetrical subjects, for example perinatal mortality studies. Another key publication is an official triennial report devoted to the detailed analysis of maternal deaths. The latest in a line of reports, first published in 1957 (covering the period 1952–54), is *Report on Confidential Enquiries into Maternal Deaths in the United Kingdom, 1985-87* (HMSO, 1991) emanating from the Department of Health, the Welsh Office, the Scottish Home and Health Department, and the Department of Health and Social Security, Northern Ireland.

Various comprehensive births surveys have taken place over the years. A survey of births in the UK took place for one week in April 1970 and the results are reported in the two published volumes of *British births 1970: a survey under the joint auspices of the National Birthday Trust Fund and the Royal College of Obstetricians and Gynaecologists*. Volume 1, entitled *The first week of life*, was published under the direction of R. Chamberlain and others (Heinemann, 1975) and contains chapters, with detailed tables, on topics such as birthweight and length of gestation, illness of the baby, and stillbirths and first-week deaths. Volume 2, *Obstetric care* by G. Chamberlain and others (Heinemann, 1978), covers aspects indicated by the title such as antenatal care, labour and labour induction. More recently, G. Chamberlain and P. Gunn have edited *Birthplace: report of the confidential enquiry into facilities available at the place of birth* (Wiley, 1987), a survey conducted under the auspices of the National Birthday Trust. *Birth counts: statistics of pregnancy and childbirth* by Alison MacFarlane and Miranda Mugford (2 vols, HMSO, 1984) remains a useful source despite its publication date as it brings together statistics collected by a number of official sources. Volume 1 contains detailed chapters on a wide range of relevant topics whilst Volume 2 devotes over 300 pages to statistical tables. Caesarean section rates is a topic which claims a great deal of attention. The Maternity Alliance produced a study in 1986 entitled *One birth in nine: a survey and discussion papers on caesarean section trends since 1978* which, although not an official publication as such, contains some statistical data of interest.

Finally *Maternity care in the world: international survey of midwifery practice and training. Report of a Joint Study Group of the International Federation of Gynaecology and Obstetrics and the International Confederation of Midwives* (2nd edn., International Federation of Gynaecology and Obstetrics International Confederation of Midwives, 1976) is a comprehensive source of international statistics, particularly on birth and infant mortality rates, although maternal and perinatal mortality figures are not given. Wherever possible figures for 1973 are quoted, but less recent or estimated statistics are substituted where 1973 figures have not been made available. A new edition has occasionally been contemplated but has not, so far, been realized.

History and biography

Numerous histories now exist, although few are readily available except for reference in a limited number of libraries. In view of the level of interest in the subject it is helpful to be aware of the most useful sources of information which can quickly be traced at need in specialist or long-established large medical collections.

Ancient history is covered by W.J.S. McKay's *The history of ancient gynaecology* (Baillière, 1901) which deals with the Egyptian, Hindu, Greek and Roman periods; it contains a list of works consulted but lacks an index. Several anthropological studies are available, of which, the most comprehensive is easily H. H. Ploss, M. Bartels and P. Bartels' *Woman: an historical, gynaecological and anthropological compendium* translated and edited by E. J. Dingwall (3 vols, Heinemann, 1935), which covers all aspects of womanhood in all races and cultures. It contains 1000 illustrations and an extensive bibliography, but unfortunately no index, although material is arranged in a logical sequence.

As far as general histories of the subject are concerned H. Speert has produced *Iconographia gyniatrica: a pictorial history of gynecology and obstetrics* (Davis, 1973) in which there is rather more emphasis on illustrative material than text, and the same author has also produced an earlier volume entitled *Essays in eponymy: obstetric and gynecologic milestones* (Macmillan, 1958). J.V. Ricci's books are comprehensive studies with extensive lists of references, and quotations from original sources: *One hundred years of gynaecology, 1800-1900* (Blakiston, 1945); *The genealogy of gynaecology; history of the development of gynaecology throughout the Ages. 2000* B.C. to 1800 A.D. (2nd edn., Blakiston, 1950); and *The development of gynaecological surgery and instruments: a comprehensive review of the evolution of surgery and surgical instruments for the treatment of female diseases from the Hippocratic Age to the antiseptic period* (Blakiston, 1949) while T. Cianfrani's *A short history of obstetrics and gynecology* (C. C. Thomas, 1960) sets the subject in a background of social, economic and general medical history. A popular, readable narrative without documentation but with a selective bibliography was provided by I. H. Flack under the pseudonym H. Graham in *Eternal Eve* (Heinemann, 1950), of which a revised, abridged edition was published in 1960; a short but authoritative little book by W. Radcliffe called *Milestones in midwifery* (Wright, 1967) has general appeal. Those more interested in socio-political aspects are likely to find the following of interest: *With child: birth through the ages* by J. Carter and T. Duriez (Mainstream Publishing, 1986); *A history of women's bodies* by Edward Shorter (Allen Lane, 1983); *The politics of maternity care: services for childbearing women in twentieth century Britain*, edited by J. Garcia, R. Kilpatrick and M. Richards (OUP, 1990) is a collection of studies on associated topics; Ann Oakley's *The captured womb: a history of the medical care of pregnant women* (Basil Blackwell, 1984) which contains numerous figures and tables, and O. Moscussi's *The science of woman: gynaecology and gender in England 1800-1829* (CUP, 1990) covering the period up to the founding of the Royal College of Obstetricians and Gynaecologists.

As far as British obstetrical and gynaecological practice is concerned the two basic information sources are H. R. Spencer's *The history of British midwifery from 1650 to 1800* (Bale, 1927) which is continued by J. M. Munro Kerr, R. W. Johnstone and M. H. Phillips' *Historical review of British obstetrics and gynaecology, 1800-1950* (Livingstone, 1954), a well-documented volume with indexes of personal names and subjects. A translation from Middle English of a mediaeval manuscript (Sloane 2463), so far the earliest known reference source in obstetrics in the vernacular to be made freely available in printed form, has been published. Translated by B. Rowland, it is entitled *Medieval woman's guide to health* (Croom Helm, 1981). For information on the development of midwifery as a profession, as distinct from obstetrics, a useful source is J. Donnison's *Midwives and medical men: a history of inter-professional rivalries and women's rights*, 2nd. edn. Heinemann, 19xx); also *Midwives in history and society* (Croom Helm, 1986) by J. Towler and J. Bramall, containing an appendix on statutory bodies and legislation.

J. Dewhurst's *Royal confinements* (Weidenfeld and Nicolson, 1980) spans two centuries from the Restoration Stuarts to Queen Victoria and is a publication which has appealed greatly to the taste of both medical men and the lay public. The history of the specialty in America is the subject of H. Speert's *Obstetrics and gynecology in America: a history* (American College of Obstetricians and Gynecologists, 1980).

On more specialized topics are the invaluable *Obstetric forceps; its history and evolution* (Art Press, 1929) by Sir Kedarnath Das, while the Chamberlen family and their famous forceps are the subject of W. Radcliffe's *The secret instrument: the birth of the midwifery forceps* (Heinemann, 1947) and J. H. Aveling's *The Chamberlens and the midwifery forceps. Memorials of the family and an essay on the invention of the instrument* (Churchill, 1882). B. M. Hibbard has recently compiled a short, but authoritative, account of the history of midwifery forceps in his *The obstetric forceps: a short history and descriptive catalogue of the forceps in the Museum of the Royal College of Obstetricians and Gynaecologists* (RCOG, 1988) which museum also houses the aforementioned Chamberlen instruments.

J. H. Young's *Caesarean section: the history and development of the operation from earliest times* (Lewis, 1944) is the main source of information on this very topic. This may be supplemented by D. Trolle's *The history of caesarean section* (Copenhagen: Reitzel, 1982) which comprises Volume 33 of *Acta Historica Scientarum Naturalium et Medicinalium.*

Various efforts have been made to document the life and work of some of the more notable obstetricians and gynaecologists, although few of these biographies are outstanding. Most worthy of mention are:

Memoir of Sir James Y. Simpson by J. Duns (Edmonstone and Douglas, 1873)

Simpson and Syme of Edinburgh by J. A. Shepherd (Livingstone, 1969)

Dr. William Smellie and his contemporaries by J. Glaister (Maclehose, 1894)

William Smellie, the master of British midwifery by R. W. Johnstone (Livingstone, 1952), which is shorter but nonetheless authoritative

Spencer Wells. The life and work of a Victorian surgeon by J. A. Shepherd (Livingstone, 1965)

Semmelweis: his life and doctrine by Sir W. J. Sinclair (Manchester University Press, 1909)

Mea culpa and the life and work of Semmelweis by L. P. Celione (Little, Brown, 1937), translated from the French by R. A. Parker

Woman's surgeon: the life story of J. Marion Sims by S. Harris; reprinted 1968 (Macmillan, 1950)

The story of my life by J. M. Sims (Appleton, 1884 and 1888)

William Blair-Bell – father and founder by John Peel (RCOG, 1986)

The life and times of Ephraim McDowell by L. A. Gray Sr. (privately printed, 1987)

There is, as yet, no definitive biography of William Hunter (1718-1783), but the following studies may be useful:

William Hunter, anatomist, physician, obstetrician ... with notices of his friends Cullen, Smellie, Fothergill and Baillie by R. H. Fox (Lewis, 1901)

Two Great Scotsmen; the brothers William and John Hunter by G. R. Mather (Maclehose, 1893)

Memoir of William and John Hunter by G. C. Peachey (privately printed, 1924)

James Douglas of the Pouch and his pupil William Hunter by K. B. Thomas (Pitman, 1964)

William Hunter and the eighteenth century medical world, edited by W.F. Bynum and R. Porter (CUP, 1985)

In this connection a biography by J. L. Thornton entitled *Jan van Rymsdyk: medical artist of the eighteenth century* (Oleander, 1982) documents what is so far known of the life and work of this great illustrator who was largely responsible for illustrating Hunter's *Gravid uterus* (1774) and other eighteenth-century texts and papers. Finally, there is available a collection of short biographies of eminent figures of this century in the form of Sir John Peel's *The Lives of the Fellows of the Royal College of Obstetricians and Gynaecologists, 1929-1969* (Heinemann, 1976).

Other texts which should perhaps be mentioned are: *Records and curiosities in obstetrics and gynaecology* compiled by I.L.C. Fergusson, R. W. Taylor and J. M. Watson (Baillière Tindall, 1981) by B. Cowell and

D. Wainwright; *Abortion in England, 1900-1967* by Barbara Brookes (Croom Helm, 1988); *A history of embryology*, edited by T.J. Horder, J.A. Witkowski and C.C. Wylie (CUP, 1986) which covers the history of developmental embryology from 1880 and comprises the Eighth Symposium of the British Society for Developmental Biology, and Sir William Fletcher Shaw's *Twenty-five years: the story of the Royal College of Obstetricians and Gynaecologists, 1929-1954* (Churchill, 1954), which has been updated by Sir John Peel in an article entitled *The Royal College of Obstetricians and Gynaecologists, 1929 to 1979* published in the *British Journal of Obstetrics and Gynaecology*, 1979, **86**, 673-692. *Super Ardua: The Royal College of Obstetricians and Gynaecologists in Australia 1929-1979* by I.A. McDonald, I. Cope and F.M.C. Forster (Australia Council, RCOG, 1981) traces the development of what is now the Royal Australian College of Obstetricians and Gynaecologists.

Acknowledgement

I am most grateful to my colleague, Gillian Edwards, for her assistance in the preparation of this chapter.

CHAPTER TWENTY

Paediatrics

ELAINE S. BROOKE

Paediatrics is concerned with the prevention, cure and alleviation of diseases and disorders of infants and children, and with the development, health and welfare of the normal child. Children are no longer considered to be 'little adults', so paediatrics is a branch of medicine in its own right. In recent years the development of many specialties within the field has produced a significant increase in the literature.

Indexes, abstracts and bibliographies

Paediatric literature is included in the *Index Medicus* and the *NLM Current Catalog* (see Chapter 3). For current awareness three of the sections of *Current Contents* may be useful, depending on the bias of the research; these are *Current Contents, Clinical Medicine, Current Contents: Life Sciences*; and *Current Contents: Social and Behavioral Sciences*.

Excerpta Medica (Section 7) covers *Pediatrics and Pediatric Surgery* from 1947. *International Abstracts of Pediatric Surgery* is published in the *Journal of Pediatric Surgery* (Saunders, 1966–). The development of the child is covered by *Child Development Abstracts and Bibliography* (University of Chicago Press, 1930–). Each year the *Bibliography of Developmental Medicine and Child Neurology* appears as a supplement to *Developmental Medicine and Child Neurology* (Blackwell, 1962–). A set of six bibliographies from the National Children's Bureau, prepared by Rosemary Dinnage covers cerebral palsy (1986a), chronic medical problems (1986b), epilepsy (1986c), spina bifida

(1986d), the orthopaedically handicapped child (1986e) and asthma (Dinnage and Gooch, 1986).

Reference books

Most reference books, such as dictionaries, directories and pharmacopoeias, used by paediatricians are those that are used generally, but S.I. Magalini *et al. Dictionary of medical syndromes* (3rd edn., Lippincott, 1990) is particularly useful. The *Catalog of teratogenic agents* by T.H. Shepard (6th edn., Johns Hopkins University Press, 1989) should be consulted when birth defects are being considered.

Fiona Macdonald has compiled *The parents' directory* (Bedford Square Press, 1989). This lists about 800 voluntary organizations, with addresses and contacts; the sections on handicap and health are the most useful. The annual British Paediatric Association (BPA) *Handbook* includes a list of members with addresses and positions, as well as information about the Association. The BPA has produced the *BPA classification of diseases* (2 vols, BPA, 1979) which list the codes for use in the classification of paediatric and perinatal disorders, and is compatible with the *WHO international classification of diseases* (WHO, 1977).

Statistics of morbidity, mortality and the well-being of the, child are always in demand. The following sections of the Office of Population Censuses and Surveys statistical publications are applicable: *DH3 Mortality Statistics: perinatal and infant* (this also includes birthweight statistics), *DH6 Mortality Statistics: childhood, FMI Birth Statistics* and *MB3 Congenital Malformation Statistics. The World Health Statistics* (WHO, annual) and UNICEF's *The State of the World's Children* (OUP, annual) contain much information.

Reviews

With subject fields expanding so rapidly, review volumes are most helpful. Paediatric subjects appear in many such volumes, but the following are worth particular mention: *Advances in Child Development and Behavior* (Academic Press, 1963–), *Advances in Pediatrics* (Year Book Medical Publishers, 1942–), *Progress in Pediatric Surgery* (Springer, 1970–) and *Year Book of Pediatrics* (Year Book Medical Publishers, 1933–).

Journals

Articles on child health and disease appear in general medical journals, and also in journals for specific subjects, e.g. pathology or surgery. There are many journals devoted to children, some highly specialized, so only a select list can be included here.

Acta Paediatrica Scandinavica (Almqvist and Wiksell, 1921–)

American Journal of Diseases of Children (American Medical Association, 1911–)

Archives of Disease in Childhood (British Medical Association, 1926–)

Child; Care, Health and Development (Blackwell, 1975–)

Child Development (University of Chicago Press, 1930–)

Current Opinion in Pediatrics (Current Science, 1989–)

Developmental Medicine and Child Neurology (Blackwell, 1962–)

Early Human Development (Elsevier, 1977–)

European Journal of Pediatrics (Springer, 1976–; formerly *Zeitschrift für Kinderheilkunde,* 1911–1975)

Journal of Child Psychology and Psychiatry (Pergamon, 1960–)

Journal of Pediatric Surgery (Saunders, 1966–)

Journal of Pediatrics (Mosby-Year Book, 1932–)

Journal of Tropical Pediatrics (OUP, 1955–)

Pediatric Clinics of North America (Saunders, 1954–)

Pediatric Research (Williams and Wilkins, 1967–)

Pediatrics (American Academy of Pediatrics, 1948–)

Series

There are several monographic series which are important to the paediatrician:

Birth Defects, Original Article Series (A.R. Liss, 1964–)

Child Health and Development (Karger, 1982–)

Clinics in Developmental Medicine (Blackwell, 1964–)

Monographs of the Society for Research in Child Development (University of Chicago Press, 1936–)

Pediatric and Adolescent Medicine (Karger, 1990–; formerly *Modern Problems in Pediatrics,* 1954–1989 and *Monographs in Pediatrics,* 1971-1986)

Recent Advances in Paediatrics (Churchill Livingstone, 1954–)

Surveys and studies

Surveys of groups of children, at birth and as they grow up, give much valuable information. A national survey of all the children born during the first week of March 1946 is documented by J.W.B. Douglas and J.M. Blomfield in *Maternity in Great Britain* (OUP,1948) and *Children under five* (Allen and Unwin, 1958). In 1958 there was a British Perinatal Mortality Survey and from this came two reports, *Perinatal mortality* by N.R. Butler and D.G. Bonham (Livingstone, 1963) and *Perinatal problems* by N.R. Butler and E.D. Alberman (Livingstone, 1969). The National Child Development Study (1958 Cohort) has produced three reports *From birth to seven* by R. Davie *et al.* (Longman, 1972), *11 000 seven year olds* by M.L. Pringle *et al.* (Longman, 1966) and *Britain's sixteen year olds* by K. Fogelman (National Children's Bureau, 1976). These have been followed by articles at regular intervals, a selection of which have been published with an introduction and overview as *Growing up in Great Britain*, edited by K. Fogelman (Macmillan, 1983). Under the auspices of the National Birthday Trust Fund and the Royal College of Obstetricians and Gynaecologists, the British Births Survey 1970 took place including children born between 5 and 11 April 1970. The two volumes are entitled *British births, 1970, vol. 1: the first week of life* (Heinemann, 1975), *vol. 2: Obstetric Care* (Heinemann, 1978). A report of the British Births Child Study (1970) is *The prevalence of illness in childhood* by R.N. Chamberlain and R.N. Simpson (Pitman, 1979), which surveys approximately 10 per cent of the children in the original survey. In 1975 a follow-up survey of the 1970 cohort was carried out by the Department of Child Health, Bristol and called the Child Health and Education Study. Two volumes have been produced from the study *The social life of Britain's five-year-olds* by A.F. Osborn *et al.*, (Routledge and Kegan Paul, 1984) and *From birth to five* edited by N.R. Butler and J. Golding (Pergamon, 1986).

A study of health and illness in children in Newcastle has been the subject of three volumes: *A thousand families in Newcastle upon Tyne* by J. Spence *et al.* (OUP, 1954); *Growing up in Newcastle upon Tyne* (OUP, 1960); and *The school years in Newcastle upon Tyne* (OUP, 1974) both by F.D.W. Miller *et al.* John and Elizabeth Newson studied 700 infants in Nottingham in *Infant care in an urban community* (Allen & Unwin, 1963). The second phase of the project was a study of children at four years old, *Four years old in an urban community* (Allen & Unwin, 1968) which particularly emphasized parent/child relations, and the third phase was at seven years old, *Seven years old in the home environment* (Allen and Unwin, 1976). A study by a general practitioner in Brixton is recorded in M. Pollak's *Today's three year olds in London* (Heinemann, 1972) and *Nine years old* (MTP Press, 1979), and gives an insight into the experiences of children, living side by side, but being reared in different cultural life styles.

The 'Isle of Wight Survey' was a series of three surveys carried out in 1964 and 1965 including all children 9–12 years old living on the island, noting intellectual, educational, psychiatric and physical handicap, and reported in *Education, health and behaviour* by M. Rutter *et al.* (Longman, 1970). The progress of over 2000 pupils was followed during secondary education in inner London by M. Rutter *et al.* in *Fifteen thousand hours* (Open Books, 1979). *My mother said ...* by C. Farrell (Routledge and Kegan Paul, 1978) is based on over 1500 interviews in 1974/5 to establish how young people learned about sex and birth control.

Monographs and textbooks

General

There are many textbooks of paediatrics, some having appeared in several editions; of particular note are the *Nelson Textbook of pediatrics*, edited by R.E. Behrman *et al.* (13th edn., Saunders, 1987) and *Textbook of paediatrics*, edited by J.O. Forfar and G.C. Arneil (3rd edn., 2 vols, Churchill Livingstone, 1984). The influence of medical advances and altered patterns of society stimulated the BPA to produce *Child health in a changing society*, edited by J.O. Forfar (OUP, 1988) to mark its diamond jubilee. Also reflecting our changing society is John Black's *Child health in a multicultural society* (2nd edn., BMJ, 1989) which helps the health worker understand differences in culture and language. All paediatricians should have access to *Medical research with children; ethics, law and practice*, edited by R.H. Nicholson (OUP, 1986).

Two volumes which appeal to undergraduate students are *Jolly's Diseases of children* edited by M.I. Levene (6th edn., Blackwell, 1990) and *Essential paediatrics* by D. Hull and D. I. Johnstone (2nd edn., Churchill Livingstone, 1987). Postgraduate students find J.H. Hutchison's *Practical paediatric problems* (6th edn., Lloyd-Luke, 1986) useful, and all students like M. Dynski-Klein's *A colour atlas of paediatrics* (Wolfe, 1975, reprinted 1986). The management of paediatric problems by the young physician within the hospital is outlined in *Hospital paediatrics* by A.D. Milner and D. Hull (Churchill Livingstone, 1984). T.L. Chambers aims to explain the physiology of fluid and electrolyte balance in a simple way as an aid to clinical management in *Fluid therapy in childhood* (Blackwell, 1987). As treatment becomes more complex Davis and Dobbing's *Scientific foundations of paediatrics* (2nd edn., Heinemann, 1981) and Godfrey and Baum's *Clinical paediatric physiology* (Blackwell, 1979) help with understanding some of the background mechanisms. A new development is sports medicine, and O. Bar-Or brings together information from physiological principles to clinical applications in *Paediatric sports medicine for the practitioner* (Springer, 1983).

During recent years the three strands of child health care, the hospital paediatric service, general practice and the community and school health services, have become an integrated child health service and community paediatricians are being trained. The Diploma of Child Health (DCH) has reverted to being the examination for GPs and community paediatricians and *Harvey and Kovar's Child health; textbook for the DCH* (2nd edn., Churchill Livingstone, 1991) is not only a basic book for candidates, but also for family doctors in everyday practice. *Child care in general practice*, edited by C. Hart and J. Bain (3rd edn., Churchill Livingstone, 1989) is written by general practitioners for general practitioners, and *Community paediatrics* by D. Hull and L. Polnay (Churchill Livingstone, 1985) covers the care of the child within the home, school and community. Planned alterations in primary health care have emphasized prevention of disease and health surveillance. D.M.B. Hall edited a working party report on the subject *Health for all children* (OUP, 1989). J.R. Butler has reviewed the different opinions about who, what and when in a Department of Health publication *Child health surveillance in primary care* (HMSO, 1989).

Genetics and inherited disease

A short introduction to genetics is A.E.H. Emery and R.F. Mueller's *Elements of medical genetics* (7th edn., Churchill Livingstone, 1988). D.J. Weatherall has written an introduction to human molecular genetics for the non-specialist in *The new genetics and clinical practice* (3rd edn., OUP, 1991). A.E.H. Emery and D.L. Rimoin have edited a comprehensive text, *Principles and practice of medical genetics* (2 vols, Churchill Livingstone, 2nd edn., 1990). Photographs illustrate clinical manifestations in *A colour atlas of clinical genetics* (Wolfe, 1983) by M. Baraitser and R.M. Winter. An essential reference book is V. A. McKusick's *Mendelian inheritance in man* (9th edn., Johns Hopkins University Press, 1990).

The standard work on inherited metabolic disease now edited by C.R. Scriver *et al.* is entitled *Metabolic basis of inherited disease* (2 vols, 6th edn., McGraw Hill, 1989). The genetic causes of metabolic disease feature in *Genetic and metabolic disease in pediatrics*, edited by J.K. Lloyd and C.R. Scriver (Butterworths, 1985). For all clinicians involved in the management of inborn errors of metabolism *Genetic biochemical disorders* by P.F. Benson and A.H. Fensom (OUP, 1985) gives clinical and biochemical features of the disorders and also basic data for genetic counselling. Clinicians with little knowledge of genetics will find P.S. Harper's *Practical genetic counselling* (3rd edn., Wright, 1988) helpful when dealing with patients and parents.

Congenital malformations by J. Warkany (Year Book Medical Publishers, 1971) is a standard work and W.L. Nyhan and N.O. Sakati's *Genetic and malformation syndromes in clinical medicine* (Year Book Medical Publishers, 1976) and D. Bergsma's *Birth defects compendium* (2nd edn., Macmillan, 1979) are also important. K.L. Jones has revised *Smith's Recognizable patterns of human malformation* (4th edn., Saunders, 1988) and J.M. Graham has revised *Smith's Recognizable patterns of human deformation* (2nd edn., Saunders, 1988) and both are profusely illustrated. Robin Winter and Michael Baraitser have developed LONDON DYSMORPHOLOGY DATABASE (OUP) containing 1800 malformation syndromes. New information is being added continuously and updates are available.

Newborn infant

Just as the child is not treated as a 'little adult', the newborn infant is not treated as a 'little child', and there is a wide-ranging literature especially for the neonate. N.R.C. Roberton's *Textbook of neonatology* (Churchill Livingstone, 1986) covers the subject in depth. Clinical and radiological illustrations have been gathered by R. D. G. Milner and S. M. Herber in *A colour atlas of the newborn* (Wolfe, 1984). A small practical guide to the care of the newborn is *A neonatal vade-meum*, edited by P.J. Fleming *et al.*, (2nd edn., Arnold, 1991). Brazleton 's assessment scale for evaluation of the behaviour of the newborn infant is described in *Neonatal behavioral assessment scale* (2nd edn., Blackwell, 1984) and Dubowitz's scoring system based on neurological and superficial characteristics is described in *Gestational age of the newborn* (Addison-Wesley, 1977). Pathology is contained in G. B. Reed *et al. Diseases of the fetus and newborn* (Chapman and Hall, 1989). N. R. C. Roberton's *Manual of neonatal intensive care* (2nd edn., Arnold, 1986) covers the practical management of acute medical and surgical problems. J. Lister and I.M. Irving edit *Neonatal surgery* (3rd edn., Butterworths, 1990), a comprehensive textbook. In *The surgical neonate* (2nd edn., Appleton-Century-Crofts, 1985) H.C. Filston and R.J. Izant cover the general management, congenital anomalies and common paediatric surgical problems. Anaesthesia for the newborn is particularly difficult owing to the rapidly developing physiology and D.J. Hatch and E. Sumner devote a section to perinatal physiology in *Neonatal anaesthesia and perioperative care* (2nd edn., Arnold,, 1986).

Improved care and technological advances have helped save many infants. The care of the premature and sick neonate is contained in *Care of the high risk neonate*, edited by M.H. Klaus and A.A. Fanaroff (3rd edn., Saunders, 1986). Immaturity of sucking, swallowing and absorption cause difficulties for feeding, and the European Society of Paediatric Gastroenterology and Nutrition's committee on nutrition, chaired by B.A. Wharton, prepared guidelines entitled *Nutrition and feeding of preterm infants* (Blackwell, 1987). Very preterm babies are different so David Harvey *et al.* have edited *The baby under 1000g* (Butterworths, 1989). In *Born too soon or born too small* (Heinemann, 1976) G.A. Neligan *et al.* have followed, for seven years, the development of a group of high-risk infants from Newcastle upon Tyne, and in *Sequelae of low birthweight* (Blackwell, 1986) H.G. Dunn *et al.*, have followed 500 infants from the nursery of Vancouver General Hospital up to school age, particularly studying neurological and ophthalmological defects.

Infection can be damaging to the neonate and P.A. Davies and L.A. Gothefors have written *Bacterial infections of the fetus and newborn infant* (Saunders, 1984) for those responsible for newborn babies. *Viral diseases of the fetus and newborn* by J.B. Hanshaw *et al.* (2nd edn., Saunders, 1985) is concerned with both short- and long-term effects of viral infections, their effect on normal fetal development and upon the child after birth. Rapid diagnosis of disease is important; many techniques use blood analysis, and F.A. Oski and J.L. Naiman cover this field with *Hematologic problems in the newborn* (3rd edn., Saunders, 1982). The subtle signs of neonatal neurological disorders are included in *Neurology of the newborn* by J.J. Volpe (2nd edn., Saunders, 1987).

Sudden infant death syndrome continues to be a puzzle and J. Golding *et al.* in *Sudden infant death* (Open Books, 1984) use information from a retrospective study of parents in a survey by the Foundation for the Study of Infant Deaths and from a survey of sudden infant death in Oxfordshire and West Berkshire in 1971–75, to analyse various factors in an attempt to build up an accurate picture. The medical aspects and psychological management are covered in *Sudden infant death syndrome*, edited by J.L. Culbertson *et al.* (Arnold, 1988).

Growth and development

The normal growth of the child has to be studied before the abnormal, and the three-volume work *Human growth*, edited by F. Falkner and J.M. Tanner (2nd edn., Plenum Press, 1986) covers the subject in depth. Tanner's *Foetus into man* (2nd edn., Castlemead, 1989) is a basic and easily understood book. J.M. Tanner and R.H. Whitehouse's *Atlas of children's growth* (Academic Press, 1982) illustrates normal variation in growth, and also growth disorders. *Worldwide variation in human growth* by Phyllis Eveleth and J.M. Tanner (2nd edn., CUP, 1990) includes height, weight, skinfold and other body measurements from all over the world, many previously unpublished. Noel Cameron is the expert on the technical aspects of measurement of the growing individual and his book *The measurement of human growth* (Croom Helm, 1984) explains the skills. Normal data is presented for quick use by J.M.H. Buckler in *A reference manual of growth and development* (Blackwell, 1979). A child's height, whether too short or too tall, can be a problem, and in this context, *Assessment of skeletal maturity and prediction of adult height (TW2 method)* by J.M. Tanner *et al.* (2nd edn., Academic Press, 1983) is useful.

R.S. Illingworth's *The normal child* (10th edn., Churchill Livingstone, 1991) and *Development of the infant and young child* (9th edn., Churchill Livingstone, 1987) remain the standard texts. *Child development and child health* by Martin Bax *et al.* (Blackwell, 1990) is written for community paediatricians and the text deals primarily with development of the infant and young child, but also includes normal health care and childhood disorders encountered in clinics, and is particularly good on social and environmental factors. A brief and simple handbook for use in assessing the child in clinic or surgery is *Basic developmental screening: 0-4 years* by R.S. Illingworth (4th edn., Blackwell, 1988). In *Development disabilities*, edited by M. Lewis and L.T. Taft (MTP, 1982) there is an interdisciplinary approach to the study, assessment and treatment of developmentally disabled preschool children. S. Levitt outlines the contributions of physiotherapists, occupational and speech therapists in the care of the handicapped child in *Paediatric development therapy* (Blackwell, 1984).

Nutrition

A small practical guide to the nutritional needs of infants and children is *Nutrition for children* by D.E.M. Francis (Blackwell, 1986). *MacKeith's infant feeding and feeding difficulties*, edited by C.B.S. Wood and J.A. Walker-Smith (6th edn., Churchill Livingstone, 1981) and *Textbook of paediatric nutrition*, edited by D.S. McLaren *et al.*, (3rd edn., Churchill Livingstone, 1991) are valuable texts. Two publications from the former Department of Health and Social Security are reports of working parties chaired by Professor T.E. Oppé. First, *Artificial feeds for the young infant* (HMSO, 1980) which gives guidelines for nutrient composition of foods to be used when human milk is not available, and secondly *Present-day practice in infant feeding: Third Report* (HMSO, 1988). The dietary habits of British schoolchildren were measured using a 7-day record in 1983, and the results published by the Department of Health entitled *Diets of British schoolchildren* (HMSO, 1989).

Breast feeding is being actively encouraged and an international symposium was published under the title *Human milk; its biological and social value*, edited by S. Freier and A.I. Eidelman (Excerpta Medica, 1980). A multinational study on breast feeding resulted in two WHO reports, *Contemporary patterns of breast feeding* (WHO, 1981) and *The quantity and quality of breast-milk* (WHO, 1985).

The sick child needs special attention and Dorothy Francis' book *Diets for sick children* (4th edn., Blackwell, 1987) gives great help, especially where specialized dietetic advice is not available. A clinician (Donald Bentley) and a nutritionist (Margaret Lawson) have combined to produce *Clinical nutrition in paediatric disorders* (Baillière Tindall, 1988) covering a range of childhood disorders where nutritional management plays an important part in treatment. *A colour atlas of nutritional disorders* compiled by D.S. McLaren (Wolfe, 1981) gives a vivid picture of disorders caused by faulty feeding.

Diagnosis and therapy

Green and Richmond's *Pediatric diagnosis* (4th edn., Saunders, 1986) aids interpretation of symptoms and signs at various ages. *Pediatric decision making* by S. Berman (Decker, 1985) clearly outlines decision lines for clinical management of children. An atlas containing 1200 colour pictures to aid diagnosis by instant recognition is edited by B.J. Zitelli and H.W. Davis and entitled *Atlas of pediatric physical diagnosis* (Arnold, 1987).

Isky Gordon's *Diagnostic imaging in paediatrics* (Chapman & Hall, 1987) guides paediatricians and radiologists to choose the most relevant type of imaging in order to reach a diagnosis. X-ray diagnosis is dealt with in depth in *Caffey's Pediatric X-ray diagnosis*, edited by F.N. Silverman (2 vols, 8th edn., Year Book Medical Publishers, 1985).

C.H. Kempe *et al.* cover treatment as well as diagnosis in *Current pediatric diagnosis and treatment* (10th edn., Lange, 1987), and Gellis and Kagan's *Current pediatric therapy* (12th edn., Saunders, 1986) is a standard text. A practical handbook for doctors treating children in hospital or at home is Jack Insley's *A paediatric vade-mecum* (12th edn., Arnold, 1990).

Alleviation of pain has stimulated interest in the use of hypnotherapy and Olness and Gardner's book *Hypnosis and hypnotherapy with children* (2nd edn., Grune and Stratton, 1988) discusses applications in various psychological, medical and surgical problems. *Physiotherapy in paediatrics* by R. Shepherd (2nd edn., Heinemann, 1980), *Hydrotherapy in paediatrics* by M.R. Campion (Heinemann, 1985) and *Occupational therapy for children* by P.N. Pratt and A.S. Allen (2nd edn., Mosby, 1989) describe other methods of treatment.

Pathology

Paediatric pathology, edited by Colin Berry (2nd edn., Springer, 1989) and Dehner's *Pediatric surgical pathology* (2nd edn., Williams & Wilkins, 1987) are the most important books in the field. Chemical pathology is essential in diagnosis and treatment of many diseases, and to help general paediatricians and those who work in chemical pathology departments, B. Clayton and J. Round have edited *Chemical pathology and the sick child* (Blackwell, 1984). Clayton *et al.* have also compiled a handbook of clinical tests and reference ranges entitled *Paediatric chemical pathology* (Blackwell, 1980). *Paediatric forensic medicine and pathology*, edited by J.K. Mason (Chapman and Hall, 1989) is the first book to cover forensic aspects of childhood.

Hematology of infancy and childhood, edited by D.G. Nathan and F.A. Oski (2 vols, 3rd edn., Saunders, 1987) encompasses haematology and oncology, whilst *Blood diseases of infancy and childhood*, edited by D.R. Miller *et al.* (6th edn., Mosby, 1989) is a comprehensive text on diseases of the blood. Microscopic appearances of blood and bone marrow, including normal appearances are pictured in *Colour atlas of paediatric haematology* by I.M. Hann *et al.* (2nd edn., OUP, 1990). Cancer in childhood is covered by W.W. Sutow *et al.* in *Clinical pediatric oncology* (3rd edn., Mosby, 1984) and clinical management by P.A. Voute *et al.* in *Cancer in children* (2nd edn., Springer, 1986). Surgery is an integral part of combined therapy of cancer and D.M. Hays has edited *Pediatric surgical oncology* (Grune and Stratton, 1986).

Immunology is a growing subject and E.R. Steihm's *Immunologic disorders in infants and children* (3rd edn., Saunders, 1989) covers the development and function of the immune system as well as immunological disorders. J.F. Soothill *et al.* in *Pediatric immunology* (Blackwell, 1983) take the organ-based approach to immunology. C.W. Bierman and D.S. Pearlman have edited a book on *Allergic diseases from infancy to adulthood* (2nd edn., Saunders, 1988). There are many theories about allergies to food; in *Food intolerance* (Baillière Tindall, 1987), edited by John Dobbing, the group of authors met to discuss the subject before writing their chapters, and they also had the opportunity to comment on all the chapters, thus this book presents information from experts from which conclusions can be drawn.

R.D. Feigin and J.D. Cherry's *Textbook of pediatric infectious diseases* (2 vols, 2nd edn., Saunders, 1987) covers the subject according to organ systems with explicit instructions for treatment, and Saul Krugman's *Infectious diseases of children* (8th edn., Mosby, 1985) is a concise and practical text. The BPA *Manual on infections and immunizations in children*, edited by Peter Rudd and Angus Nicoll (2nd edn., OUP, 1991) is for primary care and hospital staff giving information on specific problems, and also includes immunization schedules and guidance for going abroad. This is similar in content to the 'Red book' which is produced by the American Academy of Pediatrics (1988).

Gastroenterology

Abdominal pain can be elusive to diagnose and Barry O'Donnell's small book *Abdominal pain in children* (Blackwell, 1985) covers acute and recurrent pain. *Pediatric clinical gastroenterology* by A. Silverman and C.C. Roy (3rd ed., Mosby, 1983) gives information about gastro-intestinal function in health and disease as well as the clinical management of gastrointestinal diseases. *Harries' Paediatric gastroenterology* (2nd edn., Churchill Livingstone, 1988) has been edited by P.J. Milla and D.P.R. Muller, and is for the general paediatrician and postgraduate student. J. Walker-Smith's *Diseases of the small intestine in childhood* (3rd edn., Butterworths, 1988) and A.P. Mowat's *Liver disorders in childhood* (2nd edn., Butterworths, 1987) are written with a specific area in mind. Walker-Smith and McNeish cover chronic diarrhoea in developed and developing countries in *Diarrhoea and malnutrition in childhood* (Butterworths, 1986).

Nephrology and urology

Pediatric nephrology, edited by M.A. Holliday *et al.* (2nd edn., Williams & Wilkins, 1987) is a comprehensive text containing information on kidney diseases for nephrologists, paediatricians, urologists and family physicians. Covering the essentials rather than being comprehensive is *Clinical paediatric nephrology*, edited by R.J. Postlethwaite (Wright, 1986).

In *Clinical pediatric urology* edited by P.P. Kelalis *et al.* (2 vols, 2nd edn., Saunders, 1985) all aspects of paediatric urology are covered. D. Innes Williams and J.H. Johnston edited *Paediatric urology* (2nd edn., Butterworths, 1982) and J.D.Frank and J.H. Johnston wrote *Operative paediatric urology* (Churchill Livingstone, 1990).

Cardiology and pulmonology

R.H. Anderson *et al.* in *Paediatric cardiology* (2 vols, Churchill Livingstone, 1987) have edited a multi-author comprehensive text applicable throughout the world. A short textbook is *Heart disease in paediatrics* (3rd edn., Butterworths, 1989) in which S.C. Jordan and O. Scott present a simple and practical introduction for cardiologists who occasionally see children, GPs and community paediatricians. 'The outcome of successful surgery depends on careful planning and precise execution of a series of technical steps', say J. Stark and M. de Leval in their introduction to *Surgery for congenital heart defects* (Grune and Stratton, 1983). R.H. Anderson and A.E. Becker have written *Cardiac anatomy* (Churchill Livingstone, 1980) and also *Cardiac pathology; an integrated text and colour atlas* (Churchill Livingstone, 1983). M.K. Park and W.G. Guntheroth's book *How to read pediatric ECGs* (2nd edn., Year Book Medical Publishers, 1987) is a practical guide to electrocardiographs illustrating both normal and deviations from normal.

R. Dinwiddie has produced a basic overview in *The diagnosis and management of paediatric respiratory disease* (Churchill Livingstone, 1990). *Kendig's Disorders of the respiratory tract in children* (5th edn., Saunders, 1991) edited by Victor Chernick contains a comprehensive account of illnesses of the respiratory tract. Many cystic fibrosis patients are surviving into adolescence and adult life. *Cystic fibrosis*, edited by M.E. Hodson *et al.* (Baillière Tindall, 1983) covers the patient from birth to adult and aims to be particularly helpful to physicians taking over care from the paediatrician. A manual of diagnosis and management entitled *Cystic fibrosis* has been prepared for the Cystic Fibrosis Research Trust by M.C. Goodchild and J.A. Dodge (Baillière Tindall, 1985). *Childhood asthma* by A.D. Milner (Martin Dunitz, 1987) covers diagnosis, treatment and management and is a highly practical book.

Endocrinology

In *Clinical paediatric endocrinology*, edited by C. G. D. Brook (2nd edn., Blackwell, 1989) growth disorders are included as well as endocrine diseases. Appropriate tests for suspected endocrine disorders are contained in I.A. Hughes' *Handbook of endocrine tests in children* (Wright, 1986). The quotation 'Diabetics are people first', comes from *Diabetes mellitus in children and adolescents* by L.B. Travis *et al.* (Saunders, 1987) which is a clinically orientated text with a scientific base. Management from the point of view of the child and the family is contained in J.D. Baum and A.L. Kinmonth's *Care of the child with diabetes* (Churchill Livingstone, 1985) and includes social and educational aspects as well as medical. D.K. Edwards has updated *Dewhurst's Practical paediatric and adolescent gynaecology* (2nd edn., Butterworths, 1989) and gives guidance to paediatricians, gynaecologists and GPs.

Dermatology

Pediatric dermatology, edited by L.A. Schachner and R.C. Hansen (2 vols, Churchill Livingstone, 1988) contains the scientific foundations as well as the clinical approach to skin diseases in the neonate, child and adolescent. Illustrations are particularly useful in skin conditions and S.

Weinberg's *Color atlas of pediatric dermatology* (2nd edn., McGraw Hill, 1989) is not a textbook but a collection of annotated pictures.

Ophthalmology

The care of the child with eye problems has changed from being only a surgical discipline to the consideration of the 'whole child', his education and social life as well as medical and surgical care. David Taylor *et al.* in *Pediatric ophthalmology* (Blackwell, 1990) have produced such a text. Crawford and Morin's *The eye in childhood* emphasizes surgical techniques but also includes children's diseases with ocular involvement, contact lenses and education of visually-handicapped children.

Otolaryngology

J.F. Birrell's *Pediatric otolaryngology* has been revised by D.L. Cowan and A.I.G. Kerr (2nd edn., Wright, 1986) and is an overview particularly for paediatricians with little knowledge of the subject. When the 5th edition of *Scott-Brown's Otolaryngology* was produced, it was decided a whole volume should be devoted to children and J.N.G. Evans edited *Paediatric otolaryngology* (Butterworths, 1987). A comprehensive presentation of disorders of head, neck and air and food passages is C. D. Bluestone and S. E. Stool's *Pediatric otolaryngology* (2 vols, 2nd edn., Saunders, 1990). Management and care of deaf children requires the combined skills of medical and non-medical professions and *Childhood deafness*, edited by F.H. Bess (Grune and Stratton, 1977) should be valuable to all. An introductory text to all facets of audiology is Joyce Tweedie's *Children's hearing problems* (Wright, 1987).

Rheumatology

Victor Dubowitz is the expert on muscle disorders and two of his books are *Muscle disorders in childhood* (Saunders, 1978) and *A colour atlas of muscle disorders in childhood* (Wolfe, 1989). A practical guide to rheumatic problems likely to confront paediatricians is B.M. Ansell's *Rheumatic disorders in childhood* (Butterworths, 1980).

Surgery

Clinical paediatric surgery, edited by P.G. Jones and A.A. Woodward (3rd edn., Blackwell, 1986) is a good basic introduction to diagnosis and management; the standard work is *Pediatric surgery*, edited by K.J. Welch *et al.* (2 vols, 4th edn., Year Book Medical Publishers, 1986). Two atlases are L. Spitz and H.H. Nixon's *Paediatric surgery* which is a volume in the fourth edition of Rob and Smith's *Operative surgery* (Butterworths, 1988) and *A colour atlas of paediatric surgical condi-*

tions, edited by L. Spitz *et al.* (Wolfe, 1981). S.L. Gans' *Surgical pediatrics; nonoperative care* (2nd edn., Grune and Stratton, 1980) gives total management and care of the infant or child needing surgery, rather than operative technique. In *Complications of pediatric surgery* (Saunders, 1982) K.J. Welch advises on prevention and management of complications which occur during the operation or in the postoperative period. J.C. Mustarde and I.T. Jackson edit *Plastic surgery in infancy and childhood* (3rd edn., Churchill Livingstone, 1988).

Orthopaedics is a branch of surgery which M.O. Tachdjian covers in his comprehensive *Pediatric orthopedics* (4 vols, 2nd edn., Saunders, 1990). An introductory text has been written by G.C. Lloyd-Roberts and J.A. Fixsen *Orthopaedics in infancy and childhood* (2nd edn., Butterworths, 1990). Management of the patient, with chapters on specific age groups, is contained in *Orthopaedic management in childhood*, edited by P.F. Williams (Blackwell, 1982). Developmental skeletal disorders, with clinical histories and treatment, appear in *Atlas of skeletal dysplasias*, edited by R. Wynne-Davies *et al.* (Churchill Livingstone, 1985).

Emergencies

With the advances in paediatric surgery the anaesthetist is expected to deal with increasingly complex clinical problems. E. Sumner and D.J. Hatch edit *Textbook of paediatric anaesthetic practice* (Baillière Tindall, 1989). M.C. Rogers' *Textbook of pediatric intensive care* (2 vols, Williams and Wilkins, 1987) is comprehensive and *A practical guide to pediatric intensive care*, edited by D.L. Levin *et al.* (2nd edn., Mosby, 1984) is a book to have at hand when dealing with life-threatening situations.

Paediatric emergencies, edited by J.A. Black (2nd edn., Butterworths, 1987) aims to help in the treatment of a child injured or suddenly taken ill; it is a large book but has short concise entries. A practical manual for the general practitioner or casualty officer is C. M. Illingworth's *The diagnosis and primary care of accidents and emergencies in children* (2nd edn., Blackwell, 1982). E.K. Alpar and R. Owen edit a practical reference book of management of childhood injuries in *Paediatric trauma* (Castle House, 1988). The emergency of poisoning is covered by G.N. Volan *et al.* in *Handbook of poisoning in childhood* (Blackwell, 1989).

Psychology and psychiatry

The effect of environment, social factors and family relationships make us the sort of people we are; this subject is explored in *Early influences shaping the individual*, edited by S. Doxiadis (Plenum, 1989). Normal human development is covered in J. Kahn and S.E. Wright's *Human growth and the development of personality* (3rd edn., Pergamon, 1980). P.H. Mussen's *Handbook of child psychology* (4 vols, 4th edn., Wiley, 1983) is a comprehensive survey of contemporary theory.

Abnormal behaviour manifests itself in many ways and books on specific problems are numerous. Jo Douglas introduces the assessment and management in *Behaviour problems in young children* (Tavistock, 1989) and H.C. Quay and J.S. Werry edit *Psychopathological disorders of childhood* (3rd edn., Wiley, 1986). John Bowlby's work on maternal deprivation and its short- and long-term effects in *Attachment and loss* (3 vols, Hogarth Press, 1969-1980) has influenced the care of children, particularly in hospital and institution. L.A. Sroufe (1986) assessed Bowlby's contribution to psychoanalytic theory and developmental psychology. The understanding and management of children's illness, both physical and emotional, for which tests reveal no diagnosis is outlined by B. Lask and A. Fosson in *Childhood illness; the psychosomatic approach* (Wiley, 1989). In *The child's world of illness* by S.R. Wilkinson, many aspects of illness are described including their views of illness from children from 3 to 13 years. Emotional stress as well as behaviour problems affect a child's schooling and P.H. Dworkin looks at these implications in *Learning and behavioral problems in school children* (Saunders, 1985). Truancy and school refusal from the medical, legal and welfare points of view, including practical management, is covered by Hersov and Berg's *Out of school* (Wiley, 1980). R. Lansdown and W. Yule attempt to provide a balanced account of *The lead debate* (Croom Helm, 1986) and the effect that lead pollution has on children's IQ and behaviour.

An introduction to psychiatry is P. Barker's *Basic child psychiatry* (5th edn., Granada, 1988). Philip Graham's book *Child psychiatry; a developmental approach* (OUP, 1986) is for all doctors dealing with children and their families. *Child and adolescent psychiatry*, edited by M. Rutter and L. Hersov (2nd edn., Blackwell, 1985) is a comprehensive text containing developmental theories as well as clinical applications. Two books edited by Michael Rutter are *Scientific foundations of development psychiatry* (Heinemann, 1980) which covers development psychology and child psychiatry, and *Developmental neuropsychiatry* (Guilford Press, 1983) which covers the psychological sequelae following injury to the developing brain. A.M. Clarke *et al.* edit a multidisciplinary volume entitled *Mental deficiency, the changing outlook* (4th edn., Methuen, 1985). J.W. Varni has a biobehavioural approach to disease prevention and management in *Clinical behavioral pediatrics* (Pergamon, 1983). P. Barker introduces family therapy in *Basic family therapy* (2nd edn., Collins, 1986). A. Bentovin *et al.* have edited, on behalf of the Institute of Family Therapy (London), *Family therapy* (2 vols, Academic Press, 1982).

Neurology and neurosurgery

K. Swaiman's *Pediatric neurology; principles and practice* (Mosby, 1989) is in two volumes that cover the subject extensively. *Paediatric neurology*, edited by E.M. Brett (2nd edn., Churchill Livingstone, 1991) emphasizes the clinical assessment of the child and his symptoms as the foundation for treatment, prognosis and genetic counselling. The neurologically handicapped (chronic disorders) and the neurologically sick (acute and complex disorders) are covered by the respective volumes of *Children with neurological disorders*, edited by N. Gordon and I. McKinlay (2 vols, Blackwell, 1986). These are helpful to all health professionals involved with sick children. Stephenson and King's *Handbook of neurological investigations in children* (Butterworths, 1989) should make selection of the correct tests easier. H.F.R. Prechtl's *The neurological examination of the full term newborn infant* (2nd edn., Heinemann, 1977) is a practical guide.

Migraine is increasingly recognized, in its various presentations, in children; all aspects are covered in *Migraine in childhood*, edited by J.M. Hockaday (Butterworths, 1988). J. Aicardi writes on *Epilepsy in children* (Raven, 1986).

Atlas of pediatric neurosurgical operations (Saunders, 1982) was conceived and begun by D.D. Matson and completed by J. Shillito. Surgery of the developing nervous system is discussed by R. McLaurin *et al.* in *Pediatric neurosurgery* (2nd edn., Saunders, 1989).

Social aspects

Much concern is now shown for the rights of the child and there is a wealth of legislation contained in Hall and Morrison's *Law relating to children and young persons*, edited by N. Harris and R.A.H. White (2 vols, 10th edn., Butterworths, 1985). An easy-to-use book on how the law affects children in all aspects of life is Maggie Rae's *Children and the law* (Longman, 1986) which includes a helpful section on the ages at which rights are acquired. A small book of interest is M.L.K. Pringle's *The needs of children* (2nd edn., Hutchinson, 1980) outlining how these needs are normally met and the consequences if they are not met. E. de H. Lobo defines the particular health and social problems of *Children of immigrants to Britain* (Hodder and Stoughton, 1978).

Henry Kempe was a pioneer in recognizing child abuse and the book he edited with Helfer in 1968, *The battered child*, is now edited by R.E. Helfer and R.S. Kempe (4th edn., University of Chicago Press, 1987). Clear guidance and advice on the recognition and detection of all forms of child abuse, is given in *ABC of child abuse*, edited by R. Meadow (BMJ, 1989). Although many books have been written on sexual abuse, Mrazek and Kempe's *Sexually abused children and their families* (Pergamon, 1981) remains a standard work. A. Bentovim *et al.* have edited *Child sexual abuse within the family* (Wright, 1988) which gives methods of assessment and treatment for the children and their families. In *Lasting effects of child sexual abuse*, edited by G.E. Wyatt and G.J. Powell (Sage, 1988) research with adults molested as children is included as well as research with child victims.

The care of the handicapped and chronically ill child involves much understanding of the child and the family. Lindy Burton has produced two helpful books, *Care of the child facing death* (Routledge and Kegan Paul, 1974) and *The family life of sick children* (Routledge and Kegan Paul, 1975). Everyday needs of sick children are dealt with by Richard Lansdown in *More than sympathy* (Tavistock, 1980). The impact of acute and chronic illness on the patient and the family, and how terminal illness and bereavement are coped with is the subject of *Health, illness and families*, edited by D.C. Turk and R.D. Kerns (Wiley, 1985). Most children with chronic disorders live with their families and a handbook for the doctor responsible for continuing care is *Chronic childhood disorders*, edited by G. Hosking and R. Powell (Wright, 1985). P.J. McGrath and A.M. Unruh deal with all types of pain in *Pain in children and adolescents* (Elsevier, 1987). A well-illustrated book by M.L. Batshaw and Y.M. Perrett entitled *Children with handicaps* (2nd edn., Brookes, 1986) includes information on how handicaps occur at various stages of development as well as studies of particular handicapping conditions. S.G. Garwood emphasizes the development, physical, cognitive and social, of the child with a handicap in *Educating young handicapped children* (Aspen, 1983). The Office of Population Censuses and Surveys, Social Survey Division, has produced six reports on disability in the UK, three of which concern children, on prevalence of disability by Bone and Meltzer (1989), on financial circumstances by Smyth and Robus (1989) and on services, transport and education by Meltzer *et al.*, (1989). Going into hospital can have dramatic effects on children, as reviewed by R. Zetterstrom (1984) and Petrillo and Sanger's book *Emotional care of hospitalized children* (2nd edn., Lippincott, 1980) gives helpful guidance.

Tropical medicine and developing countries

Diseases of children in the subtropics and tropics, edited by J.P. Stanfield *et al.* (4th edn., Arnold, 1990) is the standard work. *Macmillan tropical community health manuals* is a series of books for health personnel in the tropical and subtropical countries, for example on care of the newborn (Ebrahim, 1979), mother and child health (Ebrahim, 1978) and mother and child nutrition (Ebrahim, 1983).

David Morley was a pioneer in improving health for children; he developed under-five clinics and charts for monitoring growth, illustrated in Morley and Woodland's *See how they grow* (Macmillan, 1979). He was also the first to draw attention to the health problems of the child in developing countries in *Paediatric priorities in the developing world* (Butterworths, 1973). The concept of primary health care has been endorsed by WHO (1978) as the way to 'Health for All by the Year 2000' emphasizing disease prevention and community participation in health care. *Practising health for all* (OUP, 1983), edited by D.C. Morley *et al.* presents problems from around the world arising from health care implementation and suggests how these can be overcome.

G.J. Ebrahim in *Social and community paediatrics in developing countries* (Macmillan, 1985) shows the links between causes of poverty and the level of ill health and the need for effective community health provision in rural and urban areas, and gives ideas for improvements to move towards 'Health for All'. Ebrahim and Ranken's book *Primary health care* (Macmillan, 1988) was written for those administrating, planning and delivering health services with principles to be applied to differing situations.

Maternal and child health is an area of preventive medicine among a large proportion of the population of any country. Basic information is given in C.D. Williams *et al. Mother and child health; delivering the services* (2nd edn., OUP, 1985). Experts share their experience in *Maternal and child health around the world*, edited by H.M. Wallace and G.J. Ebrahim (Macmillan, 1981). *Child health in a changing society* by G.J. Ebrahim (Macmillan, 1982) outlines the basic requirements of children for growth and development, the influences of family and community and how available services can be used to provide necessary health care.

Tape/slide presentations for health personnel in developing countries can be obtained from TALC (Teaching Aids at Low Cost, P.O. Box 49, St. Albans, Herts, AL1 4AX).

History and biography

Specialized books on paediatrics did not appear until the sixteenth century, but earlier writers had made observations on children's diseases. J. Ruhräh's anthology *Pediatrics of the past* (Hoeber, 1925) gives a fascinating glimpse into writings from Hippocrates (460–370 BC) to Friedrich Ludwig Meissner (1796–1860). Ruhräh followed this with his *Pediatric biographies*, reprinted from the *American Journal of Diseases of Children*, where they were originally between January 1928 and December 1931. The biographies continued to be published monthly in the *Journal* until the end of 1935.

G.F. Still wrote *The history of paediatrics* (OUP, 1931) and this covers the subject from earliest times up to the end of the eighteenth century. Abt-Garrison's *History of pediatrics* (Saunders, 1965) contains chapters on more recent times. T.E. Cone has written *History of American pediatrics* (Little, Brown, 1979) and *History of the care and feeding of the premature infant* (Little, Brown, 1985). V.A. Fildes uses letters, diaries, poetry and fiction as well as medical literature in *Breasts, bottles and babies; a history of infant feeding* (Edinburgh University Press, 1986). The everyday care of babies, including such things as swaddling, babywalkers and christenings, is contained in D. Dick's *Yesterday's babies* (Bodley Head, 1987). Linda Pollock reviews the work that has been written on the history of childhood, including Aries (1973), De Mause (1976), Shorter (1976) and Stone (1977), and then quotes from diaries and autobiographies to present her view of the status of the child in *Forgotten children; parent–child relations from 1500 to 1900* (CUP, 1983). An interesting study which examines the contemporary sources is Dwork's *War is good for babies and other young children* (Tavistock, 1987) which is a history of the infant and child welfare movement in England 1898–1918. A special issue of the *American Journal of Diseases of Children* published in July 1976 to mark the American bicentennial was entitled *Children and child care in the United States.* Volume 20 of *Progress in Pediatric Surgery* contains historical aspects of paediatric surgery and also some biographical sketches of eminent surgeons. G.J. Rees (1987) has written about the history of paediatric anaesthesia and Von Gontard (1988) and Hersov (1986) about the history of child psychiatry. J.M. Tanner has researched the *History of the study of human growth* (CUP, 1981).

Pioneers in pediatrics by A. Levinson (2nd edn., Froben Press, 1943) and B.S. Veeder's *Pediatric profiles* (Mosby, 1975; originally published in the *Journal of Pediatrics*) give biographical sketches of many famous paediatricians. *The man behind the syndrome* by P. and G. Beighton (Springer, 1986) presents doctors who have achieved eponymous immortality, 100 with picture, biography and commentary on the syndrome, and a further 110 with brief biographical details.

The American Pediatric Society published a *Semi-centennial volume* in 1938. This contains biographical sketches of the founders and members, as well as an historical account of the Society. A brief centennial history of the American Pediatric Society was published in *Pediatric Research* by Howard Pearson (1990). J.O. Forfar *et al.*, wrote *The British Paediatric Association 1928-1988* (BPA, 1989) for the diamond jubilee. This contains a recapitulation of the two earlier volumes published to mark the 25th anniversary, Cameron's *The British Paediatric Association 1928-1952* (BPA, 1955), and the 40th anniversary, Neale's *The British Paediatric Association 1952-1968* (Pitman, 1970), and then covers in greater detail the last 20 years. All three volumes contain biographies and photographs of BPA members.

To mark the diamond jubilee of the *Archives of Disease in Childhood* a special issue was produced in October 1986. G. Fanconi wrote on the international scene in *The history of the International Paediatric Association* (Schwabe, 1968).

S.X. Radbill (1955) wrote about the history of hospital care for children beginning from ancient times. There were no hospitals limited to the care of sick children before the nineteenth century, although out-patient care had a beginning when, in 1769, George Armstrong opened the Dispensary for the Infant Poor in London (Bloch, 1989). This was followed by the foundation of the Universal Dispensary for Children by John Bunnell Davis in 1816 (Loudon, 1979). Charles West worked at the Universal Dispensary but was frustrated by the lack of accommodation for in-patients. He resigned and turned to the foundation of the Hospital for Sick Children, Great Ormond Street, a centennial history of which was written by Thomas Twistington Higgins, entitled *Great Ormond Street 1852-1952* (Odhams, 1952).

The biographies of Abraham Jacobi (1830–1919) and Mary Jacobi (1842–1906), who were both professors of children's diseases, are told in R. Truax's book *The doctors Jacobi* (Little, Brown, 1952). M. and J. Rendle Short record the life of William Cadogan (1711–1797) in *The father of child care* (Wright, 1966) and W. Craig records the story of *John Thomson, pioneer and father of Scottish paediatrics, 1856-1926* (Livingstone, 1968). Cicely Williams, famous for her work in tropical child health has her life story told by A. Dally in *Cicely; the story of a doctor* (Gollancz, 1968) and by Sally Craddock in *Retired except on demand* (Green College, 1983). Also in Cicely Williams' honour there was a special issue of *Nutrition Reviews* in November 1973, reprinting several of her important articles as well as biographical and bibliographical details. Anna Freud (1895–1982) is remembered by Elisabeth Young-Bruehl in *Anna Freud* (Macmillan, 1989). In a commemorative issue for William Osler in *Journal of the American Medical Association*, McGovern and Davison (1969) outline Osler's contribution to paediatrics and the example he set in his relations with young people. P.G. Jones (1972) gave a lecture on Charles Dickens' literary children, which reviewed his own childhood experiences and which influenced the children he created in his books, and incidentally provided a glimpse of the life of children in Dickens' day.

References

American Academy of Pediatrics (1991) *Report of the Committee on Infectious Diseases*, 22nd edn. Elk Grove Village, IL: AAP.

Aries, P. (1973) *Centuries of childhood*. Harmondsworth: Penguin.

Bloch, H. (1989) George Armstrong (1719-1787); founder of the first dispensary for children. *American Journal of Diseases of Children*, **143**, 239-241.

Bone, M. and Meltzer, H. (1989) *The prevalence of disability among children*. London: HMSO.

De Mause, L. (1976) *The history of childhood*. London: Souvenir Press.

Dinnage, R. (1986a) *The child with cerebral palsy*. Windsor: NFER-Nelson.

Dinnage, R. (1986b) *The child with a chronic medical problem; cardiac disorders, diabetes, haemophilia*. Windsor: NFER-Nelson.

Dinnage, R. (1986c) *The child with epilepsy*. Windsor: NFER-Nelson.

Dinnage, R. (1986d) *The child with spina bifida*. Windsor: NFER-Nelson.

Dinnage, R. (1986e) *The orthopaedically handicapped child*. Windsor: NFER-Nelson.

Dinnage, R. and Gooch, S. (1986) *The child with asthma*. Windsor: NFER-Nelson.

Ebrahim, G.J. (1978) *Practical mother and child health in developing countries*. London: Macmillan.

Ebrahim, G.J. (1979) *Care of the newborn in developing countries*. London: Macmillan.

Ebrahim, G.J. (1983) *Nutrition in mother and child health*. London: Macmillan.

Hersov, L. (1986) Child psychiatry in Britain; the last 30 years. *Journal of Child Psychology and Psychiatry*, **27**, 781-801.

Jones, P.G. (1972) Dickens' literary children. *Australian Paediatric Journal*, **8**, 233-245.

Loudon, I.S. (1979) John Bunnell Davis and the Universal Dispensary for Children. *British Medical Journal*, **1**, 1191-1194.

McGovern, J.P. and Davison, W.C. (1969) Osler and children. *Journal of the American Medical Association*, **210**, 2241-2244.

Meltzer, H. *et al.* (1989) *Disabled children: services, transport and education*. London: HMSO.

Pearson, H.A. (1990) Centennial history of the APS. *Pediatric Research*, **27**, S4-S7.

Radbill, S.X. (1955) A history of children's hospitals. *American Journal of Diseases of Children*, **90**, 411-416.

Rees, G.J. (1987) Paediatric anaesthesia: past, present and future. *Zeitschrift für Kinderchirurgie*, **42**, 67-80.

Shorter, E. (1976) *The making of the modern family.* London: Collins.

Smyth, M. and Robus, N (1989) *The financial circumstances of families with disabled children living in private households.* London: HMSO.

Sroufe, L.A. (1986) Bowlby's contribution to psychoanalytic theory and developmental psychology; attachment; separation; loss. *Journal of Child Psychology and Psychiatry,* **27,** 841-849.

Stone, L. (1977) *The family, sex, and marriage in England, 1500-1800.* London: Weidenfeld and Nicolson.

Von Gontard, A. (1988) The development of child psychiatry in 19th century Britain. *Journal of Child Psychology and Psychiatry,* **29,** 569-588.

WHO (1978) *Primary health care; Report of the International Conference on Primary Health Care, Alma-Ata.* Geneva: WHO.

Zetterstrom, R. (1984) Responses of children to hospitalization. *Acta Paediatrica Scandinavica,* **73,** 289-295.

CHAPTER TWENTY-ONE

Dentistry

MARGARET A. CLENNETT

The modern literature of dentistry has developed since the mid-nineteenth century, when the dentist began to achieve professional status and to strive towards systematic instruction and qualification. Dental books have been published in increasing numbers since the sixteenth century, but historical works are not covered in this chapter. Similarly, the journals mentioned are confined to those providing a means of communication between dentists and their co-workers.

Journals

General

All the developed countries have national bodies representing the dental profession, and most issue a journal publishing scientific articles on all aspects of dentistry.

The leading British publication is the *British Dental Journal (BDJ)*, which is the official organ of the British Dental Association, a body that furthers the interests of all branches of the profession. The *BDJ* is published twice a month, and has papers describing research work, clinical cases and epidemiological surveys. Series of articles are regularly commissioned from leading authorities, on such subjects as orthodontics and occlusion.

Foremost among foreign associations' periodicals is the *Journal of the American Dental Association* (monthly), other important titles being the *Australian Dental Journal* (bi-monthly), *New Zealand Dental*

Journal (quarterly), *Journal of the Canadian Dental Association* (monthly) and *Swedish Dental Journal* (bi-monthly). Leading journals from Europe, publishing in their own language, are: *Österreichische Zeitschrift für Stomatologie; Chirurgien-Dentiste de France; Tandlaegebladet* (Denmark); *Deutsche Zahnärztliche Zeitschrift* (Germany); *Stomatologie der DDR* (East Germany); *Nederlands Tijdschrift voor Tandheelkunde; Norske Tannlaegeforenings Tidende* (Norway); *Schweizer Monatsschrift für Zahnmedizin; Stomatologiia* (USSR).

Although most other titles are in specialist fields, there is still a need and demand for journals general in scope. *The International Dental Journal* (bimonthly) is the organ of the International Dental Federation (FDI), an organization whose annual congress produces a number of important papers, many of which are published in the *Journal*. An important contribution is made by the *Journal of Dental Research* (USA, monthly), published under the auspices of the International Association for Dental Research (IADR). Special supplements are issued which contain abstracts of the IADR annual congress and other significant meetings.

The *Scandinavian Journal of Dental Research* (bi-monthly, Denmark) is published by Munksgaard, a firm renowned for the quality of its dental publications. This journal comprises chiefly papers from Scandinavian authors, but has international interest, and is the official publication of the Scandinavian Division of the IADR. *Acta Odontologica Scandinavica* (bi-monthly, Norway) publishes scientific and clinical papers in English and has issued over 70 supplements on specific topics, many of which have become classics.

Commercially published general dental journals include *Compendium of Continuing Education in Dentistry* (USA), *Dental Update* (UK), *Journal of Dentistry* (UK) and *Quintessence International* (USA).

Specialist

Most titles appear under the auspices of specialist societies, being published either by a society itself, or by a commercial publisher on the society's behalf. Core English-language titles for the various specialties are listed in Table 21.1.

Textbooks and monographs

With the growth in specialization, the general textbook covering the whole of dentistry is the exception, rather than the norm. Introductory

Table 21.1

PERIODONTOLOGY

*Journal of Clinical
    Periodontology* (Denmark)
Journal of Periodontal Research
    (Denmark)
Journal of Periodontology (USA)

PUBLIC HEALTH DENTISTRY

Community Dental Health (UK)
*Community Dentistry and Oral
    Epidemiology* (Denmark)
*Journal of Public Health
    Dentistry* (USA)

CHILDREN'S DENTISTRY (PAEDODONTICS)

*International Journal of
    Paediatric Dentistry (USA)*
Journal of Clinical Paediatric
    Dentistry (USA)
Journal of Dentistry for Children
    (USA)
Journal of Paediatric Dentistry
    (UK)
Paediatric Dentistry (USA)

ORAL SURGERY

*British Journal of Oral and
    Maxillofacial Surgery*
*International Journal of Oral and
    Maxillofacial Surgery*
    (Denmark)
*Journal of Craniomaxillofacial
    Surgery* (Germany)
*Journal of Oral and Maxillofacial
    Surgery* (USA)
*Oral and Maxillofacial Surgery
    Clinics of North America*

*Oral Surgery, Oral Medicine,
    Oral Pathology* (USA)

ORTHODONTICS

*American Journal of
    Orthodontics and Dentofacial
    Orthopedics*
Angle Orthodontist (USA)
British Journal of Orthodontics
*European Journal of
    Orthodontics* (UK)
Journal of Clinical Orthodontics
    (USA)

RESTORATIVE DENTISTRY

*International Journal of
    Prosthodontics* (USA)
Journal of Prosthetic Dentistry
    (USA)
Restorative Dentistry (UK)

ENDODONTICS

*Endodontics and Dental
    Traumatology* (Denmark)
International Endodontic Journal
    (UK)
Journal of Endodontics (USA)

OTHER SPECIALIST JOURNALS

Archives of Oral Biology (UK)
Caries Research (Switzerland)
*International Journal of Oral and
    Maxillofacial Implants
    (Denmark)*
*Oral Microbiology and
    Immunology* (Denmark)

and revision material is found in R.A. Cawson's *Essentials of dental surgery and pathology* (5th edn., Churchill Livingstone, 1992) which is much wider in scope than its title suggests. *Scientific foundations of dentistry*, edited by B. Cohen and I.R.H. Kramer (Heinemann, 1976), which is intended for those studying for higher dental qualifications, is a magnificent resume of knowledge by nearly 70 authors. For the general dental practitioner, J. Manning has edited *General dental practice* (Kluwer, 1978–) a multi-volume, loose-leaf work to which updates are added twice a year. A.H. Rowe and R.B. Johns have edited *A companion to dental studies* (Blackwell, 1981–1988) a three-volume (but four-book) production, covering all aspects of dentistry for student and practitioner. Volume 3, *Clinical dentistry* provides an invaluable overview of current techniques; other volumes discuss anatomy, biochemistry, physiology and embryology (Volume 1, in two parts), clinical methods, pathology and pharmacology (Volume 2).

Anatomy, histology, physiology, microbiology

The most concise books on dental anatomy are J.H. Scott and N.B.B. Symons's *Introduction to dental anatomy* (9th edn., Churchill Livingstone, 1982) and J.H. Scott and A.D. Dixon's *Anatomy for students of dentistry* (6th edn., Churchill Livingstone, 1986). A larger, more detailed American work is *Oral anatomy* by H. Sicher and E.L. Dubrul (8th edn., Mosby, 1988). For illustrations are recommended the pocket-sized *Dental morphology: an illustrated guide* by G.C. Van Beek (2nd edn., Wright, 1983) and the comprehensive *Colour atlas and textbook of oral anatomy* by B.K.B. Berkovitz and B.J. Moxham (2nd edn., Wolfe, 1991). This book includes comparative anatomy within its scope, but at long last there is a currrent definitive and scholarly text on this specialized topic, C.F. Colyer's *Variations and diseases of the teeth of animals*, revised edition by A.E.W. Miles and C. Grigson (Cambridge University Press, 1990).

A standard text on maxillofacial development is by D.H. Enlow entitled *Facial growth* (3rd edn., Saunders, 1990) and a more concise American text is D.M. Ranly's *Synopsis of craniofacial growth* (2nd edn., Appleton-Century-Crofts, 1988).

C.L.B. Lavelle's *Applied oral physiology* (2nd edn., Wright, 1988) and *Biochemistry and oral biology* by A.S. Cole and J.E. Eastoe (2nd edn., Wright, 1988) are excellent works for students at all levels. Comprehensive reviews of ultrastructure for the researcher are given in Volumes 5 and 6 of *Handbook of microscopic anatomy: the periodontium* by H.E. Schroeder (Springer, 1986) and *Teeth* by B.K.B. Berkovitz and others (Springer, 1989).

The best known book on histology is *Orban's Oral histology and embryology*, edited by S.N. Bhaskar (11th edn., Mosby, 1991). Briefer coverage is given by J.W. Osborn and A.R. Ten Cate in *Advanced dental histology* (4th edn., Wright, 1983), while the latter author has also written *Oral histology: development, structure and function* (3rd edn., Mosby, 1989), a highly regarded text.

Embryology is well described in D. Permar's *Oral embryology and microscopic anatomy* by R.C. Melfi (8th edn., Lea and Febiger, 1988), while G.H. Sperber's *Craniofacial embryology* (3rd edn., Wright, 1981) is a useful British book. W.A. Nolte's *Oral microbiology* (4th edn., Mosby, 1982) is a most detailed work on this subject, and a concise account is provided by T.W. MacFarlane and C.P. Samaranayake's *Clinical oral microbiology* (Wright, 1989).

Occlusion and temporomandibular joint

The standard book on occlusion is P.E. Dawson's *Evaluation, diagnosis and treatment of occlusal problems* (2nd edn., Mosby, 1989). A concise, practical work is *Occlusion in clinical practice* by H. Thomson (2nd edn., Wright, 1990), H.D. Ogus and P.A. Toller have the requirements of the British general practitioner in mind in *Common disorders of the temporomandibular joint* (2nd edn., Wright, 1986), while an American viewpoint is provided by J.P. Okeson in *Management of temporomandibular disorders and occlusion* (2nd edn., Mosby, 1989). Yet another colour atlas well received by clinicians is *A textbook and colour atlas of the temporomandibular joint* by J.E. de B. Norman and Sir P. Bramley (Wolfe, 1990).

Oral medicine, pharmacology

The authoritative, wide ranging work on oral medicine is L.W. Burket's *Oral medicine*, edited by M.A. Lynch (8th edn., Lippincott, 1984). Clinical conditions are well illustrated in the large format *Atlas of stomatology* by C. Scully and S. Flint (Martin Dunitz, 1989), which has colour photographs of oral diseases and oral manifestations of systemic diseases, and in the pocket-sized *Oral medicine*, a revision guide by P.J. Lamey and M.A.O. Lewis (Gower, 1988).

The dental implications of systemic disease are ably covered by C. Scully and R.A. Cawson in *Medical problems in dentistry* (2nd edn., Wright, 1987), while the wider significance of mouth lesions is discussed in *Oral manifestations of systemic disease* by J.H. Jones and D.J. Mason (2nd edn., Baillière, 1990). C.E. Barr and M.Z. Mander cover the clinical aspects of AIDS, and implications of the disease for dentists treating HIV-positive patients in *AIDS: a guide for dental practice* (Quintessence, 1987).

Drugs chargeable to the National Health Service which dentists may prescribe are listed in the *Dental practitioners' formulary 1988-90*, which is issued with the *British national formulary No. 16* (British Medical Association and Pharmaceutical Press, 1988). A detailed account of drugs is presented by J.G. Walton, J.W. Thompson and R.A. Seymour in *A textbook of dental pharmacology and therapeutics* (OUP, 1989).

Pathology and radiography

The standard text is W.G. Shafer, M.K. Hine and B.M. Levy's *Textbook of oral pathology* (4th edn., Saunders, 1983). For undergraduates, J.V. Soames and J.C. Southam have written *Oral pathology* (OUP, 1985). A complement to that sparsely illustrated book is K.W. Lee's *Colour atlas of oral pathology* (Wolfe, 1985), with over 450 histopathological photographs, each accompanied by brief descriptive notes. Intended for the practising pathologist and postgraduate student, R.A. Cawson and J.W. Eveson's *Oral pathology and diagnosis* (Heinemann, 1987) is a colour atlas of histopathological and clinical photographs with an accompanying text. R.A. Cawson has also produced *Oral pathology* (Churchill Livingstone, 1987), a small revision aid with brief notes and colour illustrations of common disorders. Oral cancer is covered in detail by R.B. Lucas in *Pathology of tumours of the oral tissues* (4th edn., Churchill Livingstone, 1984).

For the student, *Dental radiography* by N.J.D. Smith (2nd edn., Blackwell, 1988) is suitable, while practitioners will find R. Mason's *Guide to dental radiography* (3rd edn., Wright, 1988) a useful and practical book. From the USA comes *Oral radiology* by P.W. Goaz and S.C. White (2nd edn., Mosby, 1987). O.E. Langland, R.P. Langlais and W.D. McDavid have produced an important work in a specialized field, *Panoramic radiology* (2nd edn., Lea and Febiger, 1989).

Dental caries and preventive dentistry

L.M. Silverstone's *Dental caries* (Macmillan, 1981) is a general text for student and practitioner which emphasizes the disease process, whilst *Essentials of dental caries* by E.A.M. Kidd and S. Joyston-Bechal concentrates on management and prevention of the disease. G. Nikiforuk's *Understanding dental caries* (Karger, 1985) is a detailed two-volume work, although each can be used alone. Volume 1 covers the basic and clinical aspects of the aetiology and mechanisms of caries, Volume 2 deals with clinical aspects of prevention.

Excellent texts devoted to preventive dentistry are J.J. Murray's *The prevention of dental disease* (2nd edn., OUP, 1989) and *A textbook of preventive dentistry* by R.E. Stallard (2nd edn., Saunders, 1982). Authoritative guidance on the use of fluorides, for public health bodies and practitioners is given by J.J. Murray's *Appropriate use of fluorides for human health* (WHO, 1986), general texts on the subject being *Fluoride in dentistry* by J. Ekstrand, O. Fejerskov and L.M. Silverstone (Munksgaard, 1988) and *Fluorides in caries prevention* by J.J. Murray, A.J. Rugg-Gunn and G.N. Jenkins (3rd edn., Wright, 1991).

Restorative dentistry and endodontics

Basic undergraduate books are T.R. Pitt-Ford's *The restoration of teeth* (Blackwell, 1985) and H.M. Pickard's *Manual of operative dentistry* by E.A.M. Kidd (6th edn., OUP, 1990). For senior students and the newly qualified, P.M. Jacobsen's *Conservative dentistry: an integrated approach* (Churchill Livingstone, 1990) discusses clinical techniques and materials in the context of constraints imposed by the oral environment and actual patient, and the ability and facilities of the dentist. D.R. Kennedy's *Paediatric operative dentistry* (3rd edn., Wright, 1986) concentrates on the treatment of children.

F.S. Weine's *Endodontic therapy* (4th edn., Mosby, 1989) is a standard American work; a highly regarded and practical British book is F.J. Harty's *Endodontics in clinical practice* (3rd edn., Wright, 1990). Popular with students and practitioners is *A colour atlas of endodontics* by J.J. Messing and C.J.R. Stock (Wolfe, 1988).

Prosthetic dentistry, crown and bridgework

Standard British textbooks are *Fenn's clinical dental prosthetics* by A.R. McGregor (3rd edn., Wright, 1989) and *Partial dentures* by J. Osborne and G.A. Lammie (5th edn., Blackwell, 1986), by Lammie and W.R.E. Laird. The American viewpoint is given in W.L. McCracken's *Removable partial dentures* (8th edn., Mosby, 1989) by G. P. McGivney and D.J. Castleberry, and C.O. Boucher's *Prosthetic treatment for edentulous patients* (10th edn., Mosby, 1990 by J.C. Hickey, G.A. Zarb and C.L. Bolender). A concise account is provided by J.A. Hobkirk in *Complete dentures* (Wright, 1986). Special types of prostheses are discussed in H.W. Preiskel's two-volume *Precision attachments in prosthodontics* (Quintessence, 1984). Volume 1 covers intra- and extracoronal attachments, and Volume 2 overdentures and telescopic prostheses.

A popular book on crown and bridgework is B.G.N. Smith's *Planning and making crowns and bridges* (2nd edn., Martin Dunitz, 1990) complementing the standard texts by D.H. Roberts, *Fixed bridge prostheses* (2nd edn., Wright, 1980) and *Fundamentals of fixed prosthodontics* by H.T. Shillingburg, S. Hobo and D. Whitsett (2nd edn., Quintessence, 1981). Concise guidance is given in G.F. Kantorowicz's *Inlays, crowns and bridges* (4th edn., Wright, 1985). Specialized texts on new techniques are *Porcelain laminate veneers* by D.A. Garber, R.E. Goldstein and R.A. Feinman (Quintessence, 1988) and *A colour atlas of resin bond retained prostheses*, by R.T. Walker and others (Excerpta Medica, 1989). Practitioners and postgraduate students are the readership for J.H.N. Pameijer's *Periodontal and occlusal factors in crown and bridge procedures* (Dental Centre for Postgraduate Courses, 1985).

Children's dentistry

This subject is covered by many large American textbooks. Among the best are *Dentistry for the child and adolescent* by R.E. McDonald and D.R. Avery (5th edn., Mosby, 1987), *Textbook of pediatric dentistry* by R.L. Braham and M.E. Morris (2nd edn., Williams and Wilkins, 1985) and S.H.Y. Wei's *Pediatric dentistry: total patient care* (Lea and Febiger, 1988). Standard, more concise works are P.J. Holloway and J.N. Swallow's *Child dental health* (3rd edn., Wright, 1982) and R.J. Andlaw and W.P. Rock's *Manual of paedodontics* (2nd edn., Churchill Livingstone, 1987). R. Rapp and G.B. Winter have produced the excellent *Colour atlas of clinical conditions in paedodontics* (Wolfe, 1979). The condition of children's teeth is surveyed in *Child Dental Health in the UK*, a report prepared by J.E. Todd and T. Dodd for the Office of Population, Censuses and Surveys (HMSO, 1985). An important aspect of paedodontics is discussed in detail in J.O. Andreasen's *Traumatic injuries of the teeth* (2nd edn., Munksgaard, 1981).

Orthodontics

An exhaustive work is that by T.M. Graber and B.F. Swain, *Orthodontics: current principles and techniques* (Mosby, 1985). T.D. Foster's *A textbook of orthodontics* (2nd edn., Blackwell, 1990) and *Textbook of orthodontics* by W.J.B. Houston and W.J. Tulley (Wright, 1986) are recommended British texts for undergraduates and practitioners, while postgraduates will wish to study *Principles and practice of orthodontics* by J.R.E. Mills (2nd edn., Churchill Livingstone, 1987) and *Contemporary orthodontics* by W.R. Proffit and H.W. Fields (Mosby, 1986). The most detailed work on removable appliances is T.M. Graber and B. Neumann's *Removable orthodontic appliances* (2nd edn., Saunders, 1984). Useful texts for students and practitioners are *The design, construction and use of removable orthodontic appliances* by C.P. Adams and W.J.S. Kerr (6th edn., Wright, 1990) and *Introduction to fixed appliances* by K.G. Isaacson and J.K. Williams (3rd edn., Wright, 1984).

Special techniques are discussed in R.C. Thurow's *Edgewise orthodontics* (4th edn., Mosby, 1982), G.G.T. Fletcher's *The Begg appliance and technique* (Wright, 1981) and *Rapid maxillary expansion* by D.W. Timms (Quintessence, 1981).

Periodontology

A concise account of current practice and the concepts on which it is based are given by W.M. Jenkins, C.J. Allan and W.J. Collins in *Guide to periodontics* (2nd edn., Heinemann, 1988). There is more detail in *Periodontal disease* by S. Schluger, R. Yuodelis, R.C. Page and R.H. Johnson (2nd edn., Lea and Febiger, 1990) and J. Lindhe's *Textbook of clinical periodontology* (2nd edn., Munksgaard, 1989). An authoritative work for clinicians and postgraduates is *J.B. Kieser's Periodontics: a practical approach* (Wright, 1990). Popular atlases illustrating clinical conditions, therapy and surgical procedures are by I.M. Waite and J.D. Strahan, *Colour atlas of periodontology* (2nd edn., Wolfe, 1990) and *Colour atlas of periodontal surgery* (Wolfe, 1987).

Oral surgery

The two-volume *Outline of oral surgery* by H.C. Killey and L.W. Kay has been justly popular for many years. G.R. Seward, M. Harris and D.A. McGowan have produced a new edition of Part I (2nd edn., Wright, 1987), describing procedures and clinical conditions especially relevant to general practice. Part II (Wright, 1975) is devoted to conditions which would usually be treated in a hospital oral surgery department. D.A. McGowan has written *Atlas of minor oral surgery* (Martin Dunitz, 1989) for general practitioners and students, while more detailed coverage is provided by J.R. Moore's *Surgery of the mouth and jaws* (Blackwell, 1985). The long-awaited successor to Rowe and Killey's classic *Fractures of the facial skeleton* is N.L. Rowe and J.L. Williams' *Maxillofacial injuries* (Churchill Livingstone, 1987). This comprehensive, two-volume set is an essential reference work for the postgraduate student and practising oral surgeon. Special aspects are discussed in *Cancer of the face and mouth* (Churchill Livingstone, 1986) by I.A. McGregor and F.M. McGregor, who cover pathology and management of oral cancer, and by D.A. Keith with *Surgery of the temporomandibular joint* (Blackwell, 1988).

Anaesthesia

All methods used in dental practice are discussed in G.D. Allen's *Dental anesthesia and analgesia* (3rd edn., Williams and Wilkins, 1984). Standard British guides on local anaesthesia are *Local analgesia in dentistry* by G.L. Howe and F.I.H. Whitehead (3rd edn., Wright, 1990) and *Local analgesia in dentistry* by D.H. Roberts and J.H. Sowray (3rd edn.,

Wright, 1987), while a well established American text is L.M. Monheim's *Local anesthesia and pain control in dental practice* by C.R. Bennett (7th edn., Mosby, 1984). C.M. Hill and P.J. Morris cover general anaesthesia and the increasingly popular relative analgesia in *General anaesthesia and sedation in dentistry* (2nd edn., Wright, 1991).

Materials and technology

Books on dental materials can be out of date by the time they are published. Nevertheless, there is a need for reference texts which deal with clinical and scientific aspects, the definitive works being *Skinner's Science of dental materials* by R.W. Phillips (9th edn., Saunders, 1991), and *Restorative dental materials* by R.C. Craig (8th edn., Mosby, 1989). A practical outline for the clinician is given by H.J. Wilson, J.W. McLean and D. Brown in *Dental materials and their clinical application* (British Dental Association, 1988), based on a series of articles published in the *British Dental Journal*. A specialized work is *Glass ionomer cement* by A.D. Wilson and J.W. McLean (Quintessence, 1988). For undergraduates, H.J. Wilson, M.A. Mansfield, J.R. Heath and D. Spence have produced *Dental technology and materials for students* (8th edn., Blackwell, 1987).

Practice management; assistants

There has been a wealth of American books on this topic, but the most detailed and useful for British purposes is still H.C. Kilpatrick's *Work simplification in dental practice* (3rd edn., Saunders, 1974). Written specifically for British dentists are J.O. Forrest's *Guide to successful dental practice* (Wright, 1984) and D.W. Crosthwaite's *Handbook of dental practice management* (Churchill Livingstone, 1982). Several textbooks are available for ancillary staff, e.g. R.G. Smith's *Dental surgery assistants' handbook* (Gower, 1988) which covers practical dentistry at an elementary level. *Law and ethics in dentistry*, by J.E. Seear and L. Walters (3nd edn., Wright, 1990) charts a way through the new regulations on advertising and other important non-clinical aspects of British practice. For foreign regulations and brief information about practice overseas, the FDI has published *Handbook of regulations of dental practice* (2nd edn., 1986).

Public health dentistry

Standard textbooks giving British and American viewpoints respectively are G.L. Slack's *Dental public health* (2nd edn., Wright, 1981) and J.M. Dunning's *Principles of dental public health* (4th edn., Harvard University Press, 1986). An approach to dental care drawing on psychology and the social sciences is offered by M.C. Jacob and D. Plamping in *The practice of primary dental care* (Wright, 1989).

The findings of the national dental survey in England and Wales in 1988 appear in *Adult dental health 1988, United Kingdom* by J.E. Todd and D. Lader (HMSO, 1991) while the most recent survey for Scotland is *Adult dental Health in Scotland 1972*, by J.E. Todd and A. Whitworth (HMSO, 1974). The children's dental health survey has already been mentioned.

With a broader remit, the World Health Organization produces documents on planning and monitoring the provision of dental services. *Oral health surveys: basic methods* (WHO, 3rd edn., 1988) is a small but invaluable document in the WHO Technical Report Series, a companion being *Monitoring and evaluation of oral health* (WHO, 1989). *Health through oral health* (Quintessence, for WHO, 1989) by the WHO and FDI gives details of criteria and formulae for manpower planning and monitoring care.

A useful report on oral conditions and dental health policies has been produced by the WHO Regional Office for Europe in *Country profiles on oral health in Europe* (WHO Regional Office for Europe, 1986).

Miscellaneous topics

Inevitably, some books cannot easily be categorized into the subject groups discussed above. *Cross infection control in general dental practice* by D. Croser and J. Chipping (Quintessence, 1989) covers microbiology, sterilization and other procedures which have come into prominence since the AIDS epidemic.

Geriatric dentistry is covered by several books now, one of the most useful being *Dental care for the elderly* by B. Cohen and H. Thomson (Heinemann, 1986). B. Hunter deals with adults and children in *Dental care for handicapped patients* (Wright, 1987).

There has been a renewed interest in forensic dentistry, which will be further stimulated by *A colour atlas of forensic dentistry* by D.K. Whittaker and D.G. Macdonald (Wolfe, 1989).

Dental implants had been regarded as a fringe topic until the early 1980s when Branemark demonstrated high success rates with his unique technique. T. Albrektsson and G.A. Zarb have written a definitive text, *The Branemark osseointegrated implant* (Quintessence, 1989), and the subject will doubtless be well documented by several other authors within the near future.

Indexes, abstracts, current awareness

Index Medicus, although it includes the leading dental periodicals, is not the chief tool to be used in searching the literature for dental subjects. The *Index to Dental Literature* is similar in format, although it appears in quarterly instead of monthly parts, each cumulating with the previous issues for the year until the bound annual volume appears. The creation of the *Index* began in 1898 as the brain-child of Arthur Black, who worked retrospectively back to 1839, when the first regular dental journal made its debut. The *Index* covered five-year periods up to 1950, when the first annual volume was published; its subject arrangement was at first based on a modification of the Dewey classification with an author index. An outline of and an index to the classification is printed on the centre pages. In 1939 the classified arrangement was abandoned in favour of author and subject entries published in one alphabetical sequence, but they separated once again in 1965 when the MEDLARS production methods of the National Library of Medicine were adopted. In addition to periodical publications, the *Index* now lists dental dissertations and theses, and also new dental books.

The principal abstracting journal in dentistry is *Dental Abstracts*, published monthly by the American Dental Association. Some 200 journals are covered, with dental titles from the USA predominating, but with occasional excursions into medical and scientific periodicals and lay journalism. There are about 25 subject headings, each with four or five abstracts every month, and an annual index of authors and subjects. *Oral Research Abstracts*, which ceased publication in 1978, included about 7000 abstracts each year. It gave a more comprehensive coverage of research publications from a considerably wider range of sources, being particularly valuable for abstracts of foreign-language papers.

The *Year Book of Dentistry* (Year Book Medical Publishing) appears annually, giving a retrospective review of some 200 articles, one-third from non-American sources, under about 20 headings. The abstracts are signed and include brief comments by the abstractors, with illustrations, diagrams and tables reproduced from the original papers.

The *Journal of the Western Society of Periodontology Periodontal Abstracts* (USA, quarterly) devotes about half the pages of each issue to a critical appraisal of the literature of one special subject, the rest comprising abstracts of articles in the specialty, grouped under various headings.

Until 1962, when foreign-language articles first began to be included, only articles in English were cited in the *Index to Dental Literature*. Articles published after 1934 in foreign journals may sometimes be traced in the bibliographical half of *Deutsche Zahn- , Mund- und Kieferheilkunde*, which still gives short abstracts of papers from the world's dental literature in subject groupings, with author and subject indexes. Foreign-language articles published between 1925 and 1933 may be traced in *Fortschritte der Zahnheilkunde*, which has a similar arrangement, and those published between 1902 and 1932 in *Index der Deutschen und Ausländischen Literatur*, which lists articles under authors in broad subject groups and has author and subject indexes but no abstracts. The 1902 volume notes articles published since 1847.

Current Titles in Dentistry (Munksgaard) is a monthly listing of original articles in major international journals published in English, French and German. Articles of dental interest from journals in other fields are included.

Reviews

Oral Sciences Reviews, published in Copenhagen by Munksgaard, is a series of 10 volumes published during the years 1972 to 1977. Each volume is devoted to a particular topic, and provides comprehensive analytical review articles, with extensive bibliographies, by leading authorities in each field. *The Dental Clinics of North America* (USA, quarterly) may be regarded as a review journal, since it reports on current theories and practice, publishing state-of-the-art papers rather than original research.

The *Dental Annual* (Wright, 1985-1989) is an excellent source of good reviews, but its contents have not been included in the *Index to Dental Literature*.

Conferences

As in many fields, conference proceedings are published in a variety of formats, such as books, or journal supplements. The *International Dental Congresses*, once separately published, have not appeared in book form since 1936. *The International Dental Journal* now publishes selected proceedings of the Fédération Dentaire Internationale annual congress.

ORCA, the European Organisation for Research on Fluoride and Dental Caries Prevention published the proceedings of its 9th (1962) to 12th (1965) congresses as separate volumes, entitled *Advances in Fluoride Research and Dental Caries Prevention* (Pergamon). Latterly, the ORCA congresses have been reported as abstracts in the journal *Caries Research*.

The International Association of Dental Research annual meetings are abstracted in special issues of the *Journal of Dental Research*; American Association of Dental Research abstracts (the North American Division of the IADR) in one issue and Divisional Abstracts (the rest of the world) in another.

The *Journal of Dental Research* also has occasional special issues devoted to papers from other conferences, while its companion journal, *Advances in Dental Research* (twice a year) is devoted solely to the publication of conference and symposia proceedings.

Bibliographies

There has been a trend away from published bibliographies, possibly due to the availability of online services. The National Library of Medicine has produced some bibliographies of dental interest from the MEDLINE data base, e.g. *Oral complications of cancer therapy* (Washington, Government Printing Office, 1989) and *Dental implants* (Washington, GPO, 1988). J.J. Pindborg has produced two editions of *Selected and annotated bibliography on oral manifestations of the HIV infection*, covering 1981-87 and 1988 (WHO Collaborative Centre for Oral Manifestations of HIV Infection, Copenhagen, 1990). Most, but not all references are in English. Since 1981 the same publisher has issued the monthly *Dent-AIDS*.

Social sciences and dentistry: a critical bibliography, Volume 2, edited by L.K. Cohen and P.S. Bryan (Quintessence, for the FDI, 1984) gives state of the science reviews of the international research literature on behavioural and social science aspects of dentistry.

Current books are listed in a preliminary section of the *Index to Dental Literature*.

Dictionaries

There are four English-language dictionaries of dental terminology available, two British, two American. J. and G. Fairpo have produced the *Heinemann dental dictionary* (3rd edn., Heinemann, 1987), while F.J. Harty and R. Ogston have compiled a *Concise illustrated dental dictionary* (Wright, 1987). Both give brief definitions and explanations and each includes words not found in the other. C.O. Boucher's *Clinical dental terminology*, edited by T.J. Zwemer (3rd edn., Mosby, 1982) has longer explanations, but lists many words not of clinical relevance. S. Jablonski's *Illustrated dictionary of dentistry* (Saunders, 1982) includes many medical terms, also trade names and biographical entries, and gives more detail for dental entries than Boucher. The British Standards

Institution has issued a *Glossary of terms related to dentistry* (BS4492: 1983) listing terms and definitions for nine subdivisions of dentistry. Some terms are described as 'deprecated' where their use is considered undesirable.

The International Organization for Standardization has produced ISO 1942: *Dental vocabulary* (2nd edn., ISO, 1989). Definitions are given in English and French, and are in five subject groups: general and clinical terms, dental materials, dental instruments, dental equipment, and terms associated with testing.

English–foreign-language dictionaries are almost non-existent but the FDI's *Lexicon of English dental terms with their equivalents in español, deutsch, français* (2nd edn., FDI, 1985) is invaluable for the translator. Unlike the first edition (1966) this does not include Italian. A good English–German dictionary, *Dental Wörterbuch*, compiled by H. Bucksch (Verlag Neuer Merkur, 1970) has filled one of the gaps in the field.

General reference works

A general guide to the literature and other sources is M.A. Clennett's *Keyguide to information sources in dentistry* (Mansell, 1985). The book has three parts: narrative chapters on dentistry and information sources; annotated subject bibliographies and address lists of national dental associations, schools, and other organizations. Although some information is no longer current, the content for the most part has not dated. A.A. Kowitz has produced *Dental journals and serials: an analytical guide* (Greenwood Press, 1985), an alphabetical list of currently published English-language titles. For each entry is given publisher, address, editor, circulation, target audience, where indexed, and an annotation on content.

The *Dentists Register* (General Dental Council, annual) lists all registered dental practitioners, and gives names, addresses, date of registration, and qualifications. Similar lists exist for most developed countries. There is no dental equivalent to the *Medical Directory*.

The Dental Laboratory Yearbook and Directory gives much technical information. Particularly useful are the sections listing trade names, equipment and materials, manufacturers and suppliers. The *FDI's Basic facts sheets* (FDI, 1990) give information about dentistry in over 120 countries, with particular reference to manpower, education, and licensure, surveys of oral conditions, dental practice and fluoridation. The FDI has issued a *World directory of dental schools* (FDI, 1990) with addresses, phone numbers, and names of deans.

History and biography

W. Hoffmann-Axthelm's *History of dentistry* (Quintessence, 1981) is a detailed and scholarly work, with numerous black-and-white illustrations, and an emphasis on European developments. M.E. Ring has produced the accurate and readable *Dentistry: an illustrated history* (Abrams, 1985) with many good quality colour photographs. For the lay reader, C. Hillam's *The roots of dentistry* (British Dental Journal, 1990) gives a general introduction. A classic text still of value today is *A history of dentistry* by V. Guerini (Lea and Febiger, 1909), a work of great accuracy and careful scholarship which traces developments up to the end of the eighteenth century. H. Prinz's *Dental chronology* (Kimpton, 1945) gives notes on persons and developments from ancient times to the mid-twentieth century. For the study of British dental history, there are A. Hill's *The history of the reform movement in the dental profession in Great Britain during the last twenty years* (Trubner, 1877) and *The advance of the dental profession: a centenary history, 1880–1980* (BDA, 1979). B.W. Weinberger covers developments on the other side of the Atlantic in his two-volume book *An introduction to the history of dentistry in America* (Mosby, 1948). International aspects of the growth of dentistry are traced in *The story of the Fédération Dentaire Internationale 1900–1962* by J. Ennis (FDI, 1967) and, more briefly, by G.H. Leatherman in *The FDI — 1900–1980* (Quintessence 1981).

Two pictorial books of great interest are *The dentist in art* by J. J. Pindborg and L. Marvitz (Munksgaard, 1960), which depicts works of art with dental features, and *A pictorial history of dentistry* by C. Proskauer and F.H. Witt (Dumont Schauberg, 1962), which uses contemporary art to illustrate dental developments. Sir Frank Colyer's *Old instruments used for extracting teeth* (Staples, 1952) is a well-illustrated and accurate work of great value to students of historical instruments. E. Bennion has produced the beautifully illustrated *Antique dental instruments* (Sotheby's 1980), which shows tools used for a variety of procedures, and includes a list of instrument makers.

B. W. Weinberger's two-volume *Orthodontics: a historical review of its origin and evolution* (Mosby, 1926) covers this specialized subject up to 1870, but with some errors. *The strange story of false teeth* by J. Woodforde (Routledge and Kegan Paul, 1968) gives an exact and entertaining history of prosthetic dentistry. An authoritative history of another specialty is given by A.J. Held in *Periodontology: from its origins up to 1980: a survey* (Birkhauser, 1989).

There are several useful works for identifying dental writings of historical interest. B.W. Weinberger compiled his *Dental bibliography* (Part I, 1929, Part II, 1932) from his own library and that of the New York Academy of Medicine. Books, monographs, theses and reprints are arranged in alphabetical order of authors and Part II has a subject index to both bibliographies. Part I lists dental periodicals by geographical subdivision as well as noting medical classics containing references to dentistry, while in Part II is found a list of dental books published between 1530 and 1810. Weinberger claimed to have included every important dental work to have been published and, although there are omissions, his work is highly regarded. C. G. Crowley's *Dental bibliography* (S.S. White, 1885) was a pioneer effort in comprehensiveness, listing dental books published from 1536 to 1885, chronologically arranged in five geographical groups. *A dental bibliography* by J. Menzies Campbell (David Low, 1949), lists British and American dental books and pamphlets published between 1682 and 1880 in a chronological arrangement with an author index; it is widely used by collectors and historians. The *Catalogue of the J. Menzies Campbell Collection presented to the Royal College of Surgeons of England* (RCS, 1970) lists pre-1860 books alphabetically by author.

H.L. Stromgren's *Index of dental and adjacent topics in medical and surgical works before 1800* (Munksgaard, 1955) is arranged in two sections, the first alphabetically by author, the second by subjects. In the author section annotations indicate the references of dental importance.

Biographical works of a dental nature are scarce. The supreme example is Sir Zachary Cope's *Sir John Tomes: a pioneer of British dentistry* (Dawson, 1961). J. Menzies Campbell's *Dentistry then and now* (3rd edn., privately printed, 1981), a revision of his *From a trade to a profession* (privately printed, 1958), opens with a description of the author's experience of 50 years of dental practice and continues with a fascinating miscellany of historical topics.

Conclusion

Despite the growth of specialization in the different fields of dentistry, its interactions with other medical and scientific disciplines are many. Although not discussed here, these links must be remembered and sources in other relevant areas should be used when appropriate.

CHAPTER TWENTY-TWO

General practice

MARGARET HAMMOND and D.J. PEREIRA GRAY

Introduction

General medical practice is simultaneously the oldest and one of the newest branches of medicine. It is the oldest because all practising doctors were originally doctors for all parts of the body, all ages, and all problems; it is one of the newest because it is relatively recently that it has been recognized as an independent academic discipline with a research base and a defined body of knowledge of its own (Gray, 1989).

The literature can be seen to be the life of any academic discipline. Without a literature, there is no discipline. With it, the breadth, dynamism and intellectual capacity of the activists in the field are clearly set out and revealed. The literature of general practice provides an interesting case study of the development of the discipline. By tracing its history, the literature provides the evidence for such development, and it provides a good guide as to how it will develop further in the future.

In most fields of academic study, both inside and outside medicine, evidence of academic life lies in the research literature. It is research reports which describe new findings and new developments and the absence of research in effect implies that the discipline is not alive. Accompanying research reports come, of course, a variety of articles commenting, interpreting and underlining different aspects of the subject and these can consist of separate articles or books.

An emerging literature

The history of the discipline of general practice started in the eighteenth and nineteenth centuries, with research reports from Jenner and Budd, and Findley. Some of the most important early books were those by Sir

James Mackenzie who is rightly regarded as one of the giants of general practice. *Principles of diagnosis and treatment in heart affections* (Henry Frowde and Hodder & Stoughton, 1916) is a good example.

In the first half of the twentieth century William N. Pickles stood out with his classic work *Epidemiology in country practice* (Wright, 1939), although it was not until after World War II that the literature really emerged. Early books tended to focus on the difference between medicine outside hospital as opposed to medicine inside. R.J.F.H. Pinsent's *An approach to general practice* published in 1953 by E. & S. Livingstone and D. Craddock's *Introduction to general practice* published in the same year by H.K. Lewis drew attention to the work of general practitioners outside hospitals. The main stimulus to the academic development of general practice was the formation of the (Royal) College of General Practitioners in November 1952, which effectively unlocked the energy and ideas of the largest branch of the profession. Since then the early trickle of publications has turned into a flood.

A notable feature over the years has been the greater specificity of content in the books which have moved from general themes about general practice as a whole to specific themes such as the management of particular diseases in general practice. The earliest was probably D. Craddock's (1969) *Obesity and its management* (Churchill Livingstone) and an important recent example is J. Tudor Hart's *Hypertension* (Churchill Livingstone, 1980).

Practice library

An important development in recent years has been the encouragement of general practitioners, particularly those who are appointed as trainers, to build up a library in their own practices. Practice libraries have several important advantages, particularly in bringing the literature close to hand and providing an information base for doctors, particularly trainees, in training practices. A useful introduction to the organization of the practice library, written by Margaret Hammond (1988) will hopefully kindle closer awareness of the joys of having a small library on the surgery premises and lead to greater use of the existing network of medical libraries.

Problem of classification

When books intended for general practice refer to some age group or disease group there is a danger of them being classified separately within specialist fields of practice, so that general practitioners visiting libraries can find that there is apparently no section on general practice at all. It is important to generalists that they are recognized as generalists and therefore it is preferable that all books from, and about, general practice be grouped together in a medical library.

Classics

There are about half a dozen books on general practice which stand out from the rest of the extensive literature, either because the impact at the time was of special historical importance or because the message they brought has proved of permanent importance. The following are books which both made a major impact at the time of publication and are still highly relevant and topical today.

The doctor, his patient and the illness by M. Balint, first published in 1957 (Pitman), was certainly the most influential book on general practice written at that time. It provided a new theoretical basis for the generalist in medicine, placed a new significance on the interpretation of multiple pathology and symptoms, and described a new role for the generalist in establishing personal relationships and a deep understanding of the patient as a person.

As general practice began to grapple with the significance of behaviour, E. Berne's *Games people play* (Deutsch, 1968) described many subtle forms of behaviour and offered a deep psychoanalytical interpretation of them. Several of these 'games' are in fact serious disturbances of relationships and behaviour in society and several are directly medical. The analysis illuminated the understanding of doctors, especially general practitioners, throughout the world.

Family medicine. A medical life history of families by F.J.A. Huygen (Dekker and van de Vegt) was published in 1978. In most parts of the world general practitioners are known as family doctors or family physicians and the family as a unit of care has special significance in the front line of the health service. Professor Huygen from the Netherlands wrote the most important book on the family in medicine and moreover illustrated it beautifully himself. There had been some difficulties in obtaining this book, and it was republished by the Royal College of General Practitioners in 1990.

The first book on research in general practice of importance was T. Eimerl and A.J. Laidlaw's *Handbook for research in general practice* (Churchill Livingstone, 1962) which came from the research committee of the then new College of General Practitioners. Now out of print, it has been overtaken by Professor J.G.R. Howie's *Research in general practice* now in its second edition (1989). Although the subject is not of great interest outside general practice, the book's emphasis on research as an integral part of general practice, its claim that it can and should be done by general practitioners, and its description of appropriate techniques gives it special importance.

The future general practitioner — learning and teaching written by a working party of the Council of the Royal College of General Practitioners (1972) sought to define the content of general practice, to classify this into useful divisions, and to provide educational objectives for some of the content. It was a landmark book, a book of its time, which is still relevant today. It has been translated into several different languages and remains an important text for the MRCGP examination.

A fortunate man by J. Berger and J. Mohr (Penguin, 1967) is a fascinating analysis of the role of the general practitioner seen through the eyes of a country doctor and illustrated by some striking and poignant photographs. Some fundamental theoretical problems of general practice, namely the difficulty in being everyone's personal doctor, are sensitively treated and the book has had an important influence in the development of the understanding of the generalist role in medicine.

Indexes and bibliographical lists

The major international *Index Medicus* and *Cumulated Index Medicus* first listed general practice as a separate heading in 1963. Currently general practice literature is cross referenced to the heading Family practice with a related reference to 'Physicians, family'. Coverage is limited to the listed periodicals and does not include book material. The online version of *Index Medicus*, MEDLINE, therefore also includes substantial amounts of relevant information and is described in Chapter 5.

Starting in 1980, after a long development, the World Organization of National Colleges, Academies and Academic Associations of General Practitioners (WONCA) produced in cooperation with the National Library of Medicine, — *FAMLI* (*Family Medicine Literature Index*). This appeared quarterly with an annual cumulation until 1985, but since 1986 has been an annual volume only. *FAMLI* is arranged in two sections. The first section is taken from *Index Medicus*/MEDLINE and includes all citations to international general practice material and covers all material appearing in certain general practice periodicals. The second section the supplement — contains references to general practice periodicals not included in *Index Medicus*/MEDLINE. Both sections follow the established *Index Medicus* format of separate author and subject sequences. *FAMLI* includes a list of books on general practice. *FAMLI* has been sponsored since the first issue (1980) by the College of Family Physicians of Canada and in 1987 they replaced WONCA as joint publisher. Circulation has always been small but the 1989 volume supplement section was also produced as a floppy disc in an effort to make the transmission to personal bibliographic databases easier.

Research projects by general practitioners (1950–1967) published by the Royal College of General Practitioners was the cumulation of a project started at the Usher Institute to review research work in general practice. Some 724 UK references and 35 foreign-language references were arranged in author and subject sequences. A second edition covering 1968–1973, detailing 962 entries of which 39 were in a foreign language, gives some indication of the rapid growth of material.

New reading for general practice published by the Royal College of General Practitioners, first produced in 1975 was a follow-up to the *Research projects* listings. Produced quarterly with an annual cumulation, it gave details of books, articles and reports with a general practice content, in subject and author sequences. Content covered mainly UK material with an attempt to include some of the more important foreign publications. 389 entries in 1975 grew to some 620 in 1980, and the amount of material to be looked at was becoming unmanageable when set against the available resources. Increased selectivity with less frequent publication resulted in Volume 14, No. 1 being the last issue in 1988. Although *Research projects* and *New reading* have ceased publication both contain valuable information which is not easily accessible elsewhere. An attempt to identify research material, to give a one or two line inclusion of many 'grey area' publications (for example theses) made these publications different from *FAMLI*.

Booklists giving only bibliographical details are printed annually in *FAMLI* (since 1981) and in the Royal College of General Practitioners' *Members' reference book* (since 1983). The Information Resources Centre of the RCGP list of book acquisitions 1989, arranged under subject headings, gives contents listings and descriptive annotations to many of the entries.

A selection of recent important titles appears with comment under the heading *General practice medicine* in *Medical textbook review: books for medical libraries* by V.G. Daniels (Cambridge Medical Books, 10th edn., 1990).

Reviews, yearbooks and abstracts

The only major review of general practice is still *Primary health care* by D. Hicks, commissioned by the Operational Research Service of the Department of Health and Social Security and published in 1976 by HMSO. The review describes and analyses work done over a 20-year period; 430 publications are cited. The tremendous growth of general practice literature since the 1970s makes a later review a daunting task. However, a yearly review has been included in *The Medical Annual*. This publication, started in 1882, was the most important yearly review of current UK work and trends. The 1966 edition, edited by R. Bodley

Scott and R.M. Walker (John Wright) contained a section on general practice which was continued until 1982. The content of the whole publication was then changed to reflect the development of primary medical care and *The Medical Annual: the Year Book of General Practice*, edited by D.J. and J. Pereira Gray (Wright) was published from 1983 to 1987. Aimed at general practitioners and trainees it included an analysis of the main events of the year and a précis of important publications, together with articles of current importance grouped in five sections — Health and disease, Human development, Human behaviour, Medicine and society, and Practice organization. *The General Practitioner's Yearbook: an Advisory Guide* published by Winthrop Laboratories from 1974 to 1987, gives information on matters of concern to a GP's daily routine, for example, medical ethics, legal matters, finance and an outline of major reports and Acts of Parliament affecting the medical practitioner. The *Members' reference book* of the RCGP, published annually since 1982, contains the College's annual report and a number of articles of current interest.

There is currently no major abstracting publication for UK general practice. The wide range of interests that general practitioners have may contribute to the difficulty of sustaining a viable publication. *Archives of family practice*, edited by J.P. Geyman (Vols 1–3, Appleton-Century-Crofts, 1980–82) attempted to fill the gap. Although an American publication, *Archives* reprinted and abstracted articles from world literature in subject groups. Volume 3, for example, included a section 'Clinical research in family practice'. The papers within this section, however, were published between 1969 and 1981 giving the volume a bibliographical rather than an abstracting function. Volume 3 was the last in this series.

1989 Year Book of Family Practice, edited by R.E. Rakel *et al.* (Year Book Medical Publishers) (No. 13 in this series) covers all the major clinical specialties. This U.S. publication is a collection of 400 abstracts of clinical research picked from 650 periodicals appearing in the previous 12 months. The chapters are organized according to body systems. A number of UK general practice periodicals have sections of 'current literature'. *Medical Monitor* (1988–) abstracts papers from 200 clinical periodicals each week. The majority of the abstracts are clinical papers of interest to GPs rather than papers from general practice.

Series

The publishers' role in the propagation of literature is often overlooked, but together with mainly general practitioner editorial boards, three series of books have developed in the 1980s. Many authoritative texts have already emerged as potential standard textbooks of the future. The *Library of general practice* series published by Churchill Livingstone started in 1980. Each volume deals with an important aspect of general practice, written by a GP well known for his work in that field, often in association with a leading specialist. The first volume of the *Oxford general practice series* (OUP) was produced in 1982. This series is written mainly by general practitioners. The third series, *Management of common diseases in family practice*, published by MTP under the editorship of J. Fry and M. Lancaster-Smith, has each book written by a family doctor and a consultant physician. This series which was started in 1985, superseded the *Problems in practice series*, which, although intended for general practitioners, was written by specialists working in district general hospitals. All three series are currently adding to their lists and details of individual volumes are noted in the subject areas.

There are two major series of pamphlets. The *Occasional papers* published by the Royal College of General Practitioners started in 1976. Originally educational in context they now include any topic of importance to general practice. They do not reflect College policy unless this is specifically stated. On average three papers are produced a year. A newer series of pamphlets, *Practical guides for general practice*, was inaugurated by OUP in 1985.

The RCGP also produces an *Information folder* series. Starting with practice organizational folders in 1985, the range was extended to include clinical topics in 1986.

Journals

Many general practitioners would say that they are saturated by the amount of unsolicited free periodicals and newspapers they receive. Nevertheless, this type of material is, according to readership surveys, amongst the most widely read (Cowhig, 1982; Owen, 1989).

Three examples of medical newspapers are *Pulse* (Morgan-Grampian, 1960–), *GP General Practitioner* (Haymarket Publications, 1963–) and *Doctor* (Reed Healthcare Communications, 1971–). All give a very up-to-date résumé on what is going on in general practice as well as covering topical clinical situations.

Therapeutics is dealt with by *Prescribers' Journal* (DHSS, 1961–) formerly *Prescribers' Notes* (1952–1960), *MIMS* (1959–) with the associated *MIMS Magazine* (Haymarket Publications, 1959–) and *Drug and Therapeutics Bulletin* (Consumers' Association, 1963–).

Practice organization is reported on in *Medeconomics* (Haymarket Publications, 1980–) and *Financial Pulse* (Morgan-Grampian, 1986–). *Practice Computing* published in association with the RCGP (Modern

Medicine Group, 1982–) and the *British Journal of Healthcare Computing* (1984–) have established themselves with authoritative coverage of a practical nature.

Health Bulletin (Scottish Home and Health Department, 1941–) and *Health Trends* (DHSS, 1969–) provide 'semi-official' information.

General clinical periodicals include *Practitioner* (Morgan-Grampian, 1868–), *Modern Medicine* (1956–), *Update* (Reed Health Care Communications, 1968–), *Physician* (Mark Allen, 1983–) and *Horizons: Continuing Education in Primary Care* (1987–) and *Medical Monitor* (1988–) both published by Medicom (UK) Ltd.

Examples of journals on specific subjects are *Geriatric Medicine* (Edgell Communication, 1979–) formerly *Modern Geriatrics* (1970–1978), *British Journal of Sexual Medicine* (Medical Tribune, 1973–) and *Maternal and Child Health: The Journal of Family Medicine* (Barker Publications, 1985–) formerly *Journal of Maternal and Child Health* (1975–1984). There is inevitably a good deal of change in this category of publication and two titles which ceased in the 1980s were *World Medicine* (IPC Business Press, 1965–1984) and *Trainee* (Update Group, 1981–1985).

Subscription journals of direct relevance include the *British Medical Journal*. The specific coverage of general practice was initiated in 1981 by a Practice Observed version which was subsequently modified to a separate section. *Postgraduate Education for General Practice* (Radcliffe, 1990–) is also of direct interest, incorporating the former *Journal of the Association of Course Organisers* (1985–1989).

Journals for medical and non-medical staff working in practice settings have multiplied in recent years and this expansion is likely to continue. *AMSPAR Magazine* (Association of Medical Secretaries, Practice Administrators and Receptionists, 1986–) formerly *Medical Secretary and Receptionist* (1964–1985) is distributed to members of the Association, as is *Practice Outlook* (Association of Health Centre and Practice Administrators, 1975–). *Stuart Management Review* (BOMPA, 1989–) formerly *Stuart Reception Review* (1985–1988) is distributed free to all practices. *Practice Nurse* (Reed Healthcare Communications, 1988–) is a subscription journal. *The Practice Receptionist* (Radcliffe Medical Press, 1988-1989) published by the Joint Committee for Receptionists' Continuing Education has been superseded by *PACE* (Radcliffe, 1990–) published for the Joint Committee for the Continuing Education of Practice Administrative Staff. This is distributed free to all practices as is *Practice Team: Shared Care in the Community* (Medicom, 1989–).

Publications of general practice organizations

Another category of interest is the official journal of an association or college of general practice. These show the development of the discipline throughout the world. Most of the publications include information of the host organization and many include articles of original research in general practice. The format and style vary enormously, but many publications starting as cyclostyled sheets have developed into respected academic journals. The selected list below is in chronological order. '(R)' indicates research content.

American Family Physician (formerly *GP* 1950–1969) (American Academy of Family Physicians, 1970–)

Florida Family Physician (Florida Academy of Family Physicians, 1951–)

British Journal of General Practice (formerly *Journal of the College of General Practitioners*, 1952–1967, renamed *Journal of the Royal College of General Practitioners*, 1967–1989) (1990–) (R)

Canadian Family Physician (formerly *Journal of the College of Family Physicians of Canada*, 1954–1967) (1967–)

Australian Family Physician (formerly *Annals of General Practice*, 1956–1971) (Royal Australian College of General Practitioners, 1972–) (R)

Huisarts en Wetenschap (Netherlands College of General Practitioners, 1958–) (R)

Filipino Family Physician (Philippine Academy of Family Physicians, 1963 (R)

Médecin du Québec (Federation of General Practitioners of Quebec, 1965–)

Family Medicine (formerly *Family Medicine Teacher* and *Family Medicine Times*, 1967–1980) (Society of Teachers of Family Medicine and North American Primary Care Research Group, 1981–) (R).

Medicus Universalis (Hungarian Association of General Practice, 1968–)

Family Physician Israel (Kupat Holim Health Insurance Institution of the General Federation of Labour, 1970–) (R)

Allgemein Medizin: Journal for Research and Methodology in General Practice (formerly *Allgemeinmedizin International General Practice* 1971–1984) (International Society for General Medicine *et al.*, 1985–) (R)

Singapore Family Physician (formerly *GP Singapore*, 1973–1975) (College of General Practitioners Singapore, 1975–) (R)

Family Physician, Malaysia (formerly *Family Practitioner, Malaysia,* 1974–1988) (College of General Practitioners of Malaysia, 1989–)

New Zealand Family Physician (New Zealand College of General Practitioners, 1974–) (R)

Journal of General Practice, India (General Practitioners' Association Greater Bombay, 1974–)

Journal of Family Practice (Association of Departments of Family Medicine, North American Primary Care Research Group and the Society of Teachers of Family Medicine, 1974–)

WONCA News (World Organization of National Colleges, Academies and Academic Associations of General Practitioners/Family Physicians, 1975–)

Hong Kong Practitioner (Hong Kong College of General Practitioners, 1978–) (R)

Japanese Journal of Primary Care (Japanese Medical Society of Primary Care, 1978–)

Sri Lankan Family Physician (College of General Practitioners of Sri Lanka, 1979–)

SA Family Practice (formerly *Southern African Family Practice, 1980– 1983)* (South African Academy of Family Practice/Primary Care, 1984–) (R)

Family Physician Korea (Korean Academy of Family Medicine, 1980–)

Family Practice Research Journal (Michigan, Minnesota and Ohio Academies of Family Physicians, 1981–) (R)

Jamaican Practitioner (Association of General Practitioners of Jamaica, 1981–)

MF International Journal of Family Medicine (International Centre for Family Medicine Buenos Aires, 1982–)

Scandinavian Journal of Primary Health Care (National Colleges or Societies of General Practice in Denmark, Finland, Iceland, Norway and Sweden, 1983–)

Atención Primaria (Spanish Society of Family and Community Medicine, 1984–) (R)

Revista Portuguesa de Clinica Geral (Association of Portuguese General Practitioners, 1984–)

Family Practice (OUP: WONCA links, 1984–) (R)

Journal of the American Board of Family Practice (1988–) (R)

Government and official statements

While any policy document on the health service is likely to have implications for general practice, the items listed below are of particular relevance for general practice.

1981

The Primary Health Care Team. Report of the Standing Medical Advisory Committee and the Standing Nursing and Midwifery Advisory Committees by Joint Working Group (Chairman W.G. Harding, HMSO)

Primary Health Care in Inner London by London Health Planning Consortium Primary Health Care Study Group (Chairman E.D. Acheson, DHSS)

1982

Informal Working Group on Effective Prescribing (Chairman P.R. Greenfield, DHSS)

1983

Report of the DHSS/NHS Audit Working Group (Chairman P. Salmon, DHSS)

NHS Management Inquiry. Report by DHSS (Chairman R. Griffiths, HMSO)

Mental Health Act (HMSO)

1984

Report of the Working Party on Section 63 Courses for General Medical Practitioners in England by DHSS (Chairman A. Walford, DHSS)

Committee of Inquiry into Human Fertilisation and Embryology. Report. (Chairman M. Warnock, HMSO)

Deputising Services. Revised circular and code of practice by DHSS (HC (FP) (84) 2)

Data Protection Act (HMSO)

Health Services Information by DHSS Steering Group (Chairman E. Körner, HMSO, 1982–1984). Six reports issued

Report of a Study of Family Practitioner Services Administration and the Use of Computers commissioned by DHSS and Welsh Office (Arthur Andersen) (*Appendices* 1985)

1985

Community Care with Special Reference to Adult Mentally Ill and Mentally Handicapped People by Social Services Committee (HMSO)

Management Arrangements for Family Practitioner Committees by DHSS (DHSS (HC(FP)85)10)

Family Practitioner Services, Travel and Subsistence Payments in Respect of Approved Study Courses for General Medical Practitioners (Principals, Assistants and Trainees) by DHSS (HN(FP)(85)11)

A Guide to the Registration Requirements for Doctors of the European Communities and Information Concerning Access to Medical Practice in the Social Security Systems by European Union of General Practitioners (BMA)

1986

The Position of the General Medical Practitioner and General Practice in the Health Care Systems of the European Community by European Union of General Practitioners

Primary Health Care: an Agenda for Discussion by DHSS (HMSO)

Neighbourhood Nursing — a Focus for Care, a report by the Community Nursing Review (Chairman J. Cumberlege, HMSO)

Charter for Action: Health for All 2000 by Faculty of Community Medicine (RCP)

Project 2000: A New Preparation for Practice by the United Kingdom Central Council for Nursing, Midwifery and Health Visiting

1987

Promoting Better Health: the Government's Programme for Improving Primary Health Care by Secretaries of State for Social Services (HMSO)

The Front Line of the Health Service, response by the RCGP

Single European Act (HMSO)

Hospital Medical Staffing: Achieving a Balance: Plan for Action a report issued on behalf of the UK Health Departments, the Joint Consultants Committee and Chairman of Regional Health Authorities

Deprivation and Ill Health by BMA Board of Science and Education

District Health Authority Use of Family Practitioner Committee Patient Registration Data by DHSS and Welsh Office

1988

Access to Medical Reports Act (HMSO)

Community Care: an Agenda for Action by DHSS (Chairman R. Griffiths, HMSO)

Report of the Inquiry into Child Abuse in Cleveland by E. Butler-Sloss (HMSO)

Priorities in Medical Research by House of Lords Select Committee on Science and Technology (HMSO)

Violence to Staff by DHSS

Public Health in England by Committee of Inquiry into the Future Development of the Public Health Function (Chairman D. Acheson, HMSO)

1989

Working for Patients. The Health Service: Caring for the 1990s and Working Papers 1–11 by Secretaries of State for Health (HMSO)

Services of Medical Practitioners: A Report on the Supply of the Services of Registered Medical Practitioners in Relation to Restrictions on Advertising by Monopolies and Mergers Commission (HMSO)

General Practice in the National Health Service: A New Contract by DoH and Welsh Office (HMSO)

Caring for People: Community Care in the Next Decade and Beyond by Secretaries of State for Health and Social Security (HMSO)

Textbooks and monographs

Clinical

GENERAL

It is very difficult to categorize books to fall neatly within defined subject areas. The books in this section are those which cover a range of clinical information. They are arranged in chronological order to show development of UK literature from 1980. A small amount of foreign material is included. Education, research and material appertaining to the practice setting are in separate sections.

Tutorials in general practice by M. Mead and H. Patterson (Pitman, 1983) is the earliest text and covers 30 case studies of the most common problems encountered in general practice. The book arose from joint discussions between a trainer and his trainee.

Common dilemmas in family medicine is edited by J. Fry (MTP, 1983) and presents arguments for and against a number of clinical and non-clinical situations.

General practice medicine is edited by J.H. Barber (Churchill Livingstone, 1984) and is the second edition of a mainly Scottish multi–author book on clinical 'system based' topics written for trainees.

Lecture notes on medicine in general practice by C.M. Harris (2nd edn., Blackwell, 1984) intended for students and trainees, looks at routine morbidity, psychosocial aspects, resources, special skills and the clinical aspects of general practice.

Textbook of family practice is edited by R.E. Rakel (3rd edn., Saunders, 1984) and is a very comprehensive American text of 71 chapters.

Presentation in primary care. An illustrated introduction to patient management in general practice by J.D.E. Knox (Butterworths, 1985) is intended for the new trainee. The first section gives 36 presentations, followed by a series of questions answered at length in the second section. A third section deals with teaching in general practice.

Towards earlier diagnosis, a guide to primary care, by K. Hodgkin (5th edn., Churchill Livingstone, 1985) is the longest and most established textbook (770 pages). Aimed at new and established general practitioners it is concerned with the principles of primary care and the early diagnosis of important disorders.

Common diseases: their nature, incidence and care, by J. Fry (MTP, 1985), is a longevity runner-up with a fourth edition. Diseases are grouped in broad subject areas with relevant statistical information.

Primary health care 2000: global challenges edited by J. Fry and J. Hasler (Churchill Livingstone, 1986) was published to coincide with the WONCA conference in London.

A guide to general practice by the Oxford GP Group, edited by S. Street and A. Wilkinson (2nd edn., Blackwell, 1987) gives details of recent legislation, vocational training regulations, and data for everyday use for the young general practitioner.

Essential primary care by S. Street and K. Burch (Blackwell, 1987) presents the fundamentals of primary care with the emphasis on diagnosis and management of the most commonly seen problems in general practice.

Clinical method: a general practice approach edited by R.C. Fraser (Butterworths, 1987) is written by members of the Department of General Practice at the University of Leicester. Intended for medical students, it contrasts the difference between hospital practice and general practice covering problem solving, patient management, communication and anticipatory care.

Textbook of general medicine and primary care, edited by J. Noble

(Little, Brown, 1987) is another comprehensive U.S. text (2376 pages) providing a commentary of problems of interest to the UK situation. *A colour atlas of general practice* by John Cohen (Wolfe, 1988) containing about 300 full colour photographs covers practical problems as well as practice characteristics, morbidity data, techniques and illness and social groups.

Student reviews–primary care by B. Jarman (Heinemann, 1988) begins with an account of the development of general practice in the UK, covers social and economic factors in health, epidemiology and prevention, the consultation, and holistic medicine. Although written for students, there is much up-to-date information for trainees and established practitioners.

Practical general practice. Guidelines for logical management by A. Knot and A. Polmear (Butterworth, 1988) provides a summary of management strategies for common areas of general practice. *Aids to general practice* by M. Mead (Churchill Livingstone, 1988) summarizes the essentials of good practice both in terms of clinical conditions, practice management and prescribing.

Practice. Clinical management in general practice, edited by J. Cormack, Marshall Marinker and D. Morrell (Kluwer Medical, 1976–88) provides a loose-leaf updating service designed to solve the common presenting problems of practice. The multi-author text is divided into four sections: the diagnostic process, management, the complaint (the largest section) and continuing care. A bound version of *Practice* (2nd edn., 1987) is also available.

Family medicine; principles and practice edited by R.B. Taylor *et al.* (3rd edn., Springer-Verlag, 1988) identifies core problems and procedures, and provides an overview of the nature and scope of family practice in the USA.

A textbook of family medicine by I.R. McWhinney (OUP, 1989) defines the basic principles illustrated with a number of clinical problems.

SPECIFIC AREAS

Infective and Parasitic

Infectious diseases: management of common diseases in family practice by D. Brooks and E.M. Dunbar (MTP, 1986) is a practical guide to the management of patients presenting to a doctor. An analysis of morbidity from the author's own practice is given.

Infective disease in primary care by R. Hull (Chapman and Hall, 1987) is arranged on symptom basis and is a ready reference for general practitioners and students.

Endocrinology

Endocrinology by P. Marsden and A.C. McCullagh (MTP, 1985) is one of the Management of Common Diseases in Family Practice Series.

Diabetes in practice, edited by H. Connor and A.J.M. Boulton (Wiley, 1989) covers all aspects of diabetic care that the general practitioner and practice need to know in order to care for their patients.

Psychiatry and Psychology

Psychiatric illness in general practice by M. Shepherd, B. Cooper, A.C. Brown, G. Kalton and A. Clare (2nd edn., OUP, 1981) is the account of research undertaken by the General Practice Research Unit at the Institute of Psychiatry. The first edition published in 1966 was a milestone in describing the role of general practitioners in the diagnosis and treatment of mental disorders. The second edition reviews developments since 1966.

Psychiatry in general practice, edited by A.W. Clare and M. Lader (Academic Press, 1982) is based on the proceedings of a conference and covers counselling, classification problems and the recognition of psychological illness. *Psychosocial disorders: management of common diseases in family practice* by R.M. Turner and P. Williams (MTP, 1986) adopts a problem-oriented approach.

A matter of interest: clinical notes of a psycho-analyst in general practice by K. Sanders (Clinical Press, 1986) and *Behaviour therapy in primary care: a practical guide* by R. France and M. Robson (Croom Helm, 1986) deal with management.

Alcohol: A balanced view. Report from general practice 24, by the Royal College of General Practitioners (1986) gives guidelines on what ought to be recorded in the patient's record and offers an analysis of the problems posed by alcohol.

The presentation of depression: current approaches by P. Freeling, L.J. Downey and J. C. Malkin (RCGP, 1987) — the proceedings of a meeting held in 1986 — discusses the nature of depression in general practice, perceptions held by patients and doctors and the relationship between physical and psychological problems.

Psychiatric emergencies in family practice, edited by J.D. Pollitt (MTP, 1987) provides practical advice to general practitioners and specialists on the assessment and management of psychiatric emergencies.

To heal or to harm: the prevention of somatic fixation in general practice, edited by R. Grol (3rd edn., RCGP, 1988) emphasizes the influence of home and the family on the behaviour of individual patients.

Drug misuse: a practical handbook for GPs by A. Banks and T.A.N. Waller (Blackwell, 1988) covers all drugs of dependence except tobacco and alcohol and brings together the historical, theoretical, attitudinal, medical, social, psychological, psychiatric and spiritual aspects of this contemporary problem.

Alcohol problems: practical guides for general practice by P. Anderson, P. Wallace and H. Jones (OUP, 1989) is an introductory management guide as is *Depression: recognition and treatment in general practice* by G. Wilkinson (Radcliffe, 1989).

Psychological problems in general practice by A.C. Marcus, C. Murray Parkes, P. Tomson and M. Johnston (OUP, 1989) covers psychiatric diseases as well as those problems with no clear diagnostic labels. Incidence, prevention, management, influence of family life, psychosomatic disorders are presented to help general practitioners and other members of the primary health-care team.

Finally in this section *Family problems* by P.R. Williams (OUP, 1989) deals with conditions attributable to stress in families, recognition of these symptoms and techniques to deal with them.

Nervous System and Sense Organs

The eye in general practice by C.R.S. Jackson and R.D. Finlay (Churchill Livingstone, 1985) has been completely rewritten for the eighth edition. *ENT disorders* by G.W. Hickish (Churchill Livingstone, 1985) is written by a general practitioner. *Neurology* by T.J. Fowler and R.W. May (MTP, 1985) is one of the Management of Common Diseases in Family Practice Series and *Stroke* by D. Wade (OUP, 1988) is a practical guide.

Cardiovascular Disorders

Cardiovascular problems in practice by R. Blackwood (Beaconsfield) and *Cardiology* by C.P.F. Wharton and A.R. Archer (MTP) were both published in 1986 and the second edition of *Hypertension: community control of high blood pressure* by J.T. Hart (Churchill Livingstone) was published in 1987.

Respiratory System

Epidemiology and research in a general practice by G.I. Watson (RCGP, 1982) published posthumously, consists of 16 chapters on respiratory-tract infections and reprints on the impact of viral diseases in general practice.

Respiratory disorders by J. Fry, R. White and M. Whitfield (Churchill Livingstone, 1984) and *Respiratory diseases* by G. Jariwalla and J. Fry (MTP, 1985) are textbooks and *Practical management of asthma* by T. Clark and J. Rees (Martin Dunitz) and *Asthma: its management in general practice* by I. Gregg (Update) were both published in 1985.

Digestive, Urinary Systems and Sexual Medicine

Gastroenterology, edited by J. Fry and M. Lancaster-Smith (MTP,

1985) and *Gastrointestinal disorders* by D.A. Coffman, J. Chalstrey and G. Smith-Laing (Churchill Livingstone, 1986) present similar information. *Urinary tract infections*, edited by D. Brooks (MTP, 1987) is the only text to cover this subject separately.

Sexual Medicine by G.R. Freedman (Churchill Livingstone, 1983) and *Understanding sexual medicine* by I. Feldstein (MTP, 1986) complete this section.

Gynaecology and Obstetrics

Modern obstetrics in general practice, edited by G.N. Marsh (2nd edn., OUP, 1985) is a collection of essays written by different authors intended to reflect current thinking.

Booking for maternity care by M. Klein, D. Elbourne and I. Lloyd (RCGP, 1985) is a study from the National Perinatal Epidemiology Unit in Oxford reporting on the views of mothers booked for delivery in a general practitioner unit and shared care. *Cervical screening* by A. McPherson (OUP, 1985) is a practical guide for all the team.

Obstetrics and gynaecology in general practice by J. Eddy and J. Owen (Churchill Livingstone, 1987) follows the pattern of this series of textbooks in being written by a general practitioner and a specialist.

Breast cancer screening by J. Austoker and J. Humphreys (OUP, 1988) a practical guide explaining the National Screening Programme, is issued as part of an information pack.

Women's problems in general practice, edited by A. McPherson (2nd edn., OUP, 1988) written by 21 contributors covers many areas of women's health not dealt with in other general practice books. *Health promotion in primary care* by the English National Board for Nursing, Midwifery and Health Visiting (1989) is the first distance-learning package funded by the Government to promote training for practice nurses. Its subject is cervical screening.

Skin Diseases

Dermatology — management of common diseases in family practice by L. Fry and M.N.P. Cornell (1985) is one of the MTP series.

Musculoskeletal System and Connective Tissue

Rheumatology in general practice by M. Rogers and N. Williams (Churchill Livingstone, 1982), *Locomotor disability in general practice*, edited by M.I.V. Jayson and R. Million (OUP, 1983), *Rheumatology* by H. Berry and A.S.M. Jawad (MTP Series, 1985), *Orthopaedic disorders in general practice* by R.L.M. Newell and J.G. Turner (Butterworths, 1985) and *Rheumatology for general practitioners* by H.L.F. Currey and S. Hull (OUP, 1987) are all comprehensive texts reflecting the importance of these subjects.

Children

Healthier children — thinking prevention by the RCGP (1982) is one of the five policy statements on prevention issued by the College. *Commonsense paediatrics* by M. Pollak and J. Fry (MTP, 1986), *Paediatrics: management of common diseases in family practice* by A.N.W. Evans and C.A. McCarthy (MTP, 1986) and *Paediatric problems in general practice* by M. Modell and R. Boyd (2nd edn., OUP, 1988) cover clinical problems as well as normal development and the place of children within the family and society.

The importance of screening and preventive medicine are represented by *Handbook of preventive care for preschool children* by RCGP and GMSC (2nd edn., 1988), *Health for all children: the Report of the Joint Working Party of Child Health Surveillance*, edited by D.M.B. Hall (OUP, 1989) (which analyses the existing schemes and includes a guide to recommended screening procedures), and two pamphlets in the Practical Guide Series — *Child health: the screening tests* by A. Macfarlane, S. Sefi and M. Cordeiro and *Immunizing children* by S. Sefi and A. Macfarlane — both OUP series (1989).

Child care in general practice, edited by C. Hart and J. Bain (Churchill Livingstone, 1989) is the third edition of a multi-author book providing practical advice and management for day-to-day practice.

Elderly and Geriatrics

The care of the elderly in general practice by M.K. Thompson (Churchill Livingstone, 1984) discusses epidemiology, resources, psychosocial problems as well as disorders and care. *Geriatrics* by A. Martin and E.C. Gambrill (MTP, 1986) is more disease orientated.

Preventive care of the elderly, edited by R.C. Taylor and E.G. Buckley (RCGP, 1987) presents a review of current developments from the National Workshop on the Role of the Primary Care Team. *Elderly people, their medicines and their doctors* by A. Cartwright and C. Smith (Routledge, 1988) is the first account of a national study of 778 people.

Caring for elderly people in the community by E.I. Williams (2nd edn., Chapman and Hall, 1989) and *Commonsense geriatrics* by K. Thompson (Clinical Press, 1990) cover the subject comprehensively.

Therapeutics, investigations and procedures: surgery and emergencies

Treatment; a handbook of drug therapy, edited by V.W.M. Drury, O.L. Wade, L. Beeley and P. Alesbury (Kluwer, 1984/5) is a loose-leaf add-on handbook for GPs.

Practical prescribing by M.J. Brodie and I. Harrison (Churchill Livingstone, 1986) reviews prescribing in a London practice and identifies important areas for the practitioner. *Prescribing – what, when and why?* by J. Fry, M. Godfrey and B. Prichard (Churchill Livingstone, 1986) presents everyday clinical situations and prescribing responses.

Three formularies for general practice are: *Practice formulary 1988–1990* by RCGP Northern Ireland Faculty, the *Lothian formulary 1989: No. 2*, by the Liaison Committee and an OUP Practical Guide – *A basic formulary for general practice* by G.B. Grant, D.A. Gregory and T.D. van Zwanenberg.

Diagnostic techniques are covered in *Laboratory: a manual for the medical practitioner*, edited by H.W.K. Acheson (Kluwer, 1983), first issued in 1978 in a loose-leaf format. *The ECG in general practice* by J.R. Hampton (Churchill Livingstone, 1986), *An atlas of bedside microscopy* by J.M. Longmore (RCGP, 1986) and *Radiology* by R.F. Bury (OUP, 1988) cover specific areas.

Surgical procedures are covered by *Minor surgery: a text and atlas* by J. S. Brown (Chapman and Hall, 1986), *Surgical problems in clinical practice*, edited by J. Fry and H.E. Berry (Arnold, 1987) which, co-authored by a general practitioner and a surgeon, presents views on the diagnosis and management of selected conditions from two points of view, and *Surgery for general practitioners* by B.A. Maurice (Castle House, 1989) is an extension of talks given to trainees.

An introduction to acupuncture: a practical guide for GPs and other medical personnel by P. Pearson (MTP, 1987), *Emergencies in general practice* by A.J. Moulds, P.B. Martin and T.A.I. Bouchier-Hayes (MTP, 1983) and *Handbook of emergencies in general practice* by N. Lawrence and J. Watts (OUP, 1989) complete this section.

Education for general practice

General

The nature of general family practice: an alternative to syllabus development, edited by W.E. Fabb and J.R. Marshall (MTP, 1983) presents 583 clinical vignettes describing the discipline of general practice. *The assessment of clinical competence in general family practice* by W.E. Fabb and J.R. Marshall (WONCA/MTP, 1983) presents examples and tests used by colleges and academies worldwide.

Working together: learning together by R.V.H. Jones (RCGP, 1986) reports on several years' study of multidisciplinary training. *The stem doctor* by A. Chant (Chant, 1989) describes an alternative to the present position of provision and training of general practitioners.

Undergraduate

Undergraduate medical education in general practice by the Association of University Teachers in General Practice (RCGP, 1984) is an analysis of the GMC recommendations to medical schools about the content of courses leading to medical qualifications and the contribution general practice can play in meeting them.

The Mackenzie Report: general practice in the medical schools of the United Kingdom — 1986 (Mackenzie Fund, 1986) is an account of visits to 24 undergraduate departments of general practice. The structure and work of departments is detailed, together with a discussion on academic issues and funding.

The contribution of academic general practice to undergraduate medical education by R.C. Fraser and E. Preston-Whyte (RCGP, 1988) presents the questionnaire reply findings from 25 university departments discussing contributions made to the curriculum, involvement in assessment procedures and teaching preparation and methods.

Vocational training

Training for general practice by D.J. Pereira Gray (MacDonald and Evans, 1982) is the first comprehensive account of the history, organization and progress of vocational training of general practitioners. *The influence of trainers on trainees in general practice* by J. Freeman, J. Roberts, D. Metcalfe and V. Hillier (RCGP, 1982) compares two groups of trainees in the North of England. *A workbook for trainees in general practice* by P. Freeling (Wright, 1983) suggests tutorial topics for the vocational year. *Milestones, the diary of a trainee GP* by P. Stott (Pan, 1983) is a readable account of the problems and day-to-day working of a practice.

The Joint Committee on Postgraduate Training of General Practice (JCPTGP) who are responsible for standards of vocational training in England and Wales, Northern Ireland and Scotland issued *Recommendations to regions for the establishment of criteria for the approval and reapproval of trainers in general practice* in 1985.

Trainee Projects: Syntex Award winners 1981–1984 (RCGP) was published in 1985. The Syntex Award Scheme was set up to provide a stimulus to research in general practice through vocational training. Summaries of award-winning projects are also included.

Course organizers in general practice by A.H.E. Williams (RCGP, 1986), a national survey covers all aspects of their work, responsibilities and support. *Assessment and vocational training for general practice: final report* by a working party of the JCPTGP (1987) includes a GP job specification.

Running a course by K. Bolden, D. Dwyer, R. Leete and R. Steele

(Radcliffe, 1988), a guide for course organizers, is based on work carried out from the Department of General Practice, University of Exeter. *Priority objectives for general practice vocational training* by the Oxford Region Course Organizers and Regional Advisers Group (2nd edn., RCGP, 1988) was achieved after consultation within the region.

Rating scales for vocational training in general practice developed by the University of Manchester Department of General Practice has been updated (RCGP, 1988) and *The assessment of vocational training in general medical practice* by D. and J. Taylor (Centre for Health Economics, 1988) calls for independent assessment of vocational training recommending the use of the Manchester rating scales.

Vocational training in general practice: Proceedings of a Workshop, 15-18th October 1987, organized by the New Leeuwenhorst Group, edited by J. Heyrman and C. Spreevwenbergh (1988) reviews the situation of vocational training in Europe in preparation for the new EEC rules. Many of the books mentioned in the monographs section are written to help candidates prepare for the MRCGP examination, but the *MRCGP study book* by E. Gambrill, A. Moulds, J. Fry and D. Brooks (2nd edn., Butterworths/Update, 1988) and *Notes for the MRCGP* by K.T. Palmer (Blackwell, 1988) have that specific purpose.

Learning general practice: a structured approach for trainee GPs and trainers by J. Sandars and R. Baron (Pastest, 1988), *A guide for trainees in general practice* by J. Fry, P. Martin, E. Gambrill, A. Moulds, M. Godfrey and G. Strube (2nd edn., Heinemann, 1989) and *A GP training handbook*, edited by M.S. Hall (2nd edn., Blackwell, 1989) all provide practical advice for the trainee year and preparation for the MRCGP examination. *Trainee-centred assessment*, edited by P. Sackin, J. Henry, R. Leete, R. Seiler and J. Terry is a booklet produced in 1989 by a working party of the Association of Course Organisers which reviews methods of assessment of trainees currently in use in the UK.

Continuing education

The most important development in further education of GPs has been the *Continuing Learning in Practice Project (CLIPP)*, a distance-learning project, developed by the RCGP in association with the Centre for Medical Education (Donald, 1984). The first programme, modelled on the Australian College's Family Medicine Programme (1973–) CASE (Clinical Assessment for Systematic Education) launched in 1984, has been distributed to over 10 000 general practitioners in the UK.

The other important educational development which also encompasses research and organizational change is the growing importance of looking at the quality of general practice. Material on this aspect has been collected together in a separate section.

Continuing education for general practitioners by A. Branthwaite, A. Ross, A. Henshaw and C. Davie (RCGP, 1988) reports a study investigating the patterns of attendance at meetings. In-depth interviews with 32 GPs reveal problems in attending courses.

Quality assessment, audit and peer review

Quality in general practice by the RCGP (1982) is a policy statement for the 1982 position with future strategy. *Medical audit in general practice* by M.G. Sheldon (RCGP, 1982) reviews the literature, analyses the key issues and suggests a protocol for carrying out audit based on personal experience. *The principles of quality assurance* by WHO is published as EURO Reports and Studies 94 (1983).

Clinical knowledge and education for general practice by H.W.K. Acheson and M.H. Henley (RCGP, 1984) is the account of a postal questionnaire study asking groups of GPs and consultants what action they would take in relation to seven common clinical conditions. *Prescribing — a suitable case for treatment* by C.M. Harris, B. Jarman, E. Woodman, P. White and J.S. Fry (RCGP, 1984) documents a survey carried out by London GPs.

What sort of doctor?: assessing quality of care in general practice (RCGP Report Series, 1985), the findings of two working parties, describes a system of performance review based on work done by GPs in their own practices.

Explorations in quality assessment and monitoring by A. Donabedian (Health Administration Press in three volumes, 1980, 1982 and 1985) is the core work on its stated subject.

In pursuit of quality: approaches to performance review in general practice, edited by D. Pendleton, T. Schofield and M. Marinker (RCGP, 1986) is a collection of essays.

Quality improvement by quality assessment, is a statement by the New Leeuwenhorst Group (1986). *Practice activity analysis* by the RCGP Birmingham Unit (RCGP, 1988) promotes PAA as a means of facilitating audit by self-evaluation. *Practice assessment and quality of care* by R. Baker (RCGP Series, 1988) assesses the current position.

Two important books from the Netherlands — *Peer review in general practice: methods, standards, protocols*, edited by R.P.T.M. Grol, P.J.R. Mesker and F.G. Schellevis (Nijmegen University, 1988) and *Peer group performance review for general practitioners: a handbook for counsellors* by A.H.J. van de Rijdt-van de Ven, A.M. Tovw, M.J. Vermue, R.I.M. Kluver and J. Bide Groot (Netherlands Institute for Development and Support of General Practice and Primary Health Care, 1988) — detail experience gained from large-scale projects.

Who killed Susan Thompson? by S. Irvine, M. Marinker and A.

Wright (MSD Foundation and RCGP, 1990) is a video and course book package designed to demonstrate the link between clinical practice and medical audit.

The analysis of prescribing in general practice by C.M. Harris, P.L. Heywood and A.D. Clayden (HMSO, 1990) is a guide to audit and research based on the data from the Prescription Pricing Authority and *Managing for quality in general practice*, by D. Irvine (1990) is the second in the King's Fund Centre Medical Audit Series.

Statistics, research and epidemiology

Statistics

Disease data book by J. Fry, G. Sandler and D. Brooks (MTP, 1986) presents morbidity statistics in a popular way. *Morbidity statistics from general practice 1981–82: third national study* by the RCGP, Office of Population Censuses and Surveys and the Department of Health (HMSO, 1986) is the main source of morbidity information in the UK. This third study completes a recording period of over 30 years. The survey period of one year from July 1981 involved 332 270 patients registered with 48 practices.

Mortality, morbidity and health by M. Alderson (Stockton Press, 1988) cites important sources. The *Compendium of health statistics* by the Office of Health Economics (7th edn., 1989) presents non-clinical information from Family Practitioner Services.

The General Household Survey from the Social Survey Division of the Office of Population Censuses and Surveys, published annually is based on interviews from the general population. The 1987 *Survey* published in 1989 includes statistics on morbidity and services in the section on health. Of a similar status to the UK morbidity survey has been a study involving sentinel stations in the Netherlands. Starting in 1969 with findings presented in annual reports *The Dutch sentinel practice network: relevance for public health policy*, edited by A.I.M. Bartelds, J. Fracheboud and J. Van der Zee (Netherlands Institute of Primary Care, 1989) reviews the work of the network by the presentation of clinical areas. A second socio-economic analysis from the UK study *Morbidity statistics from general practice 1981–82* by the RCGP/OPCS/DoH (HMSO) was published in 1990. Finally, statistics about the working and services of general practitioners are presented annually in *Health and Personal Social Services Statistics* published by the Department of Health (HMSO).

Research and epidemiology

Epidemiology in country practice by W. Pickles (3rd impression, RCGP, 1984) is a classic example of original research in general practice. *Practice-based research in family medicine* by A.D. Berg, M.J. Gordon and D.C. Cherkin (American Academy of Family Physicians, 1986) is written for beginners, as is *Epidemiology in general practice*, edited by D. Morrell (OUP, 1988).

Research in general practice by J. Howie (2nd edn., Chapman and Hall, 1989) updates the thinking on the use of technology and the data-gathering mechanisms pioneered by the social sciences, and discusses the widening scope of work done in general practice. *User surveys of general practice. 1. Some suggestions about how to do such surveys by post* by A. Cartwright and *2. Some findings from a postal survey of users' views and experiences of general practice* by A. Jacoby (Institute for Social Studies in Medical Care, 1989) elaborate, in booklet form, the comments made by J. Howie.

Research methods for general practitioners by D. Armstrong, M. Calnan and J. Grace (OUP, 1989) aims to take a GP through the research process from initial idea to final publication.

Research intelligence by the RCGP (No. 19, 1989) lists ongoing projects in general practice before they reach publication.

Classification

The actual and potential growth in the use of computers in general practice has emphasized the importance of being able to compare data nationally or internationally. *The classification and analysis of general practice data* by the RCGP (2nd edn., 1986) has evolved from usage in the RCGP, OPCS and DHSS morbidity surveys.

ICPC: international classification of primary care, edited by H. Lamberts and M. Wood (OUP, 1988) for WONCA (World Organization of National Colleges, Academies and Academic Associations of General Practitioners/Family Physicians) in collaboration with NAPCRG (North American Primary Care Research Group), although based on the RCGP's first code, has developed in a different direction. This classification, which has been field tested for ten years, combines *ICHPPC2-2 defined* and *IC-PROCESS-PC*, and enables encounters with a patient to be classified according to presenting reason, diagnosis and action taken.

The classification of general practice data, the final report of the GMSC/RCGP Joint Computing Technical Working Party (GMSC, 1988) recommends a third classification as a basis for UK standardization. This is the *Read clinical classification* by J.D. Read (Loughborough Computer-Aided Medical Systems, 1989) developed as a thesaurus of medical terms with a computerized medical language. It includes data from the RCGP and WONCA systems. The classification codes not only diseases but also history and symptoms, examination, diagnostic, preventive, therapeutic and administrative procedures as well as occupational and social information.

Practice setting

The material discussed in this section shows considerable change from that in the last edition. There is very little about premises as buildings. *Practical guidance to achieve cost effective new or improved surgery premises for the 1990s* by M.S. Valins (1990) is an exception. The emphasis has been on the organizational aspects of practices, the training of team members and, of course, computers.

Management of buildings and services

Organising a practice (BMA, 1983), a collection of articles published in the *British Medical Journal* and *Management in general practice*, by P. Pritchard, K. Low and M. Whalen (OUP, 1984), still provides useful information. *Principles of practice management*, edited by W. Fabb and J. Fry (MTP, 1984) prepared on behalf of WONCA provides an international perspective.

Running a practice: a manual of practice management by R.V.H. Jones, K.J. Bolden, D.J.P. Gray and M.S. Hall (3rd edn., Croom Helm, 1985) and *Towards better practice* by P. Martin, A.J. Moulds and P.J.C. Kerrigan (Churchill Livingstone, 1985) give comprehensive coverage.

The emperor's new clothes: family practitioner committees in the 1980s by J. Allsop and A. May (King Edward's Hospital Fund for London, 1986) reviews the range of work and the role and functions of the bodies who administer GP contracts.

Guidance to general practitioners on data protection registration by the BMA General Medical Services Committee was published in 1986. *Tax and financial planning for medical practitioners* by N. Eastaway and S. Burwood (Butterworths, 1987) gives current information.

A video programme, with additional course book, *Management in practice* (1987) by J. Huntington, S. Irvine and M. Marinker is produced jointly by the RCGP and the MSD Foundation. A second CLIPP (Continuing Learning in Practice Project) programme developed by the RCGP and the Centre for Medical Education, Dundee, called *If only I had the time*, was produced in 1989 as an eighteen month distance learning course. *Systemed — an information system for general practice* by B.

Essex (BMJ, 1989) is a loose-leaf information system designed to be used by the whole practice team.

Family doctors and economic incentives by N. Bosanquet and B. Leese (Dartmouth Publishing, 1989) is the account of a study which attempts to determine how economic considerations influence practice decisions.

In addition to the books mentioned above, a number of items in the Monographs section (p. 525) are also of interest.

Computers

Publications about computers go out of date so quickly that this section covers a proportion only of what has been published since 1980.

A Government-sponsored scheme initiated in 1982 to promote awareness of information technology was reported in *General practice computing: evaluation of the 'Micros for GP's scheme'* (HMSO, 1985) and *Micros in practice: report of an appraisal of GP microcomputer systems*, both by the former DHSS (HMSO, 1986). *A prescription for change: a report on the longer term use and development of computers in general practice* by M.J. Fitter, J.R. Garber, G.A. Herzmark and D. Robinson (HMSO, 1986) examined further progress of the same scheme.

Computing survey 1989 by the Statistics and Management Information Division (DoH, 1989) targeted the estimated quarter of all partnerships in England and Wales owning computers. The survey analysed the types of hardware and software packages in practices and the uses to which they were put.

Computers — a guide to choosing and using by A. Willis and T. Stewart (OUP Practical Guides Series, 1989), *Computers in general practice* by R. Peckitt (Sigma, 1989), *The use of computers in general practice* by J. Preece (2nd edn., Churchill Livingstone, 1990) and *Computers in general practice: guidance notes* by RCGP (1990) have all been written to advise and help those practices yet to choose and install a computer system.

Two books looking at computer functions in a wider sense than that of dealing with practice routines are *Decision making in general practice*, edited by M. Sheldon, J. Brooke and A. Rector (Macmillan Press, 1985) and *Information handling in general practice*, edited by R. Westcott and R.V.H. Jones (Croom Helm, 1988).

Staff: role and training

Nurses working in the community by K. Dunnell and J. Hobbs (DHSS, 1982) is an account of a national survey. *The medical secretary's and receptionist's handbook* by M. Drury and M. Collin (5th edn., Baillière) was published in 1986.

The work of counsellors in general practice by J. McLeod (RCGP, 1988) describes the position in several practices and discusses the advantages and disadvantages for doctors, patients and counsellors.

Team-work in general practice by D.N.H. Greig (Castle House, 1988) is based on the author's own experience.

The practice receptionist programme, by M. Drury (Radcliffe, 1988) is part of the practice receptionist course and *A handbook for medical receptionists* by D. Hallsworth (Parthenon, 1988) covers similar information.

The nurse in family practice: practice nurses and nurse practitioners in primary health care, edited by A. Bowling and B. Stilwell (Scutari, 1988) outlines the history and role of the nurse in primary care and presents research findings of the activities of practice nurses in various parts of England. It is complemented by *Practice nurse handbook* by K.J. Bolden and B.A. Takle (2nd edn., Blackwell, 1989) which is a guide to professional duties and responsibilities.

Employing staff by N. Ellis (3rd edn., BMA, 1989) needs no explanation. *We need a practice manager* by J. Huntington, S. Irvine and M. Marinker is the second in the Practice Management video series (RCGP/MSD, 1989). Book Two in *The practice receptionists' programme* edited by M. Whalen (Radcliffe, 1989) builds upon the knowledge and attitudes developed in book One.

The practice nurse: theory and practice edited by P. Jeffree (Chapman and Hall) and *Nursing in general practice: clinical care*, edited by B. Stilwell and R. Hobbs (Radcliffe) are both published in 1990 as is *The new practice manager* edited by M. Drury (Radcliffe).

Non-clinical management of patients

A survey of primary care in London by B. Jarman (RCGP, 1981) provides detailed documentation both on the illnesses and social conditions of patients and the characteristics of their general practitioners and other health services.

Rethinking general practice. Dilemmas in primary health care by M. Jeffreys and H. Sachs (Tavistock, 1983) is a major research project, funded by the former DHSS. Carried out from 1970 to 1982 it investigates the changes in practice management, staffing and attitudes after a move into a health centre.

General practitioners and consultants: a study in outpatient referrals by R. Dowie (King Edward's Hospital Fund, 1983) describes a study based on referrals to a district general hospital in 1977. *General practi-*

tioner hospitals, edited by R. Jones (RCGP, 1983) reviews the history and literature of that subject.

Access to GPs by the Consumers' Association (1983) is another review of the literature and records the results of a telephone survey undertaken by the Association. *Social class and health status: inequality or difference*, by D.L. Crombie (RCGP, 1984) uses data taken from the second morbidity survey and compares it with Census data for the year 1970–71 showing general practitioner care. *Access to GPs: a fair share for all?* by R. Leavey (Manchester University Centre for Primary Care Research, 1985) compares GP utilization in relation to levels of ill health and the accessibility and acceptability of GP services to users. Data are taken from existing surveys with original information from 1897 interviews in a 1982 Manchester population survey. *Telephone access to GPs in the UK: a study of London* by J. Allsop and A. May (King Edward's Hospital Fund, 1985) looks at patient use and doctor attitude.

Too many patients? A study of the economy of time and standards of care in general practice by J. Butler and M. Calnan (Gower, 1987) presents work done by the Health Services Research Unit at Kent University. *General medical practitioner's workload* by the former DHSS (1987) analyses returns from 1224 GPs in a one-year period 1985–1986. *Anatomy of urban general practice* by D. Wilkin, L. Hallam, R. Leavey and D. Metcalfe (Tavistock, 1987) based on three large scale research projects in the Greater Manchester area, studies GPs and their practices, illnesses and the patterns of work. *Primary health care in Newcastle upon Tyne. A report on the GP facilitator project* by T.D. van Zwanenberg (Newcastle Medical School, 1989) is a similar survey of 51 practices. *On-Call: out-of-hours telephone calls and home visits* by J.D.E. Knox (OUP, 1989) is one of the *Practice Guides* series.

Doctor–patient communication and consultation

The doctor–patient relationship by P. Freeling and C.M. Harris (2nd edn., Churchill Livingstone, 1983) presents a number of case histories to illustrate patient types. *Doctor–patient communications*, edited by D. Pendleton and J. Hasler (Academic, 1983) is written by a number of authors from different disciplines.

Primary health care: bridging the gap between theory and practice by N.C.H. Stott (Springer-Verlag, 1983) propounds a philosophy of communication and behaviour skill in the consultation process. *Doctor to doctor: writing and talking about patients*, edited by J. Walton and G. McLachlan (Nuffield Provincial Hospitals Trust, 1984) approaches the subject in yet another way, that of consultation between professionals. *Doctors talking to patients*, by P.S. Byrne and B.E.L. Long, first published in 1976 and reprinted by the RCGP in 1984 is a study of the verbal behaviour of general practitioners in their surgeries, where 100 doctors taped interviews with 2500 patients. *The consultation: an approach to learning and teaching* by D. Pendleton, T. Schofield, P. Tate and P. Havelock (OUP, 1984) is a review of current research and theories about consultation management and monitoring.

Treatment or diagnosis: a study of repeat prescriptions in general practice by M. Balint, J. Hunt, D. Joyce, M. Marinker and J. Woodcock (Tavistock, 1970 reprinted 1984) evolved from the 'Balint Group' work.

Meetings between experts by D. Tuckett, M. Boulton, C. Olson and A. Williams (Tavistock, 1985) is the account of research on more than 1000 consultations by four social scientists and follows on from the work of Byrne and Long.

Partners in care: the consultation in general practice by P.G. Livesey (Heinemann, 1986) reveals the author's philosophy. *Ethical issues in family medicine* by R.J. Christie and C.B. Hoffmaster (OUP, 1986) illustrates problems of doctor-patient relationships from North American situations. *While I'm here doctor: A study of the doctor–patient relationship*, edited by A. Elder and O. Samuel (Associated Book Publishers, 1987) is a multi-author text written from a Balint background. *Encounters between doctors and patients*, edited by J.D. Stoeckk (MTP, 1987) brings together some of the basic texts on doctor–patient interactions, especially ones from the USA. *Skills and management in family medicine*, by K.K. Koh, L.G. Goh and P. Kee (PG Publishing, 1988) brings together much material which is currently spread over a number of different publications. *The inner consultation* by R. Neighbour (MTP, 1988) is a practical manual for trainees.

Patients

An example of a book for the patient is *Making the most of your doctor* by J. King, D. Pendleton and P. Tate (Thames Methuen, 1986). *Patients' charter: guidelines for good practice* by the Association of Community Health Councils (1987), *Patient information: advice on the drafting of leaflets* by ABPI (1988) and *Patients' rights* by the National Consumer Council and the Association of Community Health Councils for England and Wales (1989) have been written to further improve doctor–patient relationships.

Health promotion

Preventive medicine in general practice, edited by J.A.M. Gray and G.H. Fowler (OUP, 1983) is a multi-author volume covering the principles and practicalities of prevention. *Practising prevention* (BMA, 1983) is a collection of articles from the *British Medical Journal*.

Promoting prevention by the RCGP (1983) brings together the themes of five major reports — *Combined reports on prevention* (reprinted 1984). *Prevention and the primary care team* by the RCGP and the Royal College of Nursing (1986) is the report of a multidisciplinary working party. *Promoting health through participation* by A. Richardson and C. Bray (Policy Studies Institute, 1987) reports on the experience of 63 patient participation groups in general practice. *Prevention of coronary heart disease and stroke* by J.T. Hart, B. Stilwell and J.A. Muir Gray (Faber, 1988) is a workbook for primary care teams. *Health checks in general practice: why some people attend and others do not*, by N.C.H. Stott and R.M. Pill (University of Wales, 1988) is based on a study carried out in a Cardiff general practice.

Literature on the prevention of particular conditions can be found. pp. 527–531.

Care of special categories of patients

Terminal care at home, edited by R. Spilling (OUP, 1986), *Domiciliary terminal care* by D. Doyle (Churchill Livingstone, 1987) and *Teamwork in palliative care* by R. Hull, M. Ellis and V. Sargent (Radcliffe, 1989) reflect the importance placed on this subject.

Transcultural medicine by B. Qureshi (Kluwer, 1989) and *Health care for Asians in general practice*, edited by B. McAvoy and L.J. Donaldson (OUP, 1990) highlight another important area and the second edition of *Continuing care: The management of chronic disease*, edited by J. Hasler and T. Schofield (OUP, 1990) illustrates the importance of this aspect of care.

History, biography, general philosophy

General medical history is dealt with in Chapter 24 but the following titles are of specific interest.

Doctors: the lives and work of GPs by J. Gathorne-Hardy (Weidenfeld and Nicolson, 1984) is an account of general practice from 1890 to the present day illustrated by personal interviews with doctors. Although there are many autobiographical accounts by practitioners, *Sir James Mackenzie* MD 1853–1925 by A. Mair (RCGP, reprinted 1986) is a biography of one of the most important general practitioners of his day. A new chapter in the reprint describes important academic developments since Mackenzie's death.

Medical care and the general practitioner 1750–1850 by I. Loudon (Clarendon, 1986) deals with the rank-and-file practitioners, the surgeon-apothecaries and the successors — the general practitioners. This study is based on manuscript sources. *General practice and primary health care 1940s–1980s* by J. Fry (Nuffield, 1988) recounts, from his own experience the development of a discipline from before the introduction of the National Health Service and logically follows I. Loudon's study. *A new kind of doctor: the general practitioner's part in the health of the community* by J.T. Hart (Merlin Press, 1988) is an historical and personal observation drawn from 30 years' work in a Welsh practice.

References

Cowhig, J. (1982) The medical newspaper. *British Medical Journal*, **285**, 109–111.

Donald, A.G. (1984) Continuing Learning in Practice Project (CLIPP). *Journal of the Royal College of General Practitioners*, **39**, 242–245.

Gray, D.J.P. (1989) The emergence of the discipline of general practice, its literature, and the contribution of the College Journal. McConaghey Memorial Lecture 1988. *Journal of the Royal College of General Practitioners*, **39**, 228–233.

Hammond, M. (1988) *The practice library*. London: Royal College of General Practitioners and Stuart Pharmaceuticals.

Owen, P.A., Allery, L.A., Harding, K.G. and Hayes, T.M. (1989) General practitioners' continuing medical education within and outside their practice. *British Medical Journal*, **299**, 238–240.

CHAPTER TWENTY-THREE

Consumer health information

R. GANN

The third edition of this book was the first to include a chapter on information for patients and the public. At that time it was observed that medical libraries are largely concerned with the information needs of health-care professionals and health-care consumers are largely excluded. In the intervening years, a significant change has taken place. Medical libraries have had an increasing inclination and ability to provide information to patients. There has been a blossoming in new consumer health information services in centres like Southampton, Stevenage and Milton Keynes, combining the subject expertise of the medical library with the accessibility of the public library. At the same time there has been an unprecedented expansion in the amount of published literature on health topics for lay people. Consumer health information services are described in more detail in *The health information handbook* by R. Gann (Gower, 1986) and the literature is reviewed in *Informing health consumers* by E. Kempson (British Library/College of Health, 1987). The U.S. scene is comprehensively covered by *Managing consumer health information services* by Alan Rees (2nd edn., Oryx Press, 1990). This new edition also includes chapters on Canada, Australia, New Zealand and the UK.

There are a number of reasons for the above developments. One is undoubtedly an increasing consumerism in society generally, which is reflected in our behaviour as patients. People are no longer content to be told what is good for them; they want access to information which enables them to weigh up risks and benefits, and to make informed choices between options in health care. This new health consumerism has been encouraged by government health policies which emphasize consumer choice. The NHS White Paper *Working for patients* (HMSO, 1989 Cm 555) urged health authorities to provide to patients 'clear information about the facilities available ... and clear and thoughtful explanations of what is happening — on practical matters such as where to go and who to see, and on clinical matters such as the nature of the illness and its proposed treatment'. The subsequent NHS and Community Care Act 1990 aims to introduce a 'reformed' NHS in which 'provider units' (hospitals) attract patients through quality health care provision, which involves a greater level of patient information and education provision than ever before. GPs are being encouraged to 'shop around' for treatment where waiting times are shortest, leading to a demand for opening up previously closed areas of information on waiting lists. In turn the intention is that GPs will attract patients to their practices with practice information brochures, health promotion clinics and easier ways of changing doctor. The NHS reforms are deeply unpopular in many parts of the National Health Service, but there is no doubt that they have produced a fertile climate for the development of better information for patients.

The new health consumerism may in part be politically inspired but there is also a growing body of research evidence which is demonstrating that the provision of information to patients can have significant benefits. Giving patients information can lead to more truly informed consent, increased patient understanding and satisfaction, increased compliance with treatment, and quicker and less stressful recovery from illness and surgery. The most comprehensive overview of the topic, which analyses over 300 studies, is *Communicating with patients* by P. Ley (Croom Helm, 1988).

A further factor in the increased availability of health information for lay people has been a growing realization of the limitations of high-tech medicine in producing further real advances in the health status of the population. This has been recognized in a series of statements from the World Health Organization, supporting the goal of 'Health for All by the year 2000'. WHO's *Targets for health for all* (World Health Organization, 1985) sets 38 measurable targets for member states, covering not only medical concerns (reducing disease and disability) but also the promotion of healthy environments and personal healthy lifestyles. 'Health for all will be achieved by people themselves. A well-informed, well-motivated and actively participating community is a key element for attainment of the common goal.'

The global AIDS pandemic has been a grim reminder of the limitations of medical science. Doctors and scientists are as yet powerless in the face of a grave threat to the health of the population. The most effective weapon we have in the fight against HIV infection and AIDS is information — ensuring that ordinary people are informed about the real and imagined risks to their health, and that they adopt healthy and responsible life styles. The increasing importance of health information for the public was underlined most dramatically in 1987 by the delivery to every home in the UK of a government leaflet entitled, *AIDS: don't die of ignorance.*

Primary sources

Guides to services

In an increasingly diversified system of health and welfare provision, health-care consumers need guidance through the maze of rights, services and benefits. Two standard works were published in 1983: *A patient's guide to the National Health Service* (Consumers Association, 1983) and *Patients' rights: a guide for NHS patients and doctors* (National Consumer Council, 1983). Both are now in need of updating, although *Patients' rights* was made available in revised leaflet form in 1989. The British Medical Association book *Rights and responsibilities of patients and doctors* (BMA, 1988) provides a more academic view, but a second edition (to be published in 1992) promises to take more of a patient standpoint. The most up to date users' guide to the Health Service is now *The health care consumer guide* by R. Gann (Faber, 1991). This covers social welfare, self help and self care, and library and information sources, as well as health care under the NHS. For patients and GPs who wish to shop around for short waiting lists for treatment, the *Guide to hospital waiting lists* (College of Health, 1990) is a unique source. The guide simply suggests District Health Authorities with comparatively short waiting lists for particular specialties. For addresses of hospitals within those Districts consumers will need to use the *Hospitals and Health Services Yearbook* (Institute of Health Services Management, annual). *Why are we waiting: an analysis of hospital waiting lists* by J. Yates (OUP, 1987) is a fascinating exploration of why waiting lists occur. Those wishing to consult a practitioner of complementary medicine will find *The handbook of complementary medicine* by S. Fulder (2nd edn., OUP, 1988) the most comprehensive guide to the different therapies and their regulating bodies.

Looking beyond the NHS to social services and community care, the *Guide to the Social Services* (Family Welfare Association, annual) has been a standard reference book for over 100 years, covering personal social services, social security and health care. The most detailed guide to services and opportunities for disabled people is *Directory for dis-*

abled people by A. Darnbrough and D. Kinrade (5th edn., Woodhead-Faulkner, 1988), with sections on topics such as holidays, leisure, sex and legislation, as well as the usual information on benefits and statutory services. The *Disability rights handbook* (Disability Alliance, annual) is an indispensable and comprehensive guide to welfare rights and benefits for people with disabilities and their carers, which is updated with the benefit changes each year. Aids and equipment for disabled people are comprehensively described and illustrated in the *Equipment for disabled people* series of handbooks (Oxford Regional Health Authority). *Social Services Yearbook* (Longman, annual) is worth the expense as a directory of statutory agencies (health, social services, social security, education, etc.) as well as some voluntary bodies.

Directories of voluntary organizations and self-help groups abound. The most up to date is *The health directory* (Bedford Square Press, 1990) although *The voluntary agencies directory* (Bedford Square Press, 1989) is still useful for its wider coverage beyond health. *The self help guide: a directory of self help organisations in the UK*, edited by S. Knight and R. Gann (Chapman and Hall, 1988) is the most recent edition of the directory originally edited by S. Knight and called *Help! I need somebody*. *Charities digest* (Family Welfare Association, annual) is most useful for benevolent associations. The *Directory of British associations* (CBD Research, 1990) is expensive but comes into its own for more recondite queries.

Popular health books

Popular medical publishing is a boom area, with publications ranging from home medical encyclopaedias to slim self-help guides on specific disorders. Looking at the home doctor books, the *BMA complete family health encyclopaedia* (Dorling Kindersley, 1990) inevitably carries authority and is very comprehensive. The *New Macmillan guide to family health* (Macmillan, 1987) has the same editor (Tony Smith) and is not very different. An interesting alternative to the encyclopaedic approach is provided by *Take care of yourself* by D. M. Vickery and others (Unwin, 1980) which uses flow charts to aid self diagnosis and provide guidance on when professional advice should be sought. A new edition is long overdue. Another interesting format is provided by the U.S. patient education classic *Instructions for patients* by H. W. Griffith (4th edn., Saunders, 1989). This is a loose-leaf binder of single-page patient education sheets which can be removed and photocopied for patient use. Similar information is more cheaply presented for popular consumption in *The complete guide to symptoms, illness and surgery* by H. W. Griffith (Equation, 1985) but not in loose-leaf form. A cheap alternative to the weighty home doctor tomes for basic self-care advice is the practical little *Home doctor: an A–Z guide* by V. G. Daniels (Cambridge Medical Books, 1986).

A growing body of research is demonstrating that patients who have information about what to expect from medical treatment experience less stress and anxiety, and make a better recovery. Going into hospital for surgery is one of the most stressful experiences we face. There are two popular guides to surgery, both ten years old and surprisingly still not updated: *A dictionary of operations* by A. Stanway (Granada, 1981) and *A patient's guide to operations* by D. Delvin (Penguin, 1981). Unfamiliar tests and investigative procedures can be equally anxious experiences. The *Thorsons guide to medical tests* by J. Trevelyan and D. Dowson (Thorsons, 1989) fills a gap in the popular market. Before the appearance of the Thorsons book, *Handbook of investigations* by J. A. Booth (Harper and Row, 1983) was the only comparatively simple guide to tests and this still offers more detail than Trevelyan and Dowson.

Although most people receive hospital care at some time in their lives, most everyday health care is self care. The most common form of self care is self medication and many patients will seek information about side effects, contraindications etc. The standard popular work is *Medicines: a guide for everybody* by P. Parish (6th edn., Penguin, 1989). Now in its sixth edition, Parish is up to date, easy to use and affordable. A new addition to the field is the *British Medical Association guide to medicines and drugs* (Dorling Kindersley, 1988). As with the BMA's *Complete family health encyclopaedia*, this popular pharmacopoeia combines authority with an attractive design. Single page summaries use clear pictograms to present information on adverse effects, precautions and interactions in a standard format. Single-sheet summaries are also used in a new loose-leaf guide *A–Z of medicines: a carer's guide* (North East Thames RHA, 1989). *A consumer's guide to prescriptive medicines* by B. Copper and L. Gerlis (Hamlyn, 1990) is a straight forward alphabetical listing of drugs under trade and non-proprietary names.

There are literally thousands of popular health titles currently in print and this review could not, of course, list them all. The library, consumer health information service or patient collection in general practice would need access to some major titles on topics such as women's health and child care in addition to the more general books listed above. *Our bodies ourselves* was an early milestone in patient empowerment when it was first published by the Boston Women's Health Collective in 1971. The latest UK edition is *The new our bodies ourselves*, edited by A. Phillips and J. Rakusen (Penguin, 1989). It remains the definitive guide to self care for women. There is a wide range of books on child care, and parents will make their choice according to their personal approaches and values. Many will want to have *Baby and child* by P. Leach (Michael Joseph, 1988). There are probably almost as many books on HIV/AIDS as on child care by now. The most comprehensive and accessible book for the general reader, person with HIV or carer is *Caring for someone with AIDS*, edited by D. Yelding (Consumers' Association, 1990). Library and information services dealing with HIV enquiries on a regular basis will need the huge and all-embracing *National AIDS manual* (NAM Publications, 1990 and regular updates). The best general guide to the different cancers, screening and treatment is *Cancer: a guide for patients and their families* by C. and S. Williams (Wiley, 1986). On mental health there are two useful books: *Not on your own: the MIND guide to mental health* by S. Burningham (Penguin, 1989) and *Understanding mental health* by A. Gibbs (Consumers Association, 1986).

Several publishers now have impressive lists of titles on health topics. Series worth looking for are the Churchill Livingstone *Patient handbooks*, *The facts*, from Oxford University Press, Sheldon Press's *Overcoming common problems* series, and the *Positive health guides* published by Macdonald Optima. These series are reviewed in more detail in 'Health information — in everyone's good books' by R. Gann, *Self Health*, December 1987, 26–27.

Journals

Health stories abound in the general press, and the 'quality' newspapers all have their regular health pages. Problem pages of women's magazines probably provide health information to a wider audience than any other print medium. In 1979, 'agony aunt' Claire Rayner reported that she receives 40 000 letters a year (*Journal of Advanced Nursing*, 1979, **4**, 69–77). Several popular magazines deal entirely with health topics and are widely available in newsagents, supermarkets and health food shops: look for *Practical health* (South Bank Publishing) and *Here's Health* (Emap). The best health periodical for lay people is undoubtedly *Which Way to Health?* (Consumers' Association), which started life as the College of Health magazine *Self Health*. Published every two months, it includes medical news, consumer reports and practical health advice, and is mercifully free of advertising. The sister periodical from the Consumers' Association, *Which?*, includes a health feature in most monthly issues. *Health Matters* (Health Matters Publications) provides a more political perspective on current health issues. Although primarily designed for community health councils, *Community Health News* (Association of Community Health Councils for England & Wales) is of interest to a wider readership for its health news, parliamentary round-up, and reviews of publications.

For updates on community health initiatives and projects *Community Health Bulletin* (National Community Health Resource) is required reading. The bulletin comes with the equally useful *Women's Health Network News*. The bulletin of the National Self Help Support Centre, *Mutual Aid and Self Help*, includes articles, news and reviews on self-help activities in the UK and abroad. The wider issues of volunteering, both on an individual basis and through voluntary agencies, are covered in *Volunteers* (Volunteer Centre).

For news of health promotion and health education activities get on the mailing list for the Health Education Authority's free newspaper *Health Education News*. *Positive Health* (World Health Organization/Health Promotion Authority for Wales) has a more international view and also covers public health issues, healthy cities, etc. *Public Health News* (Bureau of Hygiene and Tropical Diseases) gives short reports on contemporary public and environmental health topics, such as salmonellosis, bovine spongiform encephalopathy and drinking water quality, based on articles in the general and medical press. On the philosophies and politics of health promotion, *Radical Health Promotion* (Radical Health Promotion Cooperative) is usually stimulating.

Most voluntary organizations and self-help groups issue journals or at least newsletters. There are several hundred of these but the following are some of the most generally useful. On disability topics, *Caring* (incorporating *Handicapped Living* and published by A.E. Morgan) is of interest partly because it is the one disability magazine to appear in newsagents. The Spastics' Society newspaper *Disability Now* is relevant beyond the specific area of cerebral palsy, as is *Spinal Injuries Association Newsletter* beyond spinal injuries. For mental health topics *Open Mind* (MIND) is indispensable.

The rights of parents and the quality of care of children in hospital are covered attractively and sympathetically in *NAWCH Update* (National Association for the Welfare of Children in Hospital). Parents of children with rare syndromes and the professionals working with them will realize the great value of *In Touch* (produced by Mrs Ann Worthington of the In Touch Trust from her own home). *In Touch* contains information not easily found elsewhere, including shared advice on coping with handicapped children and contacts for many rare conditions. The National Childbirth Trust magazine *New Generation* treats its readers particularly intelligently, with well-referenced book reviews and research summaries. Enquiring women will also find *Women's Health and Reproductive Rights Newsletter* (WHRRIC) stimulating and informative.

Of the many new periodicals on HIV/AIDS, the most useful for professionals and interested lay people alike are *AIDS Newsletter* (Bureau of Hygiene and Tropical Diseases) and *AIDS Letter* (Royal Society of Medicine). Both include summaries of articles from other journals as well as their own editorial features. On cancer, *BACUP News* (BACUP) is a particularly good example of a patient newspaper, covering developments in treatment and prevention. *Link-up* (Cancerlink) has a particular emphasis on cancer and self help.

Secondary sources

Printed indexes and current awareness

The unique UK index to health literature at a lay level is *Popular Medical Index* (Mede Publishing), edited by Sally Knight of the Health Information Service in Stevenage. Issued quarterly with an annual cumulation, it indexes popular medical books, selected professional journals (*BMJ, The Lancet, Nursing Times, Scientific American*, etc.), and popular periodicals including women's magazines. The U.S. equivalent is *Consumer Health and Nutrition Index* (Oryx Press), edited by Alan Rees. This also covers specialized and general sources of consumer health information. For access to the literature of voluntary activity, the best source is *Community Currents* (Community Development Foundation). Described as 'the community development information digest', this bimonthly publication provides abstracts for items in over 180 journals, books and unpublished reports.

For current awareness, the Health Education Authority library lists are invaluable. Three current awareness lists are available: *Recent Additions to the Library, Recent Additions to the Resource Centre* and *Journal Articles of Interest to Health Educators*. There are also HEA resource lists available on a range of individual topics. The quarterly journal *Health Libraries Review* (Blackwell) includes a regular column 'Consumer Health Information' (formerly 'Patient Information'). The column provides updates on consumer health information activities in Britain and abroad, and reviews new publications. Consumer health information has many of the characteristics of grey literature and keeping up to date requires a good deal of scanning of diverse sources. Voluntary organization bulletins and newsletters are particularly fruitful sources, in particular *RADAR Bulletin* (Royal Association for Disability and Rehabilitation) and *Age Concern Information Circular*. Another good source is the current-awareness newsletter which accompanies the *Disabled Living Foundation Information Service*.

Bibliographies and source books are published less frequently than current-awareness services but provide important overviews of the literature. A particularly noteworthy British example is *Reflections: a subject guide to fiction and biography on illness and disability*, edited by R. Tabor and J. Stephenson (3rd edn., Wessex Regional Library and Information Service, 1989). First published in 1981, *Reflections* provides annotated entries for over 900 works of fiction, biography and autobiography which provide an insight into the experience of illness and disability. Unmatched in Britain, the entire American consumer health information literature scene is reviewed in *The consumer health information source book*, edited by A.M. Rees and C. Hoffman (3rd edn., Oryx Press, 1990). The source book includes descriptive evaluations of 750 books, over 700 pamphlets, 70 popular periodicals, and several hundred hotlines, information services and other organizations. The full texts of many of the pamphlets listed are available in microform in *Consumer health information service* (University Microfilms).

Electronic sources

Online

When this chapter first appeared in *Information sources in the medical sciences* 3rd edn., there were no online or other databases for consumer health information. The fact that this section appears in the fourth edition is due not only to developing technologies but also to the growing scale and respectability of the subject area.

The major online bibliographic database is CHID: COMBINED HEALTH INFORMATION DATABASE. Available through BRS since 1985, CHID contains references to consumer health information and health promotion materials, including formally published and grey literature and audio-visual materials. Also included are health promotion projects currently in progress in the USA. Managed by agencies of the United States Public Health Service, the database contains 13 sub-files (on subjects including AIDS, Alzheimer's disease, arthritis, diabetes, digestive diseases, eye care, hypertension, kidney disease, health promotion and patient education). Although there are a few British references, the coverage is unfortunately very largely American. Other BRS databases which index material of relevance to consumer health information and health promotion are ALCOHOL INFORMATION FOR CLINICIANS AND EDUCATORS, CONSUMER DRUG INFORMATION, CANCERLIT, HAZARDLINE, TOXLINE AND NURSING AND ALLIED HEALTH. Some of the databases are also available via other hosts, and most British health-care librarians will be familiar with using Data-Star. There are some references to consumer health information on the major medical databases like MEDLINE, particularly under the *MeSH* term 'Patient education'. Consumer health information services are unlikely to be able to afford subscriptions to many of the major medical journals, so the availability of full-text databases like the COMPREHENSIVE CORE MEDICAL LIBRARY (CCML) is likely to prove attractive for occasional use.

Online coverage of UK consumer health information is still limited. Health stories in the general press are covered by BMA PRESS CUTTINGS on Data-Star. The BUREAU OF HYGIENE AND TROPICAL DISEASES AIDS DATABASE is available via DIMDI, and the Bureau's PUBLIC HEALTH NEWS is expected to be similarly available before long. Two important UK databases are available online direct from their producers: VOLNET UK and DLF-DATA. VOLNET is produced jointly by the Volunteer Centre and the Community Development Foundation. It consists of over 18 000 references to books, journal articles, reports, etc. on community development and voluntary action, including a reasonable health coverage. VOLNET is geared to the needs of the community and voluntary sector so charges are kept low, with an annual subscription giving unlimited access. DLF-DATA is the online version of the Disabled Living Foundation Information Service. The major file is the equipment database containing details of over 15 000 technical aids and daily living equipment for disabled people. There is also an 'Equipment mart' which offers a unique facility for sale and purchase of second-hand equipment. The DLF Library database is also available on DLF-DATA and there are plans to add new files including a directory of organizations and holiday information. A CD-ROM version of DLF-DATA is being developed which allows high-quality illustrations to accompany descriptions of aids and equipment. DLF-DATA is also a major element of Handynet, the European multi-lingual information on disability.

Portable databases

Some of the most interesting developments in access to consumer health information today are in the area of 'portable databases' (information on floppy disc or CD-ROM). The most comprehensive coverage of British consumer health information is provided by HELPBOX, the database developed by Help for Health. Sub-files provide details of national self-help organizations, popular health books, and self help leaflets. Available on subscription as a set of floppy discs, HELPBOX is in use in over 80 libraries, health promotion departments and similar organizations throughout the UK. Most subscribers are using Helpbox with the database management package CARDBOX-PLUS (Business Simulations), but there is a dBase version called HELPBASE (developed by Health Matters in Milton Keynes) and it is also available on some health authority networks.

The American *Consumer Health and Nutrition Index* (see above) is now also available on CD-ROM through the NISC DISC CONSUMERS INDEX. Alan Rees's *Consumer health information source book* is also available on CD-ROM as part of the HEALTH REFERENCE CENTER (Information Access). The HEALTH REFERENCE CENTER may point the way forward for easy access to consumer health information. One disc contains a shelf of consumer health reference books (a medical dictionary, a home medical encyclopaedia, a book of medical tests, and a pharmacopoeia), an index to several hundred popular health and professional journals many of them in full text, and a directory of support groups and information services. At the moment the high cost and almost exclusively U.S. coverage makes the HEALTH REFERENCE CENTER of limited interest to UK consumer health information providers. But as CD-ROM technology becomes increasingly cheaper the potential for swift and comprehensive access to information for patients and the public is enormous.

CHAPTER TWENTY-FOUR

Historical, biographical and bibliographical sources

E.J. FREEMAN

History

There is no hope of compressing a complete or even reasonably comprehensive survey of writing on the history of medicine into the space of a single chapter. All that is attempted here is to provide the neophyte and particularly the amateur historian and the busy medical student with a bibliographical *entrée* to a fast-growing subject. What follows may also be of use to those medical librarians who are required by sentiment and tradition to maintain a 'history corner' in their libraries.

Professionals, and those with serious scholarly aspirations, are well served by a sister-title in this series, *Information sources in the history of medicine and science*, edited by Pietro Corsi and Paul Weindling (Butterworth Scientific, 1983). A new edition of this valuable book is much needed.

The 'social history of medicine' was described in the last edition of this guide as the 'dominant trend'. It is now the dominant mode, although there are signs, welcome to some, of a resurgence of interest in narrative history and biography, albeit both transformed by the social history experience.

No one has yet produced an uncontroversial definition of what is, precisely, the social history of medicine. The product is easier to recognize than to describe. Its distinguishing marks are the assumption that medicine is always relative to the society and culture that produces it. Further, that medicine, society and culture are best studied, described and explained in terms of patterns, structures and models. Above all, the medicine of the past, or of other cultures, must not be described in categories derived exclusively from the (Western) science of the present day. 'History in context' is the basis of the social historian's creed. At its worst a passing fashion (the 'constipation and society' mode, as one critic put it), the social history of medicine more usually sins by promising more than it can deliver. In the hands of its finest practitioners, the social approach to medical history is an illuminating and exciting entry to the medicine of the past.

The standard source books for the history of medicine, such as *Morton's Medical bibliography* (5th edn., revised by J. Norman, Gower, 1991) and Blake and Roos' *Medical reference works, 1679-1966* (MLA, 1967), *Supplement 1, 1967–68* compiled by M.V. Clarke (1970); *Supplement 2, 1969–72* (1973) and *Supplement 3, 1973–74* (1975) both compiled by J.S. Richmond, do not reflect the particular interests of the social history of medicine in their selection of either primary or secondary sources. The student must take into account the bibliographies of general history and the social sciences in order to ensure contact with the latest and best work. (See also sections on Bibliography and Indexes above.) A recent and solid guide, although appealing more perhaps to librarians than to historians, is *Thornton's Medical books, libraries and collectors: a study of bibliography and the book trade in relation to the medical sciences* (3rd revised edition by Alain Besson *et al.*, Gower, 1990). The ten chapters vary somewhat in quality but all have extensive bibliographic annotation. This book has been plundered unmercifully for present purposes.

General

Single-author general histories of medicine are now unusual and examples are often the result of amateur as opposed to professional endeavours. Professionalization of history of medicine has inevitably produced specialization and historians no longer care to attempt single-handed the grand general syntheses of their forebears. The older English-language one-volume histories are best avoided. Attempts are still made to survey the whole field and the results can have value as appetizers. Recent examples include Philip Rhodes', *An outline history of medicine* (Butterworths, 1985) and Vernon Coleman's, *The story of medicine* (Hale, 1985). For primary orientation in the field the student is referred to the essays in Pietro Corsi and Paul Weindling (*Information Sources in the history of medicine and science*, Butterworth Scientific, 1983). A useful contrast of two 'how to do it' collections of essays published 15 years apart can be made: Edwin Clarke's *Modern methods in the history of medicine* (Athlone Press, 1971) and Roy Porter and Andrew Wear's edition of essays, *Problems and methods in the history of medicine* (Croom Helm, 1987). Two histories of science retain their value as general introductions to the field, S.F. Mason's *A history of the sciences* (rev. edn., Collier, 1962) and A.C. Crombie's *Augustine to Galileo*, last printed in a one-volume edition (Heinemann, 1979). Not a comprehensive history, W.P.D. Wightman's *The emergence of scientific medicine* (Oliver and Boyd, 1971) is a trim paperback masterpiece which traces the evolution of medical concepts from classical times to the seventeenth century. Also well worth consulting are Erwin H. Ackerknecht, *A short history of medicine* (rev. edn., Johns Hopkins University Press, 1982) and F.F. Cartwright, *A social history of medicine* (Longman, 1977, reprinted 1983), both available in paperback. Readers of European languages should consider: in German, C. Lichten-thaeler, *Geschichte der Medizin* (2 vols, 3rd edn., Deutscher Ärzte-Verlag, 1982), available also in French (A. Fayard, 1978); E. Fischer-Homberger, *Geschichte der Medizin* (2nd edn., Springer, 1977); in Italian, V. Busacchi, *Storia della medicina* (2nd edn., Patron, 1978); A. Pazzini, *Storia dell'arte sanitaria dalle origini a oggi* (2 vols, Minerva Medica, 1973–74). P.T. Durbin has edited *A guide to the culture of science, technology and medicine* (Free Press, 1980), a valuable introduction to seventies' historiography which would be well worth revision and up-dating. Chapter 3 is on the history of medicine. An unusual (for modern times) approach is reflected in H.L. Coulter's *Divided legacy: a history of the schism in medical thought* (3 vols, Wehawken Book Co., 1973–77; Vol. 3 has imprint McGrath). The author maintains that 'medical thinkers in western culture may be divided into two traditions — those who attribute primary importance to the sensory data of experience being opposed to those who seek the reality assumed to lie behind the sensory data'.

Of the specialist varieties of history, J. Barzun's *Clio and the doctors: psycho-history, quanto-history and history* (Chicago University Press, 1974) is an interesting survey. L. Demause has edited a collection of essays on a particularly controversial type of historical investigation, *The new psychohistory* (Psychohistory Press, 1975). His *Foundations of psychohistory* (Creative Roots, 1982) should also be consulted. No longer new, a recent representative of the genre is Peter Loewenberg, *Decoding the past: the psychohistorical approach* (Alfred A. Knopf, 1982; reprinted. 1983). This book explores 'the frontier between the humanistic, social, political, analytic, and narrative crafts of history and the clinical art of psychoanalysis'.

Collections of essays by acknowledged masters may be suggestive alternatives to survey histories. Examples from each side of the Atlantic are Owsei Temkin, *The double face of Janus and other essays in the history of medicine* (Johns Hopkins University Press, 1977) and two volumes of the writings of Walter Pagel, edited by Marianne Winder, *From Paracelsus to Van Helmont: studies in Renaissance medicine and science* (Variorum Reprints, 1986) and *Religion and neoplatonism in Renaissance medicine* (Variorum Reprints, 1985).

The gap left by the virtual demise of one-volume histories has been overfilled by multi-volumed, many-authored histories, affordable only by libraries and of value chiefly for their often magnificent illustrations. Examples are *Historia universal de la medicina* edited by P. Lain Entralgo (7 vols, Salvat, 1972–75), and *Histoire de la médecine, de la pharmacie, de l'art dentaire, et de l'art vétérinaire* by J.C. Sournia *et al.* (A. Michel, etc., 1978), available also in German (8 vols, plus index volume, Andreas, 1980); and A.S. Lyons and R.J. Petrucelli, *Medicine: an illustrated history* (Abrams, 1978).

Period histories and special topics

PREHISTORY

Diseases in antiquity by D. Brothwell and A.T. Sandison (C.C. Thomas, 1967) is complemented by D. Brothwell's *Digging up bones. The excavation, treatment and study of human skeletal remains* (2nd edn., British Museum Natural History, 1972). *Human palaeopathology*, edited by Saul Jarcho (Yale University Press, 1966) is the proceedings of a symposium and the findings described are mostly from digs in the USA. *Bones, bodies and disease* by C. Wells (Thames and Hudson, 1964) comprises essays on different types of abnormalities, cannibalism, vital statistics, etc. *History of medicine, Vol. 1, Primitive and archaic medicine* by Henry E. Sigerist (OUP, 1951, available since 1987 in paperback) is still useful but needs supplementing by later work, such as *Mummies, disease and ancient cultures* by A. and E. Cockburn (CUP, 1980) L.R. Binford, *Bones: ancient man and modern myths* (Academic Press, 1981); Keith Manchester, *The archaeology of disease* (Bradford University Press, 1983) a fairly technical treatment of diagnostic signs; and A. Stirland, *Human bones in archaeology* (Shire Publications, 1986). The most famous palaeopathological investigation of the century is recorded in I.M. Stead *et al.* (eds.), *Lindow Man: the body in the bog* (British Museum, 1986) and D. Brothwell, *The Bog Man and the archaeology of people* (British Museum, c. 1986).

ANCIENT

F. Köcher, *Die babylonisch-assyrische Medizin in Texten und Untersuchungen* (W. de Gruyter, 1963–) is a continuing series (6 vols to date, 1980) reproducing texts with commentary. A.P. Leca, *La Médecine Egyptienne au temps des Pharaons* (R. Dacosta, 1971) is an attractively produced book as, on similar topics, is P. Ghaliounghi, *The house of life. Magic and medical science in Ancient Egypt* (2nd edn., B.M. Israël, 1973). H.E. Sigerist, *History of medicine, Vol. 2, Early Greek, Hindu and Persian Medicine* (OUP, 1961, available since 1987 in paperback) encroaches on the classical period, as does G. Majno, *The healing hand: man and wound in the Ancient World* (Harvard University Press, 1975), an extraordinary *tour de force* by an eminent American surgeon. Manchester University has become a leading centre for the scientific study of mummies, hence *Evidence embalmed: modern medicine and the mummies of Ancient Egypt* (Manchester University Press, 1984), edited by Rosalie David and Eddie Trapp and the conference papers edited also by Rosalie David, *Science in egyptology* (Manchester University Press, *c.* 1986). Marshall Clagett has produced what promises to be a useful guide in *Ancient Egyptian science: a source book* (American Philosophical Society, 1989). Volume 1 is entitled *Knowledge and order* and he promises to deal with medicine and biology in a forthcoming Volume 3.

CLASSICAL

Fine general introductions to Greek science and medicine are G.R. Lloyd's two volumes, *Early Greek science: Thales to Hippocrates* (Chatto and Windus, 1970) and *Greek science after Aristotle* (Chatto and Windus, 1973) both now in paperback, which are supplemented by his later books, *Magic, reason and experience: studies in the origin and development of Greek science* (CUP, 1979) and *The revolutions of wisdom: studies in the claims and practice of ancient greek science* (University of California, *c.* 1987) also available in paperback. Older, but still useful, is L. Edelstein, *Ancient medicine* (Johns Hopkins University Press, 1967, paperback in 1987), the essays of a profoundly learned scholar, now dead. M.D. Grmek's survey is available in English as *Diseases in the Ancient Greek world* (Johns Hopkins University Press, 1988). The Loeb texts of Hippocrates, with English translations (Vols 1–4, edited by W.H.S. Jones, Heinemann, 1923–31; Vols 5–6, edited by Paul Potter, Heinemann, 1988) have a useful, selected, complement in *Hippocratic writings* (new edition, with additional material, Penguin, 1978, much reprinted) edited by G.E.R. Lloyd. Paul Potter has also produced a useful *Short handbook of Hippocratic medicine* (Québec, Editions du Sphinx, 1988). John Scarborough's *Roman medicine* (Thames and Hudson, 1969) is now joined by Ralph Jackson's *Doctors and diseases in the Roman Empire* (British Museum, 1988) which lays particular stress on archaeological evidence. E.D. Phillips' *Greek Medicine* (Thames and Hudson, 1973) has been re-issued as *Aspects of Greek medicine* (Croom Helm, 1987) but without the revision its author might have given it had he lived. Phillips' relative neglect of Galen may be compensated for by the excellent introduction on Greco-Roman anatomy and physiology which prefaces M. Tallmadge May's translation of *De usu partium* (2 vols, Cornell University Press, 1968). Scholarly research on Galen may be sampled in *Galen: problems and prospects*, edited by Vivian Nutton (Wellcome Institute for the History of Medicine, 1981) whose collected essays *From Democedes to Harvey: studies in the history of medicine* (Variorum, 1988) may be studied with profit. The importance of the so-called School of Alexandria in the transmission of Ancient medical thought is a lively area of research. A profound study by Heinrich van Staden appeared in 1988, *Herophilus: the art of medicine in early Alexandria* (CUP). The pervasive influence of classical medicine on later times may be studied in J. Scarborough's edition of papers on *Byzantine medicine* (Dumbarton Oaks Papers, Vol. 38, 1985) and particularly in O. Temkin, *Galenism: rise and decline of a medical philosophy* (Cornell University Press, 1973) and Wesley D. Smith, *The Hippocratic tradition* (Cornell University Press, 1979).

MEDIEVAL

In spite of the fact that George Sarton loathed everything characteristically medieval, his *Introduction to the history of science* (3 vols in 5, Williams and Wilkins, 1927–48) is now, and is likely to remain, the basic, indispensable bio-bibliographic guide to the period. General histories of medieval medicine in English have the general limitation of relying too exclusively on UK materials. The best are still C.H. Talbot, *Medicine in Medieval England* (Oldbourne, 1967) and S. Rubin, *Medieval English medicine* (David and Charles, 1974). E.J. Keeley's medieval medicus. *A social history of Anglo-Norman medicine* (Johns Hopkins University Press, 1981) is an attractively written book, marred by the author's use of anachronistic concepts. The Early English Text Society provides, for readers of Anglo-Saxon, a text of *The Old English herbarium and medicina de quadrupedibus* (OUP, 1984), edited by H.J. de Vriend. Tony Hunt has contributed to our understanding of a slightly later period in *Plant names of medieval England* (D.S. Brewer, 1989) and *Popular medicine in thirteenth-century England* (D.S. Brewer, 1990). A great deal may be gleaned from the work of Peter M. Jones, most conveniently in his *Medieval medical miniatures* (British Library, *c.* 1984) and 'Medical Books before the Invention of Printing', being chapter 1 of *Thornton's Medical books, libraries and collectors* (3rd revised edition, Alain Besson *et al.*, Gower, 1990), see p. 556. Two profoundly learned works are by Brian Lawn, *Salernitan questions* (Clarendon Press, 1963) and *The prose Salernitan Questions* (OUP, 1979) which are brilliant analyses of medical question-and-answer texts.

Special topics are handled in S.N. Brody, *The disease of the soul: leprosy in medieval literature* (Cornell University Press, 1974); P. Richards, *The medieval leper and his northern heirs* (D.S. Brewer, 1977) and F. Bériac, *Histoire des lépreux au moyen age: une société d'exclus* (Imago, 1988). Danielle Jacquart, a French historian, has an interesting study (with Claude Thomasset) of *Sexuality and medicine in the Middle Ages* (Polity, 1988). The standard work on plague, medieval and later, is J.N. Biraben, *Les hommes et la peste en France et dans les Pays Européens et Méditerranéans* (2 vols, Mouton, 1975). The effect of plague on British history may be studied with the help of J. Hatcher, *Plague, population and the English economy, 1348–1530* (Macmillan, 1977). G. Twigg has a controversial solution to what the plague was in *The Black Death: a biological reappraisal* (Batsford, 1984). A fine study of a late medieval teacher is N.G. Siraisi, *Taddeo Alderotti and his pupils* (Princeton University Press, 1981). The same author has now produced *Medieval and Early Renaissance medicine: an introduction to knowledge and practice* (University Press of Chicago, 1990). Finally, the important topic of the medicine of the Islamic civilisation may be approached through E.G. Browne, *Arabian medicine* (CUP, 1921, reprinted 1962) which is now rather old-fashioned, and M. Ullmann, *Islamic medicine* (Edinburgh University Press, 1978) which is beginning to look rather conservative.

RENAISSANCE TO THE EIGHTEENTH CENTURY

Primary bibliographic orientation is provided by chapters 3-5 of *Thornton's Medical books* (see above) as revised by Yvonne Hibbott, Christine English and Patricia Want respectively. Nancy G. Siraisi spans the medieval–modern divide in her *Avicenna in Renaissance Italy: the canon and medical teaching in Italian universities after 1500* (Princeton University Press, *c.* 1987). The popular format of collected essays is a good way to get a feel of scholarly research in this period. Examples are: *Health, medicine and mortality in the 16th century*, edited by Charles Webster (CUP, 1979); *The medical Renaissance of the 16th century*, edited by Andrew Wear *et al.* (CUP, 1984); *Patients and practitioners: lay perceptions of medicine in pre-industrial society*, edited by Roy Porter (Cambridge U. P., 1985); *Famine, disease, and the social order in early modern society*, edited by John Waite and Roger Schofield (CUP, 1989) and Roger French and Andrew Wear's *The medical revolution of the 17th century* (CUP, 1989).

A.G. Debus, *The chemical philosophy. Paracelsian science and medicine in the 16th and 17th centuries* (2 vols, Neale Watson, 1977) offers a view of an important anti-Galenic movement. Anything by Walter Pagel is worth reading, although rarely easy going, for example his *Paracelsus: an introduction to philosophical medicine in the era of the Renaissance* (Karger, 1958) or his *William Harvey's biological ideas: selected aspects and historical background* (Karger, 1967). The latter study (and the subject is European, rather than merely British, in importance) may be supplemented by a collection of essays edited by J.J. Bylebyl, *William Harvey and his age* (Johns Hopkins University Press, 1979).

Charles Webster's *The great instauration: science, medicine and reform, 1626–1660* (Duckworth, 1975) is a good, though densely written, example of 'history in context'. Lester S. King's books are essential reading for students of eighteenth-century medicine. His *The road to medical enlightenment, 1650–1695* (Macdonald, 1970) examines the transition from Galenism to iatrochemistry and iatrophysics, whereas *The medical world of the 18th century* (Chicago University Press, 1958, reprinted by Krieger, 1971) and *The philosophy of medicine: the early 18th century* (Harvard University Press, 1978) both develop King's essential history of ideas view of the century.

NINETEENTH AND TWENTIETH CENTURIES

Many general studies draw their evidence from sources in particular countries so this section (and indeed the one preceding) need to be read in conjunction with those immediately following. One general work and one collection of essays provide a good beginning: Richard H. Shryock, *The development of modern medicine: an interpretation of the social and scientific factors involved* (Knopf, 1947, Wisconsin University Press, 1979 in paperback), and Charles Webster (ed.), *Biology, medicine and society, 1840–1940* (CUP, 1981).

Most of the following references draw their evidence from British or American sources:

Doctors and the state: the British medical profession and government action in public health, 1870-1912 by J.L. Brand (Johns Hopkins University Press, 1965)

Health care and popular medicine in 19th century England, edited by J. Woodward and D. Richards (Croom Helm, 1977) is a not entirely successful attempt to exemplify the social history approach

Half a century of medical research by Sir A.L. Thomson (2 vols, HMSO, 1973, 1975, reprinted by the Medical Research Council in 1987) deals with the rôle of government-funded research in terms of the history of the Medical Research Council

Antivivisection and medical science in Victorian society by R.D. French (Princeton University Press, 1975)

The division in British medicine. A history of the separation of general practice from hospital care, 1911-68 by F. Honigsbaum (Kogan Page, 1979)

Profession and monopoly: a study of medicine in the United States and Great Britain by J.L. Berlant (University of California Press, 1975)

The return of the plague: British society and cholera 1831-32 by M. Durey (Gill and Macmillan, 1979)

The scientific revolution in Victorian medicine by A.J. Youngson (Croom Helm, 1979)

The people's health 1830-1910 by F.B. Smith (Croom Helm, 1979) is a controversial but stimulating study notable for its 'anti-doctor' emphasis

Doctors in science and society: essays of a clinical scientist, by Sir Christopher Booth (BMJ, 1987)

Sexual visions: images of gender in science and medicine between the 18th and 20th centuries, by L.J. Jordanova (Harvester, 1989), a well-reviewed study which exemplifies the flourishing of women's studies within the history of medicine

By country and region

GREAT BRITAIN AND THE REPUBLIC OF IRELAND

Professional study of the medical history of Britain has burgeoned during the 1970s and 1980s. The social historian's concern to avoid anachronistic categorization is exemplified in the essays edited by W.F. Bynum and R. Porter, *Medical fringe and medical orthodoxy 1750–1850* (Croom Helm, 1982). Other collected essay volumes which give the flavour of recent research include the previous editors' *William Hunter and the 18th century medical world* (CUP, 1985) and *Urban disease and mortality in 19th century England* (Batsford Academic, (1984) edited by R. Woods and J. Woodward. The enormous output of Roy Porter, mostly on eighteenth-century matters, may be exemplified by his *Disease, medicine and society in England 1550–1860* (Macmillan Education, 1987); *Health for sale: quackery in England, 1660–1850* (Manchester University Press, 1989), and, with Dorothy Porter, *In sickness and in health: the English experience 1650–1850* (Fourth Estate, 1988) and *Patient's progress: doctors and doctoring in 18th century England* (Polity/Blackwell, 1989). Make of the disclaimer what you will, but the authors deny that the last title is either a history of medicine, nor even a social history of medicine ... rather, 'an exploration of the relations between sick people and their doctors in the premodern era'.

Among the many studies of the British experience in medicine may be noted: Lucinda M. Beier, *Sufferers and healers: the experience of illness in 17th century England* (Routledge, 1987); Paul Slack, *The impact of plague in Tudor and Stuart England* (Routledge, 1985); Harold J. Cook, *The decline of the old medical regime in Stuart England* (Cornell University Press, 1986); T. Forbes, *Surgeons at the Bailey: English forensic medicine to 1878* (Yale University Press, 1985); Ivan Waddington, *The medical profession in the Industrial Revolution* (Gill and Macmillan, 1984); Irvine Loudon, *Medical care and the general practitioner 1750–1850* (Clarendon Press, 1987); Ruth Richardson, *Death, dissection and the destitute* (Routledge, 1987) on the social context of the Anatomy Act 1832, and, as an example of many local studies, Hilary Marland's *Medicine and society in Wakefield and Huddersfield, 1780–1870* (CUP, 1987). The Celtic regions of Britain may be studied in: *Wales and medicine. An historical survey*, edited by John Cule (J.D. Lewis, 1975) which contains papers given at the 9th British Congress on the History of Medicine held at Swansea and Cardiff in 1973; David Hamilton, *The healers: a history of medicine in Scotland* (Canongate, 1981; reprinted 1987); E. O'Brien *et al.*, *Portrait of Irish medicine* (Royal College of Surgeons in Ireland, 1984); and J.F. Fleetwood, *The history of medicine in Ireland* (2nd edn., Skelling Press, 1983).

USA

Publications include:

Public health in the town of Boston, 1630–1822 by J.B Blake (Harvard University Press, 1959)

Medicine and society in America, 1660–1860 by R.H. Shryock (New York University Press, 1960)

American Medicine and the public interest by R. Stevens (Yale University Press, 1971), studies the effects of specialization and government medical care in the twentieth century

Medicine in New England 1790–1840 by B. Riznik (2nd edn., Old Sturbridge Village, 1969)

Medical men at the Seige [sic] of Boston, April 1775–April 1776: problems of the Massachusetts and Continental armies by P. Cash (American Philosophical Society, 1973)

Theory and practice in American medicine: historical studies from the Journal of the History of Medicine, edited by G.H. Brieger (Science History Publications, 1976)

Two centuries of American medicine (1776–1976) by J. Bordley and A.M. Harvey (Saunders, 1976)

Advances in American medicine: essays at the bicentennial, edited by J.Z. Bowers and E.F. Purcell (2 vols, J. Macy, 1976)

Adventures in medical research: a century of discovery at Johns Hopkins by A.M. Harvey (Johns Hopkins University Press, 1976)

A centennial history of medicine at Johns Hopkins by A.M.Harvey *et al.* (2 vols, Johns Hopkins University Press, 1989)

The healers: the rise of American medicine by J. Duffy (McGraw-Hill, 1976)

The Therapeutic Revolution. Essays in the social history of American medicine edited by M.J. Vogel and Charles E. Rosenberg (University of Pennsylvania Press, 1979)

The above titles should now be supplemented by:

The structure of American medical practice, 1875-1941 by George Rosen (University of Pennsylvania Press, 1983)

The therapeutic perspective: medical practice, knowledge and identity in America, 1820–1885 by J.H. Warner (University of Illinois Press, 1986)

Medicine in the New World: New Spain, New France and New England, essays edited by R.L. Numbers (University of Tennessee Press, 1987)

The College of Physicians of Philadelphia: a bicentennial history, by Whitfield J. Bell (Science History Publishers, 1987)

Yellow fever in the North: the methods of early epidemiology, by William Coleman (University of Wisconsin Press, 1987)

EUROPE

E.H. Ackerknecht's *Medicine at the Paris Hospital, 1794–1848* (Johns Hopkins University Press, 1967) is on the rise of clinical medicine in Europe. John E. Lesch has a complementary text in his *Science and medicine in France: the emergence of experimental physiology, 1790-1855* (Harvard University Press, 1984). Also on the French experience and influence are: E. Haigh, *Xavier Bichat and the medical theory of the 18th century* (Wellcome Institute for the History Medicine, 1984); M. Ramsey, *Professional and popular medicine in France, 1770-1830: the social world of medical practice* (CUP, 1988), and A.C. Saucerotte, *Les médecins pendant la Révolution* (new edition, L. Pariente, *c.* 1989). Carlo M. Cipolla, *Public health and the medical profession in the Renaissance* (CUP, 1976) is drawn from Italian local archive sources. Also on Italian themes are: Katharine Park, *Doctors and medicine in early Renaissance Florence* (Princeton University Press, *c.* 1985) and Ann G. Carmichael, *Plague and the poor in early Renaissance Florence* (CUP, 1986). Recent work on Germany may be represented by Richard J. Evans' brilliant study, *Death in Hamburg: society and politics in the cholera years*, 1830–1910 (Clarendon Press, 1987). Other, earlier studies on European medicine include:

Medicine and society in France, edited by R. Forster and O. Ranum (Johns Hopkins University Press, 1980) which reprints translated essays from the French history journal *Annales*

Histoire de la médecine Belge by F.A. Sondervorst (Elsevier Librico, 1981)

Medical revolution in France 1789–1796 by D.M. Vess (University of Florida Press, 1975)

Geschichte der medizinischen Wissenschaften in Deutschland by A. Hirsch was published as long ago as 1893, but reprinted by Johnson Reprint Corp., New York, 1966, and is a still useful and detailed history of the eighteenth and nineteenth centuries, with a brief review of earlier periods

The Vienna Medical School of the 19th century by E. Lesky (translated by L. Williams and I.S. Levij, Johns Hopkins University Press, 1976)

Historia social de la medicina en la España de los siglos XIII al XVI, Vol. 1, La Minoria Musulmana y Morisca by L. Garcia Ballester (Akal, 1976)

Storia della medicina e della sanitá in Italia ... 1348–1918 by G. Cosmacini (Laterza, 1987)

AFRICA

Work on the indigenous, as well as the European-influenced, medical history of Africa is a growth industry:

Religion and healing in Mandari by J.C. Buxton (Clarendon Press, 1973)

A service to the sick. A history of the health services for Africans in Southern Rhodesia, 1890–1953 by M. Gelfand (Mambo Press, 1976), also his *Christian doctor and nurse: the history of medical missions in South Africa from 1799–1976* (Mariannhill Mission, 1984)

Body and soul in Zulu medicine by H. Ngubane (Academic Press, 1977)

African folk medicine. Practices and beliefs of the Bambara and other peoples by P.J. Imperato (York Press, 1977)

Disease in African history. An introductory survey and case studies, edited by G.W. Martwig and K.D. Patterson (Duke University Press, 1978)

Pestilence and disease in the history of Africa by J.N.P. Davies (Witwatersrand University Press, 1979)

African pioneers of modern medicine by A. Adeloye (OUP, 1982)

Medicine and power in Tunisia, 1780–1900, by N.E. Gallagher (CUP, 1983).

Yoruba medicine, by Anthony D. Buckley (Clarendon Press, 1985)

Medicine, tradition and development in Kenya and Tanzania, 1920–1970, by A. Beck (Crossroads Press, 1982)

Imperial medicine and indigenous societies, essays edited by David Arnold (Manchester University Press, 1988)

ORIENT

Islamic

For Arabic medicine reference should be made to the titles listed under the medieval period (above), supplemented by S.H. Nasr's *Islamic science — an illustrated study* (World of Islam Festival, 1976), which, along with other studies by the same author, presents an interesting though controversial view of traditional Arabic medicine through the eyes of a prominent modern Islamic thinker. Cyril Elgood's *Safavid medical practice* (Luzac, 1970) covers medicine, surgery and gynaecology in Persia from AD 1500 to AD 1750. Elgood's more general account, *A medical history of Persia and the Eastern Caliphate from the earliest times ... until 1932*, was published in 1951 and reprinted (APA-Philo, 1979). D. Brandenburg's *Priesterärzte und Heilkunst im alten Persien* (J. Fink, 1969) discusses medicine in the writings of Zarathustra and Firdausi, while Volume 2, Part 2 of C.A. Storey's *Persian literature: a bibliographical survey* (Royal Asiatic Society., 1958–1971) is basic for the serious student.

Z.M. Agha has produced a valuable *Bibliography of Islamic medicine and pharmacy* (Brill, 1983).

China

For China, P. Huard and Ming Wong's *Chinese medicine* (World University Library, 1968), translated from the French, emphasizes the continuity of Chinese medicine down to modern times. R.C. Crozier's *Traditional medicine in modern China* (Harvard University Press, 1968) looks at the relationship of medicine to cultural and intellectual developments in China since 1800. Joseph Needham's *Clerks and craftsmen in China and the West* (CUP, 1970) includes essays on protoendocrino-logy in medieval China, elixir poisoning, hygiene and examinations. Needham's *Science and civilization in China* (6 vols in 15, CUP, 1954–) is a definitive account by a brilliant scientist and scholar leading a team of Chinese experts. (*A Shorter science and civilization in China*, 1980– is now available; Vols 1–3 edited by C.A. Ronan, in hard cover and paperback.) *Modern China and traditional Chinese medicine*, edited by G.B. Risse (C.C. Thomas, 1973) and *Medicine and society in China*, edited by J.Z. Bowers and E.F. Purcell (J. Macy Jr. Fnd., 1974) are col-lections of essays with complementary emphases.

Paul U. Unschuld has produced a series of works of high scholarship, including: *Medicine in China: a history of pharmaceutics* (University of California Press, 1985) *Medicine in China: a history of ideas* (Univer-sity of California Press, 1985); *Introductory readings in classical Chinese medicine* (Kluwer, 1988); and *Approaches to traditional Chinese medical literature* (Kluwer, 1988). For the modern period S.M. Hillier and J.A. Jewell's *Health care and traditional medicine in China 1800–1982* (Routledge, 1983) is available, while Yasuyori Tamba links China with its main medical beneficiary in *The essentials of medicine in Ancient China and Japan* (translated with introduction and annotation by E.C.H. Hsia, Ilsa Veith and R.H. Geertsma, 2 vols, Brill, 1986). Japanese medicine is described in M. Wong, P. Huard and Z. Ohya's *La médecine japonais des origines ä nos jours* (R. Dacosta, 1974). W.W. Farris deals with the remote past in his *Population, disease and land in early Japan, 645–900* (Harvard University Press, 1985) while Hugh Cortazzi, erstwhile British Ambassador in Tokyo, has written about an interesting European episode in *Dr. Willis in Japan, 1862-1877* (Ath-lone Press, 1985).

Tibetan medicine is best studied in E. Finckh's *Foundations of Tibet-an medicine* (Vol. 1, Watkins, 1978; Vol. 2, Robinson Books, 1985).

India

Much writing on traditional Indian medicine is of a disappointingly poor quality. J. Jolly's *Indian medicine*, translated from the original German and supplemented by C. G. Kashikar (2nd rev. edn., Munshir-am Marshareal, 1977), although an old book, is still one of the best accounts. O.P. Jaggi's *History of science and technology in India* (15 vols to date, 1973–) is the most ambitious modern account, also closely rivalled in bulk by a similarly titled work in 12 volumes, edited by G. Kuppuram and K. Kumudamani (Sundeep Prakashan, 1990). Perhaps the best introduction to current scholarship is through the essays col-lected by Dominik Wujastyk, *Studies on Indian medical history* (E. Forster, 1987), a volume which has valuable bibliographic references.

AUSTRALIA

For Australia, E. Fordis' *Bibliography of Australian medicine, 1790–1900* (Sydney University Press, 1976) is now joined by *Annotated bibliography of the history of medicine and health in Australia [to 1980]* (Royal Australasian College of Physicians, 1984), edited by B. Gandevia *et al.*

Nursing

The history of nursing, as that of hospitals (see below), was cursed with dull narrative and anecdotal accounts. Recently, there has been something of a minor renaissance in this blighted corner of medical history. The older works before Brian Abel-Smith's *A history of the nursing profession* (Heinemann, 1960, reprinted in paperback 1982) are best ignored. Bibliographic orientation is provided by Alice M.C. Thompson's *A bibliography of nursing literature, 1859–1960* (Library Association, 1968; *Supplement 1961–70*, 1974), supplemented by Frances Walsh's *A bibliography of nursing literature: the holdings of the Royal College of Nursing 1971–1975; 1976–1980* (Library Association, 1985–86). Christopher Maggs has carved a niche in the subject with his *Sources for the history of nursing in Great Britain* (King's Fund, 1984), *The origins of general nursing* (reprinted with corrections, Croom Helm, 1985), and his edition of essays *Nursing history: the state of the art* (Croom Helm, 1987). Robert Dingwall, Anne M. Rafferty and Charles Webster have produced *An introduction to the social history of nursing* (Routledge, 1988), while from S.M. Sparks comes a useful *Index to nursing photographs in the Manuscripts and Prints and Photographs Section of the History of Medicine Division, National Library of Medicine* (N.L.M., 1988). B. Ehrenreich and D. English's *Witches, midwives and nurses: a history of women healers* (Feminist Press, 1973) presents another side of nursing history. Grace L. Deloughery, *History and trends of professional nursing* achieved eight editions (Mosby, 1977). R. White's *Social change and the development of the nursing profession. A study of the Poor Law nursing service, 1848–1948* (Kimpton, 1978) and the volume of essays edited by C. Davis, *Rewriting nursing history* (Croom Helm, 1980), in their different ways blow a fresh breeze into a musty corner of medical history.

There is a flourishing modern Florence Nightingale industry, to which bear witness:

Florence Nightingale: reputation and power (Croom Helm, 1982) by F.B. Smith

Florence Nightingale and the nursing legacy (Croom Helm, *c.* 1986) by Monica E. Baly

Useful reproductions of F.N. texts in *Florence Nightingale on hospital reform*, edited by C.E. Rosenberg (Garland, 1987), include her *Notes on hospitals*, 3rd edn, 1863, and *Introductory notes on lying-in institutions*, 1871

Dear Miss Nightingale: a Selection of Benjamin Jowett's letters to F.N., 1860–1893 (Clarendon Press, 1987), edited by Vincent Quinn and John Prest

Letters from Egypt: a journey on the Nile 1849–1850 (Barrie and Jenkins, 1988) edited by A. Sattin

Ever yours: F.N.: selected letters (Virago, 1989), edited by Martha Vicinus and Ben Nergaard

Hospitals

The very early history of hospitals is being actively researched, threatens to overturn much of received opinion, but is as yet unpublished in accessible form. T.S. Miller's *The birth of the hospital in the Byzantine Empire* (Johns Hopkins University Press, 1985) has been criticized adversely by competent reviewers, so should be used with caution.

The evolution of hospitals in Britain, edited by F.N.L. Poynter (Pitman, 1964) includes a bibliography of secondary works by Eric Gaskell which is comprehensive to its date. Brian Abel-Smith, *The Hospitals, 1880–1948* (Heinemann, 1964) has, as a companion volume, R. Pinker, *English hospital statistics, 1861–1938* (Heinemann, 1966). G.M. Ayer's England's *First state hospitals ... 1867–1930* (Wellcome Institute for the History of Medcine, 1971) is massively documented. J.D. Thompson and Grace Goldin's *The hospital: a social and architectural history* (Yale University Press, 1975) is perhaps the best and certainly the most beautifully illustrated general account, although Dieter Jetter's *Geschichte des Hospitals* (6 vols, F. Steiner, 1966–86) is the standard European history. John Woodward's *To do the sick no harm. A study of the British voluntary hospital system to 1875* (Routledge, 1974) is a far better book than its misleading title would lead one to expect. Recent works of note include: John Pickstone, *Medicine and industrial society: a history of hospital development in Manchester and its region, 1752–1946* (Manchester University Press, *c.* 1985); Geoffrey Rivett, *The development of the London hospital system 1823–1982* (King Edward's Hospital Fund, 1986); and Gunther B. Risse, *Hospital life in enlightenment Scotland: care and teaching at the Royal Infirmary of Edinburgh* (CUP, 1986).

Histories of individual hospitals are legion and almost always excruciatingly dull. Fortunately there are comprehensive references in the later chapters of a far from dull collection of essays, *Hospitals in history*

(Routledge, 1988) edited by L. Granshaw and R. Porter. Indeed Lindsay Granshaw's *St. Mark's Hospital, London: a social history of a specialist hospital* (King Edward's Hospital Fund, 1985) set new standards of meticulous research and documentation in a field where casual sloppiness had reigned too long.

Medical Education

Education is a corner of medical history which is remarkably underdeveloped, at least so far as English-language monographs are concerned. The student will need to search the periodical literature and its indexes (see below).

T. Puschmann's *A history of medical education* was translated from the German edition of 1889 (H.K. Lewis, 1891) and is useful, as is C. Newman's *The evolution of medical education in the 19th century* (OUP, 1957). *The history of medical education*, edited by C.D. O'Malley (University of California Press, 1970) contains papers (some now a little outdated) on each of the main countries. T.N. Bonner's *American doctors and German universities: a chapter in intellectual relations 1870-1914* (University of Nebraska Press, 1963) examines a period when a high proportion of the most talented and ambitious of American medical men studied ... in German universities'. *Oxford medicine* edited by K. Dewhurst (Sanford, 1970) has papers on the rise of the Oxford clinical school. Also useful are M. Kaufman's *American medical education: the formative years, 1765-1910* (Greenwood Press, 1976) and W.S. Craig's *History of the Royal College of Physicians of Edinburgh* (Blackwell, 1976). M.J. Peterson's *The medical profession in mid-Victorian London* (University of California Press, 1978) is a sociological study of an important, formative period.

Biography

The shelves of historical medical libraries groan under an accumulated load of biographies built up from the strong hagiographical tradition in medicine. During the 1960s and 1970s, the social historians made the 'great man' approach to history less than respectable. During the 1980s there have been signs of biography regaining some new status as a proper mode of history.

The seeker after medical biography has a convenient and up-to-date guide in Leslie T. Morton and Robert J. Moore's *A bibliography of medical and biomedical biography* (Scolar Press, 1989). This indispensable book lists the biographies of individuals, collective biographies, has an index of biographees by discipline, and even a useful short list of books on the history of medicine and related subjects. Brief indications are given of the whereabouts of archival sources. The book's sole serious limitation is its restriction to English-language publications.

The most useful general dictionary of medical biography is A. Hirsch's *Biographisches Lexikon der hervorragenden Ärzte aller Zeiten und Völker* (2nd edn., 5 vols, with a supplement, Urban and Schwarzenberg, 1929–34) which was continued in 2 vols covering 50 years more (1932–33). Four of its predecessors which have not been entirely superseded are N.F.J. Eloy's *Dictionnaire historique de la médecine ancienne et moderne* (4 vols, H. Hoyois, 1778; reprinted Brussels, 1973), with good bibliographies and biased towards France, Belgium and Italy; J.E. Dezeimeris *et al. Dictionnaire historique de la médecine ancienne et moderne* (4 vols, Bèçhet, 1828–39); A.J.L. Jourdan's *Dictionnaire des sciences médicales: biographie médicale* (7 vols, Panckoucke, 1820-1825; reprinted Amsterdam, 1967), which supplements the two preceding titles; and A.L.J. Bayle and A.J. Thillaye's *Biographie médicale* (2 vols, Delahaye, 1855; reprinted Amsterdam, 1967) the contents of which were gathered eclectically (from Eloy *inter alios*), then revised and rearranged in chronological order.

A.G. Debus' *World who's who in science* (A.N. Marquis, 1968) covers the full sweep of recorded history with brief entries. More selective is T.I. Williams' *Biographical dictionary of scientists* (3rd edn., A. & C. Black, 1982), but it contains longer entries. Authoritative, sometimes definitive, are the entries in *Dictionary of scientific biography*, edited by C.C. Gillispie (16 vols, Scribner, 1970–80), written by professional historians of science and medicine.

Two books deal exclusively with the lives of medieval practitioners, namely C.E.A. Wickersheimer's *Dictionnaire biographique des médecins en France au Moyen-Age* (2 vols, Droz, 1936), of which a new edition (actually a reprint of the two basic volumes) has recently appeared under the general editorship of G. Beaujouan, with a supplementary volume by D. Jacquart (Droz, 1979) and C.H. Talbot and E.A. Hammond's *The medical practitioners in Medieval England: a biographical register* (Wellcome Institute for the History of Medicine, 1965). Dr. Faye Getz, of the University of Wisconsin, is gathering additions and corrections to Talbot and Hammond in an electronic database.

For the period since 1518 there is W. Munk's *Roll of the Royal College of Physicians of London* (2nd edn., 3 vols plus supplementary volumes carrying the roll-call to 1985 (RCP, IRL Press 1878–1989)), a work which contains hundreds of short biographies of the UK medical élite, a short history of the College and lists of office-holders, lecturers and prize-winners.

In the difficult period before the regular run of *Medical directories* began in 1845, one has to rely on the irregularly produced volumes of the same general title published in 1779, 1780 and 1783. There are useful lists of apothecaries in C. Wall, H.C. Cameron and E. Underwood's *History of the Worshipful Society of Apothecaries of London volume 1, 1617–1815* (only one volume, OUP, 1963). Interested students may consult the unpublished typescripts of volume 2 in the Wellcome Institute for the History of Medicine, London.

Useful sources for the middle and lower social reaches of the healing professions are J.H. Bloom and R.R. James' *Medical practitioners in the Diocese of London, licensed ... 1529–1752* (CUP, 1935), J.H. Raach's *Directory of English country physicians, 1603–1643* (Dawson, 1962) and R.W. Innes Smith's *English-speaking students of medicine at the University of Leyden* (Oliver and Boyd, 1932).

The nineteenth century is better served by biographical sources. Key events were the creation in 1800 of the College of Surgeons, leading to its first printed list of members in 1805 and the passing of the Apothecaries' Act 1815. The year 1840 saw the publication of a cumulated list of apothecaries who had passed the Society's new examinations. For the higher ranks of the surgical profession one should consult V.G. Plarr's *Lives of the Fellows of the Royal College of Surgeons of England* (2 vols, Wright, 1930), continued in three volumes compiled by Sir D'Arcy Power for the years 1930–51 (RCS, 1953), by W.R. LeFanu and R.H.O.B. Robinson for 1952–64 (Livingstone, 1970), by Sir J.P. Ross and W.R. LeFanu for the years 1965–73 (Pitman Medical, 1981), and by Eustace H. Cornelius and S.F. Taylor for 1974–82 (RCS, 1988). The Royal College of Obstetricians and Gynaecologists has a biographical record in Sir John Peel's *The lives of the Fellows ... 1929–1969* (Heinemann Medical, 1976).

For military medicine the basic works are: D.G. Crawford's *Roll of the Indian Medical Service, 1615–1930* (Thacker, 1930) — an appendix and errata were issued in 1933; and W. Johnston, A. Peterkin and R. Drew's *Commissioned officers in the medical services of the British Army, 1660–1960* (2 vols, Wellcome Institute for the History of Medicine, 1968).

For countries other than Great Britain, a good selection of references would be as follows:

FRANCE

Les biographies médicales by P. Busquet and A. Gilbert (5 vols, Baillière, 1927–1936).

Biographies médicales et scientifiques: XVIIIE siècle, edited by P.A. Huard, a promised series which has not, thus far, gone beyond Volume 1 (R. Dacosta, 1972)

ITALY

Profili bio-bibliografici di medici e naturalisti celebri Italiani del sec. XV al sec. XVIII (2 vols, Serono, 1925-1928). Vol. 1 only was reissued in 1932

GERMANY

Biographisches Lexikon by A. Hirsch (see page 572)

Biographisches Lexikon hervorragender Ärzte des neunzehnten Jahrhunderts by J.L. Pagel (Urban and Schwarzenberg, 1901; reprinted Zentralantiquariat der DDR, 1989)

HOLLAND

Dutch medical biography: a biographical dictionary of Dutch physicians and surgeons, 1475-1975 by G.A. Lindeboom (Rodopi, 1984)

USA

Dictionary of American medical biography by H.A. Kelly and W.L. Burrage (Appleton, 1928) which includes Canadians

Biography of eminent American physicians and surgeons by R.F. Stone (2nd edn., Carlon and Hollenbeck, 1898)

American medical biography by J. Thacher (2 vols, with a new introduction and a bibliography by W.J. Bell, Jr., Da Capo, 1967); this is a reprint of the first edition which appeared in 1828

Dictionary of American medical biography by M. Kaufman *et al.* (2 vols, Greenwood Press, 1984). Now the best source which, apart from the usual alphabetical entries by name, has separate listings by date of birth, place of birth, state where prominent, specialty or occupation, and by medical college

Catalogues of portraits

Finally, not to be ignored are catalogues of portraits, often containing not only pictures but small masterpieces of biography based on meticulous research. The best known examples are:

Photographs of eminent men of all countries by T.H. Barker (2 vols, Churchill, 1867–68)

Royal College of Physicians of London: portraits by G.E.W. Wolstenholme (2 vols, Churchill-Elsevier, 1964-1977)

College portraits ... Royal College of Physicians of Edinburgh by R. Thin (Oliver and Boyd, 1927)

A catalogue of the portraits and other paintings, drawings and sculp-ture in the Royal College of Surgeons of England by W.R. LeFanu (Livingstone, 1960, i.e. 1959)

Catalogue of engraved portraits in the Royal College of Physicians of London by A.H. Driver (RCP, 1952)

Catalogue of portraits in the Wellcome Institute by R. Burgess (Well-come Institute for the History of Medicine, 1973)

Portrait catalog. New York Academy of Medicine (5 vols, plus supple-ments, G.K. Hall, 1959–70)

Portrait catalogue. College of Physicians of Philadelphia by J.S. Berko-witz (Philadelphia College of Physicians, 1984)

Historical library portrait file. Yale Medical Library (Yale Historical Library, 1988)

Bibliography

If medicine cannot quite claim to be the oldest profession, it can cer-tainly look back farther than most to an exceptionally well-recorded past, thanks to a long line of dedicated historians, bibliographers and li-brarians.

The starting point for the study is now John Symons' revision of chapter 8 of *Thornton's Medical books, libraries and collectors*, 1990 (see p.558) on medical bibliographies and bibliographers.

The first printed history-cum-bibliography of medicine was written by Symphorien Champier (1472–1539), a physician and polymath who devoted a large part of his energies to the rescue and transmission of classical scientific learning. His 57-leaf tract *De medicine claris scrip-toribus* (Lyons, *c.* 1506) is divided into five sections each of which has a chronological sequence of bibliographies. The story of Champier's pioneering efforts and accounts of those later bibliographers whose work is still of importance to the medical historian may be read in J.F. Fulton's *The great medical bibliographers: a study in humanism*, (University of Pennsylvania Press, 1951) and E. Brodman's *The devel-opment of medical bibliography* (MLA, 1954; reprinted 1981).

The principal older bibliographies still useful to the historian include Conrad Gesner's *Bibliotheca universalis* (3 vols, and an appendix, Zü-rich, 1545-55, reprinted Osnabrück, 1966). The section on medicine was planned but never appeared, but the other *libri* contain much of relev-ance to medicine. J. A. Van Der Linden's *De scriptis medicis* (Amsterdam, 1637; 2nd edn., 1651; 3rd edn., 1662) set a new style in medical bibliographies by combining a main alphabetical sequence of entries with subject indexes. The revision of this work by Abraham Mercklin, *Lindenius renovatus* (Nuremberg, 1686) includes entries for articles in periodicals and produces a useful list of the individual treatises of Galen and Hippocrates. Martinus Lipenius' *Bibliotheca realis universalis* (6 vols, including one on Medica, Frankfurt, 1679–85) was printed in admirably clear double columns. This subject bibliography covers the writings of *c.* 20 000 authors and has an effective system of indexes and cross-references. Cornelius à Beughem compiled two bibliographies in the late seventeenth century, both of which cover literature produced in the decades prior to publication: *Bibliographia medica et physica novissima* (Amsterdam, 1681) lists books published between 1651 and 1681 while *Syllabus recens exploratorum in re medica, etc.* (Amsterdam, 1696) indexes articles in the early volumes of such periodicals as then existed (e.g. *Journal des Sçavans*).

Albrecht von Haller (1708–77) produced an extraordinarily rich collection of bibliographies in a series of noble folio volumes. All his great *Bibliothecae* (on botany, 2 vols, Zürich, 1771–72; on surgery, 2 vols, Basle, 1774–75; on anatomy, 2 vols., Zürich, 1774–77; and on medicine, 4 vols, Berne, 1776–88) are remarkable for their thoroughness and accuracy.

Towards the end of the eighteenth century the flow of medical literature quickened. More monographs appeared and the periodical began to make its now characteristic contribution to scientific and medical publishing. Quite clearly, if scientists or doctors wished to keep abreast of the latest information in their field, they would be more likely to find it quickly and easily in a bibliography arranged by subject, rather than in the traditional author form. Two early works that fall into this category are C.W. Kestner's *Bibliotheca medica* (Jena, 1746), which has sections on pathology, therapeutics, materia medica, dietetics, etc., supplemented by an author index; and Stephanus H. de Vigilliis von Creutzenfeld's *Bibliotheca chirurgica* (2 vols, Vienna, 1781), in which annotated entries are grouped under an alphabetical sequence of heads representing the different branches of surgery.

For the same period, the best example of a subject bibliography is Wilhelm G. Ploucquet's *Literatura medica digesta, sive repertorium medicinae practicae, chirurgiae atque rei obstetricae* (4 vols, Tübingen, 1808–9).

A work that complements Ploucquet's is J.D. Reuss' *Repertorium commentationum a societatibus litterariis editarum* (16 vols, Göttingen, 1801–21; reprinted Burt Franklin, 1961). This splendid guide to the contents of learned society journals is clearly printed and well designed. Volumes 10 to 16 deal with science and medicine.

One of the finest achievements in the history of medical bibliography is Adolph C.P. Callisen's *Medizinisches Schriftsteller-Lexikon.* Published in 33 indifferently printed volumes (Copenhagen, 1830–45; reprinted B. de Graaf, 1962–65), this marvellously compendious and accurate guide names and identifies (by their places of residence) hundreds of authors active in the period from about 1750 to 1830. Under each name are given particulars of that person's literary output — journal articles included — even down to the different editions and translations. For good measure, Callisen gives references to book reviews and lists the contents of contemporary periodicals, volume by volume, from their beginnings. The reprinting of this indispensable tool of research was one of the more intelligent actions of a section of the modern publishing industry not noted for its rational choices.

Some of the new journals produced cumulative indexes and these can be useful to the historian. Four especially good examples are: *London Medical and Physical Journal*, 1799–1818; *Edinburgh Medical and Surgical Journal* (and its predecessors), 1731–1823 annexed to which is a list of Edinburgh theses from 1726 to 1823; *Medico-Chirurgical Review*, 1820–34; and *Journal de Médecine, Chirurgie et Pharmacie*, 1754–1826. All four are indexed by subject and author.

A. Hiersemann, an enterprising German publishing house, has embarked on a series of volumes ambitiously aimed at indexing German natural history and medical periodicals for the years before 1850. Entitled *Indices naturwissenschaftlich-medizinischer Periodica bis 1850*, the first volume, edited by A. Geus, covers the journal *Der Naturforscher*, 1774–1804, and has indexes for authors, subjects and illustrations. Volume 2 of this excellent series, edited by D. von Engelhardt, appeared in 1974, on the chemical journals of Lorenz von Crell, and volume 3, on eighteenth-century veterinary journals, edited by B. Wimmel and A. Geus, in 1981.

When one considers the mountain of medical literature created during the nineteenth century, it becomes obvious why no single bibliography — not even that remarkable creation the *Index-Catalogue of the Library of the Surgeon General's Office, United States Army: Authors and Subjects* (1st–5th series in 61 vols, Government Printing Office, 1880–1961) — has succeeded in mapping out the terrain completely. Current medical bibliography owes almost everything to the *Index-Catalogue* and its National Library of Medicine successors. We must also give credit to the Royal Society of London's *Catalogue of Scientific Papers, 1800–1900* which, in 19 volumes (various publishers, 1867–1925; Johnson Reprint Corporation and Kraus Reprint Corporation, 1965) lists alphabetically by author thousands of periodical articles on most branches of science, including the pre-clinical, but excluding clinical medicine. It has been continued for material published after 1900 as the *International Catalogue of Scientific Literature*.

The Royal Society's deficiencies in the listing of medicine are only

partially made good by R. Neale's very selective *Medical digest,* a bi-
zarrely classified index to the contents of fewer than 20 journals for the
period 1850 to 1877 and beyond that (in two subsequent editions) up to
1899. In E.J. Waring's *Bibliotheca therapeutica* (2 vols, New Sydenham Society, 1878–79) there are references to over 10 000 books
'arranged under 600 separate headings or articles'.

A natural response to the growth in periodical literature was the attempt to monitor it by means of abstracts. This new trend gathered force
from the middle of the nineteenth century. The most important abstracting journals were Schmidt's *Jahrbücher der in- und ausländischer
gesammten Medizin* (1834–1922), proofsheets of which were furnished
to the New Sydenham Society to act as a basis for its own annual survey
of the literature, *Year Book* (London, 1860–79), W. Braithwaite's *Retrospective of Practical Medicine and Surgery* (Simpkin and Marshall,
1846–1901), and Ranking's *Half-yearly Abstract of the Medical Sciences* (London, 1845–73). There are many other similar publications.

Students interested in the history of scientific and medical periodicals should consult B. Houghton's *Scientific periodicals: their
historical development, characteristics and control* (C. Bingley, 1975)
and D.A. Kronick's *A history of scientific and technical periodicals,*
1665–1790 (2nd edn., Scarecrow Press, 1976).

Library catalogues

It would be wrong to consider printed catalogues as mere book-finding
instruments when, at their best, they can be singularly agreeable to read
and browse upon.

The *Bibliotheca Osleriana* (Clarendon Press, 1929; reprinted McGill
University Press, 1969) is an attractive key to the older part of the historical collections of the Osler Library at McGill University, Montreal.
In spite of the subsequent reaction against the 'Oslerian view' of medical history, this catalogue retains much of interest to bibliophiles and
book dealers.

The *Bibliotheca Walleriana* (2 vols, Almqvist and Wiksell, 1955) is,
likewise, a monument to a private collection, now housed in the Royal
University, Uppsala. It records over 20 000 items, including many rare
classic texts on medicine and related subjects. Volume 2 has useful sections
on secondary works of medical history, biography and bibliography.

The Wellcome Institute for the History of Medicine's library is one
of the richest collections in the world and its catalogues are much used
by librarians, researchers and the trade:

A catalogue of incunabula by F.N.L. Poynter (OUP, 1954)

A catalogue of printed books

Vol. 1 (edited by F.N.L. Poynter) *Books printed before 1641* (1963)

Vol. 2 (edited by H.R. Denham) *Books printed from 1641 to 1850: A–F* (1966)

Vol. 3 (edited by H.R. Denham) *Books printed from 1641 to 1850: F–L* (1976)

Vol. 4 (edited by H.R. Denham and H.J.M. Symons) *Books printed from 1641 to 1850: M–R* (in preparation)

Catalogue of western manuscripts on science and medicine by S.A.J. Moorat

Vol. 1 *MSS written before AD 1650* (1962)

Vol. 2 *MSS written after AD 1650*, 2 vols (1973)

A supplementary catalogue of western MSS, by R.J. Palmer (*First cumulative supplement*, 1989. *Second cumulative supplement*, in press)

A Catalogue of Arabic MSS on medicine and science by A.Z. Iskandar (1967)

Portraits of doctors and scientists, by R. Burgess (1973)

An Annotated Catalogue of medical Americana, by R.M. Price (1983)

Contemporary Medical Archives Centre. Consolidated accessions list by J. Sheppard and L. Hall. 2nd edn. (1985)

A handlist of the Sanskrit and Prakrit MSS by D. Wujastyk (Vol. 1, 1985)

A descriptive and analytical catalogue of Persian MSS by F. Keshavarz (1986)

Catalogue of Tibetan MSS and xylographs, and catalogue of thankas, banners and other paintings and drawings by Marianne Winder (1989)

The Wellcome Institute's *Subject catalogue* of (largely) secondary literature was published in 18 volumes (comprising three series — subject, topographical and biographical) by Kraus International (1980).

The largest collection of historical medicine in the world is probably that of the Historical Division of the National Library of Medicine in Bethesda, Maryland. Published catalogues of its older materials include the following:

A catalogue of incunabula and manuscripts in the Army Medical Library by Dorothy M. Schullian and Francis E. Sommer (who contributes a section on oriental manuscripts; H. Schuman, 1948)

A catalogue of sixteenth century printed books in the N.L.M., by Richard J. Durling (Bethesda, 1967). Peter Krivatsy published a first supplement to this catalogue in 1971

A catalogue of seventeenth century printed books in the N.L.M. by Peter Krivatsy (Washington, 1989)

Short-title catalogue of eighteenth century printed books in the N.L.M. by John B. Blake (Bethesda, 1979).

Other related guides are:

Incunabula scientifica et medica by A.C. Klebs (St. Catherine Press, 1938)

Incunabula medica, 1467–1480 by W. Osler (Bibliographical Society, 1923)

Deutsche medizinische Inkunabeln by Karl Sudhoff (Barth, 1908)

The awakening interest in science during the first century of printing, 1450–1550 by M.B. Stillwell (Bibliographical Society of America, 1970), about half of which covers medicine and natural science

A catalogue of the medieval and Renaissance manuscripts and incunabula in the Boston Medical Library by J.F. Ballard (privately printed, 1944)

The Morris H. Saffron Collection of Books on Historical Medicine: a Short-title Catalogue (New Jersey College of Medicine and Dentistry, 1981)

Author–title catalog of the Francis A. Countway Library of Medicine for imprints through 1959 by Harvard Medical Library (10 vols, G.K. Hall, 1973)

Verzeichnis medizinischer und naturwissenschaftlicher Drucke 1472–1830 Wolfenbüttel, Herzog August Bibliothek (14 vols, Kraus–Thomson, 1976–78)

Useful medical library catalogues, and their characteristics are, in summary form:

LONDON

Royal College of Physicians (1912): author entries (occasionally annotated), lists of Harveian Orations and Lumleian Lectures, no serial publications

Royal Medical and Chirurgical Society (now Royal Society of Medicine) (3 vols, 1879): author entries in vols 1 and 2, including serial titles by country, subject index in vol. 3, list of Jacksonian Prize Essays

Royal College of Surgeons (1831): author entries with additional headings for 'Journal', 'Midwifery', 'Hospital', 'Academy', etc.

English books printed before 1701 (Royal College of Surgeons, 1963): author entries with coverage of English-language books by British authors published abroad

Short-title catalogue of books printed before 1851 (Royal College of Obstetricians and Gynaecologists, 2nd edn., 1968)

Medical Society of London (1829): drastically short author entries

Manuscripta Medica: W. Dawson (Medical Society of London, 1932)

Society of Apothecaries (1913): author entries for 1700 items

University College, London (1887): author entries, including sections for Reports, Academies and Periodicals

Catalogue of the printed books and manuscripts (1491-1900) in the library of St. Thomas's Hospital Medical School, by D.T. Bird (1984)

EDINBURGH

Royal College of Physicians (2 vols, 1898): author entries (many of them analytical), with headings for reports and journals, includes a chronological list of librarians and a catalogue of medical portraits, engravings, etchings and busts

A catalogue of medical incunabula in Edinburgh libraries by G.D. Hargreaves (1976)

A Catalogue of the 16th Century Medical Books in Edinburgh libraries by D.T. Bird (1982)

GLASGOW

Faculty of Physicians and Surgeons (2 vols, 1885–1901): author entries preceded by an index of subjects, includes periodicals and reports (by subject) and a two-page list of MSS

Hunterian Museum in the University of Glasgow (1930): author entries with a topographical index of books printed before 1600 and a one-page list of items in Chinese

ENGLISH PROVINCES

Manchester Medical Library (1890): author entries, with reports arranged by subjects

Manchester Medical Library (1972): extremely detailed author entries for the period 1480 to 1700, with indexes to match

Liverpool Medical Institution (1968): author entries up to the end of the nineteenth century, excludes serials

York Medical Society (1961): author entries

Cole Library, Reading University (1969): Part 2 plus supplement (1975), author entries, in a rough chronological order, with a good subject index and a generous amount of reference material

Pybus Collection, University of Newcastle Library (1981): includes letters and engravings, fifteenth to twentieth centuries, as well as medical books.

USA

Harvey Cushing Collection, Yale University (1943): author entries, including separate sections for MSS, incunabula and orientalia

H. Winnett Orr Collection, American College of Surgeons (1960): in four parts, including one for rare books and classics and one for life and literature

Reynolds Library, University of Alabama (1968): author entries, with sections on incunabula and MSS. well illustrated

University of Oklahoma Libraries (1976): sciences collections

FRANCE

Bibliothèque Nationale (3 vols, 1859–1889): classified, no index but good table of contents

HOLLAND

Nederlandsche Maatschappij tot Bevordering der Geneeskunst (2 vols, 1930–59): a remarkably good collection, classified with sections for manuscripts and autograph letters

AUSTRIA

Josephinisches Bibliothek (1974): history of medicine

There are now comprehensive and up-to-date guides in *Thornton's Medical books* (see above) viz., Alain Besson's chapter 9 on private medical libraries and Roy B. Tabor's chapter 10 on medical libraries of today.

Encyclopaedias and dictionaries

It was not until the eighteenth century that dictionaries of medicine came upon the scene permanently as a most potent means for diffusing the elements of medical knowledge among the profession and the educated public. The three best examples are S. Blankaart's *Lexicon medicum graecolatinum* (Amsterdam, 1679), of which seven editions appeared between 1684 and 1726 under the title *A physical dictionary: in which all the terms relating either to anatomy, chirurgery, pharmacy, or chemistry, are ... explain'd;* J. Quincy's *Lexicon physico-medicum* (London, 1719), which began its long career in the heyday of iatrophysics and ended it at the time of Lavoisier (11th edn., 1794); and R. James's *Medicinal dictionary* (3 vols, 1743–45), an exhaustive work to which Dr. Johnson contributed a preface. As for encyclopaedias, one thinks immediately of Diderot and D'Alembert's *Encyclopédie* (published variously in the 1770s) by reason of its magnificent illustrations and substantial sections on surgery and medicine.

For the nineteenth century a good choice of dictionaries would be R. Hooper's *Lexicon medicum* (London, 1802), which continues on from where Quincy left off, reaching an eighth edition in 1848; J. Copland's *Dictionary of practical medicine* (3 vols, London, 1832–58), which contains 'prescriptions, bibliography and formulae'; New Sydenham Society's *Lexicon of terms used in medicine and the allied sciences* edited by Power and Sedgwick (5 vols, London, 1881–99), which includes long accounts of medicine, surgery, midwifery, and pathology, and 'accurate information [on] the drugs and preparations of the Indian and of the several European pharmacopoeias, with the doses, etc.'.

The following encyclopaedias are of the first importance: *Dictionaire* [sic] *des sciences médicales* (60 vols, Paris, 1812–1922) has a two-volume subject index, and *Encyclopädisches Wörterbuch der medizinischen Wissenschaft* (37 vols, Berlin, 1828–1849) has a subject index. *Cyclopaedia of practical medicine* edited by Forbes, Tweedie and Conolly (4 vols, London, 1833–35) claims to 'rescue ancient literature from oblivion and to present the latest knowledge acquired by the French, German and Italian pathologists'. *Nouveau dictionnaire de médecine et de chirurgie* (40 vols, Paris, 1864–86) presents 'articles d'ensemble' under general headings in an alphabetico-classed order and has a complete index of subjects in the final volume where there is also a long addendum on microbes. *Dictionnaire encyclopédique des sciences médicales*, edited by Dechambre (100 vols., Paris, 1864–1889) has extraordinarily good bibliographies and numerous biographical articles, and in vol. 1 an overall survey of dictionaries.; *British encyclopaedia of medical practice*, edited by Sir H. Rolleston (12 vols by, London, 1936–1944); 2nd edn., Lord Horder (12 vols, plus index, London, 1950–1952) has historical notes scattered throughout; see especially Rolleston's introduction.

Dictionaries of eponyms, syndromes and quotations should be taken into account. The leading ones are:

Die Eigennamen in der Krankheitsterminologie by I. Fischer (M. Perles, 1931)

Die klinische Eponyme by B. Leiber and T. Olbert (Urban and Schwar-zenberg, 1968)

Die klinische Syndrome by B. Leiber and G. Olbrich (5th edn., Urban and Schwarzenberg, 1972)

Dictionary of syndromes and eponymic diseases by S. Jablonski (2nd edn., Krieger, 1989)

Dictionary of medical syndromes by S.I. Magalini *et al.* 3rd edn., Lip-pincott, 1990)

Anatomical eponyms by J. Dobson (2nd edn., Livingstone, 1962)

Familiar medical quotations by M.B. Strauss (Little, Brown, 1968)

A growing trend in modern publishing is the production of dictionaries of concepts. For the history of medicine two of the most useful are *Dictionary of the history of ideas: studies of selected pivotal ideas*, edited by P.P. Wiener (4 vols, Scribner, 1973) and *Dictionary of the history of science*, edited by W.F. Bynum, E.J. Browne and R. Porter (Macmillan, 1981), a desk-top volume, even more accessible since it is available in paperback.

Recent publications include Roderick E. McGrew, *Encyclopedia of medical history* (Macmillan, 1985) and B. Oldby *et al.* (eds) *Companion to the history of modern science* (Routledge, 1989) which, although not dealing directly with medicine, is an invaluable guide to current historiography in a closely related field. Routledge promise a companion 'Companion' on the history of medicine, to be edited by W. Bynum and R. Porter.

Indexes to the historical literature

As medical history, as a subject, has grown and expanded so has it become necessary for the student to look beyond those sources concerned specifically and narrowly with the subject itself. Recourse must be had to the indexes and serial bibliographies produced for general history, the social sciences, classics, linguistics, and so on, if the careful researcher is not to miss significant work. To list even a selection of these would, however, be beyond the scope of the present chapter.

Current Work in the History of Medicine is issued quarterly by the Wellcome Institute for the History of Medicine, London. Its editorial core is a MEDLINE printout to which are added entries derived from non-medical sources. New and forthcoming books are also listed. No cumulation has been published but all the entries in the series up to the end of 1977 are included in the Wellcome Institute Library *Subject Catalogue* described above (page 581). Gerhard Fichtner has produced a useful 3-volume *Index der Autorennamen zu 'Current Work'*, *1–107* (Tübingen, 1986).

Complementary to *Current Work* is the National Library of Medicine's annual *Bibliography of the History of Medicine*. Published since 1965, it has an alphabetical arrangement of topics under general headings such as 'Statistics and Demography' and 'Tropical Medicine', preceded by a substantial section devoted to biographies. Cumulations appear at five-yearly intervals, the latest of them being for 1980–84 (to No. 20).

From the very start of its long life, *Isis*, founded by George Sarton in 1913, and now the leading international journal in the history of science, has regularly given over one part of each annual volume to a 'critical' (i.e. annotated) bibliography of newly published work in its field. Cumulations of these have been published as follows: Isis *Cumulative Bibliography. A Bibliography of the History of Science formed from* ISIS *Critical Bibliographies 1–90, 1913–65*,, edited by M. Whitrow: Vol. 1 (Part 1): *Personalities A–J*; Vol. 2 (Part 1): *Personalities K–Z*; Part 2: Institutions; Vol. 3: *Subjects*; Vol. 4: *Civilizations and Periods — Prehistory to Middle Ages*; Vol. 5: *Civilizations and Periods — 15th to 19th Centuries* (Mansell, 1971–1982); Vol. 6: *Author Index* (Mansell, 1984). The same cumulation occurs for ISIS *Critical Bibliographies 91–100, 1966–1975*, edited by J. Neu: *Personalities and Institutions* (Mansell, 1981); Vol. 2: *Subjects, Periods and Civilizations* (Mansell, 1985).

A more restricted chronological coverage is provided by Jonathan Erlen, *The history of the health care sciences and health care, 1700– 1980: a selective annotated bibliography* (Garland, 1984), which also excludes 'individual biographical and autobiographical works' and 'studies of particular medical schools or health care facilities ... unless these institutions have a uniquely important role in the history of their specialty ... '. This work has the exceedingly odd and unhelpful policy of excluding the most recent editions of some cited works if these editions are not available on inter-library loan.

The European counterpart to the *Isis* bibliographies is the French *Bulletin Signalétique: Histoire des Sciences et des Techniques* produced by the Centre de Documentation: Sciences Humaines, Paris.

For work in particular countries, one may have recourse to (for Spain) *Indice Historico Mèdico Español*, an author list, published since 1962 as an off-shoot of the periodical *Cuadernos de Historia de la Medicina Española* and (for North America) to G. Miller's *Bibliography of the History of Medicine of the United States and Canada, 1939–1960* (2nd edn., Johns Hopkins University Press, 1964).

Of the bibliographies that are defunct or that lie fallow we need mention *Index zur Geschichte der Medizin und Biologie*, etc., for the years

1945 to 1948 edited by W. Artelt (Vol. 1, 1953) and J. Steudel (Vol. 2, 1949–52, 1966), these two volumes are crammed with nearly 20 000 entries and arranged in a way that tends to impede quick reference. J. Pagel's *Historisch-medizinische Bibliographie für die Jahre 1875–1896* (Berlin, 1898) is classified but without the indexes that this arrangement demands; it is good, however, for biographies and local histories. F.A. Pauly's *Bibliographie des Sciences Médicales* (Tross, 1874, reprinted D. Verschoyle, 1954) has excellent detailed sections on hospitals, epidemics, institutions, etc. *Mitteilungen zur Geschichte der Medizin und der Naturwissenschaften* (Leipzig, 1902–42, 1961–64) is an abstracting journal rather than a true bibliography; and all the more valuable for that reason.

For modern history (post-1450) the most general source is *Historical Abstracts* (Clio, 1955–), *Part A: Modern History Abstracts, 1450–1914*; *Part B: Twentieth Century Abstracts, 1914 to the Present*. This source is also available online via Dialog (File No. 39). Films and tapes are listed in B. Eastwood, *Directory of audio-visual sources: history of science, medicine and technology* (Science History Publications, 1979).

Guidance to databases useful to the historian may be found in J.L. Hall, *On-line bibliographic databases: a directory and sourcebook* (4th edn., Aslib, 1986).

Readings

Books of readings containing reprints of, or substantial extracts from, medical classics appear to fulfil two main consumer needs. First, they help to feed the collective nostalgia of the health professions by providing a sort of *cordon bleu* cook-book of all the 'recipes' which, from the modern point of view, appear to have stood the test of time. As such, they undoubtedly nourish the progressionist, upwards-and-onwards view of medicine's past which professional historians spend much time combating. Secondly, teachers of medical history seek to provide their pupils with easily assimilated gobbets of text in an accessible language, usually English, for the purposes of course work.

Whatever we may think of these motives, anthologies of medical classics exist and may be consulted with considerable profit as introductions to further study.

A selection of the many available titles is:

Classic descriptions of disease by R.H. Major (3rd edn., C.C. Thomas, 1945)

Selected readings in pathology by E.R. Long (2nd edn., C.C. Thomas, 1961)

A history of medicine: selected readings by I.S. King (Penguin Books, 1971)

Hippocratic writings by G.E.R. Lloyd (Penguin Books, 1978)

Medical America in the 19th century: readings from the literature by G.H. Brieger (Johns Hopkins University Press, 1972)

Greek medicine: being extracts illustrative of medical writings from Hippocrates to Galen by A.J. Brock (E.P. Dutton, 1929, reprinted by AMS, 1977)

Selected readings in the history of physiology by J.F. Fulton and L.G. Wilson (2nd edn., C.C. Thomas, 1966)

Source book of medical history by L. Clendening (Dover, 1960), a convenient paperback collection

Three hundred years of psychiatry, 1535–1860 by R. Hunter and I. Macalpine (OUP, 1963, corrected reprint Carlisle Publishers, 1982). English scene from Bartholomaeus Anglicus to 1860, with lucid and often witty editorial comments on texts which range widely beyond any narrow definition of 'psychiatry'.

Readings in pharmacy by P.A. Doyle (J. Wiley, 1962)

Readings in pharmacology by B. Holmstedt and G. Liljestrand (Macmillan, 1963), from the Ebers Papyrus and by way of the 'School of Salerno' into sections headed for example 'experimental pharmacology', 'local anaesthesia', etc.

Milestones in modern surgery by A. Hurwitz and G. Degenshein (Hoeber–Harper, 1958)

Classics of cardiology by F.A. Willius and T.A. Keys (2 vols, rev. edn., Dover, 1961; Vol. 3: new material edited by J.A. Callaghan *et al.*, published by Krieger in 1982 with a reprint of the first two volumes)

Sickness and health in America: readings in the history of medicine and public health by J.W. Leavitt and R.L. Numbers (Wisconsin, 1978)

Journals

A generous selection of the current periodicals in the history of medicine and related fields is arranged in alphabetical order in the list below.

The student of medical history cannot afford to neglect the major journals in general history and the social sciences. A growth area in recent years has been the number of new titles devoted to non-western or 'alternative' medical systems. Also to be sought out are the numerous *Newsletters*, often distributed free or at very low cost, by institutions, societies and research groups, particularly in the USA but also in the UK and continental Europe.

Ambix. The journal of the Society for the Study of Alchemy and Early Chemistry (London, 1937, Vol. 1 –)

Annals of Science. A quarterly review of the history of science since the Renaissance (London, 1936, Vol. 1 –)

Archives Internationales d'Histoire des Sciences (Paris, 1947, Vol. 1–)

British Journal for the History of Science (London, 1962, Vol. 1 –)

Bulletin of the History of Medicine. Organ of the American Society for the History of Medicine (Baltimore, Johns Hopkins University Press, 1933, Vol. 1 –)

Bulletin et Mémoires de la Société Internationale d'Histoire de la Médecine (Brussels, 1954–1961, Vols 1–8)

Comparative Medicine — East and West. Formerly *American Journal of Chinese Medicine.* This original title resumed in 1979 (New York, 1973, Vol. 1 –)

Culture, Medicine and Psychiatry (Dordrecht, Boston, 1977, Vol. 1 –)

Dynamis. Acta Hispanica ad Medicinae Scientiarumque Historiam Illustrandam (Granada, 1981, Vol. 1 –)

Gesnerus. Organ of the Swiss Society for the History of Medicine and Science (Aarau, 1943, Vol. 1 –)

Histoire des Sciences Médicales. Organ of the French Society. Before 1967 the Society's official organ was called *Histoire de la Médecine* (Paris, 1967, Vol. 1 –)

Historia Hospitalium. Mitteilungen der Deutschen Gesellschaft für Krankenhausgeschichte (Düsseldorf, 1966, Vol. 1 –)

History of Nursing Society Journal (Royal College of Nursing, 1985, Vol. 1 –)

History of Science. An annual review of literature, research and teaching (Cambridge, 1962, Vol. 1 –)

Indian Journal of the History of Science (Madras, 1956, Vol. 1 –)

Isis. An international review devoted to the history of science and its cultural influences (Philadelphia, 1913, Vol. 1 –)

Janus. Archives Internationales pour l'Histoire de la Médecine, etc. (Amsterdam, 1896, Vol. 1 –)

Journal of Ethnopharmacology. An interdisciplinary journal devoted to bioscientific research on indigenous drugs (Lausanne, 1979, Vol. 1 –)

Journal of the History of the Behavioral Sciences (Brandon, 1965, Vol. 1 –)

Journal of the History of Biology (Cambridge, 1968, Vol. 1 –)

Journal of the History of Medicine and Allied Sciences (New York, 1946, Vol. 1 –)

Journal of Medicine and Philosophy (Chicago, 1976, Vol. 1 –)

Journal of Psychohistory. Until 1976 known as *History of Childhood Quarterly* (New York, 1973, Vol. 1 –)

Koroth. A quarterly journal devoted to the history of medicine and science. Organ of the Israel Society (Jerusalem and Tel Aviv, 1952, Vol. 1 –)

Medical History. Published by the Wellcome Institute, London (London, 1957, Vol. 1 –)

Medizin Historisches Journal (Hildesheim, 1966, Vol. 1–)

Pharmaceutical Historian. Newsletter of the British Society for the History of Pharmacy (London, 1967, Vol. 1 –)

Pharmacy in History. American Institute for the History of Pharmacy. Before 1965 called *AIHP Notes* (Madison, 1955, Vol. 1 –)

Psychohistory Review. Before 1976 called *Group for the Use of Psychology in History, Newsletter* (Springfield, 1972, Vol.1 –)

Social History of Medicine (the journal of the Society for the Social History of Medicine, 1988, Vol. 1 –)

Sudhoffs Archiv. Began life as *Archiv für Geschichte der Medizin* (Leipzig, 1908, Vol. 1 –)

Tibetan Medicine (Dharamsala, 1980, Vol. 1 –)

Traditional Medical Systems (Calcutta, [1980?], Vol. 1 –)

Veterinary History. Organ of the Veterinary History Society (London, 1973, Vol. 1 –)

Index